Handbook of

SO-ACQ-034

Pediatric HIV Care

This portable and practical handbook provides a concise guide to the essentials of pediatric HIV care. During the past few years, many agents for the treatment and prophylaxis of HIV infection and the opportunistic infections that accompany HIV infection have been developed, and many new ways of monitoring HIV infection in children have been produced. These new therapies and approaches to management are complicated, but the long-term health of HIV-infected children depends on their correct application. This handbook presents the core information and guidelines necessary for effective management of infected children.

Dr. Stephen L. Zeichner received his undergraduate and graduate degrees at the University of Chicago. He trained in pediatrics and infectious diseases at the Children's Hospital of Philadelphia. An investigator in the HIV and AIDS Malignancy Branch, National Cancer Institute, NIH, and an adjunct family member of the George Washington University School of Medicine, Children's National Medical Center, Washington, DC, and the Uniformed Services University of the Health Sciences, he studies the basic biology of HIV and Kaposi's sarcoma-associated herpesvirus, and directs clinical trials of new therapies for HIV-infected children.

Dr. Jennifer S. Read trained in pediatrics and infections diseases (University of Michigan, Johns Hopkins), tropical medicine (London School of Hygiene and Tropical Medicine), and epidemiology (Harvard, MIH). Her primary research interest at the National Institute of Child Health and Human Development, NIH is the prevention of mother-to-child transmission of HIV, both in the USA and globally. Among other awards, Dr. Read received the Pediatric Infectious Diseases Society's Young Investigator Award in 2001 and the University of Michigan Medical Center Alumni Society's Early Distinguished Career Achievement Award in 2003.

Handbook of
Pediatric HIV Care
Second Edition

Edited by

STEVEN L. ZEICHNER
Bethesda, Maryland, USA

and

JENNIFER S. READ
Bethesda, Maryland, USA

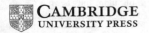
CAMBRIDGE
UNIVERSITY PRESS

CAMBRIDGE UNIVERSITY PRESS
Cambridge, New York, Melbourne, Madrid, Cape Town, Singapore, São Paulo

Cambridge University Press
The Edinburgh Building, Cambridge CB2 2RU, UK

Published in the United States of America by Cambridge University Press, New York

www.cambridge.org
Information on this title: www.cambridge.org/9780521529068

First published 2006

Printed in the United Kingdom at the University Press, Cambridge

A catalog record for this publication is available from the British Library

ISBN-13 978-0-521-52906-8 paperback
ISBN-10 0-521-52906-9 paperback

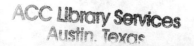

For Rachel, Sarah, and Elizabeth

For Alex, Samantha, and Geoffrey

Contents

Part I Scientific basis of pediatric HIV care

Part II General issues in the care of pediatric HIV patients

Part III Antiretroviral therapy

Part IV Clinical manifestations of HIV infection in children

Part V   Infectious problems in pediatric HIV disease

Part VI Medical, social, and legal issues

Contributors

Elaine J. Abrams, Family Care Center, Department of Pediatrics Harlem Hospital Center, 506 Lenox Avenue, MLK 16-119, New York, NY 10037, USA

Grace M. Aldrovandi, University of Alabama, Bevill Biomedical Research Building, Room 559, 845 29th Street, Birmingham, AL 35294, USA

Jane C. Atkinson, National Institute of Dental and Craniofacial Research, National Institutes of Health, Building 10, Room IN 117, Bethesda, MD 20892, USA

Andrew Blauvelt, Department of Dermatology, Oregon Health and Science University, 3181 SW Sam Jackson Park Road, Portland, OR 97239, USA

Pim Brouwers, Department of Pediatrics and Neuroscience, Baylor College of Medicine, 6621 Fannin Street, CCC 1510.12, Houston, TX, USA

Marc Bulterys, Division of HIV and AIDS Prevention National Center for HIV/STD/TB Prevention, Centers for Disease Control and Prevention, 1600 Clifton Road, Atlanta, GA 30333, USA

James M. Callahan, Department of Emergency Medicine, SUNY – Upstate Medical University, 750 East Adams Street, Syracuse, NY 13210, USA

Steven J. Chanock, Pediatric Oncology Branch, National Cancer Institute, National Institutes of Health, Bethesda, MD 20892, USA

Caroline J. Chantry, University of California Davis Medical Center, 2516 Stockton Blvd, Ticon II Suite 334, Sacramento, CA 95817, USA

Lucy Civitello, Children's National Medical Center, 111 Michigan Avenue NW, Washington, DC 20010, USA

Gul H. Dadlani, Congenital Heart Institute of Florida, All Children's Hospital and University of South Florida, St. Petersburg, FL, USA

Barry Dashefsky, Department of Pediatrics University of Medicine and Dentistry of New Jersey, Division of Pulmonary, Allergy, Immunology and Infectious Diseases, 185 South Orange Avenue, MSB F-507A, University Heights, Newark, NJ 07103, USA

Kenneth L. Dominguez, Division of HIV and AIDS Prevention, National Center for HIV/STD/TB Prevention Centers for Disease Control and Prevention, 1600 Clifton Rd, Mailstop E45, Atlanta, GA 30333, USA

Daina Dreimane, Keck School of Medicine, University of Southern California, Children's Hospital of Los Angeles, 4650 Sunset Boulevard, Mailstop 61, Los Angeles, CA 90027, USA

John Farley, Department of Pediatrics, University of Maryland School of Medicine, 685 West Baltimore St, MSTF 314, Baltimore, MD 21201, USA

Howard F. Fine Opthalmology, Wilmer Eye Institute, John Hopkins, 600N Wolfe Drive, Wilmer B-20 Baltimore, MD 21205, USA

Courtney V. Fletcher, Department of Pharmacy Practice, University of Colorado Health Sciences Center, 4200 East Ninth, Box C238 Denver, CO 80262, USA

Mitchell E. Geffner, Keck School of Medicine University of South California, Children's Hospital of Los Angeles, 4650 Sunset Boulevard, Mailstop 61, Los Angeles, CA 90027, USA

Corina E. Gonzalez, Georgetown University Hospital, Lombardi Cancer Center, 3800 Reservoir Road NW, Washington, DC 20007, USA

Heidi J. Haiken, Francois-Xavier Bagnoud Center-UMDNJ-School of Nursing, ADMC4, 30 Bergen Street, Newark, NJ 07107, USA

Teresa Hammett, Division of Viral and Rickettsial Diseases, National Center for Infectious Diseases, Centers for Disease Control and Prevention, 1600 Clifton Road, Atlanta, GA 30333, USA

Peter L. Havens, MACC Fund Research Center and Medical College of Wisconsin, 8701 Watertown Plank Road, Milwankee, WI 53226, USA

Rohan Hazra, HIV and AIDS Malignancy Branch, National Cancer Institute, National Institutes of Health Building 10, Room 10S255, Bethesda, MD 20892-1868, USA

Robert N. Husson, Division of Infectious Diseases, Children's Hospital, Enders 761, 300 Longwood Avenue, Boston, MA 02115, USA

Shirley Jankelevich, Bureau of Disease Control, Division of Acute Disease Epidemiology, South Carolina Department of Health and Environmental Control, 1751 Calhoun Street, Columbia, SC 29201, USA

Paul Jarosinski, Pharmacy Department, Clinical Center, National Institute of Health, Building 10, Room 12C440, Bethesda, MD 20892, USA

Thomas N. Kakuda, Department of Medical Affairs, Hoffman LaRoche, Nutley, NJ, USA

Jeffrey B. Kopp, Metabolic Diseases Branch, NIDDK, National Institutes of Health, Building 10, Room 3N116, Bethesda, MD 20892, USA

Paul Krogstad, Departments of Pediatrics and Molecular and Medical Pharmacology, David Geffen School of Medicine at UCLA, University of California, Los Angeles, 10833 Le Conte Avenue, Los Angeles, CA 90095, USA

Susan S. Lee, National Eye Institute, National Institutes of Health, Building 10, Room 10N202, Bethesda, MD 20892, USA

Sandra Y. Lewis, Manchester State University and François-Xavier Bagnoud Center-UMDNJ, Psychology Department One Normal Avenue Montclair, NJ 07043, USA

Mary Lou Lindegren, Office of Genomics and Disease Prevention, Centers for Disease Control and Prevention, 1600 Clifton Road, Atlanta, GA 30333, USA

Steven E. Lipshultz, Department of Pediatrics, Batchelor Children's Research Institute, Mailman Center for Child Development, Sylvester Comprehensive Cancer Center, University of Miami, Miller School of Medicine, Holtz Children's Hospital, University of Miami-Jackson Memorial Medical Center, Miami, FL, USA

Richard F. Little, HIV and AIDS Malignancy Branch, National Institute of Health, Building 10, Room 10S255, MSC 1868, Bethesda, MD 20892-1868, USA

Frank Maldarelli, HIV Drug Resistance Program, National Cancer Institute, NIH, Building 10, Room 4A12, Bethesda, MD 20892, USA

Carolyn McAllaster, Duke University School of Law, Box 90360, Durham, NC 27708, USA

Elizabeth J. McFarland, Pediatric Infectious Diseases, University of Colorado Health Sciences Center, Box C227, 4200 E Ninth Avenue, Denver, CO 80262, USA

Ross McKinney, Jr., Department of Pediatrics, Duke University of School of Medicine, P.O. Box 3461, Durham, NC 27710, USA

James G. McNamara, Clinical Immunology Branch, Division of Allergy, Immunology and Infectious Diseases, National Institutes of Health, 6700B Rockledge Drive, Bethesda, MD 20892-7620, USA

Ann Melvin, Children's Hospital and Regional Medical Center, CH-32, 4800 Sand Point Way, Seattle, WA 98105, USA

Lynne M. Mofenson, Pediatric, Adolescent and Maternal AIDS Branch, National Institute of Child Health and Human Development, National Institutes of Health 6100 Executive Boulevard, Room 4B11, Bethesda, MD 20852, USA

Rachel Y. Moon, Division of General Pediatrics and Community Health, Children's National Medical Center, 111 Michigan Avenue NW, Washington, DC 20010, USA

Jack Moye, Jr., Pediatric, Adolescent, and Maternal AIDS Branch, National Institutes of Child Health and Human Development, National Institutes of Health, Building 1E, Room 4B11, MSC 7510, Bethesda, MD 20892-7510, USA

Anne O'Connell, Dept of Public Health and Dental Health, Dublin Dental Hospital, Lincoln Place, Dublin 2, Ireland

William C. Owen, Division of Pediatric Hematology / Oncology, Children's Hospital of the King's Daughters, 601 Children's Lane, Norfolk, VA 23507, USA

Paul Palumbo, UMDNJ-New Jersey Medical School, Department of Pediatrics, 185 S Orange Avenue, F-578 Medical Science Building, Nerwark, NJ 07103, USA

Ligia Peralta, Division of Adolescent and Young Adult Medicine, Department of Pediatrics, University of Maryland School of Medicine, 120 Penn Street, Baltimore, MD 21201, USA

Stephen C. Piscitelli, Discovery Medicine-Antivirals, GlaxoSmithKline, 5 Moore Drive, Research Triangle Park, NC 27709, USA

Jennifer S. Read, Pediatric, Adolescent, and Maternal AIDS Branch, National Institute of Child Health and Human Development, National Institutes of Health, Room 4B11F, 6100 Executive Boulevard MSC 7510, Bethesda, MD 20892-7510, USA

Lisa-Gaye Robinson, Department of Pediatrics, Harlem Hospital Center and College of Physicians and Surgeons, Columbia University, New York, NY 10037, USA

Michael R. Robinson, National Eye Institute, National Institutes of Health, Building 10, Room 10N202, Bethesda, MD 20892, USA

Bret J. Rudy, The Craig Dalsimer Division of Adolescent Medicine, Children's Hospital of Philadelphia, 34th St and Civic Center Boulevard, Philadelphia, PA 19104-4399, USA

Richard M. Rutstein, Special Immunology Clinic, Children's Hospital of Philadelphia, 34th St & Civic Center Boulevard, Philadelphia, PA 19104, USA

Leslie K. Serchuck, Pediatric, Adolescent and Maternal AIDS Branch, National Institute of Child Health and Human Development, National Institutes of Health, 6100 Executive Boulevard, Room 4B11, Bethesda, MD 20892–7510, USA

Sherilyn Smith, Children's Hospital and Regional Medical Center, CH-32, 4800 Sand Point Way, Seattle, WA 98105, USA

Stuart E. Starr, Division of Immunology and Infectious Diseases, Children's Hospital of Philadelphia, 34th St & Civic Center Boulevard, Philadelphia, PA 19104, USA

Somsak Tanawattanacharoen, Metabolic Diseases Branch, NIDDK, National Institutes of Health, Building 10, Room 3N116, Bethesda, MD 20892, USA

Russell B. Van Dyke, Section of Infectious Diseases, Department of Pediatrics TB-8, Tulane University Health Sciences Center, 1430 Tulane Avenue, New Orleans, LA 70112, USA

Ellen R. Wald, Division of Allergy, Immunology and Infectious Diseases, Children's Hospital of Pittsburgh, 3705 Fifth Avenue, Pittsburgh, PA 15213, USA

Eric J. Werner, Division of Pediatric Hematology / Oncology, Children's Hospital of the King's Daughters, 601 Children's Lane, Norfolk, VA 23507, USA

Lori S. Wiener, HIV and AIDS Malignancy Branch, National Cancer Institute, National Institutes of Health, Building 20, Room 10S255, Bethesda, MD 20892-1868, USA

Harland S. Winter, Division of Pediatric Gastroenterology and Nutrition, Massachusetts General Hospital for Children, 55 Fruit Street, Boston, MA 02114, USA

Pamela L. Wolters, HIV and AIDS Malignancy Branch National Cancer Institutes and Medical Illness Counseling Center, 9030 Old Georgetown Road, Building 82 Room 109, Bethesda, MD 20892–8200, USA

Lauren V. Wood, Vaccine Branch, National Cancer Institute, National Institutes of Health, Building 10, Room 6B04, Bethesda, MD 20892, USA

Carol J. Worrell, HIV Research Branch, Therapeutic Research Program, Division of AIDS, National Institute of Allergy and Infections Diseases, 6700B Rockledge Drive, Room 5216, Bethesda, MD 20892-1868, USA

Steven L. Zeichner, HIV and AIDS Malignancy Branch, National Cancer Institute, Bldg 10, Room 10S255, 10 Center Drive, MSC1868, Bethesda, MD 20892-1868, USA

Abbreviations

AAP	American Academy of Pediatrics
ABC	abacavir
ABCD	amphotericin B colloidal dispersion
ABLC	amphotericin B lipid complex
ACCAP	AIDS Community Care Alternatives Program
ACEI	angiotensin enzyme inhibitors
ACIP	Advisory Committee on Immunization Practices
ACOG	American College of Obstetricians and Gynecologists
ACTG	AIDS Clinical Trals Group
ACTH	adrenocorticotropin hormone
ACTIS	AIDS Clinical Trials Information Service
ADCC	antibody-dependent cell-mediated cytotoxicity
ADDP	AIDS Drug Distribution Program
ADEC	Association for Death Education and Counseling
ADHD	attention deficit/hyperactivity disorder
AEGIS	AIDS Education Global Information System
AFB	acid-fast bacilli
AFXB	Association François-Xavier Bagnoud
AGCUS	atypical glandular cells of undetermined significance
AIDS	acquired immune deficiency syndrome
ALRI	acute lower respiratory tract infection
AmFAR	American Foundation for AIDS Research
AMP	amprenavir
ANC	absolute neutrophil count
ANRS	Agence Nationale de Recherches sur le SIDA
AOM	acute otitis media
ACP	antigen-presenting cell
APV	amprenavir
ARB	angiotensin blockers
ARDS	acute respiratory distress syndrome

ARF	acute renal failure
ARL	AIDS-related lymphoma
ARN	acute retinal necrosis
ART	antiretroviral therapy
ASCUS	atypical squamous cells of undetermined significance
AST	asparate aminotransferase
ATN	adolescent medicine trials network
ATP	adenosine triphosphate
ATZ	atazanavir
AUC	area under the curve
AZT	zidovudine (also known as ZDV)
BAL	broncheoalveolar lavage
BBB	blood-brain barrier
BCG	Bacille Calmette–Guerin
βHCG	serum beta human chorionic gonadotropin
BIA	bioelectrical impedance analysis
BMC	bone mineral content
BMD	bone mineral density
BMI	body mass index
BUN	blood urea nitrogen
BV	bacterial vaginosis
CARE	Ryan White (Comprehensive AIDS Resources Emergency) Act
CAT	computerized axial tomography
CBC	complete blood count
CD	cluster of differentiation
CDC	Centers for Disease Control and Prevention
CDC-GAP	Centers for Disease Control and Prevention Global AIDS Program
CHF	congestive heart failure
Cho	choline
CHOP	cyclophosphamide, doxorubicin, vincristine and prednisone
CIN	cervical intraepithelial neoplasia
CIPRA	Comprehensive International Program of Research on AIDS
C_{max}	maximum concentration/peak blood concentration
CMT	cervical motion tenderness
CMV	cytomegalovirus
CNS	central nervous system
CPAP	continuous positive airway pressure
CRF	case report form
CRH	corticotropin-releasing hormone
CRP	C-reactive protein

CSF	cerebrospinal fluid
CSOM	chronic suppurative otitis media
CT	computed tomography
CTL	cytotoxic *T*-lymphocytes **also** cytotoxic memory T-cells
CVC	central venous catheter
CXR	chest X-ray
d4T	stavudine
DC	dendritic cells
DC-SIGN	dendritic cell-specific intercellular adhesion molecule-grabbing non-integrin
ddC	zalcitabine
ddI	didanosine
DEXA	dual energy X-ray absorptiometry
DFA	direct fluorescent antibodies also direct immunofluorescence assay
DHEAS	dihydroepiandrosterone sulfate
DHFR	dihydrofolate reductase
DHPS	dihydropteroate synthase
DHSS	Department of Health and Human Services
DIC	disseminated intravascular coagulation
DLBCL	diffuse large B-cell lymphoma
DL_{co}	diffusing capacity
DLV	delavirdine
DMAC	disseminated *Mycobacterium avium* complex
DMPA	depot medroxyprogesterone acetate
DNA	deoxyribonucleic acid
dNTPs	triphosphorylated nucleosides
DOT	directly observed therapy
DOTS	directly observed therapy (short course)
DSMB	Data Safety Monitoring Board
DTH	delayed type hypersensitivity
DTP	diphtheria–tetanus–pertussis
DTaP	diphtheria–tetanus–acellular pertussis
DUB	dysfunctional uterine bleeding
EBCT	electron beam computed tomography
EBV	Epstein–Barr virus
EC	emergency contraception **also** enteric coated
ECG	electrocardiogram
ECHO	echocardiography
ED	Emergency Department **also** end diastolic

EEG	electroencephalogram
EFV	efavirenz
EGPAF	Elisabeth Glaser Pediatric AIDS Foundation
EGW	external genital warts
EIA	enzyme immunoassay
ELISA	enzyme-linked immunosorbent assays
EMEA	European Agency for the Evaluation of Medicinal Products
ENF	enfuvirtide
Env	viral envelope
EP	extrapulmonary pneumocytosis
ERCP	endoscopic retrograde cholangiopancreatography
ES	end systolic
ESR	erythrocyte sedimentation rate
ESRD	end-stage renal disease
5-FU	5-fluorouracil
FACS	fluorescent antibody cell sorting
FAMA	fluorescent antibody membrane antigen
FDA	Food and Drug Administration
FEV_1	forced expiratory volume in 1 second
FFA	free-fatty acids
FFM	fat free mass
FRS	fat redistribution syndrome
FSGS	focal segmental glomerulosclerosis
FSH	follicle stimulating hormone
FTC	emtricitabine
FTT	failure to thrive
FVT	forced vital capacity
G-6-PD	glucose-6-phosphate dehydrogenase
GCP	good clinical practices
g-CSF	filgrastim
G-CSF	granulocyte-colony stimulating factor
GER	gastroesophageal reflux
GH	growth hormone
GI	gastrointestinal
GM-CSF	granulocyte-macrophage colony-stimulating factor
GnRH	gonatropin releasing hormone
HAART	highly active antiretroviral therapy
HAIRAN	hyperandrogenic-insulin resistant acanthosis nigricans
HAMB	HIV and AIDS Malignancy Branch

HAM/TSP	HLTV-1-associated myelopathy/tropical spastic paraparesis
HAV	hepatitis A virus
HAZ	height-for-age Z-scores
hbhA	heparin-binding hemagglutinin adhesin
HBIG	hepatitis B immunoglobulin
HBV	hepatitis virus B
HCP	healthcare personnel
HDL	high-density lipoprotein
HDL-C	high-density lipoprotein cholesterol
HHV-6	human herpesvirus-6
HHV-8	human herpesvirus-8
HIB	*Hemophbilus influenzae* type B
HIV	human immunodeficiency virus
HLA	human leukocyte antigen
HMOs	health maintenance organizations
^{1}HMRS	proton magnetic resonance spectroscopy
HPA	hypothalamic-pituitary-adrenal
HPTN	HIV Prevention Trials Network
HPV	human papillomavirus
HRCT	high-resolution computerized tomography
HRIG	human rabies immunoglobulin
HSI	HIV/AIDS and sexually transmitted infections
HSV	herpes simplex virus
HTLV-1	human T-cell leukemia virus 1
HUS	hemolytic-uremic syndrome
ICASO	International Council of AIDS Services Organizations
ICD	immune complex dissociated
ICMA	immunochemiluminescent assay
IDU	injection drug use
IDV	indinavir
IFA	immunofluorescence assay
IFN	interferon
Ig	immunoglobulin
IGFPB-3	insulin-like growth factor binding protein-3
IgFBPs	IGF binding proteins
IgF-1	insulin-like growth factor 1
IL	interleukin
ILD	interstitial lung disease
IMCI	integrated management of childhood illness
INH	isoniazid

INR	international normalized ratio
In V	intravaginal
IP	interferon inducible protein
IPAA	International Partnership Against AIDS
IPI	invasive pneumococcal infections
IPV	inactivated polio vaccine
IQ	inhibitory quotient
IRB	Institutional Review Board
IRU	immune recovery uveitis
ISA	induced sputum analysis
ITP	immune thrombocytopenia purpura
IUDs	intrauterine devices
IUS	intrauterine system
IVIG	intravenous immunoglobulin
KOH	potassium hydroxide
KS	Kaposi's sarcoma
KSHV	Kaposi's sarcoma-associated herpesvirus
LBM	lean body mass
LDH	lactate dehydrogenase
LDL	low-density lipoproteins
LDL-C	low-density lipoprotein cholesterol
LFT	liver function test
LGE	linear gingival erythema
LH	iuteinizing hormone
LIFE	leadership and investment in fighting an epidemic
LIP	lymphoid interstitial pneumonitis
LIPA	line probe assays
LP	lumbar puncture
LPN	licensed practical nurse
LPV	lopinavir
LPV/r	lopinavir plus ritonavir
LTNP	long-term non-progression
LTR	long terminal repeat (HIV promotor)
LV	left ventricular
MAC	*Mycobacterium avium* complex **also** mid-arm circumference
MACS	Multicenter AIDS Cohort Study
MALT	mucosa-associated lymphoid tissue
MAMC	mid-arm muscle circumference

MCP	monocyte chemoattractant protein
MDI	Mental Developmental Index **also** metered dose inhaler
MDR	multi-drug resistance
MEMS	medication event monitoring system
MESA	myoepithelial sialadenitis
MHC	major histocompatibility complex
MI	myo-inositol
MIG	monokine induced by interferon gamma
MIP	macrophage inflammatory protein
MIRIAD	mother–infant rapid intervention at delivery
Mo	month
MMR	measles, mumps and rubella
MRI	magnetic resonance imaging
MRS	magnetic resonance spectroscopy
MRSA	methicillin-resistant *Staphylococcus aureus*
MSM	men who have sex with men
MTCs	multilocular thymic cysts
MTD	*Mycobacterium tuberculosis* direct test
MTCT	mother-to-child transmission

NAA	*N*-acetyl asparate
NAHC	National Association for Home Care
NAMs	nucleoside associated mutations
NAAT	nucleic acid amplification tests
NASBA®	nucleic acid sequence-based amplification
NCHS	National Center for Health Statistics
NCI	National Cancer Institute
NF-kappa B	nuclear factor kappa-B
NFV	nelfinavir
NHL	non-Hodgkin's lymphoma
NIAID	National Institute of Allergy and Infectious Diseases
NICHD	National Institute of Child Health and Human Development
NIH	National Institutes of Health
NK	natural killer
NMDA	*N*-methyl-D-asparate
NNRTIs	non-nucleoside reverse transcriptase inhibitors
NPA	nasopharyngeal aspirate
nPEP	non-occupational postexposure prophylaxis
NPO	nothing by mouth
NRTIs	nucleoside reverse transcriptase inhibitors
NSAIDs	non-steroidal anti-inflammatory drugs
NSS	normal saline solution

NUG	necrotizing ulcerative gingivitis
NUP	necrotizing ulcerative periodontitis
N/V	nausea/vomiting

17-OHP	17-hydroxyprogesterone
OCs	oral contraceptives
OD	optical density
OGTT	oral glucose tolerance test
OHL	oral hairy leukoplakia
OHRP	Office of Human Research Protections
OIs	opportunistic infections
OLA	oligonucleotide ligation assays
oPEP	occupational postexposure prophylaxis
OPV	oral polio vaccine
OSHA	Occupational Safety and Health Administration

PACTG	Pediatric AIDS Clinical Trials Group
PACTS	Perinatal AIDS Collaborative Transmission Study
PAHO	Pan American Health Organization
PAP	Papanicolaou (Smear)
PBLD	polymorphic B-cell lymphoproliferative disorder
PBMC	peripheral blood mononuclear cells
PCM	protein–calorie malnutrition
PCNS	primary central nervous system
PCOS	polycystic ovary syndrome
PCP	*Pneumocystitis jiroveci* pneumonia **also** primary healthcare provider
P Cr	plasma creatinine
PCR	polymerase chain reaction
PCV	pneumococcal conjugate vaccine
PCV7	heptavalent pneumococcal conjugate vaccine
PEL	primary effusion lymphoma
PENTA	The Pediatric European Network for the Treatment of AIDS
PEP	postexposure prophylaxis
PFC	persistent fetal circulation
PFTs	pulmonary function tests
PGE_2	prostaglandin E_2
PGP	p-glycoprotein
PHA	phytohemaglutinin
PHC	preventive health care
PHS	public health service
PI	pentamidine isothionate
PIs	protease inhibitors

PIC	pre-integration complex
PID	pelvic inflammatory disease
PIT	pills identification test
PJ	*P. jiroveci*
PLH	pulmonary lymphoid hyperplasia
PMDD	premenstrual dysphoric disorder
PML	progressive multifocal leukoencephalopathy
PMPA	9-[2-(R)-(phosphonylmethoxy)propyl] adenine
PMS	premenstrual syndrome
PMTCT	prevention of mother-to-child transmission
P Na	plasma sodium
PNS	peripheral nervous system
PORN	progressive outer retinal necrosis
POS	point of service
PPD	purified protein derivative
PPOs	preferred providers organizations
PPV	pneumococcal polysaccharide vaccine
PMN	polymorphonuclear leukocyte
PRA	peripheral renin activity
PRAMS	pregnancy risk assessment monitoring system
PSD	Pediatric Spectrum of Disease
PT	prothrombin time
PTH	parathyroid hormone
PTT	partial thromboplasin time
PTX	spontaneous pneumothorax
PWAs	persons with AIDS
PZA	pyrazinamide
RAD	reactive airway disease
RBC	red blood cells
RDA	recommended dietary allowance
REACH	reaching for excellence in adolescent care and health
RER	rough endoplasmic reticulum
RN	registered nurse
RNA	ribonucleic acid
ROspA	recombinant outer surface protein
RPE	retinal pigment epithelium
RR	relative risk
RRE	rev responsive element
RSV	respiratory syncytial virus
RTI	reverse transcriptase inhibitor

RT-PCR	reverse transcription-polymerase chain reaction
RTV	ritonavir
SBIs	serious bacterial infections
Sc	subcutaneous
SDF	stromal-cell derived factor
SHBG	sex hormone-binding globulin
SIADH	syndrome of inappropriate secretion of antidiuretic hormone
SILs	squamous intraepithelial lesions
siRNA	small interfering ribonucleic acids
SIV	simian immunodeficiency virus
SMM	Sooty Mangabey monkey
SOIs	sharp object injuries
SPECT	single photon emission computed tomography
SPNS	special projects of national significance
SQV	saquinavir
SSDI	Social Security Disability Income
SSI	Supplemental Security income
SSRIs	selective serotonin reuptake inhibitors
STIs	sexually transmitted infections
SUDS	single use diagnostic system
3TC	lamivudine
T4	free levothyroxine
TAMS	thymidine analogue mutations
TANF	temporary assistance for needy families
TAR	transactivation responsive
TB	tuberculosis
TCA	trichloroacetic acid
TCR	t-cell receptors
Td	tetanus and diphtheria toxoids
TDF	tenofovir disoproxil fumarate
TDM	therapeutic drug monitoring
Th	T-helper
TIG	tetanus immunoglobulin
TMP/SMX	trimethoprim-sulfamethoxazole
TNF	tumor necrosis factor
TOA	tubo-ovarian abscess
TPN	total parenteral nutrition
TREAT	treatment regimens enhancing adherence in teens
TRH	thyrotropin-releasing hormone

TSF	triceps skinfold thickness
TSH	thyroid stimulating hormone
TST	tuberculin skin test
TTP	thrombotic thrombocytopenia purpura
U Cr	urine creatinine
UDPGT	uridine diphosphoglycronyltransferase
U Na	urine sodium
URIs	upper respiratory infections
USAID	United States Agency for International Development
USPHS	United States Public Health Service
UTI	urinary tract infection
VCAM-1	vascular cell adhesion molecule-1
VGC	valganciclovir
VLA-4	very late activation antigen-4
Vif	virion infectivity factor
VLDL	very low density lipoprotein
VZIG	varicella-zoster immunoglobulin
VZV	varicella-zoster virus
WAZ	weight-for-age Z-scores
WBCs	white blood cells
VVC	vulvovaginal candidiasis
WHO	World Health Organization
WITS	Women and Infants Transmission Study
XR	extended release
ZDV	zidovudine (also known as AZT)

Foreword

Catherine M Wilfert, M.D.

Professor Emerita, Duke University Medical Center, Department of Pediatrics, Scientific Director

More than two decades have passed since this devastating infection was first identified. We have come from a time when no diagnosis could be made and there was no treatment, to an era when the development of multiple therapeutic agents and advances in the prevention of HIV infection is commonplace in the developed world. Foremost amongst these accomplishments is our ability to prevent mother-to-child transmission of HIV infection. Seldom is it possible to chronicle such advances in knowledge, which materially affect the lives of thousands of people on a daily basis. All of this speaks to the commitment of scientists and care providers and the rapid evolution of information and technology. There is, however, a pervasive recurrent theme of needing to advocate for the health of children infected and affected by HIV infection.

This handbook provides accessible information at a time when the developed world has succeeded in dramatically decreasing the number of children who acquire infection from their mothers. The need for this information is greater now than ever before. First, because the evolution of information continues at a rapid rate. Second, because the complexity of treatment requires expertise and access to the most current information. Third, because the numbers of HIV-infected children have decreased in the USA and the probability that a physician will have cumulative experience with substantive numbers of these children has diminished. It is important that pediatricians continue to be sensitive to the possibility that a child is HIV-infected and be attuned the specific medical needs and support systems required.

There is an index to Web sources of information, convenient summary tables, and eloquent discussions of antiretroviral drugs conveniently separated from therapeutic decision making. The material is readable, concise, and thorough.

I would wish that this information was accessible, in demand, and essential in the parts of the world where there is so much HIV infection of adults and children. One must reflect on the fact that as many infants are born with HIV infection in sub-Saharan Africa every day as were born in the USA in an entire year prior to the availability of interventions to prevent mother-to-child transmission. Progress is being made to bring these effective interventions to the developing world. We would hope we can entice a new generation of pediatricians, public health authorities, and other providers to devote their lives to addressing the problem as effectively in the developing world as has been done in the developed world. This handbook contributes to the knowledge, and hopefully will provide additional incentive to take these advances to the entire world of children.

Preface

When Cambridge University Press decided to undertake the publication of the second edition of the *Handbook of Pediatric Care*, they told us that they were very enthusiastic about the book, but that they thought that, while the handbook was too large to be a true "handbook," they still valued and appreciated the more comprehensive content of the book. The Press therefore asked us, for the second edition, to both shorten the material to a more manageable size to make a new handbook and to augment the material in the handbook to make an even more comprehensive *Textbook of Pediatric HIV Care*. We hope that we have achieved these goals in these two books, a second edition of the *Handbook of Pediatric HIV Care* and the first edition of the *Textbook of Pediatric HIV Care*.

Our goals for both books are to provide the clinician with the information needed to provide excellent care to children infected with HIV. Neither book is meant to be an exhaustive treatise on the subject of pediatric HIV disease, covering all the many societal and policy issues that are involved necessarily in a complete discussion of HIV and children. Rather, we aim to provide helpful management information for the frontline clinician. While we have focused on the management of pediatric HIV disease, we believe that effective management requires a solid understanding of the basic and applied virology, immunology, and pathophysiology of the disease, so that the practitioner can thoughtfully and rationally apply the management information supplied in the other chapters. Our authors have included more detailed discussions in their *Textbook* chapters, and have tried to condense their presentations in their *Handbook* chapters to include the most clinically pertinent details. Some of the information presented in more than one *Textbook* chapters has been condensed into a single chapter for the handbook, but we hope that we have been able to include the information in the handbook that will enable clinicians to provide optimum care for their HIV-infected patients.

The HIV epidemic changes quickly. The authors of the individual chapters have attempted to include a significant amount of new information, including new basic science findings, new information concerning the pathogenesis of the disease and the opportunistic infections that affect children with HIV, descriptions of recently approved drugs and recently developed drugs that may be close to approval, both for HIV and for HIV-related opportunistic infections, new information concerning the management of children infected with HIV, and information concerning the social welfare of children infected with HIV. In some fields, so much new information has become available that we included entirely new chapters in the book. There are new chapters about the evolutionary biology of antiretroviral drug resistance and the assessment and management of antiretroviral drug resistance, the interruption of mother-to-infant HIV transmission, metabolic complications of HIV infection and antiretroviral therapy, therapeutic drug monitoring for HIV infection, and the gynecology of the HIV-infected adolescent. Neither book has chapters discussing, in detail, HIV vaccines because both prophylactic and therapeutic vaccines are only in the earliest stages of clinical development, but the basic science chapters about virology, immunology, pathogenesis, and natural history describe some of the fundamental information that vaccine developers are using in their efforts. We hope that we will be able to include in a future edition chapters that outline the use of prophylactic and therapeutic vaccines for HIV infection.

The book does not include a specific chapter on the management of pediatric HIV disease in resource-poor countries. We initially contemplated including such a chapter in the book, but soon came to realize that the spectrum of resources available in 'resource-poor' countries varied tremendously from one country to another. For example, in some countries there are government-mandated commitments to essentially universal access to antiretrovirals, while in others only a tiny fraction of the population has access to the drugs, and these circumstances are changing month by month. We look forward to the day when everyone will receive the best care possible, but until then we thought it wisest to describe state-of-the-art care as practiced in the world's richer countries, and acknowledge that providers elsewhere will know best how to adapt these principles to their own local circumstances.

Part I
Scientific basis of pediatric HIV care

1 The scientific basis of pediatric HIV care

Combined from the following chapters in the *Textbook of Pediatric HIV Care: Normal development and physiology of the immune system* Sherilyn Smith and Ann Melvin. *HIV basic virology for clinicians* Steven L. Zeichner. *The immunology of pediatric HIV disease* Elizabeth McFarland. *The clinical virology of pediatric HIV disease* Paul Palumbo. *The natural history of pediatric HIV disease* Grace Aldrovandi

Normal development and physiology of the immune system

Components and function of the immune system

The immune system can be divided into two components. The "innate arm" of the immune system provides a rapid, non-specific pathogen response. It acts as a surveillance system and initiates the antigen-specific phase of the immune system. The major components of innate immunity include physical barriers, complement and other opsonins, the spleen, phagocytes and NK (natural killer) cells. Many responses are triggered by the Toll-like receptor (TLR) with the molecules they bind.

The antigen-specific phase of immunity is directed at specific pathogen antigens. The inducible portions of the immune system include cellular and humoral immune responses. These components control infection and form long-term immunity. Table 1.1 summarizes the major functions of the immune system and the infections that can result from its dysfunction.

Innate immune system

Barriers

The initial defense against microbes is an intact physical mucosal and epithelial barrier. Specialized cells (including ciliated respiratory epithelia), and localized chemical barriers (stomach acid, mucus layers in respiratory and gastrointestinal tracts, and skin

Handbook of Pediatric HIV Care, ed. Steven L. Zeichner and Jennifer S. Read.
Published by Cambridge University Press. © Cambridge University Press 2006.

Table 1.1. The immune system: functions, developmental aspects and infections associated with dysfunction

Immune system component	Function	Developmental differences	Infections associated with dysfunction
Innate			
Epithelial barriers/ mucosal defense	• Impede entrance of microorganisms • Present antigen • Sample environment	• Epithelial barriers decreased in premature infants • Decreased IgA–adult levels by 6–8 years	• Low virulence organisms: coagulase negative staphylococcus opportunistic gram negative bacteria fungi
Complement/opsonins	• Amplify the immune response • Facilitate phagocytosis • Chemoattractants	• Terminal complement levels decreased in neonates	• Encapsulated organisms • Recurrent infections with *Neisseria* species • Recurrent/recalcitrant skin infections
Phagocytes	• Engulf and kill microorganisms • Present antigens to T-cells (macrophages) • Elaborate immune active substances including cytokines and chemotactic factors	• Monocytes: decreased chemotaxis, decreased cytokine production–adult function by 6 years • Neutrophils: decreased bone marrow pool in neonates, decreased chemotaxis–adult levels by 1 year	• *S. aureus* • Low virulence organisms: other staphylococci gram negative opportunistic bacteria fungi
Spleen	• Filters intravascular organisms • Aids with opsonization • Antibody formation		• Encapsulated organisms (*S. pneumoniae*, Salmonella, *H. influenzae*) • Develop severe or recurrent infections

Cell type	Function		Clinical consequence of deficiency
Natural killer (NK) cells	• Lyse cells presenting "non-self" antigens (e.g., tumor or viral proteins)	• Decreased ADCC, decreased cytolytic activity	• Recurrent/severe viral infections with members of the Herpesvirus family
Dendritic cells	• Capture and present antigens to lymphocytes	• Decreased ability to present antigen	?
Antigen specific			
T-cells	• Cell-mediated immunity • Elaboration of cytokines • Regulation of the immune response • Cytolysis • Increases the efficiency of B-cell function by providing "help"	• Increased absolute numbers – decline to adult levels by late childhood • Naive phenotype in neonate (90%) decreased cytokine production, costimulatory molecule expression, and ability to provide "help" to B-cells – normalizes throughout infancy with antigenic exposure	• Infections with "unusual" organisms: intracellular bacteria (listeria, mycobacteria) • Fungi (aspergillus, candida) • Viruses (esp HSV, VZV, CMV, HHV-8) • Protozoa (giardia, *Pneumocystis carinii*)
B-cells	• Humoral immunity (formation of antibody to specific antigens)	• Unable to respond to polysaccharide antigens until ~ 2 years of age	• Encapsulated organisms • Enteroviral infections • Recurrent GI or sinopulmonary infections • Inability to respond to vaccines

fatty acids and cerumen) impede pathogen entry. Breaches in these barriers may result in infection by low virulence organisms.

Mucosal immunity

Mucosal-associated lymphoid tissues are located at sites close to the environment. These lymphoid aggregates (e.g., Peyer's patches) sample the environment, allowing for early initiation of antigen-specific responses [1, 2]. Secretory IgA, synthesized in these tissues, adds to the local mucosal defense.

Opsonins

Opsonins are proteins that bind to pathogen surfaces, facilitating phagocytosis. They include acute phase reactants (C-reactive protein, fibronectin), complement and antibody. Complement is a protein that is sequentially activated by proteases. Complement plays an important role in the killing of invasive bacteria. Two pathways activate complement: the classical pathway (antibody binds bacterial antigen which then is complexed with C1, a complement component), which begins a series of proteolytic reactions activating additional complement components, and the alternate pathway (bacterial antigen directly binds the C3b complement component). Both pathways produce a complex that lyses bacteria [3].

Spleen

The spleen efficiently filters opsonized bacteria and is an antibody production site. Absence or dysfunction of the spleen predisposes to overwhelming infection with encapsulated organisms.

Macrophages

Macrophages and monocytes clear invading microbes. Macrophages migrate to sites of infection and phagocytose foreign substances. Macrophages elaborate many cytokines and growth factors that modify evolving immune responses [4].

Neutrophils

Neutrophils are blood phagocytes that migrate to sites of infection and phagocytose pathogens, notably immunoglobulin- or complement-coated microbes, including bacteria and fungi. Neutrophils kill phagocytosed pathogens via the respiratory burst (reactive oxygen metabolites generation) or by degranulation with release of substances that directly kill pathogens.

Natural killer (NK) cells

NK cells are specialized lymphocytes that recognize non-self proteins, important in early responses to viral infections. Viruses often down-regulate host major histocompatibility complex molecules (see below) on infected cells surfaces, which causes NK cells to recognize them as foreign, making them targets for lysis.

Dendritic cells (DC)

DC capture antigen and present it to lymphocytes. There are three major DC populations: (a) Langerhans cells (interdigitating cells) reside in tissues and migrate to T-cell areas of lymphoid organs after antigen uptake; (b) myeloid DCs (interstitial or dermal DCs), which become germinal center DCs in lymphoid follicles; and (c) plasmacytoid DCs, which reside in T-cell lymphoid tissues areas [5]. Immature DCs take up and process antigen. Migrating to lymphoid tissues, they mature to become antigen-presenting cells [5]. Different populations of DCs have different functions. Langerhans cells activate CD8+ cytotoxic T-cells [6] and promote T-helper type 1 (Th1) responses in CD4+ T-cells. Myeloid DCs (known as DC1 cells) also promote Th1 responses; plasmacytoid DCs (DC2 cells) induce Th2 responses [7].

Toll-like receptors

Toll-like receptors are a family of transmembrane proteins that help initiate the innate immune response. Ten Toll-like receptors (TLR1–10) have been cloned. They serve as an "early warning system" for recognition of microbial antigens and molecules produced by microbes, such as lipopoly saccharides, CpG DNA, and double-stranded RNA. Activation releases chemokines and other inflammatory mediators from dendritic cells and macrophages and modulates expression of chemokine receptors on dendritic cells. Several toll-like receptors can probably act in concert [8].

Antigen-specific immunity
Cell-mediated immunity
T-cells

T-lymphocytes (thymus-dependent lymphocytes) mediate delayed-type hypersensitivity reactions, regulate the development of antigen-specific antibody responses, and provide specific defense against many organisms. Distinct T-lymphocyte subpopulations express different cell surface proteins (see Table 1.2).

T-cell receptor complex

T-cells bear antigen-specific T-cell receptors (TCR), required for foreign antigen recognition and binding. TCRs have either α- and β-chains or γ- and δ-chains. Each chain has a variable amino-terminal involved in antigen recognition and constant carboxy-terminal regions. As T-lymphocytes mature, the TCR genes rearrange [9], creating unique TCRs within T-cells with specific antigen recognition capacity, generating TCR diversity to recognize many antigens. Lymphocytes with α/β-chain TCRs (α/β-cells) locate in lymphoid organs and peripheral circulation, those with γ/δ TCR chains (γ/δ T-cells) locate in mucosa.

MHC molecules

Antigen-presenting cells present antigen to T-cells as short peptides complexed with major histocompatibility complex (MHC) molecules. These cell surface molecules were

Table 1.2. Lymphocyte function and phenotype

Lymphocyte type	Function	Type of antigen receptor	Common cell surface markers
T-lymphocytes			
Helper			
Th1	• Regulation of the immune response • Development of "memory" response to antigens • Cell mediated immunity – control of intracellular pathogens, DTH response • Activates macrophages via cytokine elaboration (IFN-γ and IL-2)	αβ T-cell receptor	CD3+,CD4+, CD8–
Th2	• Stimulates B-lymphocyte differentiation and proliferation (humoral immunity) • Elaborates cytokines involved primarily in the allergic response (IL-4, IL-5, IL-10)	αβ T-cell receptor	CD3+,CD4+, CD8–
Cytotoxic	• Lysis of tumor cells, virus-infected cells • Stimulates cell-mediated immunity via cytokine production	αβ T-cell receptor	CD3+, CD4–, CD8+
B-lymphocytes	• Production of antigen-specific immunoglobulins (humoral immune response)	Immunoglobulin molecules (IgG, IgM, IgE, IgA)	Fc receptors, MHC II molecules CD20, CD19
Natural killer (NK) lymphocytes	• Lysis of virus infected cells and tumor cells lacking MHC class I; antibody-dependent cellular cytotoxicity		CD16, CD56

initially identified as major antigens involved in transplant rejection. Cells expressing different MHC molecules are recognized as "non-self" and rejected. When foreign antigens are complexed with MHC molecules, the complex is recognized as non-self, initiating an immune response [10]. Class I MHC molecules are expressed on the surface of most cells and present intracellular antigens (e.g., antigens derived from infecting viruses). Class II MHC molecules exist primarily on "professional" antigen presenting cell (monocyte, macrophage, dendritic, and B-cell) surfaces and present proteins originating outside or within the cell (e.g., phagocytosed bacterial protein). CD4+ (helper/inducer) T-cells recognize exogenous antigen bound to class II molecules, and CD8+ (cytotoxic) T-cells recognize endogenous antigen bound to class I molecules [11].

Antigen presentation

The initiation of specific immune responses begins when the T-cell TCR recognizes short peptides processed and bound to an antigen-presenting cell (APC) MHC molecule. The TCR-associated CD3 molecule transduces a signal into the cell. Proper antigen recognition requires the TCR/CD3 complex. Other T-cell accessory molecules (CD4 and CD8) must also interact with the APC [12]. They bind the invariant regions of class I or class II MCH molecules. Other molecules, including CD28 and integrins, act as costimulatory signals to induce certain immune responses. TCR–MHC–antigen interaction produces T-cell activation and differentiation, initiating the response. T-cell surface markers change once the T-cell TCR encounters specific antigen. A subset of peripheral CD4+ T-cells (CD45RA+ CD29^{low}) includes naïve cells that have not encountered specific antigen, forming the pool of cells responding to novel antigens. After an initial antigen encounter they develop into memory T-cells (CD45RO+CD29^{hi}) [13]. These memory T-cells rapidly proliferate and produce cytokines when rechallenged with previously encountered antigens, yielding rapid, expanded secondary responses.

CD4+ T-cells

Most peripheral α/β T-cells express CD4 or CD8 antigens. CD4+ T-cells (helper/inducer cells) help regulate the immune response. CD4+ T-cells help B-cells to produce antigen-specific antibody. B-cells process antigen and present self-MHC-bound antigen fragments, activating CD4+ T-cells. During interactions between B- and CD4+ T-cells, membrane molecules that increase the efficiency of the interaction are upregulated [14]. CD40 ligand appears on the activated T-cell surface, which acts on B-cells, promoting humoral immune response [15]. CD4+ cells activate B-cells into antibody-secreting cells and help generate CD8+ T-cell cytotoxic and suppressor functions (see below). Memory T-cells (see above) are CD4+ T-cells.

T_H1 vs. T_H2 T-cells

Two functionally distinct CD4 cell subsets are distinguished by their cytokine expression [16]. T_H1 cells produce interferon-γ and IL-2, and enhance cellular immunity

Table 1.3. Selected cytokines, cell source and principal effects

Cytokine	Cell source	Target cell/principal effects
IL-2	T-cells	T-cells: proliferation and differentiation; activation of CTL and macrophages
IL-3	T-cells, stem cells	Cell colony stimulating factor
IL-4	T-cells	T/B-cells: B-cell growth factor, isotype selection
IL-6	T/B-cells	B-cells/hepatocytes: B-cell differentiation, acute phase reactant production
IL-8	Monocytes	Granulocytes, basophils, T-cells: chemotaxis, superoxide release, granule release
IL-12	Monocytes	T-cells: induction of T_H1 cells
IFN-γ	T-cells, NK cells	Leukocytes, macrophages: MHC induction, macrophage activation and cytokine synthesis
TNF-α	Macrophages, mast cells, lymphocytes	Macrophages, granulocytes: activation of monocytes, granulocytes, increase adhesion molecules, pyrexia, cachexia, acute phase reactant production

IL – interleukin; IFN – interferon; TNF – tumor necrosis factor.

and macrophage activity. T_H1 cells regulate delayed-type hypersensitivity, granuloma formation, and intracellular pathogen killing. T_H2 cells produce IL-4, IL-5, and IL-10, and regulate humoral immunity, which mediates the development of allergic diseases: IL-4 promotes IgE production; IL-5 induces eosinophil proliferation and differentiation [12, 17]. Differentiation of naïve CD4+ T-cells into T_H1 or T_H2 cells depends on the cytokine milieu, antigen dose, and the specific antigen.

CD8+ T-cells

CD8+ (cytotoxic/suppressor) T-cells act as cytotoxic T-cells and can suppress immune responses [11]. Class I MHC-bound antigen activates CD8+ T-cells to generate antigen-specific cytolytic activity. Cytolytic T-lymphocytes (CTL) respond to viral infection of most host cells [12]. CD4+ cells help CD8+ T-cells to develop a CTL response by producing several cytokines, particularly IL-2 [18].

Cytokines

Cytokines are soluble proteins that modulate immune responses. They interact with specific membrane receptors. Different cytokines may perform similar functions and affect multiple cell types. Cytokine functions include (a) regulating lymphocyte growth and differentiation, (b) mediating inflammation, and (c) regulating hematopoesis. Cytokines affecting T-cells include the interleukins (IL), interferons, growth factors, and tumor necrosis factor (TNF) [12] (Table 1.3).

Table 1.4. Selected chemokines, their receptors and target cells

Chemokine	Receptors	Target cell
MIP-1α	CCR1 – 7	Eosinophils, monocytes, activated T-cells, dendritic cells, NK cells
MIP-1β	CCR1 – 7	Monocytes, activated T-cells, dendritic cells, NK cells
RANTES	CCR1 – 7	Eosinophils, basophils, monocytes, activated T-cells, dendritic cells, NK cells
Fractalkine	CX$_3$CR1	Monocytes, activated T-cells, NK cells
SDF-1	CXCR4	Monocytes, resting T-cells, dendritic cells
MIG	CXCR3	Activated T-cells, NK cells
IL-8	CXCR1 and 2	Neutrophils
IP-10	CXCR3	Activated T-cells
MCP-1	CCR2 and 5	Monocytes, activated T-cells, dendritic cells, NK cells
Eotaxin-1	CCR1-3	Eosinophils, basophils

MIP – macrophage inflammatory protein; SDF – stromal-cell derived factor; MIG – monokine induced by interferon gamma; IL – interleukin; IP – interferon inducible protein; MCP – monocyte chemoattractant protein
Adapted from [19].

Chemokines

Chemokines are a family of cytokines that regulate chemotaxis [19]. Over 40 chemokines are grouped into four families, including the α- and β-chemokines. β-chemokines have two adjacent cysteine residues (CC); α-chemokines have one amino acid separating the first two cysteine residues (CXC). Almost all cell types produce chemokines, particularly in response to inflammation. Proinflammatory cytokines (IL-1 and TNF-α), lymphokines (INF-γ and IL-4), and bacterial LPS and viral infection stimulate chemokine production. Chemokines bind specific target cell receptors. Most chemokine receptors bind more than one chemokine; however, CC chemokine receptors bind only CC chemokines and CXC receptors bind only CXC chemokines. Different leukocyte types express different chemokine receptors. Some receptors are restricted to specific cell types; others are expressed widely (Table 1.4).

Infiltrating inflammatory cells are determined partly by chemokines in affected tissue. Chemokines link innate and adaptive immune systems. Dendritic cells internalize antigens in tissues to carry them to lymph nodes, where naïve B- and T-cells are activated. Activated cells traffic back to inflammation sites. Chemokines regulate DC and lymphocyte trafficking [19].

Humoral immunity
Immunoglobulins
Immunoglobulins (antibodies) are proteins that bind antigen with high affinity and specificity. An immunoglobulin molecule is made up of two heavy and two light chains,

aligned in parallel, and covalently linked by disulfide bonds. (IgM is a pentamer of the basic immunoglobulin). The heavy and light chains have variable (V) and constant (c) regions. The variable regions of the chains (V_H and V_L) form the antigen-binding region. During B-cell development, rearrangement of the genes within individual B-cells yields unique, specific antibodies recognizing particular antigens [20]. Heavy chain constant regions determine antibody isotype: IgG, IgM, IgA, IgE, IgD. Immunoglobulin isotype functions include: (a) opsonization or binding to a microbe or particle to facilitate phagocytosis or killing (IgM, IgG, IgA, IgE); (b) complement fixation (activated via the classical pathway) (IgM, IgG); (c) direct inactivation of toxins or viruses (IgG, IgM, IgA); (d) antigen clearance via the reticuloendothelial system (IgG, IgM); and (e) release of chemical mediators following antibody receptor binding (IgG, IgE).

B-cells

B-cells bind antigen via cell surface immunoglobulin variable regions. Naïve B-cells express both cell surface IgD and IgM before encountering cognate antigen (antigen recognized by the immunoglobulin receptor). Surface immunoglobulin is associated with two other proteins, Ig-α and Ig-β; this complex forms the signaling pathway [21]. Most B-cells require T-cell help (via cytokines, contact of B- and T-cells through co-stimulatory molecules like CD40) for activation. B-cells may differentiate terminally into plasma cells, which can produce large amounts of specific immunoglobulin [20].

The primary immune response

When the immune system first encounters an antigen, few cells specifically recognize the antigen. The primary immune response is slow and produces low affinity antibodies [20]. Antigen is endocytosed and processed by an APC (monocyte, macrophage or DC, usually not B-cells), and is then presented to an antigen-specific T-cell. The T-cell must then contact and activate B-cells specific for the antigen/TCR complex, which proliferate or differentiate into plasma cells. Low affinity, mainly IgM is produced during this immune response phase. B-cells expressing higher affinity antibody are selected for activation and differentiation. Most B-lymphocytes differentiate into plasma cells; the remainder revert to memory B-cells.

The secondary immune response

When the B-cell re-encounters its cognate antigen, the antigen is endocytosed, loaded onto MHC class II molecules, presented on the surface of the B-cell to CD4 cells, which activate the B-cell. The B-cells proliferate and differentiate further, including class switching (DNA rearrangement that results in different heavy chain isotypes linked to variable regions). These B-cells can produce different types of high affinity antigen-specific immunoglobulins – IgG, IgE or IgA. Clonal proliferation and plasma cell differentiation occur in an accelerated manner, resulting in rapid production of large amounts of high affinity antibodies when antigen is encountered [14].

Immune system development

Both innate and adaptive immune systems are less efficient in infants than in adults. Mucosal barriers are less effective, particularly in premature infants. Immunoglobulin levels are lower, and the specific immune response is decreased. Adult level immune responses are achieved within the first few years of life. Table 1.1 summarizes the major immune system developmental differences.

Innate immunity

Epithelial barriers/mucosal defenses

The epidermis increases in cell layers and thickness during gestation; infant skin is thinner than adult. Secretory IgA is undetectable at birth, but occurs in secretions by 2 weeks, reaching adult levels by 6–8 years [22]. Decreased secretory IgA permits greater adherence of pathogens to mucosa.

Complement

Complement synthesis begins early in gestation (6–14 weeks); by birth, levels and biologic activity of some complement cascade components equal adult levels. Some elements of the alternative pathway (C8, C9) are <20% adult levels, perhaps contributing to the susceptibility of infants to infection with organisms like *N. meningitides* [22]. Infants have decreased levels of C3b, contributing to increased encapsulated organism susceptibility.

Phagocytes

Macrophages and monocytes are derived from common stem cells. From bone marrow, mature monocytes migrate to peripheral blood. Monocytes circulate for 1–4 days, then migrate into tissue to differentiate into tissue macrophages. The monocytes circulating in blood vary, reflecting egress into tissues, margination along endothelial surfaces, and new cell migration from bone marrow. Tissue macrophages have long half-lives (60 days to years); they are differentiated terminally.

The number of monocytes is higher in neonates than in adults. The number decreases from the neonatal period, reaching adult levels by early childhood. Tissue macrophages from infants may not kill pathogens as successfully as adult macrophages. There are modest differences in the generation of reactive oxygen intermediates [23].

Lymphokines from activated T-cells prime monocyte function. Neonatal monocytes respond less to IFN-γ production by NK and T-lymphocytes than do adult monocytes, decreasing lymphokine production by the T-cells [23]. Neonatal monocyte/macrophages produce less of some cytokines and growth factors (TNF-α, IL-8, IL-6 and G-CSF) [22, 23]. Immature macrophages have decreased chemotaxis, which persists until approximately 6–10 years of age.

Neutrophils

Neutrophils arise from bone marrow stem cells and differentiate into granulocytes. Their development depends upon cytokines and growth factors (granulocyte-colony stimulating factor (G-CSF)). Mature neutrophils are detected by 14–16 weeks' gestation. The blood neutrophil pool has equal circulatory and marginated components. In adults, neutrophil maturation takes approximately 9–11 days, accelerated by stress or infection. The number of neutrophils in the peripheral circulation rises after birth, but the ability to expand the neutrophil pool is limited in neonates, which may contribute to the inability of infants to increase circulating neutrophils with infection. Chemotaxis of neonatal neutrophils is decreased compared with adults. This deficit is multifactorial, reflecting decreased ability to adhere to vascular endothelium, decreased monocyte cytokine production, and additional chemotactic deficiencies; chemotaxis reaches adult competence by 2 years [24].

Natural killer cells

Neonatal NK cells have reduced cytolytic activity (~50% of adults), not reaching adult levels until 9–12 months of age, and decreased antibody-dependent cell-mediated cytotoxicity (ADCC). The decreased NK cell activities may increase susceptibility to infection by herpes simplex and by cytomegalovirus [22].

Dendritic cells

The reduced ability of neonatal T- and B-cells to respond to antigens (discussed below) may partly be due to reduced ability to present antigen. Cord blood dendritic cells express fewer MHC and ICAM-1 molecules and are less effective than adult cells at supporting antigen-stimulated T-cell proliferation [25].

Cell-mediated immune response

Thymic development

The thymus descends to its position in the anterior mediastinum between 7 and 10 weeks' gestation. By 10–14 weeks' gestation, it is highly organized, and emigration of mature T-cells has been established. The thymus has a cortex, containing immature T-cells, and a medulla where mature T-cells migrate. Thymic stromal cells play a role in the differentiation, development, and selection of T-cells [26]. Proper development of T-cells bearing the $\alpha\beta$ TCR depends on an intact thymus; some T-cells bearing $\gamma\delta$ TCRs undergo thymus-independent development [22].

T-cell phenotype

Neonatal T-cells have a naive (CD45RA+ CD29^{low}) phenotype. Ninety percent of neonatal T-cells have this phenotype, compared to 60% of adult T-cells [13]. Memory T-cells (CD45RO+, CD29^{hi}) migrate to sites of inflammation, depend less on costimulatory molecules for activation, proliferate more rapidly, and produce cytokines more efficiently [27]. These attributes permit rapidly expanded T-cell responses with anti-genic rechallenge. Neonates experience delayed T-cell-dependent responses.

T-cell numbers
T-cell numbers increase from mid-gestation until 6 months of age (median CD4 cell count at 6 months is ~3000 cells/mm^3). Counts decline throughout childhood until adult levels (~1000 cells/mm^3)are reached by late childhood. Changes in CD4 percent-age are less dramatic, declining from ~50% to ~40% between infancy and adulthood. The CD4+ to CD8+ ratio changes throughout childhood, achieving the adult ratio of 2:1 at ~4 years (Fig. 1.1) [28, 29].

Cytokine production
TNF-α and GM-CSF are modestly reduced in neonates, while others, critical for a rapid integrated immune response (IFN-γ, IL-3, IL-4, IL-5 and IL-12) are markedly decreased in neonates [30]. IL-2 and TNF-β are at near adult levels [31]. Neonatal CD4+ T-cells preferentially develop a Th2 phenotype [32], but increased CD28 costimulation in high Th1 cytokine levels, suggesting that the neonatal T-cell defect is not intrinsic, but is related to activation conditions. Administration of IL-12 can induce an adult-type Th1 response in neonates. Cytokine synthetic ability increases with age. TNF-α production normalizes within the first few months of life; IFN-γ and IL-12 production normalizes by 1 year [22, 30].

T-cell help for antibody production
Infant T-cells provide less help to B-cells. This reflects reduced cytokine production and reduced expression of costimulatory molecules (CD40 ligand) [33]. Diminished T-cell help produces delayed infection and immunization.

DTH
Delayed type hypersensitivity requires the integration of T-lymphocytes with APCs. At birth, there is no detectable DTH, due to absent memory T-cells, defective monocyte chemotaxis, and/or decreased numbers of efficient APCs. A reliable DTH response exists after 1–2 years [34].

Cytotoxic T-lymphocytes (CTL)
CTL development and the magnitude of CTL activity are decreased during most natural infections in infants. CTL activity matures within the first year of life [30].

Humoral immune response
Development
The fetus can mount humoral immune responses by 6–7 months' gestation; humoral immune function reaches adult competence after 2 years of age. B-cell maturation con-tinues in bone marrow throughout life, although only a small fraction of B-lymphocytes

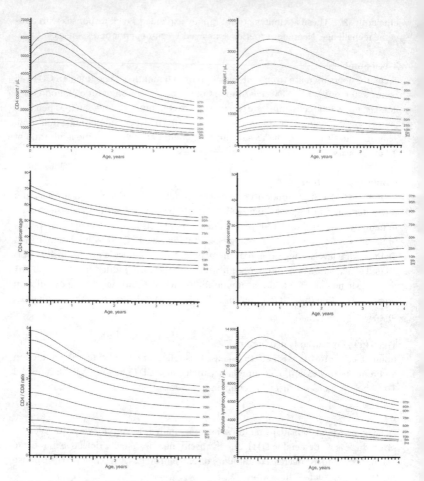

Fig. 1.1. Lymphocyte parameters as a function of age. The panels show values for the CD4+ and CD8+ lymphocyte counts and percentages, the CD4+/CD8+ lymphocyte ratio, and the absolute lymphocyte count during the first 4 years of life. Figure modified from reference [29].

circulates. An ongoing process eliminates B-cells with non-functional or self-reactive immunoglobulins [35].

Immunoglobulins

Neonatal B-cells show Ig diversity similar to adult cells. Neonatal B-cells undergo somatic mutation at the same rate as adult cells [36]. Immunoglobulin concentrations gradually rise with age (Table 1.5) although the repertoire of IgG, especially IgG2a, achieves adult phenotypes after 6–12 months [30].

B-cells

In vitro, neonatal B-cells can differentiate into plasma cells secreting IgM, but not those secreting IgA or IgG. This limitation probably reflects the lack of appropriate T-cell help (discussed above), rather than an inability of B-cells to class switch [37].

B-cell response to specific antigens

Responses to antigens that need T-cell help generally mature faster than those occurring independently of T-cells. Infants generally mount protective immune responses against protein antigens (T-cell-dependent responses, e.g., tetanus, diphtheria, polio). Thymus-dependent immune responses mature rapidly, in many cases by 2 months. IgG antibody responses to protein antigens approach adult levels after 1 year [30]. However, the response to polysaccharide antigens (e.g., *H. influenzae* or *S. pneumoniae*) (T-cell independent antigens) only matures at 2–3 years. Reduced levels of complement receptors on infant B-cells, low complement activity (C3d), reduced IgG2a production, and immaturity of the splenic marginal zone may cause these delays [30]. These differences help explain the age-specific risk for development of invasive bacterial disease.

HIV basic virology

Classification and origin of HIV

HIV-1 belongs to the *Lentivirus* genus of retroviruses (for review see [38]). The virus entered the human population in Africa about 70 years ago [39], probably as humans hunted and butchered chimpanzees. HIV-2, a less pathogenic relative of HIV-1, infects some human populations mostly in western Africa. The material in this book refers to HIV-1 (usually just "HIV") unless otherwise noted.

HIV-1 is grouped into several clades or subtypes (A, B, C, D, E, F, G, H, J, and K) [38], and three groups (M (main) group, O (outlier); N (non-M, non-O)). Certain clades predominate in certain areas. Clade B predominates in North America, and represents the major subtype in Europe and Australia. Clade A predominates in West Africa, clade D in Central Africa, and clade C in Southern and Eastern Africa and the Indian Subcontinent. Clade E is a major subtype in Thailand. Some assays optimized for one clade (clade B) may not detect other clades. Immunologic responses aimed at one clade may not affect other clades, complicating vaccine development.

HIV virion structure

The virion's capsid is composed of viral capsid (CA or p24) protein, enclosing two copies of the RNA genome, and two copies of reverse transcriptase (RT or p66/p51) (Fig. 1.2). Within the capsid, viral nucleocapsid (NC or p9) proteins are complexed with the viral

Table 1.5. Levels of immunoglobulins in normal subjects by age

Age	Total immunoglobulins mg/dl	% of adult level	IgG mg/dl	% of adult level	IgM mg/dl	% of adult level	IgA mg/dl	% of adult level
Newborn	1044±201	67±13	1031±200	89±17	11±5	11±5	2±3	1±2
1–3mo	481±127	31±9	430±119	37±10	30±11	30±11	21±13	11±7
4–6mo	498±204	32±13	427±186	37±16	43±17	43±17	28±18	14±9
7–12mo	752±242	48±15	661±219	58±19	54±23	55±23	37±18	19±9
13–24mo	870±258	56±16	762±209	66±18	58±23	59±23	50±24	25±12
25–36mo	1024±205	65±14	892±183	77±16	61±19	62±19	71±37	36±19
3–5 yr	1078±245	69±17	929±228	80±20	56±18	57±18	93±27	47±14
6–8 yr	1112±293	71±20	923±256	80±22	65±25	66±25	124±45	62±23
9–11 yr	1334±254	85±17	1124±235	97±20	79±33	80±33	131±60	66±30
12–16 yr	1153±169	74±12	946±124	82±11	59±20	60±20	148±63	74±32
Adult	1457±353	100±24	1158±100	100±26	99±27	100±27	200±61	100±31

Mean values ± one standard deviation – normal levels may vary at different reference laboratories.
Modified with permission from [299].

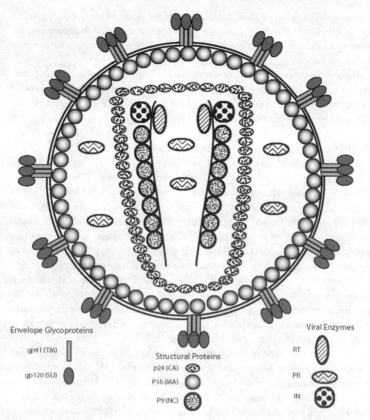

Envelope Glycoproteins

gp41 (TM)

gp120 (SU)

Structural Proteins
p24 (CA)
P16 (MA)

P9 (NC)

Viral Enzymes

RT

PR

IN

Fig. 1.2. A schematic diagram of the HIV virion. Individual viral proteins and their functions are described in detail in the text.

genomic RNA, via zinc finger domains in NC and a specific viral RNA "packaging signal" (the "Ψ-site") (see below). Also within the capsid lie viral integrase (IN or p31) and viral protease (PR or p11). RT, PR, and IN derive from gag–pol preprotein precursor (Pr160), cleaved into its subunits by PR (see below). Other core proteins derive from gag preprotein (Pr55).

The core outer region contains matrix (MA or p16) protein. MA lies inside the envelope, tethered to the interior side of the envelope via myristic acid. The envelope is a lipid bilayer, derived from host cell plasma membrane. Anchored into the lipid bilayer and extending out into extracellular space is the gp41 transmembrane portion of the viral envelope (or Env) glycoprotein (TM or gp41). TM associates non-covalently with the gp120 envelope (Env) glycoprotein (SU or gp120); gp120 and gp41, processed from a precursor, gp160, are highly glycosylated. gp120+gp41 exist as trimers on the virion surface, and mediate viral entry and syncytium formation. gp120 has constant (C) regions, with amino acid sequences remaining relatively constant among viruses, and variable (V) regions.

The virion also contains host cell macromolecules derived, and incorporated, during virion assembly [40]. Some of these (cellular lysine transfer RNA, the protein cyclophillin A) play crucial roles in viral replication. Figure 1.2 outlines virion structure. Table 1.6 lists the viral proteins.

The HIV life cycle
Viral entry into the host cell
Figure 1.3 depicts the life cycle. Infection begins when gp120 binds CD4 on the future host cell (for review see [41]). Binding triggers a change in gp120, facilitating interaction with a viral coreceptor, CXCR4 or CCR5 (which physiologically serve as chemokine receptors, see above and Table 1.4). Coreceptor binding triggers changes in gp41, inserting part of gp41, the "fusion peptide," into the host cell membrane, and the formation of a specialized structure in gp41, bringing the membranes into apposition and engendering envelope-membrane fusion [42], releasing capsid into the cytoplasm. The newly developed antiretroviral agent enfuvirtide (T-20, Fuzeon), a 36-amino acid peptide, is homologous to gp41 [43]. T-20 binds to a gp41 instead of to a native gp41 helix, preventing gp41 from forming structures producing fusion. Some small molecule inhibitors are also under development. Decreasing expression of cell surface CD4 can also block *in vitro* infection [44], but clinical utility lies far in the future.

HIV has tropisms for different host cell types: macrophage-tropic (M-tropic) and T-cell-tropic (T-tropic). Coreceptor usage determines tropism. M-tropic strains infect macrophages, monocytes, and primary T-cells, but not CD4+ T-cell lines (for review see [45]). M-tropic (or R5) viruses use CCR5 as the coreceptor. T-tropic (or X4) viruses infect CD4+ T-cells, but not macrophages and monocytes, using CXCR4 as the coreceptor. Some dual tropic (R5X4) viruses exist. Certain Env V-region envelope sequences are associated with particular tropisms. Most patients are first infected with R5 viruses. Later, the predominant virus may shift to X4, a shift associated with clinical deterioration.

The α-chemokines (or C–C chemokines, for their juxtaposed cysteines) (RANTES, MIP1-α, and MIP1-β) bind CCR5 (Table 1.4), or A β-chemokine (C–X–C chemokine, for adjacent cystein-X-cysteine residues), stromal derived factor 1 (SDF-1), or binds CXCR4. Other chemokine coreceptors may mediate HIV entry into certain cells, perhaps including the central nervous system (CNS) [46].

The coreceptors are drug development targets. Some inhibitors block viral replication *in vitro* and are currently in early stage human trials, including AMD-3100, which targets CXCR4, and Schering-C and -D, targeting CCR5 [47].

Individuals with mutant coreceptors are less likely to become HIV-infected and HIV-infected patients bearing coreceptor mutations have slower disease progression

Table 1.6. HIV viral genes and gene products: existing and potential targets for antiretroviral agents

HIV genes and gene products as targets for antiretroviral drug development. The table lists the viral genes, the proteins the viral genes encode, and the function of the proteins. The table also notes whether the proteins have been used as targets for the development of antiretroviral drugs. The proteins that are targeted by approved drugs or drugs in advanced stages of clinical development are listed in bold.

Viral protein	Gene	Function	Inhibitors
p16 (MA)	*gag*	Matrix protein; lies beneath envelope; targeted to membrane via myristoylation; recruits envelope into virion; aids in PI localization to nucleus	Nuclear localization site inhibitors; myristoylation inhibitors; transdominant negative gag mutants
p24 (CA)	*gag*	Capsid protein; viral core	
p9 (NC)	*gag*	Nucleocapsid protein; interacts with viral RNA via zinc fingers	Zinc chelators
p6 (NC)	*gag*		
Protease (PR)	*pol*	Cleaves gag (Pr55) and gag–pol (Pr160) precursor proteins during virion maturation	Protease inhibitors
Reverse transcriptase (RT)	*pol*	Catalyzes synthesis of viral cDNA from viral genomic RNA	Nucleoside analogue reverse transcriptase inhibitors (NRTIs); nucleotide analoge reverse transcriptase inhibitors (tenofovir); non-nucleoside analogue reverse transcriptase inhibitors (NNRTIs)
Integrase (IN)	*pol*	Catalyzes integration of viral cDNA into host cell genomic DNA to create provirus	Integrase inhibitors
gp120	*env*	Mediates interaction of virus with CD4 and chemokine co-receptors. Initial steps of viral binding and entry.	Chemokine co-receptor inhibitors (e.g., Schering C and D); binding inhibitors (soluble CD4)
gp41	*env*	Integral membrane envelope glycoprotein; contains fusion domain mediating virion envelope-host cell plasma membrane fusion	Fusion inhibitors (e.g., enfuvirtide (T-20)

(*cont.*)

Table 1.6. (*cont.*)

Viral protein	Gene	Function	Inhibitors
Tat	*tat*	Transactivates viral gene expression; binds to TAR structure in nascent viral RNA and cellular kinase leading phosphorylation of celluar RNA polymerase II, increasing processivity	Kinase inhibitors (cellular enzyme); Small molecule inhibitors; Tat-TAR interaction blockers; TAR decoys; antisense oligonucleotides; ribozymes, small interfering RNAs
Rev	*rev*	Mediates nuclear export of singly spliced and unspliced viral RNAs	Small molecule inhibitors, inhibitors of Rev-RRE binding (aminoglycosides); RRE decoys; transdominant Rev; antisense oligonucleotides; ribozymes; inhibitors of nuclear export, small interfering RNAs
Vif	*vif*	Viral infectivity factor	
Vpu	*vpu*	gp160/CD4 complex degradation; CD4 downregulation; virus release	
Vpr	*vpr*	Cell cycle arrest; transactivation; PIC entry into nucleus	
Nef	*nef*	CD4 downregulation; stimulates cellular signal transduction pathways	

Targets of drugs with current clinical utility (licensed drugs and drugs in advanced clinical development) are shown in **bold**.

(including some "long-term non-progressors" (LTNP)). Important mutations include a 32- base pair CCR5 gene deletion (Δ32CCR5) [48]. Δ32CCR5 does not localize to the cell membrane. Δ32CCR5 cells do not resist infection by T-tropic viruses, since they use CXCR4. Δ32CCR5 homozygotes are highly resistant to initial infection, because M-tropic viruses may be primary mediators of transmission. Δ32CCR5- individuals exhibit no discernable deleterious phenotype. Other mutations that decrease CCR5 are also seen in LTNP.

Reverse transcription

After entry, viral capsid releases the RNA genome, with proteins and the tRNA to prime reverse transcription, into the cytoplasm. RT catalyzes reverse transcription, through which it produces a cDNA of the viral genome. RT consists of a dimer, p51 and p66 (the

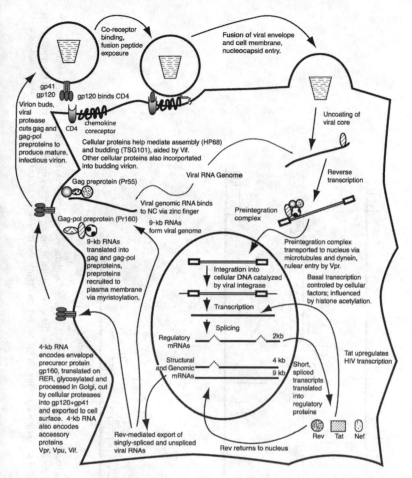

Fig. 1.3. A schematic diagram of the HIV replication cycle. The features of the viral life cycle are described in detail in the text.

catalytic subunit). Many drugs target RT, including nucleoside reverse transcriptase inhibitors (NRTIs) and non-nucleoside reverse transcriptase inhibitors (NNRTIs) (see Chapter 14).

The HIV RNA genome begins 5′ with the "R" (repeat) region, followed by the U5 (5′ unique) region, then sequences encoding viral proteins and, at the 3′ end, U3 (3′ unique) and another R (Fig. 1.4) [49]. RT synthesizes a double-stranded cDNA version of the genome, with two long terminal repeats (LTRs) at either end. Each LTR consists of the repeated versions of U3, R, and U5.

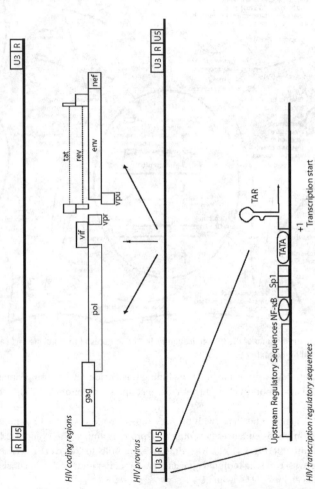

Fig. 1.4. The genomic organization of HIV. The top of the figure shows the organization of the viral genomic RNA. The middle of the figure shows the HIV provirus, with the reading frames of the different HIV genes identified. The lower portion of the figure shows the location of selected HIV transcription regulatory sites, including both selected sites active in the HIV LTR (NF-kB, Sp1, and TATA), and the TAR site as it exists in the newly transcribe viral RNA.

Reverse transcription is an essential step in replication. NRTIs were the first antiretrovirals. NRTIs are converted to the active triphosphate form by cellular kinases. The triphosphate-NRTIs compete with native nucleotide triphosphates. When RT incorporates the NRTIs into cDNA, no further nucleotides can be added, truncating the cDNA because the ribose 3'-OH is replaced by another group incapable of forming a covalent bond with the next nucleotide. For example, the 3'-OH is replaced by an azido group in zidovudine (ZDV or AZT). These drugs are termed "chain terminators."

The non-nucleoside RT inhibitors (NNRTIs) represent another class of RT inhibitors, with three licensed drugs, efavirenz, nevirapine, and delavirdine. NNRTIs act differently, binding a hydrophobic pocket near the enzyme active site (see Chapter 14).

RT is a "low fidelity" enzyme, inserting the wrong base (termed "misincorporation") in the growing cDNA chain every 1 per 1700 to 1 per 4000 bases, producing mutant virus (see Chapter 14).

Nuclear localization and entry

After reverse transcription, cDNA associates with viral proteins (IN, RT, MA, and NC, the viral accessory protein Vpr, and host cell proteins Ku, INI 1 and HMGa1 (or HMG I(Y)), to form the pre-integration complex (PIC) [50]. Some PIC components (IN) are essential for later replication cycle steps. Others (the cellular proteins) may not be essential. Following reverse transcription, cellular machinery transports PICs to the nucleus, with help from Vpr [51]. The PIC interacts with the nuclear membrane, via Vpr docking with host cell nucleoporin protein, hCG1 [52], producing nuclear entry.

Integration

After nuclear entry, HIV cDNA integrates into the host cell genomic DNA. A cDNA preintegration form with a recessed 3' end interacts with 5' overhanging ends in cellular DNA, generated by IN, which then joins the cDNA and the cellular DNA, in a process called strand transfer [53].

Since provirus formation is an essential life cycle feature and since IN is an essential enzyme in HIV replication [54], IN is a drug development target [55].

Control of viral gene expression

After integration, the provirus can either remain quiescent, or it can begin replication. *In vitro*, treatment of latently infected cells with host cell signal transduction activating or histone acetylation altering agents (phorbol esters, butyrate) [56], or certain cytokines (IL-2) can induce the infection cycle completion [57].

During lytic infection cycle progression HIV regulates its gene expression in a tightly controlled pattern of three phases (Fig. 1.5). In the initial phase, low levels of full-length transcripts are produced. Some transcripts are retained in the nucleus, spliced, and exported to the cytoplasm. These short transcripts encode viral regulatory proteins, notably Tat. Next, Tat, with cellular factors, transactivates viral gene transcription, dramatically increasing expression. Finally, Rev mediates nuclear export of unspliced

Stage 1: Initial Transcription

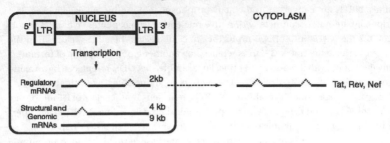

Stage 2: Tat-activated Transcription

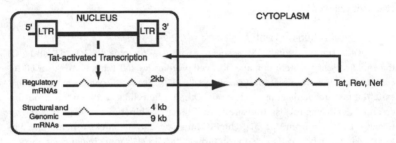

Stage 3: Late Phase Transcription

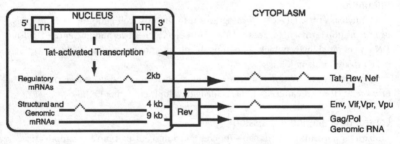

Fig. 1.5. Phases of HIV gene expression. Initially, only small amounts of transcription occur and only small quantities of short, multiply spliced viral messages encoding the viral regulatory genes Tat and Rev and the accessory gene Nef are exported to the cytoplasm. When the HIV promoter is activated, more messages are produced and sufficient Tat protein returns to the nucleus to produce a large increase in viral gene expression. Later, when sufficient quantities of Rev are present in the nucleus, the longer singly spliced and unspliced messages encoding the viral structural proteins and comprising the viral genomic RNA are exported to the cytoplasm.

and singly spliced RNAs encoding viral structural proteins, including future viral genomes.

Regulation of transcription from the HIV LTR by cellular factors

The provirus 5' HIV LTR is the viral promoter. It contains regulatory sites homologous to those in cellular promoters (Fig. 1.4) [58, 59]. Some sites regulate basal HIV expression in lymphocytic cells [60]; others may modulate expression in different cell types [61]. The critical regulatory sequences are TATA and Sp1 [62]. NF-B sequences contribute to basal expression and mediate viral promoter responses to stimulatory signals. TATA serves as the transcription machinery assembly site, including transcription factors and RNA polymerase II. Targeting certain HIV RNAs can inhibit HIV replication [44], but clinical applicability is probably distant.

Sequences 5' to the TATA, Sp1, and NF-B sites can affect HIV expression, but their function is less clear. Some 5' sequences are critically important for maximal expression in certain non-lymphocytic cell types [63].

Chromatin structure is another factor influencing HIV gene expression. The location and acetylation state of histones help control expression from the integrated provirus [64]. Altering histone acetylation can greatly increase expression [65].

Regulation of transcription by Tat

The short (2 kb) viral transcripts first produced by HIV encode three viral gene products, Tat, Rev, and Nef. Tat produces a dramatic increase in expression. Rev regulates HIV gene expression post-transcriptionally, controlling the export of HIV RNA from the nucleus. Nef has several effects on the virus and host cell.

Tat binds a distinctive stem–loop–bulge RNA secondary structure, the trans-activation responsive (TAR) region, in HIV RNAs (Figs. 1.4 and 1.6). Without Tat, RNA polymerase II stalls, producing mostly very short transcripts. If transcription is activated, so that Tat and the TAR-containing transcript are present simultaneously, Tat binds to the bulge in TAR [66], recruiting additional cellular factors, P-TEFb (or TAK, Tat-associated kinase), including the cellular protein kinase CDK9 (or PITALRE) and cyclin T [67]. CDK9 phosphorylates the RNA polymerase II C-terminal domain, making the enzyme more processive [68].

Tat can be secreted from infected cells and taken up into cells from the extracellular environment, affecting cells [69] in ways that may contribute to pathogenesis.

Inhibition of Tat activity is another potential target for drug development. Small molecule inhibitors could block Tat–TAR interaction [70]. cdk9 inhibitors can block Tat activity, inhibiting replication [71].

Post-transcriptional regulation of gene expression by Rev

Rev controls the switch from the early pattern of viral gene expression where multiply spliced 2-kb messages are expressed, to the late pattern of viral gene expression where longer 4-kb and 9-kb messages are expressed (for review see [72]) (Figs. 1.4 and 1.7).

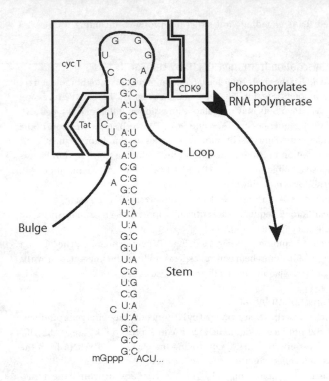

TAR, Tat, cyclin T, and CDK9

Fig. 1.6. TAR, Tat, and associated cellular factors. Tat binds to the "bulge" region of the stem–loop–bulge structure in the TAR RNA. The cellular protein cyclin T interacts with Tat and with the TAR loop region. The cellular kinase cdk9 interacts with cyclin T and then goes on to phosphorylate the C-terminal domain of RNA polymerase II, greatly increasing the processivity of the polymerase, causing a large increase in the expression of the viral RNAs.

HIV RNA is initially produced as a full-length transcript, but if introns are not spliced out of the RNA, without Rev, the 4-kb and 9-kb singly spliced and unspliced messages are not exported from the nucleus. Rev enables the nuclear export of these messages. The HIV RNA contains a region within env that forms a complicated stem–loop secondary structure, the Rev-responsive element (RRE). Revs cooperatively bind RRE RNA. With enough Rev bound, the longer unspliced messages exit the nucleus.

Rev has two regions, nuclear localization /RNA binding region, and another mediating nuclear export (Fig. 1.7). Rev, with bound HIV RNA, binds a cellular protein, CRM1. CRM1 in turn binds another cellular protein, Ran, a small GTPase, but only when Ran

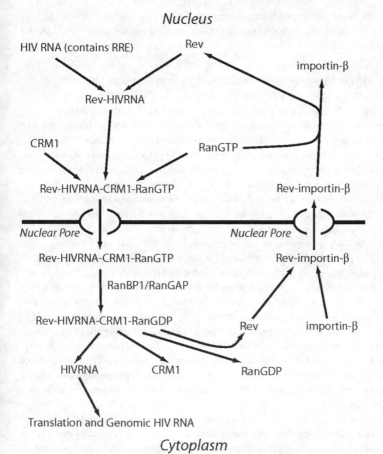

Fig. 1.7. Rev and the export of HIV RNA from the host cell nucleus. Singly spliced and unspliced HIV RNAs are exported from the host cell nucleus via a specialized host cell nuclear pore apparatus, after Rev binds to the RRE sequence in the HIV RNA. See text for details.

has bound GTP (Ran-GTP) [73]. This complex is translocated into the cytoplasm where two proteins, Ran GTPase activating protein 1 (Ran GAP1) and Ran binding protein 1 (Ran BP1) hydrolyze GTP bound to Ran, dissociating the complex bound to HIV RNA, freeing RNA [74]. Rev re-enters the nucleus by binding a cellular protein called importin-β. In the nucleus, RanGTP interacts with importin-β freeing Rev to start the cycle again.

Rev is a potential drug development target. Some small molecules inhibit Rev activity *in vitro*, but none have entered clinical development. Some Rev mutants can inhibit Rev function [75].

Translation of structural (late) viral messages and post-translational modification of the late viral proteins

The long singly spliced and unspliced RNAs encode viral structural and enzymatic proteins. A Gag preprotein, Pr55, and a Gag–Pol fusion preprotein, Pr160, are translated from full-length RNA. The capsid structural components, p16 (MA), p24 (CA), p9 (NC), and p6 (NC), are first translated in the form of Pr55 preprotein, cleaved by the viral protease during virion maturation. The Gag–Pol fusion protein is also cleaved during maturation, forming the *pol* products: RT, IN, and PR (see Chapter 14).

HIV uses a translational mechanism to regulate the relative amounts of *gag*- and *pol*-derived protein production. In the HIV virion, there are more *gag*-derived structural proteins than there are pol-derived enzymatic proteins.

The 4-kb RNA encodes the envelope preprotein gp160 and the HIV accessory proteins Vpr, Vpu, and Vif. gp160 is translated in the rough endoplasmic reticulum (RER), glycosylated, transits through the Golgi complex, and is cleaved by furin family cellular proteases, forming gp41, which remains membrane anchored, and gp120, which remains non-covalently gp41-associated [76]. The glycosylation pattern helps influence viral coreceptor usage [77]. From the Golgi, gp120/gp41 moves to the external cell surface. Blocking gp160 proteolytic processing inhibits infectious virus production.

Viral envelope glycoprotein glycosylation is essential for viral pathogenicity. Glycosylation appears to mask critical sites from host immune responses [76]. Unglycosylated glycoproteins become much more immunogenic. The resulting virus is less pathogenic, probably because the sugar residues guarding critical conserved immunogenic sites are gone [78].

gp160 and CD4 can become non-covalently associated within the RER during translation and processing, preventing the appearance of gp120 and gp41 at the surface. The viral accessory protein Vpu interacts with CD4 in the gp160/CD4 complex, inducing proteolysis [79], freeing gp 160 from the complex and for processing into envelope glycoproteins. This also causes cell surface CD4 downregulation, which may prevent host cell superinfection [80].

Virion assembly, budding, and maturation

Virion assembly occurs at the interior face of the plasma membrane, where Gag and Gag–Pol preproteins assemble beneath the envelope glycoproteins [81]. Following translation, Gag preproteins are myristoylated: a fatty acid, myristic acid targets the preprotein to the plasma membrane. The preprotein preferentially inserts into cholesterol-rich microdomains or "rafts" in the plasma membrane, where new virions bud [82]. Agents that deplete cholesterol from the plasma membrane, including approved agents like simvastatin, decrease virion production [82], but cholesterol is an obligatory component of many membranes and serves other important functions.

About 1500 Gag molecules assemble together to form a functional viral core. A cellular protein (HP68) helps assemble the Gag molecules and promotes viral core formation [83].

Other aspects of virion assembly are mediated by CA, which contains a domain enabling Gag to multimerize [84], another functioning viral core condensation, and another binding the host protein cyclophilin A [85]. Mutations in the multimerization domain or the domain involved in core condensation produce defective virions. The cyclophilin A interaction appears essential for infectious virus formation [86].

The viral RNA genome is packaged into virions by interactions with the Pr55 Gag preprotein [87]. The p9 (NC) region contains two zinc-finger amino acid motifs (cys–X_2–cys–X_4–his–X_4–cys, where X is any amino acid), distinct from cellular zinc finger domains. The full-length genomic RNA contains the RNA packaging signal sequence (Ψ site) at the 5′ end. The sequence is spliced out of the short and intermediate length viral RNAs, preventing packaging into virions. Viral RNA packaging constitutes another drug development target. Zinc chelators block zinc from binding the NC zinc finger, making it in turn unable to bind HIV RNA, blocking infectious virion formation [88].

HIV proteins are essential for budding, but the virus also uses a cellular pathway, used to form the multivesicular body (MVB), to mediate virion budding [89, 90]. Certain *env* mutations prevent Env from associating with assembling viral proteins and being incorporated into virions, implying that gp41 and MA interact to promote Env incorporation [91].

After budding, the newly formed virion undergoes maturation, required for viral infectivity, involving viral protease-catalyzed proteolytic processing. PR cleaves Pr55 (Gag) and Pr160 (Gag–Pol) proteins to produce mature virion proteins (see Fig. 1.3, and Chapter 14). PR is essential for infectious virion production and has become a favored drug development target. HIV protease inhibitors (PIs) are a remarkably effective class of antiretrovirals. PI resistance is described in more detail in Chapter 14.

HIV accessory proteins

The HIV accessory proteins, Nef, Vpu, Vif, and Vpr, have important functions in the viral life cycle. *In vitro*, mutations in the accessory genes do not abolish viral replication, but are critical *in vivo*.

Vpu enhances virus production by downregulating CD4 post-translationally by binding the cytoplasmic tail of CD4 while CD4 is in the endoplasmic reticulum (ER) [92, 93].

Vif (virion infectivity factor) is required in certain cell types during the late stages of infection for infectious virus production [94]. Some lymphocytes have innate antiretroviral activity, yielding non-infectious virus. Vif suppresses this innate antiretroviral activity. This antiretroviral activity results from a cellular gene, CEM15 (Apobec-3G), which inhibits the production of infectious virus lacking Vif [95]. APOBEC-3G

(CEM 15) deaminates cytidine to produce uracil, an activity that can cause mutations that decrease viral infectivity.

Vpr has several functions, in addition to PIC nuclear localization and import, which contribute to infection of non-dividing cells [96]. Vpr is incorporated in large amounts into virions. Vpr can modestly increase HIV gene expression and alters the expression of some cellular genes [97]. Vpr causes cell cycle arrest at G_2 [98], which may increase expression and make more precursors available for virion production.

Nef has several activities during replication and is incorporated into virions. Nef is required for the virus to be fully pathogenic. Nef augments the infectivity of HIV virions, induces downregulation of cell surface CD4 molecules [99] by targeting CD4 for incorporation into endosomes through interactions with a cellular protein, β-COP [100], and interacts with cellular signal transduction pathways [101]. Nef also decreases the surface expression of cellular MHC Class 1 [102].

Immunology of pediatric HIV disease

HIV-1 damages the immune system by harming the infected host cells, harming non-infected cells via the effects of virions and parts of virions, and by chronic cell activation. This can lead to dysfunction of other cell types, since the immune system is highly interconnected. The main target cells of HIV-1 include cells that are critical in the immune control of the virus.

Immunopathogenesis
Primary infection
Most HIV-1 infections result from exposure of HIV-1 to mucosal surfaces [103]. Mucosal dendritic cells transport HIV-1 to regional lymph nodes within 48 hours of exposure, where CD4+ T-cells become infected. Infected T-cells and virus can be found throughout the body 4–11 days after infection.

HIV in blood increases rapidly over the first weeks after infection in adults, then declines dramatically, reaching a stable set point after approximately 6 months. HIV-1-specific cytotoxic T-lymphocytes (CTL) in the peripheral blood correlate with the decline in HIV-1 (for review see [104]). Cytotoxic T-lymphocyte responses appear before antibody responses, suggesting that cell-mediated responses are the key immune activities leading to suppression of initial viremia [105].

Innate immune responses also control plasma HIV-1 levels. CD8+ T-cells produce soluble factors that suppress HIV-1 replication, including β-chemokines (RANTES, macrophage inflammatory protein-1) that compete with HIV-1 for binding to coreceptors, blocking entry [106], and the α-defensins 1, 2, and 3 [107].

The immunology of perinatal primary infection is less well understood. Most infants reach peak viremia at 1–2 months of life but, unlike adults, have only minimal declines in plasma virus over the next several months [108]. Some children with rapid disease

Table 1.7. Mechanisms used by HIV-1 to evade immune responses

---

Mutations no longer recognized by cytotoxic T-lymphocytes (CTL escape mutations)
Mutations no longer recognized by neutralizing antibodies (neutralizing antibody escape mutations)
Inherent resistance to neutralization
Downregulation of MCH class I expression (mediated by viral gene products, e.g., Nef, acting within the infected cell)
Preferential infection and destruction of HIV-1-specific CD4+ T-lymphocytes
Dysregulation of cytokine production (IL-2, IFN-γ, IL-12, IL-10)

---

progression have no decrease in viral load over the first year of life. Children with slow progression show declines in viral RNA, but usually not more than 0.5–1 $\log_{10}$.

Among proposed explanations for the absence of a significant decline in viral load in some vertically infected infants is that the infant fails to mount an effective response. HIV-1-specific CTL may be delayed in perinatally infected infants [109]. However, children who have survived to age 2 years have HIV-1-specific CTL frequencies comparable to adults [110]. The ADCC responses in infants are also less vigorous [111, 112].

Another possible explanation for the relatively high viral loads following vertical infection is transmission of virus that has mutated to escape the maternal immune response. Transmission of this type of escape mutant has been observed [113]. The observation that virus from infants with rapid progression develops fewer new mutations over time suggests that rapid progressors' virus experiences less immune pressure [114].

Chronic/progressive infection/non-progressive infection

HIV-1 replication damages the immune system. Lymph nodes harbor actively replicating HIV-1 and large quantities of antibody–virus complexes bound to follicular dendritic cells (FDC) in the germinal centers [115], which is highly infectious. In advanced HIV-1 infection, lymph node architecture becomes grossly abnormal, with complete loss of germinal center organization. Ongoing viral replication results in generalized immune activation, with higher levels of programmed cell death and T-cell turnover and, perhaps, impaired ability of the thymus to generate new T-cells. Eventually, the immune system becomes unable to respond to infectious pathogens.

HIV-1 infected adults and children can maintain detectable cytotoxic T-cell-mediated immune responses and HIV-1-specific antibody into advanced disease. However, HIV-1-specific lymphoproliferative responses are notably low or absent. This may be an indication of relative deficiency of CD4+ helper T-cell responses (for review see [104]). CD4+ T-cells that are HIV-1-specific are infected preferentially by HIV-1 [116]. Thus, HIV-1 may directly delete some of the T-cells required for generating an immune response against it.

HIV-1 uses other mechanisms to evade the immune response (Table 1.7). High mutation rates allow for outgrowth of virus with variant epitopes that escape recognition by CTL (for review see [104]). HIV-1-specific CTL have phenotypes differing from phenotypes responding to other chronic viral infections. HIV-1-specific CTL may be not fully functional effectors [117–119]. The viral accessory protein Nef downregulates expression of MHC class I on infected cells [120]. MHC class I expression is critical for CTL recognition and infected cell killing. HIV-1 is resistant to antibody-mediated neutralization due to characteristics of the HIV-1 envelope protein (for review see [121]).

A small number of HIV-1 infected adults and children have no evidence of disease progression for 10 or more years, with low levels of plasma HIV-1. This has been termed long-term non-progression (LTNP). Genetic and viral factors have been associated with LTNP. Some patients have had mutated viral co-receptors (see above); a few were infected with Nef-deleted virus (for review see [122]). Some HLA alleles are associated with slower progression. LTNP patients are more likely to have HIV-1-specific lymphoproliferative responses and many HIV-1-specific CTLs [104].

Effects of antiretroviral therapy

Antiretroviral treatment during acute infection in adults can improve the anti-HIV immune response, producing higher HIV-1-specific lymphocyte proliferative responses [123], with improvement in viral control at least temporarily. It is unclear whether this applies to infants. Infants with good viral suppression before 3 months of life do not maintain detectable HIV-1-specific immune responses [124]. Neither HIV-1-specific cell-mediated nor HIV-1 antibody responses are detected when tested at age 12–15 months. Normal responses to other antigens are found. The infants can generate HIV-1-specific responses, as interruptions of treatment result in rapid appearance of HIV-1-specific antibodies [125]. Infants beginning antiretroviral therapy after 3–6 months have higher levels of HIV-1-specific CD8+ T-cell responses and maintain HIV-1 antibodies.

Immune abnormalities associated with HIV-1 infection

Both cell-mediated and humoral immune functions are affected during HIV-1 infection (Table 1.8).

Cell-mediated immunity

Cell-mediated immunity primarily defends against intracellular pathogens, notably viral infections, and malignancies. Abnormal cell-mediated immunity in HIV-1-infected children leads to more severe or recurrent disease from pathogens such as varicella zoster virus, herpes simplex virus, cytomegalovirus (CMV), *Mycobacterium* species, and *Salmonella* species. Lymphomas and certain soft tissue malignancies are also more common. Abnormal cellular immune function contributes to abnormal humoral immunity.

Table 1.8. Immunologic abnormalities associated with HIV-1 infection

Cellular
    Decreased delayed-type hypersensitivity skin reaction
    T-lymphocytes
        Decreased absolute numbers of CD4 positive (helper) T-lymphocytes
        Increased relative numbers of CD8 positive (killer/suppressor) T-lymphocytes
        Decreased CD4/CD8 ratio
        Decreased numbers of cells with naïve phenotype (CD45RA+/CD62L+)
        Increased % cells with memory phenotype (CD45RO+)
        Increased % CD8+ cells with diminished proliferative capacity (CD28⁻; CD95+)
        Increased CD8+ T-cells with activated phenotype (CD38+/HLA-DR+)
        Decreased proliferative responses to antigen and mitogens
        Altered cytokine production (see below)
    Natural Killer (NK) cells
        Decreased number of NK cells (CD16+/CD56+)
        Decreased cytotoxic activity
    Antigen Presenting Cells (monocytes and dendritic cells)
        Decreased stimulation of T-cell proliferative response to antigen
        Decreased HLA-DR expression
        Altered cytokine production
    Phagocytes
        Monocytes
            Decreased clearance of RBC
            Decreased Fc receptor expression
            Decreased chemotaxis
            Decreased intracellular killing
            Decreased superanion production
        Polymorphonuclear cells
            Neutropenia
            Increased or decreased chemotaxis
            Decreased staphylococcus killing
            Increased or decreased phagocytosis
            Altered surface adhesion proteins and receptors
Humoral
    B-lymphocytes
        Decreased number of antigen-responsive B-cells (CD23+/CD62L+; CD21^{hi})
        Polyclonal activation of B-cells
        Increased spontaneous immunoglobulin secretion from B-cells
        Decreased immunoglobulin secretion after stimulation of B-cells
        Increased IgG, IgA, IgM
    Specific antibody responses
        Decreased antibody response to immunization: hepatitis B, HIB conjugate, measles, influenza
        Declining antibody titers after immunization: diphtheria, tetanus, *Candida*, measles
Cytokines
    Decreased production of IL-2, IFN-γ
    Decreased production of IL-12
    Decreased IFN-α
    Increased production of IL-1β, IL-6, and TNF-α
    Increased production of IL-10, transforming growth factor-β

Defects in helper T-lymphocyte cell function

Decline in the absolute number and percentage of helper T-lymphocytes (CD4+ T-lymphocytes) is the hallmark of HIV-1 disease. Since CD4 is used by HIV-1 as the receptor, helper T-lymphocytes are a main target of HIV-1 infection. Direct cytopathic and indirect effects of HIV-1 probably both contribute to the abnormalities in CD4+ T lymphocyte function and number. As CD4+ T-lymphocyte numbers decline, the risks of opportunistic infections increases.

Preceding the CD4+ T-lymphocyte decline, alterations in helper T-lymphocyte function are observed. Lymphocytes from asymptomatic, HIV-1-infected children have reduced proliferation to common antigenic stimulants [126]. As the disease progresses, reduced proliferative responses to specific antigens are followed by decreased responses to allo-antigens and, then eventually diminished responses to mitogens [127].

In HIV-1 disease, helper T-lymphocytes have an abnormal pattern of cytokine secretion (for review see [128]) and decreased post-stimulation production of IL-2 and IFN-γ, which contribute to cell-mediated function defects. Patients with advanced disease have poor DTH responses to memory antigens (e.g., tetanus, *Candida*, mumps)[129]. *Mycobacterium tuberculosis* skin testing may be unreliable.

Changes in CD4+ T-lymphocyte phenotypes also occur with HIV-1 infection. The most notable phenotypic change is an increase in proportion of memory CD4+ T-lymphocytes (CD45RO+) relative to naïve CD4+ T-lymphocytes (CD45RA+CD62L+) [130]. However, due to the overall decline in CD4+ T-lymphocyte numbers, the absolute number of both naive and memory CD4+ T-lymphocytes decreases. Loss of naïve cells may compromise the ability of the immune system to handle new pathogens.

Defects in cytotoxic/suppressor T-lymphocyte cell function

Cytotoxic/suppressor T-lymphocytes mediate direct cytotoxic activity against pathogen-infected and malignant cells, and release soluble factors that inhibit pathogens. CD8+ T-lymphocytes may play a role in downregulating the immune response after an infection has been controlled.

During acute infection, a large increase in CD8+ T-lymphocytes occurs, probably due to vigorous CD8-mediated primary immune response. Large expansions of HIV-1-specific CD8+ T-cell clones – are identified in acute and chronic infection [131, 132]. The number and percentage of CD8+ T-lymphocytes may remain high, particularly in symptomatic patients. The increased number of CD8+ T-lymphocytes can result in decreased CD4/CD8 ratios (normally > 1), even before significant declines in CD4+ T-cell number occur. In advanced disease, the absolute number of CD8+ T-lymphocytes may decline due to lymphopenia. The majority of cells accounting for the CD8+ cell increase are activated (CD38+, HLA-DR+) memory cells (CD45RO+) [133]. A higher proportion of CD8+ T-cells in HIV-1 infected people have phenotypic markers of decreased proliferative potential and increased programmed cell death [134, 135].

Defects in natural killer lymphocyte cell function

The number of NK cells is lower during HIV-1 infection, declining with disease progression [136, 137]. Early in HIV-1 infection, patients have decreased NK lytic activity and decreased production of IFN-γ [137]. Exogenous cytokines (IL-2, IL-12, IL-15) can restore these NK cell functions in vitro, suggesting that an altered cytokine milieu may account for abnormal function [138].

Defects in antigen-presenting cell function

Antigen-presenting cells (APC), including monocytes, macrophages, and dendritic cells, present antigen in the context of either MHC class I or class II antigens to lymphocytes. The presentation and the type of cytokines produced by the APC at the time of interaction with lymphocytes may determine the type of immune response. Monocytes can be directly infected with HIV-1, resulting in abnormal function and dissemination of the infection. The association of HIV-1 with dendritic cells facilitates infection of CD4+ T-cells [139]. The number of dendritic cells in peripheral blood is decreased in acute and chronic HIV-1 infection in adults [140]. Dendritic cells and monocytes from HIV-1-infected patients have a decreased T-lymphocyte proliferation capacity [141].

HIV-1 infection results in abnormal monocyte and dendritic cell cytokine secretion. Interleukin-12 is produced by antigen-presenting cells that promote cellular immune responses (for review see [142]). HIV-1 infection results in decreased IL-12 production [143]. Since IL-12 promote cellular immunity, decreased production may contribute to defective cell-mediated immunity [144]. HIV-1-infected adults have decreased dendritic cell production of interferon-α (IFN-α) [145]. Interferon-α is an important component of the innate pathogen immune response. Increased tumor necrosis factor (TNF)-α serum levels and TNF-α production have been observed, PBMC, brain, and monocytes infected *in vitro* [146]. Increased TNF-α and -β may contribute to wasting disease and encephalopathy. HIV-1 patients also have increased plasma levels of pro-inflammatory cytokines (IL-1β, IL-6) and anti-inflammatory cytokines (IL-10, transforming growth factor-β) (for review see [146]). Some cytokines enhance HIV-1 replication. Cytokine dysregulation also likely impairs normal immune development.

Defects in phagocyte cell function

Phagocytes engulf and kill extracellular pathogens, generate granulomas, and localize infection. Mononuclear phagocyte and polymorphonuclear leukocyte (PMN) defects observed during HIV-1 infection include decreased chemotaxis, diminished intracellular killing, and decreased superanion radical production; these defects may contribute to poor granuloma formation observed during HIV-1-infection [147].

PMNs defend against bacterial and fungal pathogens. Patients with advanced disease often have neutropenia resulting from drug toxicity and HIV-1 disease. HIV-1 infected patients may also have defects in PMN function (decreased phagocytosis, decreased bactericidal activity, altered superoxide production, altered chemotaxis, and altered surface adhesion molecules and activation receptors) [148].

Table 1.9. Serum immunoglobulin levels (median and upper 95% confidence limit) in uninfected, asymptomatic and symptomatic HIV-1-infected children

		Children		
	Age (mo)	Uninfected	Asymptomatic	Symptomatic
IgG (mg/dl)	0–1	554 + 757	836 + 1091	952 + 1122
	1–6	437 + 630	551 + 657	1360 + 1514
	7–12	565 + 711	615 + 918	1893 + 2422
	13–24	725 + 998	774 + 1120	2125 + 2855
IgA (mg/dl)	0–1	16 + 30	16 + 27	54 + 69
	1–6	24 + 32	27 + 39	74 + 98
	7–12	27 + 68	26 + 42	141 + 191
	13–24	42 + 69	45 + 89	149 + 188
IgM (mg/dl)	0–1	47 + 78	47 + 77	103 + 152
	1–6	59 + 89	85 + 109	134 + 159
	7–12	79 + 104	108 + 134	167 + 183
	13–24	105 + 130	120 + 177	149 + 191

Modified from [151].

Humoral immunity

Abnormal humoral immunity occurs in HIV-1-infected adults and children, but is more significant in children. Children have increased rates of minor and invasive bacterial infections. HIV-1 probably destroys the ability to produce antibodies against new antigens before the child is exposed to pathogens. An HIV-1-infected adult may have generated memory B-cells before HIV-1 infection. These adult memory cells can produce protective antibody upon repeat exposure. Hyperglobulinemia is a notable feature of the disease, particularly in many pediatric HIV-1 patients. Hypoglobulinemia can be seen in some pediatric and adult HIV-1 patients with advanced disease.

Defects in B-lymphocyte function

B-lymphocytes are not infected by HIV-1, but have abnormal function, probably because of direct effects of HIV-1 gp120, altered cytokine levels, and impaired CD4+ T-cell-mediated help. A minority of patients will have hypogammaglobulinemia, particularly with advanced disease [149]. The more common abnormality is a relatively non-specific polyclonal B-cell activation, resulting in hypergammaglobulinemia [150]. Elevated IgG, particularly IgG1 and IgG2, can be observed by age 6 months (Table 1.9). Elevated IgA and IgM are also observed, particularly in rapidly progressive disease [151]. The B-lymphocytes in vitro have increased spontaneous immunoglobulin production and cell proliferation, but decreased specific immunoglobulin production and cell proliferation in response to recall antigens or B-lymphocyte-specific mitogens [150]. Most cells produce polyclonal, low affinity antibody not directed against a discernable pathogen, although 20–40% make HIV-1-specific antibody. This HIV-1-specific antibody often does not neutralize HIV-1 found in the plasma contemporaneously, although it may neutralize HIV-1 isolated from earlier in the infection. gp120 may act as a superantigen for B-lymphocytes that bear a particular variable heavy chain, overstimulating these cells [152].

Defects in specific antibody production

Despite hypergammaglobulinemia, HIV-1-infected children have functional hypogammaglobulinemia because of diminished ability to produce specific antibody. Both T-independent and T-dependent antigens antibody responses are decreased. Asymptomatic children < 2 years have antibody responses similar to uninfected children [126]. After 2 years, untreated HIV-1-infected children have decreased antibody responses even with normal CD4+ T-lymphocyte numbers. Responses to hepatitis B, measles, influenza, and *Haemophilus influenzae* type B vaccines are decreased in untreated HIV-1-infected infants [153–156]. Disease progression is associated with decline in B-lymphocyte numbers, with preferential loss of B-lymphocytes that respond to antigen (CD23 +/CD62L+; CD21^{low}), leading to decreased antigen-specific antibody production [157, 158]. Soluble gp120 and HIV infection of CD4+ T-cells impairs T-cell help for specific B-cell responses [159].

Technique for CD4+ T-lymphocyte number and percentage determinations

CD4+ T-lymphocyte number is determined by cell surface marker (i.e., surface protein) analysis via flow cytometry, with a concurrent complete blood count (CBC) [160]. Peripheral blood cells are incubated with antibodies specific for cell surface proteins that identify the cells of interest. The monoclonal antibodies are conjugated to fluorescent molecules that fluoresce upon excitation by the flow cytometer light source. For CD4+ T-cell determinations, the fraction of total lymphocytes that express both cell surface markers CD3 (a marker shared by all T-cells) and CD4 (marker of helper T-cells) is determined. This value is reported as the CD4+ percentage (percent CD4+ T-cells). Absolute CD4+ T-lymphocyte counts are determined by multiplying the percentage of CD3+/CD4+ lymphocytes by the absolute lymphocyte count from concurrent CBC results:

Absolute CD4+ T-lymphocyte count = absolute lymphocyte count x %CD3+/CD4 + lymphocytes = WBC x % lymphocytes x %CD3+/CD4 + lymphocytes.

To standardize CD4+ T-lymphocyte determinations, the US Public Health Service has published detailed guidelines for laboratories performing the test [160, 161].

Many laboratories determine CD4+ T-lymphocyte numbers together with a larger surface marker panel, including killer/suppressor T-lymphocytes (C3+/CD8+ lymphocytes) and B-lymphocytes (CD19+ lymphocytes). This permits calculation of the CD4/CD8 ratio, which has been used as an early marker of immunologic abnormality and was once a key indicator used to diagnose AIDS.

Several biologic and analytic factors can introduce variability into CD4+ T-lymphocyte results. The absolute count depends on three separate measurements, each of which can introduce error. Biologic sources of variability include diurnal variation, acute illness, immunizations, and drug therapy, particularly corticosteroids [162]. The CD4+ T-lymphocyte values vary diurnally, with lowest values at noon and an evening peak. Between 8:00 am and 4:00 pm (usual clinic hours), an average 19% increase can occur. CD4+ T-lymphocyte determinations should be obtained at a consistent time of day. Acute illnesses and immunizations may increase or decrease total WBC, and cause transient changes in the % CD4+ T-lymphocytes. Corticosteroid therapy is associated with decreases in absolute CD4+ T-lymphocyte counts. Even stable patients may have a ±22% variation in absolute CD4+ T-cell counts [163]. CD4 T-cell percentage values fluctuate less than absolute counts, primarily because variations in total white cell count result in changes in absolute counts [164]. CD4+ T-lymphocyte values differing substantially from previous values should be evaluated critically, especially if obtained during acute illnesses or soon after immunizations.

Interpretation of CD4+ T-lymphocyte values

Interpretation of CD4+ T-lymphocyte numbers in children requires recognition that normal cell number declines over the first 6 years of life; values should be assessed relative to age-specific normal values (Fig. 1.1). The age-related change is marked for absolute CD4+ T-lymphocyte counts; % CD4+ T-lymphocyte values change less [29, 164, 165].

Pediatric guidelines recommend monitoring both percentage and absolute CD4+ T-lymphocyte counts and determining disease staging based on the lowest of the two values. Owing to CD4+ T-lymphocyte count variation, major therapeutic decisions should only be made after the changes have been confirmed and other sources of variability have been ruled out. A sustained 50% decrease in the absolute CD4+ T-cell count or percentage is evidence of disease progression. Smaller changes may also be significant if a trend is observed.

HIV-1 infection in children is associated with progressive decline in CD4+ T-lymphocyte values greater than the normal physiologic decline [29, 151, 165]. (Table 1.10) [151]. Symptomatic children have early declines, beginning by 2–3 months; by 13–24 months, CD4+ T-lymphocyte values are significantly lower even among asymptomatic children [165].

Immune restoration after highly active antiretroviral therapy

Successful treatment with highly active antiretroviral therapy (HAART) reverses most clinical and many immunologic signs of disease progression (for review see [166]). Effectively treated patients have lower incidence of opportunistic infections, resolution of HIV-1-related organ dysfunction (i.e., encephalopathy), and improved growth.

Clinical improvements correlate with CD4+ T-cell percentage and cell count increases. During the first 4 to 8 weeks after initiating HAART, the number of

Table 1.10. CD4+ and CD8+ T-lymphocyte numbers (mean ± standard deviation) in uninfected, asymptomatic and symptomatic HIV-1-infected children

		Children		
	Age (mo)	Uninfected	Asymptomatic	Symptomatic
CD4+ lymphocytes	0–1	2900 ± 1541	2580 ± 1501	2317 ± 1317
(cells/mm^3)	1–6	3278 ± 1401	3482 ± 1234	1706 ± 1215
	7–12	3051 ± 1285	2769 ± 1326	1951 ± 882
	13–24	2584 ± 1105	2030 ± 1481	1680 ± 1089
CD8+ lymphocytes	0–1	1418 ± 791	1404 ± 974	1499 ± 1046
(cells/mm^3)	1–6	1626 ± 985	1457 ± 709	1613 ± 958
	7–12	514 ± 300	394 ± 334	523 ± 266
	13–24	1374 ± 663	1902 ± 844	2242 ± 1290

Modified from [151].

CD4+ T-lymphocytes and B-lymphocytes increases rapidly (Fig. 1.10) [167, 168]. CD4+ T-lymphocytes continue to increase over the following 12–18 months. The rapid increase observed early following treatment suggests that the initial increases results from redistribution of cells from lymphoid tissue (for review see [169]). CD4+ T-cells with memory phenotype largely account for the increase [167]. Younger children have an early increase in naïve and memory cells, suggesting they may mobilize naïve cells from the thymus early after initiation of treatment [167, 170]. After the initial rise, continued increase in CD4+ T-cells is mostly composed of naïve cells [167, 168, 171]. These cells are probably newly derived from thymus, although some derive from proliferation of peripheral naïve cells [172, 173].

Since mostly naïve cells increase with HAART, children may be able to generate responses to new antigens, but be less able to reconstitute immune responses to recall antigens without renewed exposure [168, 170, 174, 175]. Proliferative responses to antigens not usually encountered (e.g., tetanus) are less likely to increase with HAART. Responses to uncommon antigens can be generated through reimmunization [168, 176]. Adults treated with HAART have decreases in quantitative IgG, IgM, and IgA levels, which are elevated during HIV-1 infection, indicating improvements toward more normal B-lymphocyte function [177]. However, not all patients achieve normal levels of immunoglobulins [178].

The number of CD8+ lymphocytes increases transiently in the first 8 weeks, but then returns to baseline by 12 weeks (Fig. 1.8) [167]. The percentage of CD8+ T-cells declines as the CD4+ T-cells increase and the CD4/CD8 ratio normalizes. There are significant changes in phenotype, with decreased numbers of cells with surface markers for activation and programmed cell death and increases in the number of CD8+ T-cells with naïve phenotype, and there is a decline in the frequency of HIV-1-specific

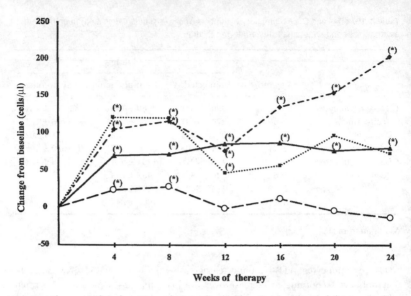

Fig. 1.8. Changes in lymphocyte populations after highly active antiretroviral therapy. Median change from entry values of CD8+ T-cell (squares), CD4+ T-cells (circles), B-cells (triangles), and NK cells (diamonds) over the course of 24 weeks. Values shown as cells per microliter. A statistically significant ($P < 0.05$) changes from baseline is identified with an asterisk. Reprinted with permission from [167].

CD8+ T-cells [179]. This probably results from decreased viral antigen levels as replication is suppressed.

In most children, HAART suppresses plasma HIV-1 RNA to low levels or below the limits of detection. However, many children will not maintain durable viral load suppression, and plasma HIV-1 RNA levels return to near pretreatment levels [168, 180, 181]. Many children will have increased CD4+ T-cell counts despite ongoing viremia. The CD4+ T-cell count increases may be as great in these virologic non-responders/immunologic responders as in children who achieve complete viral suppression [181]. Children with ongoing viremia still derive clinical benefit from HAART if their CD4+ T-cell counts are increased [182]. The explanation for partial immune restoration with continued high level viral replication is not understood. Some evidence points to decreased viral fitness or a switch of virus strain to less pathogenic phenotypes.

Adults with prolonged low CD4+ lymphocyte counts are less likely to have immune restoration following HAART. This is less apparent for children, who exhibit increases to normal ranges, even following profoundly decreased CD4+ lymphocyte counts (Fig. 1.9) [174]. Increased thymic function in children probably contributes to the

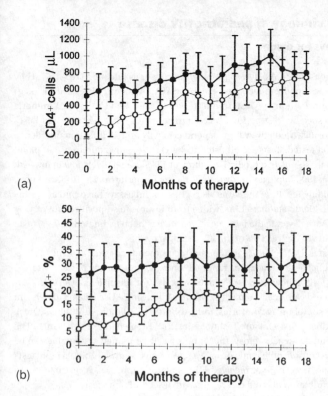

Fig. 1.9. Changes in CD4+ T-cells depend on baseline values. Changes (mean, SD) in CD4+ T-cell counts (*a*) and CD4+ T-cell percentages (*b*) in patients in CDC class 2 (filled circles) and patients in CDC class 3 (open circles) during 18 months of stavudine, lamivudine, and indinavir treatment. Reprinted with permission from [174].

greater capacity for restoration of T-lymphocytes [172, 180]. These children have a lowered incidence of opportunistic infections, indicating the recovered cells are functional.

The immune system probably cannot reconstitute completely; subtle abnormalities persist. Cell activation decreases, but remains above normal. T-cell receptors distribution may not completely normalize, a possible indication of limited T-cell diversity or persistence of expanded clones [183]. Cytokine production remains abnormal [184]. Treatment with immunologically active agents, such as IL-2, has been proposed as a possible intervention. The clinical correlates of these persistent abnormalities is unknown.

The clinical virology of pediatric HIV disease

Virologic assays for diagnosis

Serology

Enzyme immunoassays (EIAs) detect antibody responses to infection [185–187]. They are used to screen blood products and diagnose HIV infection. EIAs used for diagnosis require confirmation by Western blot to verify that the EIA-detected immune response is HIV specific. Test performance characteristics (false-negative and false-positive rates, positive predictive value) depend critically on HIV infection prevalence in the population tested. Tests are adjusted to be very sensitive due to use in blood product screening, so positive predictive values of EIAS are relatively low in low-risk populations [188–190]. Rapid antibody tests [191] can be performed in 10–30 minutes, potentially providing results at the same visit. These rapid assays have similar performance characteristics to standard EIAs, with a troublesome false-positive rate varying with HIV prevalence. Overall, the false-positive rate has been estimated as 0.4% of all persons tested and as high as 18% of initially reactive results.

The United States (US) Public Health Service recommends consideration of an alternative rapid diagnostic approach, i.e., rapid screening with reporting of results during the same clinic visit, followed by confirmatory assays for reactive assays [191]. Currently, two rapid tests are licensed by the FDA (a) Murex Single Use Diagnostic System (SUDS) HIV-1 test; Abbott Laboratories, Inc., Abbott Park, Illinois; and (b) OraQuick Rapid HIV-1 Antibody Test; OraSure Technologies, Inc., Bethlehem, Pennsylvania). The former requires an onsite laboratory; the latter is a self-contained system that can be performed at the bedside or in clinic on saliva specimens. Many additional rapid tests and assay formats have not yet received US regulatory approval. A possible future approach is confirmation of rapid test results with a second rapid test [192].

The utility of serodiagnosis is compromised in young infants due to transplacental passage of HIV antibody from their mothers. Virtually all infants born to such mothers will test positive for HIV antibody, regardless of viral transmission. Relatively rare exceptions include hypo- or agammaglobulinemia and extreme prematurity. (See also Chapter 3.)

Viral detection

Viral culture

Peripheral blood mononuclear cells are cocultivated with equal numbers of uninfected peripheral blood mononuclear cells (PBMCs). Cells are first stimulated with phytohemaglutinin (PHA) and cultured in the presence of IL-2 to enhance viral replication. Supernatant is tested periodically for p24 antigen (see below); p24 detection on two sequential samplings defines a positive. Most positive specimens will be detected by 7–14 days; declaring a culture negative requires 3–4 weeks. Culture can also be performed in a quantitative format using serial dilutions.

p24 antigen detection

p24 antigen is an HIV core protein that can be detected using commercial EIAs. Antibody to p24 is affixed to a solid phase – a bead or microtiter plate, which is incubated with the patient specimen, usually plasma or serum. If p24 antigen is present, an antigen–antibody complex forms, capturing the p24 antigen on the solid phase. The antigen–antibody complex can be detected by a second, enzyme-labeled, anti-p24 antibody. This assay is straightforward and rapid, but has two shortcomings for early pediatric diagnosis: (a) false-positives can occur in the first month of life, most probably due to placental transfer of maternal p24 antigen without infection; and (b) antibody-complexed antigen is not detectable. This is especially problematic in infancy where there is much maternal antibody. This problem can be circumvented by immune complex dissociation prior to p24 antigen detection, which can be accomplished by acid treatment or boiling [193–195] and sensitivity can be enhanced by combination with signal amplification [196, 197]. Currently, there is considerable interest in p24 assays in resource-poor settings for diagnosis and disease monitoring because it costs less and is simpler to perform than other measures, but definitive studies assessing the utility of p24 assays in such settings have not been completed.

HIV DNA PCR

HIV DNA polymerase chain reaction (PCR) to detect HIV provirus was developed in the late 1980s and is used extensively for neonatal diagnosis. Diagnostic PCR assays are optimized for extreme sensitivity, and can detect 1–10 viral targets/sample. False-positives can result from specimen contamination. Laboratory procedures and quality-controlled commercial reagent kits have been developed that greatly reduce false-positive results [198].

Heel-stick blood samples on filter paper (Guthrie cards) for newborn diagnosis by DNA PCR have been validated [199, 200]. This approach has appeal for studies conducted in technically challenging environments and may be employed for routine infant screening.

Studies have shown that virus culture and DNA PCR are sensitive and specific [201–203]. Newborn diagnosis is discussed in more detail in Chapter 3. DNA PCR assays were developed initially to detect HIV strains (clade B) prevalent in the USA. Diagnostic PCR kits have been developed that can recognize target DNAs essentially from all HIV clades. This holds true for disease-monitoring HIV RNA quantitation kits (both PCR and other non-PCR-based methodologies such as branched DNA and nucleic acid sequence-based amplification assays – see below). These disease-monitoring assays are not marketed with performance characteristics optimized for diagnostic use, but have been employed for newborn HIV diagnosis in some settings due to their widespread availability.

Table 1.11. Quantitative HIV RNA assays

Assay	Version	Dynamic range	Quantitation limit
RT-PCR	Amplicor HIV-1 Monitor	$10^{2.6}-10^{5.9}$	400
(Roche)	Amplicor HIV-1 Monitor Ultrasensitive	$10^{1.7}-10^{5.0}$	50
NASBA	HIV-1 RNA QT	$10^{2.6}-10^{7.6}$	400
(Organon-Teknika)	NucliSens	$10^{1.9}-10^{7.6}$	80
Branched DNA	Version 1	$10^{4.0}-10^{6.2}$	10,000
(Chiron/Bayer)	Version 2	$10^{2.6}-10^{6.2}$	400
	Version 3	$10^{1.7}-??$	50

(All units are copies/ml).

Viral assays for monitoring HIV infection
HIV RNA quantitation

Reverse transcription-polymerase chain reaction (RT-PCR) is commercially available as the Roche Amplicor HIV-1 Monitor and Amplicor HIV-1 Monitor Ultrasensitive® assays. In these assays, reverse transcription of viral RNA into a DNA copy is followed by DNA amplification by PCR. An internal control is co-amplified. The regular Amplicor HIV-1 Monitor assay has been in use most extensively and has a lower limit of quantitation of 400 viral copies/ml. More recently, Roche has introduced the Ultrasensitive assay, with a lower quantitation limit of 20–100 copies/ml.

A second assay, NASBA® (nucleic acid sequence-based amplification), (Organon-Teknika) also amplifies target RNA. NASBA is an isothermal amplification reaction that employs three enzymes: reverse transcriptase, RNAse H, and T7 DNA polymerase. It also utilizes internal quantitation standards, and has a lower limit of quantitation of 1000 copies/ml. A second generation assay – NucliSens® – can quantitate as little as 80–400 copies/ml of plasma, depending on sample input.

The third commercially available, quantitative assay is the branched DNA assay (Chiron/Bayer), which uses a different technique from the previous two assays: it amplifies the signal created following capture of viral RNA by nucleic acid hybridization. It is technically the easiest assay to perform, resulting in high reproducibility. Unfortunately, the standard assay requires one ml of plasma, which makes its use impractical for pediatrics. The initial version of the assay had a quantitation limit of 10 000 copies/ml, but newer versions have a lower detection limit of 200 copies/ml.

All of the assays have been tested extensively and validated (Table 1.11), but there is some sample-to-sample variation. Samples must show at least a threefold (0.5 $\log_{10}$) difference for the difference to be considered significant. For example, two samples from a child drawn 1 month apart are reported as 40 000 and 100 000 copies/ml. These two results are not significantly different from each other since they do not differ by threefold. In addition to this performance feature, clinicians should be aware that intercurrent infections and immunizations can activate viral replication and raise RNA levels briefly [204–206]. As with many laboratory tests, clinical decisions should prudently be based on reproducibility between sequential specimens over time and on a composite of clinical and laboratory observations. It would be clinically unwise to make a major change in management on the basis of a single viral load assay [207, 208].

Soon after the introduction of HIV protease inhibitors, some postulated that relatively short periods of antiretroviral therapy would be sufficient to eradicate infection. This enthusiasm has been tempered by the demonstration of long-lived cellular reservoirs in patients with long-term suppression of plasma virus [209–211]. Individuals in whom plasma virus is non-detectable for years remain positive for proviral DNA within cells and for culturable virus [212, 213]. These studies demonstrated that quiescent memory CD4+ T-lymphocytes are reservoirs of latent infection and their frequency is quite low (one in 1–10 million cells). While difficult to measure, their calculated decay rates are very slow, with elimination times measured in decades or lifetimes. Treatment methods for eliminating virus from these long-lived reservoirs will almost certainly be necessary if eradication of infection is to be achieved.

Additional quantitative assays

Newer assays that quantitate infected circulating cells have been developed. These are based on DNA PCR, with internal standards for accurate quantitation. These assays report "numbers of infected cells" or "copies of viral genomes/microgram of cellular DNA" and may help to monitor viral suppression and the amount of virus in long-lived cellular reservoirs [210, 213].

Qualitative plasma RNA assays are being developed to monitor low levels of viral replication once individuals attain a non-detectable state. Several investigators have reported that quantitative HIV RNA assays can sometimes permit earlier newborn diagnosis than DNA PCR [214–216].

Natural history of pediatic HIV infection

Natural history in adults

Infection of adults with HIV-1 is followed by three distinct virologic stages: (a) primary or acute infection, (b) clinical latency, and finally (c) progression to AIDS (see Fig. 1.10). The interval between primary infection and AIDS varies, with a mean of 10 to 11 years [217]. About 20% of individuals will progress in less than 5 years; a few (<5%) will remain immunologically normal for over 10 years [218]. The biological basis for this variability is unclear.

Soon after HIV-1infection, a non-specific clinical syndrome ("primary infection", "acute infection syndrome," or "acute retroviral syndrome"), including fever, pharyngitis, cervical adenopathy, fever, myalgias, rash, and lethargy, and sometimes neurologic or gastrointestinal symptoms is observed in some adults. Symptomatology may have prognostic significance [219–221]. These symptoms resolve spontaneously over days

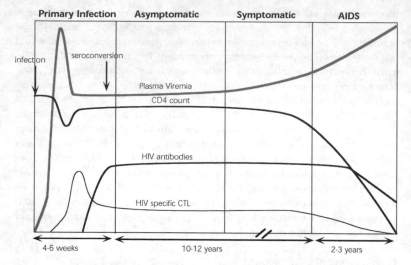

Fig. 1.10. Schematic diagram of the changes in plasma viremia, CD4+ lymphocyte count, and humoral and cellular immune response in an HIV-infected patient during the time following infection.

to weeks. These persons may be antibody negative, but have detectable plasma p24 antigen or HIV RNA. During primary infection, patients may have extremely high levels of plasma viremia (viral load) ($>10^7$ copies/ml), dropping to 100 000 copies/ml or less after several weeks [222, 223]. During this period of high viremia, CD4+ lymphocyte numbers decrease, occasionally to below 200 cells/µl. As viremia declines, the CD4+ lymphocyte count increases, often to normal levels. Decreasing viral loads precede development of antibody response and coincide with a measurable cytotoxic lymphocyte (CTL) response directed against HIV [224]. After some fluctuation, the viral load stabilizes around a "set point," usually between 10 000 and 100 000 copies/ml, frequently remaining fairly constant for many years [220], a period termed "clinical latency." However, much viral replication and CD4+ lymphocyte destruction occurs during clinical latency. An estimated 10 billion virions, with estimated half-lives of less than 6 hours, are produced daily [225]. Eventually, plasma viral levels increase and CD4+ lymphocytes decrease, heralding advancing immunodeficiency and AIDS [220]. The onset of the rapid fall in CD4+ cells is known as the "inflection point."

Plasma viral concentration, CD4+ cell level and disease progression in adults

Plasma viral load measurements offer imprecise assessments of viral replication, since the largest viral replication compartment, the lymphoid tissue, is not directly sampled

Table 1.12. Relationship between baseline HIV-1 RNA copy number and absolute CD4+ lymphocyte number and probability of developing AIDS

Baseline RNA (copies/ml)	Absolute CD4+ lymphocyte number (cells/μl)	% with AIDS		
		by 3 years	by 6 years	by 9 years
<500	>750	0	1.7	3.6
	<750	3.7	9.6	22.3
501–3000	ND	2	16.6	35.4
3001–10 000	>750	3.2	14.2	40.4
	<750	8.1	37.2	59.7
10 001–30 000	>750	9.5	36.7	62.4
	351–750	16.1	54.9	76.3
	<750	40.1	72.9	86.2
>30 000	>500	32.6	66.8	76.3
	351–500	47.9	77.7	94.4
	201–350	64.4	89.3	92.9
	<200	85.5	97.9	100

HIV-1 RNA was quantified using the bDNA system. Data are derived from [230], with permission.

[226]. Virus produced in lymphoid tissues is released into plasma; plasma viral load appears to sample lymphoid tissue viral replication indirectly [227]. Other organ systems where HIV replication occurs (central nervous system, genital tract, breast milk) may behave as distinct compartments. Plasma viral RNA levels may not reflect viral replication accurately in these compartments; virus present in these compartments may be genotypically distinct from virus found in plasma. These distinct viral genotypes may have differing pathogenic properties and differing sensitivities to antiretroviral agents [228, 229]. Since antiretroviral agents may not penetrate well into these compartments, they represent a potential source of resistant virus.

Absent antiretroviral therapy (ART), plasma viral RNA levels vary widely. There is an inverse, but variable, correlation between plasma viral RNA and CD4+ lymphocyte counts. Viral load and CD4+ count are independent prognostic markers. Before HAART, the steady-state level of plasma viral RNA after initial infection ("set point") was the best single predictor of progression to AIDS and death [230]. Combining plasma RNA levels and CD4+ count more accurately predicts prognosis than either alone [231] (see Table 1.12).

ART often produces decreases in plasma RNA and increases in CD4+ lymphocyte number. These changes have clinical and prognostic significance. After beginning ART, decreases in viral load or increases in CD4+ lymphocyte count predict the development of AIDS better than baseline values [232, 233]. For each tenfold decrease in plasma RNA, the risk of disease progression decreases by 56%; for every twofold increase in absolute CD4+ cell count it decreases by 67% [233].

Although ART has dramatic effects on plasma viremia, a small pool of long-lived latently infected CD4+ lymphocytes persist (for review see [234]). Replication-competent virus can be recovered from these latently infected cells. This reservoir is established early in infection and is relatively impervious to the effects of current ART. The rate of turnover of these cells is controversial, with estimates ranging from 6 months to 43 months. The persistence of this compartment represents a major obstacle to the eradication of HIV.

Factors associated with progression in adults

The determinants of the viral "set point" and "inflection point" are poorly understood, but factors may include effectiveness of the host immune response, including CD8+ CTL responses, and patient age. Certain combinations of HLA genes are associated with either relatively rapid (HLA B35) or delayed progression to AIDS (HLA B27 or −57) [235, 236], and HLA locus heterozygosity appears to be protective, perhaps because HLA heterozygotes are able to present a greater variety of antigenic peptides to cytotoxic T-lymphocytes. Inheritance of genes other than HLA have also been implicated in disease progression (for review see [237, 238]), notably including mutations in the HIV co-receptors and their promoters (see above).

Other host factors influence disease progression, including co-infection and other sources of immune activation. Factors leading to immune activation increase viral replication and hasten immune deterioration [239]. Infections and exposure to antigens have been associated with plasma viremia increases [240–242]. Some, but not all studies have shown that immunizations (influenza, tetanus toxoid) lead to transient bursts of viremia followed by return to baseline levels [204, 205, 243], but with no apparent long-term effects [244]. The benefits of vaccination preventing infection, which would undoubtedly result in much higher levels of immune activation, outweigh the unproven risks of transient increases in plasma RNA.

Viral factors have also been associated with disease progression. HIV-1 strains have been broadly classified as being M-tropic/NSI (non-syncytium-inducing) strains or T-tropic/SI (syncytium-inducing). The syncytium-inducing classification refers to production syncytia during *in vitro* growth of virus under certain conditions. M-tropic strains replicate in primary CD4+ T-cells and macrophages and use the β-chemokine receptor CCR5 (less often CCR3) as their coreceptors (for review see [245]). The T-tropic viruses can also replicate in CD4+ T-cells but can also infect established CD4+ T-cell lines *in vitro* via the α-chemokine receptor CXCR4 (fusin). Regardless of the transmission mode, over 90% of transmitted strains are M-tropic; transmission or systemic establishment of CXCR4-using (T-tropic) strains is rare. However, CXCR4-using strains are especially virulent and, once they emerge within an infected person, disease progression is accelerated [246]. At the inflection point, about 50% of adults infected with subtype B will have a switch in the phenotype of the virus from M-tropic viruses to T-tropic viruses [247]. Most of our understanding of HIV pathogenesis is based on subtype B, the predominant strain in developed countries. Whether different subtypes differ in transmissibility, infectivity and pathogenicity is an important area of active research.

Classification of pediatric HIV-1 infection

The Center for Disease Control and Prevention (CDC) has established a classification system for HIV-infected children according to clinical and immunologic status (Tables 1.13, 1.14, 1.15).

The classification system is based on signs, symptoms, or diagnoses. Children are assigned to one of four mutually exclusive clinical categories: N, no signs or symptoms; A, mild signs or symptoms; B, moderate signs or symptoms; C, severe signs or symptoms [248]. The AIDS-defining illnesses in the 1987 CDC definition of pediatric AIDS are included in stage C, except lymphoid interstitial pneumonitis (LIP), a stage B illness. Although most children pass from N to A, B, and C in order, others can pass directly from N to B or N to C (see below).

The immunological classification uses the CD4+ lymphocyte count. Patients are assigned to mutually exclusive categories numbered 1 through 3, with lower CD4+ lymphocyte counts having higher numbers (Table 1.15). The normal CD4+ lymphocyte count changes dramatically during the first few years of life (Fig. 1.1). Assessing immune suppression is complicated because children may develop opportunistic infections at higher CD4+ cell counts than adults [249].

The current CDC immunologic classification system is based on age, on the absolute CD4+ cell count, and on the percentage of CD4+ lymphocytes [248] (see Table 1.14). If CD4+ cell count and percentage place a child in different immunologic categories, the more severe category is used. Currently, children with immune reconstitution following therapy are not reclassified to a less severe category. Values that result in a classification change should be confirmed. Since CD4+ lymphocyte values can vary with even mild illness, values are best obtained when children are clinically well.

HIV-1 natural history in children

The pace of HIV disease progression in children is accelerated compared with adults, presumably because of infection during immunologic immaturity, and/or the availability of increased numbers of target cells. Older children infected via non-vertical routes may have a course more similar to adults [250, 251].

Vertically infected children exhibit a bimodal pattern of disease progression [252–254]. About 10–25% of infected children develop profound immunosuppression, significant symptoms, and opportunistic infections within the first year; without treatment few of these children survive more than 2 years [255]. The majority of children have a slower progression to AIDS (mean time 6–9 years) [252, 254, 256, 257]. Investigators hypothesize that children with rapid progression may acquire their infection in utero and are therefore less able to mount effective immune responses [258, 259]. A working definition has been proposed wherein in utero transmission is defined as viral detection at less than 48 hours and intrapartum transmission is defined as viral detection

Table 1.13. Conditions associated with clinical categories according to the CDC 1994 Revised HIV Pediatric Classification System

Category A	Category B	Category C
Have two or more of the conditions listed below but no category B and C conditions • Lymphadenopathy (>0.5 cm at more than two sites) • Hepatomegaly • Splenomegaly • Dermatitis • Parotitis • Recurrent or persistent upper respiratory infection, sinusitis, or otitis media	Examples of conditions in clinical category B • Anemia (<8 g/dl), neutropenia (<1000/mm^3), or thrombocytopenia (<1 000 000/mm^3) persisting >30 days • Bacterial meningitis, pneumonia or sepsis (single episode) • Candidiasis, oropharyngeal (thrush), persistent (>2 m) in a child >6 m • Cardiomyopathy • Cytomegalovirus infection, with onset >1 m of age • Diarrhea, recurrent or chronic • Hepatitis • HSV stomatitis, recurrent (>2 episodes within 1 yr) • HSV bronchitis, pneumonitis, or esophagitis with <1 month of age • Herpes zoster involving a > 2 distinct episodes or > 1 dermatome • Leiomyosarcoma • LIP or pulmonary lymphoid hyperplasia • Nephropathy • Nocardiosis • Persistent fever (lasting > 1 m of age) • Toxoplasmosis, onset < 1 m of age • Varicella, disseminated	• Multiple or recurrent serious bacterial infections (septicemia, pneumonia, meningitis, bone or joint infection, or abscess of an internal organ) • Candidiasis, esophageal or pulmonary • Coccidiomycosis, disseminated • Cryptococcosis, extrapulmonary • Cryptosporidiosis or Isosporiasis with diarrhea persisting for >1 month • Cytomegalovirus disease with onset of symptoms prior to 1 month of age • Cytomegalovirus retinitis (with loss of vision) • Encephalopathy in the absence of a concurrent illness other than HIV infection that could explain the findings • HSV infection causing a mucocutaneous ulcer persisting for >1 month; or as the etiology of bronchitis, pneumonitis or esophagitis • Histoplasmosis, disseminated • Kaposi's sarcoma • Primary CNS lymphoma • Lymphoma, Burkitt's, large cell, or immunoblastic • *M. tuberculosis*, disseminated or extrapulmonary • Mycobacterium infections other than tuberculosis, disseminated • *Pneumocystiis jiroveci* pneumonia • Progressive multifocal leukoencephalopathy • Toxoplasmosis of the brain with onset at >1 m of age • Wasting syndrome in the absence of a concurrent illness other than HIV infection

Adapted from [248], with permission.

Table 1.14. Immunologic categories according to the CDC 1994 Revised HIV Pediatric Classification

Age of child	No evidence of immune suppression		Evidence of moderate immune suppression		Evidence of severe immune suppression	
	CD4+ lymphocytes (cells/µl)	% CD4+ lymphocytes (cells/µl)	CD4+ lymphocytes (cells/µl)	% CD4+ lymphocytes (cells/µl)	CD4+ lymphocytes (cells/µl)	% CD4+ lymphocytes (cells/µl)
<1 year	≥ 1,500	≥5	750–1499	15–24	<750	<15
1–5 years	≥1,000	≥25	500–999	15–24	<500	<15
6–12 yrs	≥500	≥25	200–499	15–24	<200	<15

Adapted from [248].

Table 1.15. HIV Pediatric classification incorporating both clinical and immunologic categories

Immunologic categories	Clinical categories			
	N: No signs/ symptoms	A: Mild signs/ symptoms	B: Moderate signs/ symptoms	C: Severe signs/ symptoms
1. No evidence of suppression	N1	A1	B1	C1
2. Evidence of moderate suppression	N2	A2	B2	C2
3. Severe suppression	N3	A3	B3	C3

Adapted from [248], with permission.

Table 1.16. Proportion of children progressing to Category C disease or death within a 5-year period from the beginning of each stage (before the availability of highly active antiretroviral therapy)

Stage	Percent developing category C disease within a 5-year period from the beginning of each stage	Percent mortality within 5 years from the beginning of each stage
N	50%	25%
A	58%	33%
B	60%	35%
C	-	83%

Adapted from [256], with permission.

at greater than 7 days [260]. Approximately 10–30% of children have detectable virus in the first 2 days of life and these children may have a shorter median time to onset of symptoms and death [253, 261] and higher levels of virus, but not all studies agree on this. The most striking characteristic of vertically infected infants is the extremely high levels of plasma viremia observed during the first few months of life. The viremia declines substantially in the first year of life and then more slowly over several years [108, 262, 263] (see below). At approximately 4–6 years of age, RNA levels appear to stabilize at lower levels.

The pediatric classification system (Table 1.15) has been used to describe the natural history of HIV-1 disease in the absence of ART. Most perinatally infected children remain relatively asymptomatic for the first year of life. In the second year, most progress to moderate symptoms (category B), typically remaining at this stage for over 5 years. After entering stage C, mean and median survival times are 34 months and 23 months, respectively [256] (see Table 1.16).

Natural history of HIV-1 infection in children in Africa

The vast majority of HIV-1 infected persons live in sub-Saharan Africa, where sero-prevalence rates of over 25% are increasingly common. Over 80% of children infected with HIV live in this region and over 90% of new pediatric infections occur in this region. Although children account for less than 8% of those infected with HIV worldwide, 20% of deaths due to AIDS have been in children less than 15 years [264]. HIV infection has reversed the significant gains in child survival that had been achieved during the last few decades.

It has been hypothesized that HIV progression rates are more rapid in Africa than in industrialized countries. The immune activation associated with chronic infection, and the immunosuppression accompanying malnutrition have been postulated to result in higher levels of viremia and in a more rapid disease course. Differences in HIV subtype and host genetic factors have also been considered to be important variables. However, more recent data strongly argue that the natural history of HIV infection among adults in Africa is not fundamentally distinct from that of adults in resource-rich settings prior to the advent of ART [265, 266]. Africans, like members of disadvantaged groups in rich countries, tend to present for care later and have much higher levels of general morbidity. Moreover, the burden of infectious diseases such as tuberculosis is much higher. Nevertheless, the median time from seroconversion to AIDS in HIV-infected African adults is 9.4 years, and most die severely immunosuppressed, with clinical features of AIDS [267]. Pathophysiologically, HIV in Africa is not unique.

HAART and HIV natural history

HAART dramatically reduced disease progression in children and adults. When pro-tease inhibitors were introduced, the annual mortality rate among US children enrolled in Pediatric AIDS Clinical Trials Group (PACTG) studies decreased from 5.3% to 0.7% [268]. Two ART drugs decreased the risk of death by 30%, three ART drugs resulted in a 71% decrease [269]. Progression to AIDS is also significantly reduced with HAART [270].

Unfortunately, many children who begin HAART are unable to achieve and/or sustain viral suppression, perhaps because of higher levels of viremia, sequential use of insufficiently potent ART, inability to achieve adequately high ART levels, and problems with adherence. Many of these children have viruses resistant to all available classes of antiretrovirals. The prognosis for these children will be significantly worse than for children who achieve good viral suppression unless new therapies become available. As many as 40% of children treated with HAART who do not achieve virologic suppression appear to derive some immunologic benefit from therapy, as judged by sustained CD4+ lymphocyte count increases, perhaps because resistant virus is "less fit."

Natural history of horizontally acquired HIV infection in pediatrics

Children and youth who acquire HIV infection horizontally appear to have a disease course more similar to adults than perinatally infected infants, but the pathogenesis

Table 1.17. Relationship between baseline RNA copy number and percentage CD4 and mortality in HIV-1 infected children

Baseline HIV RNA (copies/ml)	Baseline CD4+ cell percentage	Number deaths per number patients	Percent mortality
≤100 000	≥15%	15/103	15%
≤100 000	<15%	15/24	63%
>100 000	≥15%	32/89	36%
>100 000	<15%	29/36	81%

HIV RNA was quantified using the NASBA HIV-1 QT amplification system on samples obtained during the NICHD intravenous immunoglobulin clinical trial. Mean age of subjects was approximately 3 years, and mean follow-up was about 5 years. Data was taken from [274], with permission.

of other viral infections in HIV-infected adolescents appears to be distinct. Adolescent girls appear to be more susceptible to human papilloma virus (HPV) infection than older women. HPV strains persist longer in HIV-infected adolescents and the incidence of squamous intraepithelial lesions is higher (see Chapter 8). The seroprevalence of hepatitis B in HIV-infected youth in the USA is much higher than in the population at large [271]. Moreover, the serologic response to hepatitis B vaccine appears to be suboptimal in adolescents [272].

Relationship between viral load CD4+ cell level and disease progression in children

Plasma RNA concentration appears to be a critical determinant of pediatric disease progression [273]. Plasma viral RNA kinetics in the first few months of life correlates with disease course. Rapid progressors have marked increases in viral RNA, which do not decline [262]. Infants with plasma RNA levels above the median had an increased risk of disease progression and death. There was a 44% rate of progression by 24 months for children with an early peak value above 300 000 copies/ml and only a 15% rate of progression for children below this value [108]. Nevertheless, considerable overlap exists in RNA values between rapid and non-rapid progressors, and no threshold value could be identified in the first 2 years of life. However, no infant with less than 70 000 copies/ml in the first 4 months of life had rapidly progressive disease [108, 274] (see Table 1.17). The association of mortality with HIV-1 RNA levels varied with age. For children under 2 years of age, mortality is increased only when the baseline RNA is over 1 million copies/ml; for children over 2 years of age, mortality increases when plasma RNA exceeds 100 000 copies/ml [273, 274] (see Table 1.18). A linear relationship independent of age exists between plasma RNA levels and risk for disease progression. For example, an 8-month-old and an 8-year-old, both with plasma RNA values of 100 000 copies/ml, would have similar risks for future disease progression. Studies have

Table 1.18. Relationship between baseline HIV RNA copy number and risk of disease progression or death stratified by age

Baseline HIV RNA (copies/ml)	Number with disease progression or death/ number patients	Percent with disease progression or death
Age <30 months at entry		
<1000–150 000	9/79	11%
150 001–500 000	13/66	20%
500 001–1 700 000	29/76	38%
>1 700 000	42/81	52%
Age ≥30 months at entry		
<1000–15 000	0/66	0%
15 001–50 000	7/54	13%
50 001–150 000	13/80	16%
>150 000	22/64	34%

HIV RNA was quantified using NASABA HIV-1 QT amplification on samples obtained from children participating in Pediatric AIDS Clinical Trials Group protocol 152. Mean age of children in the <30 months group was 1.1 years. Mean age of children in the group >30 months was 7.3 years. All children received ART. Data taken from [273], with permission.

demonstrated that high peak levels attained during infancy and long duration of high levels predict poor outcomes [108, 275]. Although plasma RNA is a strong independent predictor of the clinical course, additional variables such as CD4+ lymphocyte count. Use of CD4+ lymphocyte count and plasma RNA together for prediction surpasses using either alone [273, 274, 276–278, 279, 280].

Factors associated with disease progression

Several clinical factors are associated with disease progression. Age at the time of infection is probably an important factor (see above) [281]. Route of infection during the perinatal period may be a significant factor. Infants infected by vertical transmission tend to progress more rapidly than those who acquire infection by blood products [250, 251, 282]. Infants born to women with advanced disease and higher viral loads also tend to be rapid progressors [283–285]. Whether this results from emergence of more virulent strains in persons with advanced disease and/or is a reflection of shared immunogenetic factors is unknown. Certain clinical manifestations of HIV-1 disease appear to be important prognostically. Children who present at a young age with PCP or encephalopathy have a worse prognosis than those presenting with lymphoid interstitial pneumonia (LIP) or bacterial infections [255, 286–288]. Infants with enlarged lymph nodes, hepato- and/or splenomegaly at birth have almost a 40% chance of developing category C disease by 1 year compared with a 15% risk without these signs [253]. Growth failure is another clinical sign of poor prognostic import [289], and has recently been correlated with viral load [290]. Although none of these clinical findings has been found to be as predictive as the combination of plasma RNA concentration and CD4+ cell percentage, the information is easy and inexpensive to obtain [291].

Transient infection

A few pediatric centers prospectively following HIV-1 seroreverting children have described infants who had transient evidence of HIV infection, including positive DNA and RNA PCR and viral culture, in the immediate postpartum period [292–295]. Others have described the detection of cell-mediated immune responses in seroreverting infants (for review see [296]). Studies of macaques infected with Simian immunodeficiency virus (SIV) would suggest that transient infection is possible [297]. However, a detailed phylogenetic analysis of such putative human cases could not confirm transient infection [298], suggesting that, if transient HIV infection occurs, it is rare.

Conclusions

Vast amounts of information about HIV and the immune system have been accumulated since the beginning of the HIV epidemic. Advances in basic knowledge of the immune system and its development, HIV virology, and the responses of the host to HIV infection, constitute the foundation upon which the remarkable therapeutic advances of the last decade have been built. A thorough knowledge of the basic science of HIV virology and immunology will help clinicians provide the best care to their patients.

Acknowledgments

Dr. Zeichner thanks KT Jeang, Frank Maldarelli, and Rachel Moon for reading the manuscript and providing helpful comments.

Dr. McFarland thanks Tina Yee and Paul Harding for assistance in preparation of the manuscript.

Dr. Aldrovandi thanks Katherine Semrau for helpful discussion and review of the manuscript. Supported in part by grants UO1 AI41025, R01 AI40951, R01 HD39611, RO1 HD4775 and RO1 HD 40777 from the National Institute of Health, and Contract Number 97PVCL05 from Social & Scientific Systems.

REFERENCES

1. Goldblum, R., Hanson, L., Brandtzaeg, P. The mucosal defense system. In Steihm, E., ed. *Immunologic Disorders in Infants and Children*. Philadelphia: W. B Saunders; 1996: 159–200.

2. Neutra, M. R., Pringault E., Kraehenbuhl, J. P. Antigen sampling across epithelial barriers and induction of mucosal immune responses. *Annu. Rev. Immunol.* 1996;**14**:275–300.

3. Johnston, R. B., Jr. The complement system in host defense and inflammation: the cutting edges of a double edged sword. *Pediatr. Infect. Dis. J.* 1993;**12**(11):933–941.

4. Johnston, R. B., Jr. Current concepts: immunology. Monocytes and macrophages. *N. Engl. J. Med* 1988;**318**(12):747–752.

5. Gluckman, J. C., Canque B., Rosenzwajg M. Dendritic cells: a complex simplicity. *Transplantation* 2002;**73**(1 Suppl):S3–6.

6. Ferlazzo, G., Wesa, A., Wei, W. Z. S., Galy, A. Dendritic cells generated either from CD34+ progenitor cells or from monocytes differ in their ability to activate antigen-specific CD8+ T cells. *J. Immunol.* 1999;**163**(7):3597–3604.

7. Banchereau, J., Pulendran, B., Steinman, R., Palucka, K. Will the making of plasmacytoid dendritic cells in vitro help unravel their mysteries? *J. Exp. Med.* 2000;**192**(12): F39–F44.

8. Vasselon, T., Detmers, P. A. Toll receptors: a central element in innate immune responses. *Infect. Immun.* 2002;**70**(3):1033–1041.

9. Williams, A. F., Barclay, A. N. The immunoglobulin superfamily – domains for cell surface recognition. *Annu. Rev. Immunol.* 1988;**6**:381–405.

10. Berkower, I. The T cell, maestro of the immune system: receptor acquisition, MHC recognitiion, thymic selection and tolerance. In Sell S., ed. *Immunology, Immunopathology and Immunity*. Stamford, Connecticut: Appleton & Lange; 1996: 168–187.

11. Bierer, B. E., Sleckman, B. P., Ratnofsky, S. E., Burakoff, S. J. The biological roles of CD2, CD4, and CD8 in T-cell activation. *Annu. Rev. Immunol.* 1989;**7**:579–599.

12. Clement, L. Cellular interactions in the human immune response. In Stiehm, E. R., ed. *Immunologic Disorders of Infants and Children*. Philadelphia: W. B. Saunders; 1996: 75–93.

13. Sanders, M. E., Makgoba, M. W., Shaw, S. Human naïve and memory T cells: reinterpretation of helper-inducer and suppressor-inducer subsets. *Immunol. Today* 1988;**9**(7–8):195–199.

14. Berkower, I. How T cells help B cells to make antibodies. In Sell, S., ed. *Immunology, Immunopathology and Immunity*. Stamford, Connecticut: Appleton & Lange; 1996.

15. Noelle, R. J., Ledbetter, J. A., Aruffo, A. CD40 and its ligand, an essential ligand-receptor pair for thymus-dependent B-cell activation. *Immunol. Today* 1992;**13**(11):431–433.

16. Mosmann, T. R., Cherwinski, H., Bond, M. W., Giedlin, M. A., Coffman, R. L. Two types of murine helper T cell clone. I. Definition according to profiles of lymphokine activities and secreted proteins. *J. Immunol.* 1986;**136**(7):2348–2357.

17. Gelfand, E. Finkel, T. The T-lymphocyte system. In Stiehm, E. R., ed. *Immunologic Disorders of Infants and Children*, 4th ed. Philadelphia: W. B. Saunders; 1996: 14–34.

18. Biddison, W. E., Sharrow, S. O., Shearer, G. M. T cell subpopulations required for the human cytotoxic T lymphocyte response to influenza virus: evidence for T cell help. *J. Immunol.* 1981;**127**(2):487–491.

19. Luster, A. D. Chemokines – chemotactic cytokines that mediate inflammation. *N. Engl. J. Med.* 1998;**338**(7):436–445.

20. Cooper, M. D. Current concepts. B lymphocytes. Normal development and function. *N. Engl. J. Med.* 1987;**317**(23):1452–1456.

21. Reth, M., Hombach, J., Wienands, J., *et al.* The B-cell antigen receptor complex. *Immunol. Today* 1991;**12**(6):196–201.

22. Wilson, C. Lewis, D. Penix, L. The physiologic immunodeficiency of immaturity. In Stiehm, E. R., ed. *Immunologic Disorders in Infants and Children*. 4th edn. Philadelphia: W. B. Saunders; 1996: 253–295.

23. Johnston, R. B., Jr. Function and cell biology of neutrophils and mononuclear phagocytes in the newborn infant. *Vaccine* 1998;**16**(14–15):1363–1368.

24. Rao, S., Olesinski, R., Doshi, U., Vidyasagar, D. Brief clinical and laboratory observations. Granulocyte adherence in newborn infants. *J. Pediatr.* 1981;**98**(4):622–624.

25. Petty, R. E., Hunt, D. W. Neonatal dendritic cells. *Vaccine* 1998;**16**(14–15):1378–1382.

26. Haynes, B. F., Martin, M. E., Kay, H. H., Kurtzberg, J. Early events in human T cell ontogeny. Phenotypic characterization and immunohistologic localization of T cell precursors in early human fetal tissues. *J. Exp. Med.* 1988;**168**(3):1061–1080.

27. De Paoli, P., Battistin, S., Santini, G. F. Age-related changes in human lymphocyte subsets: progressive reduction of the CD4 CD45R (suppressor inducer) population. *Clin. Immunol. Immunopathol.* 1988;**48**(3):290–296.

28. Denny, T., Yogev, R., Gelman, R. *et al.* Lymphocyte subsets in healthy children during the first 5 years of life. *J. Am. Med. Assoc.* 1992;**267**(11):1484–1488.

29. European Collaborative Study. Age-related standards for T lymphocyte subsets based on uninfected children born to human immunodeficiency virus-1 infected women. *Pediatr. Infect. Dis. J.* 1992;**11**:1018–1026.

30. Siegrist, C. A. Neonatal and early life vaccinology. *Vaccine* 2001;**19**(25–26):3331–3346.

31. Ehlers, S., Smith, K. A. Differentiation of T cell lymphokine gene expression: the in vitro acquisition of T cell memory. *J. Exp. Med.* 1991;**173**(1):25–36.

32. Delespesse, G., Yang, L. P., Ohshima, Y., *et al.* Maturation of human neonatal CD4+ and CD8+ T lymphocytes into Th1/Th2 effectors. *Vaccine* 1998;**16**(14–15):1415–1419.

33. Nonoyama, S., Penix, L. A., Edwards, C. P. *et al.* Diminished expression of CD40 ligand by activated neonatal T cells. *J. Clin. Invest.* 1995;**95**(1):66–75.

34. Kniker, W. T., Lesourd, B. M., McBryde, J. L., Corriel, R. N. Cell-mediated immunity assessed by Multitest CMI skin testing in infants and preschool children. *Am. J. Dis. Child.* 1985;**139**(8):840–845.

35. Burrows, P. D., Kearney, J. F., Schroeder, H. W., Jr., Cooper, M. D. Normal B lymphocyte differentiation. *Baillieres. Clin. Haematol.* 1993;**6**(4):785–806.

36. Duchosal, M. A. B-cell development and differentiation. *Semin. Hematol.* 1997;**34**(1 Suppl 1):2–12.

37. Splawski, J. B., Lipsky, P. E. Cytokine regulation of immunoglobulin secretion by neonatal lymphocytes. *J. Clin. Invest.* 1991;**88**(3):967–977.

38. Freed E., Martin M. HIVs and their replication. In Roizman, B., ed. *Fields Virology*. Philadelphia: Lippincott Williams and Wilkins; 2001: 1971–2041.

39. Korber, B., Muldoon, M., Theiler, J. *et al.* Timing the ancestor of the HIV-1 pandemic strains. *Science* 2000;**288**(5472):1789–1796.

40. Arthur, L. O., Bess, J. W. J., Sowder, R. C. I. *et al.* Cellular proteins bound to immunodeficiency viruses: implications for pathogenesis and vaccines. *Science* 1992;**258**:1935–1938.

41. Eckert, D. M., Kim, P. S. Mechanisms of viral membrane fusion and its inhibition. *Annu. Rev. Biochem.* 2001;**70**:777–810.

42. Golding, H., Zaitseva, M., de Rosny, E. *et al.* Dissection of human immunodeficiency virus type 1 entry with neutralizing antibodies to gp41 fusion intermediates. *J. Virol.* 2002;**76**(13):6780–6790.

43. Wild, C. T., Shugars, D. C., Greenwell, T. K., McDanal, C. B., Matthews, T. J. Peptides corresponding to a predictive alpha-helical domain of human immunodeficiency virus type 1 gp41 are potent inhibitors of virus infection. *Proc. Natl. Acad. Sci. USA* 1994;**91**(21):9770–9774.

44. Novina, C. D., Murray, M. F., Dykxhoorn, D. M. *et al.* siRNA-directed inhibition of HIV-1 infection. *Nat. Med.* 2002;**8**(7):681–686.

45. Berger, E. A., Murphy, P. M., Farber, J. M. Chemokine receptors as HIV-1 coreceptors: roles in viral entry, tropism, and disease. *Annu. Rev. Immunol.* 1999;**17**:657–700.

46. Feng, Y., Broder, C. C., Kennedy, P. E., Berger, E. A. HIV-1 entry cofactor: functional cDNA cloning of a seven-transmembrane, G protein-coupled receptor. *Science* 1996;**272**(5263):872–877.

47. Strizki, J. M., Xu, S., Wagner, N. E. *et al.* SCH-C (SCH 351125), an orally bioavailable, small molecule antagonist of the chemokine receptor CCR5, is a potent inhibitor of HIV-1 infection *in vitro* and *in vivo*. *Proc. Natl. Acad. Sci. USA* 2001;**98**(22):12718–12723.

48. Kostrikis, L. G., Huang, Y., Moore, J. P. *et al.* A chemokine receptor CCR2 allele delays HIV-1 disease progression and is associated with a CCR5 promoter mutation. *Nat. Med.* 1998;**4**(3):350–353.

49. Gotte M., Li X., Wainberg, M. A. HIV-1 reverse transcription: a brief overview focused on structure-function relationships among molecules involved in initiation of the reaction. *Arch. Biochem. Biophys.* 1999;**365**(2):199–210.

50. Farnet, C. M., Bushman, F. D. HIV-1 cDNA integration: requirement of HMG I(Y) protein for function of preintegration complexes *in vitro*. *Cell* 1997;**88**(4):483–492.

51. McDonald, D., Vodicka, M. A., Lucero, G., *et al.* Visualization of the intracellular behavior of HIV in living cells. *J. Cell Biol.* 2002;**159**(3):441–452.

52. Le Rouzic, E., Mousnier, A., Rustum, C. *et al.* Docking of HIV-1 Vpr to the nuclear envelope is mediated by the interaction with the nucleoporin hCG1. *J. Biol. Chem.* 2002;**277**(47):45091–45098.

53. Roth, M. J., Schwartzberg, P. L., Goff, S. P. Structure of the termini of DNA intermediates in the integration of retroviral DNA: dependence on IN function and terminal DNA sequence. *Cell* 1989;**58**(1):47–54.

54. Englund, G., Theodore, T. S., Freed, E. O., Engleman, A., Martin, M. A. Integration is required for productive infection of monocyte-derived macrophages by human immunodeficiency virus type 1. *J. Virol.* 1995;**69**(5):3216–3219.

55. Condra, J. H., Miller, M. D., Hazuda, D. J., Emini, E. A. Potential new therapies for the treatment of HIV-1 infection. *Annu. Rev. Med.* 2002;**53**:541–555.

56. Laughlin, M., Zeichner, S., Kolson, D. *et al.* Sodium butyrate treatment of cells latently infected with HIV-1 results in the expression of unspliced viral RNA. *Virology* 1993;**196**:496–505.

57. Rothe, M., Sarma, V., Dixit, V. M., Goeddel, D. V. TRAF2-mediated activation of NF-kappa B by TNF receptor 2 and CD40. *Science* 1995;**269**(5229):1424–1427.

58. Nabel, G., Baltimore, D. An inducible transcription factor activates expression of human immunodeficiency virus in T cells [published erratum appears in *Nature* 1990;**344**(6262):178]. *Nature* 1987;**326**(6114):711–713.

59. Jones, K. A., Kadonaga, J. T., Luciw, P. A., Tjian, R. Activation of the AIDS retrovirus promoter by the cellular transcription factor, Sp1. *Science* 1986;**232**(4751):755–759.

60. Zeichner, S. L., Kim, J. Y., Alwine, J. C. Linker-scanning mutational analysis of the transcriptional activity of the human immunodeficiency virus type 1 long terminal repeat. *J. Virol.* 1991;**65**(5):2436–2444.

61. Kim, J., Gonzalez-Scarano, F., Zeichner, S., Alwine, J. Replication of type 1 human immunodeficiency viruses containing linker substitution mutations in the -201 to -130 region of the long terminal repeat. *J. Virol.* 1993;**67**:1658–1662.

62. Ross, E. K., Buckler-White, A. J., Rabson, A. B., Englund, G., Martin, M. A. Contribution of NF-kappa B and Sp1 binding motifs to the replicative capacity of human immunodeficiency virus type 1: distinct patterns of viral growth are determined by T-cell types. *J. Virol.* 1991;**65**(8):4350–4358.

63. Zeichner, S. L., Hirka, G., Andrews, P. W., Alwine, J. C. Differentiation-dependent human immunodeficiency virus long terminal repeat regulatory elements active in human teratocarcinoma cells. *J. Virol.* 1992;**66**(4):2268–2273.

64. He, G., Margolis, D. M. Counterregulation of chromatin deacetylation and histone deacetylase occupancy at the integrated promoter of human immunodeficiency virus type 1 (HIV-1) by the HIV-1 repressor YY1 and HIV-1 activator Tat. *Mol. Cell. Biol.* 2002;**22**(9):2965–2973.

65. Sheridan, P. L., Mayall, T. P., Verdin, E., Jones, K. A. Histone acetyltransferases regulate HIV-1 enhancer activity *in vitro*. *Genes Dev.* 1997;**11**(24):3327–3340.

66. Berkhout, B., Silverman, R. H., Jeang, K. T. Tat trans-activates the human immunodeficiency virus through a nascent RNA target. *Cell* 1989;**59**(2):273–282.

67. Wei, P., Garber, M. E., Fang, S. M., Fischer, W. H., Jones, K. A. A novel CDK9-associated C-type cyclin interacts directly with HIV-1 Tat and mediates its high-affinity, loop-specific binding to TAR RNA. *Cell* 1998;**92**(4):451–462.

68. Parada, C. A., Roeder, R. G. Enhanced processivity of RNA polymerase II triggered by Tat-induced phosphorylation of its carboxy-terminal domain. *Nature* 1996;**384**(6607):375–378.

69. Barillari, G., Sgadari, C., Fiorelli, V. *et al.* The Tat protein of human immunodeficiency virus type-1 promotes vascular cell growth and locomotion by engaging the alpha5beta1 and alphavbeta3 integrins and by mobilizing sequestered basic fibroblast growth factor. *Blood* 1999;**94**(2):663–672.

70. Mischiati, C., Jeang, K. T., Feriotto, G., *et al.* Aromatic polyamidines inhibiting the Tat-induced HIV-1 transcription recognize structured TAR-RNA. *Antisense Nucl. Acid Drug Dev.* 2001;**11**(4):209–217.

71. Chao, S. H., Fujinaga, K., Marion, J. E. *et al.* Flavopiridol inhibits P-TEFb and blocks HIV-1 replication. *J. Biol. Chem.* 2000;**275**(37):28345–28348.

72. Pollard, V. W., Malim, M. H. The HIV-1 Rev protein. *Annu. Rev. Microbiol.* 1998;**52**:491–532.

73. Askjaer, P., Jensen, T. H., Nilsson, J., Englmeier, L., Kjems, J. The specificity of the CRM1-Rev nuclear export signal interaction is mediated by RanGTP. *J. Biol. Chem.* 1998;**273**(50):33414–33422.

74. Gorlich, D., Mattaj, I. W. Nucleocytoplasmic transport. *Science* 1996;**271**(5255):1513–1518.

75. Malim, M. H., Bohnlein, S., Hauber, J., Cullen, B. R. Functional dissection of the HIV-1 Rev trans-activator-derivation of a trans-dominant repressor of Rev function. *Cell* 1989;**58**(1):205–214.

76. Decroly, E., Wouters, S., Di Bello C., Lazure, C., Ruysschaert, J. M., Seidah, N. G. Identification of the paired basic convertases implicated in HIV gp160 processing based on in vitro assays and expression in CD4(+) cell lines [published erratum appears in *J Biol Chem* 1997 Mar 28;272(13):8836]. *J. Biol. Chem.* 1996;**271**(48):30442–30450.

77. Ogert, R. A., Lee, M. K., Ross, W., Buckler-White A., Martin, M. A., Cho, M. W. N-linked glycosylation sites adjacent to and within the V1/V2 and the V3 loops of dualtropic human immunodeficiency virus type 1 isolate DH12 gp120 affect coreceptor usage and cellular tropism. *J. Virol.* 2001;**75**(13):5998–6006.

78. Mori, K., Yasutomi, Y., Ohgimoto, S. *et al.* Quintuple deglycosylation mutant of simian immunodeficiency virus SIVmac239 in rhesus macaques: robust primary replication, tightly contained chronic infection, and elicitation of potent immunity against the parental wild-type strain. *J. Virol.* 2001;**75**(9):4023–4028.

79. Schubert, U., Anton, L. C., Bacik, I. *et al.* CD4 glycoprotein degradation induced by human immunodeficiency virus type 1 Vpu protein requires the function of proteasomes and the ubiquitin-conjugating pathway. *J. Virol.* 1998;**72**(3):2280–2288.

80. Willey, R. L., Maldarelli, F., Martin, M. A., Strebel, K. Human immunodeficiency virus type 1 Vpu protein induces rapid degradation of CD4. *J. Virol.* 1992;**66**(12):7193–7200.

81. Conte, M. R., Matthews, S. Retroviral matrix proteins: a structural perspective. *Virology* 1998;**246**(2):191–198.

82. Ono, A., Freed, E. O. Plasma membrane rafts play a critical role in HIV-1 assembly and release. *Proc. Natl Acad. Sci. USA* 2001;**98**(24):13925–13930.

83. Zimmerman, C., Klein, K. C., Kiser, P. K. *et al.* Identification of a host protein essential for assembly of immature HIV-1 capsids. *Nature* 2002;**415**(6867):88–92.

84. Gamble, T. R., Yoo, S., Vajdos, F. F. *et al.* Structure of the carboxyl-terminal dimerization domain of the HIV-1 capsid protein. *Science* 1997;**278**(5339):849–853.

85. Franke, E. K., Yuan, H. E., Luban, J. Specific incorporation of cyclophilin A into HIV-1 virions. *Nature* 1994;**372**(6504):359–362.

86. Grattinger, M., Hohenberg, H., Thomas, D., Wilk, T., Muller, B., Krausslich, H. G. *In vitro* assembly properties of wild-type and cyclophilin-binding defective human immunodeficiency virus capsid proteins in the presence and absence of cyclophilin A. *Virology* 1999;**257**(1):247–260.

87. Berkowitz, R., Fisher, J., Goff, S. P. RNA packaging. *Curr. Top. Microbiol. Immunol.* 1996;**214**:177–218.

88. Basrur, V., Song, Y., Mazur, S. J. *et al.* Inactivation of HIV-1 nucleocapsid protein P7 by pyridinioalkanoyl thioesters. Characterization of reaction products and proposed mechanism of action. *J. Biol. Chem.* 2000;**275**(20):14890–14897.

89. Pornillos, O., Garrus, J. E., Sundquist, W. I. Mechanisms of enveloped RNA virus budding. *Trends Cell. Biol.* 2002;**12**(12):569–579.

90. Demirov, D. G., Ono, A., Orenstein, J. M., Freed, E. O. Overexpression of the N-terminal domain of TSG101 inhibits HIV-1 budding by blocking late domain function. *Proc. Natl Acad. Sci. USA* 2002;**99**(2):955–960.

91. Freed, E. O., Martin, M. A. Domains of the human immunodeficiency virus type 1 matrix and gp41 cytoplasmic tail required for envelope incorporation into virions. *J. Virol.* 1995;**70**:341–351.

92. Bour, S., Geleziunas, R., Wainberg, M. A. The human immunodeficiency virus type 1 (HIV-1) CD4 receptor and its central role in promotion of HIV-1 infection. *Microbiol. Rev.* 1995;**59**(1):63–93.

93. Geraghty, R. J., Panganiban, A. T. Human immunodeficiency virus type 1 Vpu has a CD4- and an envelope glycoprotein-independent function. *J. Virol.* 1993;**67**(7):4190–4194.

94. Khan, M. A., Aberham, C., Kao, S. *et al.* Human Immunodeficiency virus type 1 Vif protein is packaged into the nucleoprotein complex through an interaction with viral genomic RNA. *J. Virol.* 2001;**75**(16):7252–7265.

95. Sheehy, A. M., Gaddis, N. C., Choi, J. D., Malim, M. H. Isolation of a human gene that inhibits HIV-1 infection and is suppressed by the viral Vif protein. *Nature* 2002;**418**(6898):646–650.

96. Cohen, E. A., Dehni, G., Sodroski, J. G., Haseltine, W. A. Human immunodeficiency virus vpr product is a virion-associated regulatory protein. *J. Virol.* 1990;**64**(6):3097–3099.

97. Felzien, L. K., Woffendin, C., Hottiger, M. O., Subbramanian, R. A., Cohen, E. A., Nabel, G. J. HIV transcriptional activation by the accessory protein, VPR, is mediated by the p300 co-activator. *Proc. Natl Acad. Sci. USA* 1998;**95**(9):5281–5286.

98. He, J., Choe, S., Walker, R., Di Marzio, P., Morgan, D. O., Landau, N. R. Human immunodeficiency virus type 1 viral protein R (Vpr) arrests cells in the G2 phase of the cell cycle by inhibiting p34cdc2 activity. *J. Virol.* 1995;**69**(11):6705–6711.

99. Garcia, J. V., Miller, A. D. Serine phosphorylation-independent downregulation of cell-surface CD4 by nef. *Nature* 1991;**350**(6318):508–511.

100. Piguet, V., Gu, F., Foti, M. *et al.* Nef-induced CD4 degradation: a diacidic-based motif in Nef functions as a lysosomal targeting signal through the binding of beta-COP in endosomes. *Cell* 1999;**97**(1):63–73.

101. Collette, Y., Dutartre, H., Benziane, A. *et al.* Physical and functional interaction of Nef with Lck. HIV-1 Nef-induced T-cell signaling defects. *J. Biol. Chem.* 1996;**271**(11):6333–6341.

102. Schwartz, O., Marechal, V., Le Gall S., Lemonnier, F., Heard, J. M. Endocytosis of major histocompatibility complex class I molecules is induced by the HIV-1 Nef protein. *Nat. Med.* 1996;**2**(3):338–342.

103. Spira, A. I., Marx, P. A., Patterson, B. K. *et al.* Cellular targets of infection and route of viral dissemination after an intravaginal inoculation of simian immunodeficiency virus into rhesus macaques. *J. Exp. Med.* 1996;**183**(1):215–225.

104. McMichael, A. J., Rowland-Jones, S. L. Cellular immune responses to HIV. *Nature* 2001;**410**(6831):980–987.

105. Schmitz, J. E., Kuroda, M. J., Santra, S., *et al.* Control of viremia in simian immunodeficiency virus infection by CD8+ lymphocytes. *Science* 1999;**283**(5403):857–860.

106. Barker, E., Bossart, K. N., Levy, J. A. Primary CD8+ cells from HIV-infected individuals can suppress productive infection of macrophages independent of beta-chemokines. *Proc. Natl Acad. Sci. USA* 1998;**95**(4):1725–1729.

107. Zhang, L., Yu, W., He, T. *et al*. Contribution of human alpha-defensin 1, 2, and 3 to the anti-HIV-1 activity of CD8 antiviral factor. *Science* 2002;**298**(5595):995–1000.

108. Shearer, W. T., Quinn, T. C., LaRussa, P. *et al*. Viral load and disease progression in infants infected with human immunodeficiency virus type 1. Women and Infants Transmission Study Group. *N. Engl. J. Med.* 1997;**336**(19):1337–1342.

109. Luzuriaga, K., Holmes, D., Hereema, A., Wong, J., Panicali, D. L., Sullivan, J. L. HIV-1-specific cytotoxic T lymphocyte responses in the first year of life. *J. Immunol.* 1995;**154**(1):433–443.

110. McFarland, E. J., Harding, P. A., Luckey, D., Conway, B., Young, R. K., Kuritzkes, D. R. High frequency of Gag- and envelope-specific cytotoxic T lymphocyte precursors in children with vertically acquired human immunodeficiency virus type 1 infection. *J. Infect. Dis.* 1994;**170**(4):766–774.

111. Pugatch, D., Sullivan, J. L., Pikora, C. A., Luzuriaga, K. Delayed generation of antibodies mediating human immunodeficiency virus type 1-specific antibody-dependent cellular cytotoxicity in vertically infected infants. WITS Study Group. Women and Infants Transmission Study. *J. Infect. Dis.* 1997;**176**(3):643–648.

112. Pollack, H., Zhan, M. X., Safrit, J. T. *et al*. CD8+ T-cell-mediated suppression of HIV replication in the first year of life: association with lower viral load and favorable early survival. *Aids* 1997;**11**(1):F9–F13.

113. Goulder, P. J., Brander, C., Tang, Y., *et al*. Evolution and transmission of stable CTL escape mutations in HIV infection. *Nature* 2001;**412**(6844):334–338.

114. Ganeshan, S., Dickover, R. E., Korber, B. T., Bryson, Y. J., Wolinsky, S. M. Human immunodeficiency virus type 1 genetic evolution in children with different rates of development of disease. *J. Virol.* 1997;**71**(1):663–677.

115. Haase, A. T. Population biology of HIV-1 infection: viral and CD4+ T cell demographics and dynamics in lymphatic tissues. *Annu. Rev. Immunol.* 1999;**17**:625–656.

116. Douek, D. C., Brenchley, J. M., Betts, M. R. *et al*. HIV preferentially infects HIV-specific CD4+ T cells. *Nature* 2002;**417**(6884):95–98.

117. Appay, V., Nixon, D. F., Donahoe, S. M. *et al*. HIV-specific CD8(+) T cells produce antiviral cytokines but are impaired in cytolytic function. *J. Exp. Med.* 2000;**192**(1):63–75.

118. Champagne, P., Ogg, G. S., King, A. S. *et al*. Skewed maturation of memory HIV-specific CD8 T lymphocytes. *Nature* 2001;**410**(6824):106–111.

119. Migueles, S. A., Laborico, A. C., Shupert, W. L. *et al*. HIV-specific CD8+ T cell proliferation is coupled to perforin expression and is maintained in nonprogressors. *Nat. Immunol.* 2002;**3**(11):1061–1068.

120. Collins, K. L., Chen, B. K., Kalams, S. A., Walker, B. D., Baltimore, D. HIV-1 Nef protein protects infected primary cells against killing by cytotoxic T lymphocytes. *Nature* 1998;**391**(6665):397–401.

121. Letvin, N. L., Barouch, D. H., Montefiori, D. C. Prospects for vaccine protection against HIV-1 infection and AIDS. *Annu. Rev. Immunol.* 2002;**20**:73–99.

122. Hogan, C. M., Hammer, S. M. Host determinants in HIV infection and disease. Part 2: genetic factors and implications for antiretroviral therapeutics. *Ann. Intern. Med.* 2001;**134**(10):978–996.

123. Rosenberg, E. S., Altfeld, M., Poon, S. H. *et al*. Immune control of HIV-1 after early treatment of acute infection. *Nature* 2000;**407**(6803):523–526.

124. Luzuriaga, K., McManus, M., Catalina, M. *et al.* Early therapy of vertical human immunodeficiency virus type 1 (HIV-1) infection: control of viral replication and absence of persistent HIV-1-specific immune responses. *J. Virol.* 2000;**74**(15):6984–6991.

125. Hainaut, M., Peltier, C. A., Gerard, M., Marissens, D., Zissis, G., Levy, J. Effectiveness of antiretroviral therapy initiated before the age of 2 months in infants vertically infected with human immunodeficiency virus type 1. *Eur. J. Pediatr.* 2000;**159**(10):778–782.

126. Borkowsky, W., Rigaud, M., Krasinski, K., Moore, T., Lawrence, R., Pollack, H. Cell-mediated and humoral immune responses in children infected with human immunodeficiency virus during the first four years of life. *J. Pediatr.* 1992;**120**(3):371–375.

127. Roilides, E., Clerici, M., DePalma, L., Rubin, M., Pizzo, P. A., Shearer, G. M. Helper T-cell responses in children infected with human immunodeficiency virus type 1. *J. Pediatr.* 1991;**118**(5):724–730.

128. Breen, E. C. Pro-and anti-inflammatory cytokines in human immunodeficiency virus infection and acquired immunodeficiency syndrome. *Pharmacol. Ther.* 2002;**95**(3):295–304.

129. Raszka, W. V., Moriarty, R. A., Ottolini, M. G. *et al.* Delayed-type hypersensitivity skin testing in human immunodeficiency virus-infected pediatric patients. *J. Pediatr.* 1996;**129**(2):245–250.

130. Ibegbu, C., Spira, T. J., Nesheim, S. *et al.* Subpopulations of T and B cells in perinatally HIV-infected and noninfected age-matched children compared with those in adults. *Clin. Immunol. Immunopathol.* 1994;**71**(1):27–32.

131. Pantaleo, G., Demarest, J. F., Schacker, T. *et al.* The qualitative nature of the primary immune response to HIV infection is a prognosticator of disease progression independent of the initial level of plasma viremia. *Proc. Natl Acad. Sci. USA* 1997;**94**(1): 254–258.

132. McFarland, E. J., Harding, P. A., Striebich, C. C., MaWhinney, S., Kuritzkes, D. R., Kotzin, B. L. Clonal CD8+ T cell expansions in peripheral blood from human immunodeficiency virus type 1-infected children. *J. Infect. Dis.* 2002;**186**(4):477–485.

133. Gallagher, K., Gorre, M., Harawa, N. *et al.* Timing of lymphocyte activation in neonates infected with human immunodeficiency virus. *Clin. Diagn. Lab. Immunol.* 1997;**4**(6):742–747.

134. Vigano, A., Pinti, M., Nasi, M. *et al.* Markers of cell death-activation in lymphocytes of vertically HIV-infected children naive to highly active antiretroviral therapy: the role of age. *J. Allergy Clin. Immunol.* 2001;**108**(3):439–445.

135. Bohler, T., Wintergerst, U., Linde, R., Belohradsky, B. H., Debatin, K. M. CD95 (APO-1/Fas) expression on naive CD4(+) T cells increases with disease progression in HIV-infected children and adolescents: effect of highly active antiretroviral therapy (HAART). *Pediatr. Res.* 2001;**49**(1):101–110.

136. Bruunsgaard, H., Pedersen, C., Skinhoj, P., Pedersen, B. K. Clinical progression of HIV infection: role of NK cells. *Scand. J. Immunol.* 1997;**46**(1):91–95.

137. Douglas, S. D., Durako, S. J., Tustin, N. B. *et al.* Natural killer cell enumeration and function in HIV-infected and high-risk uninfected adolescents. *AIDS Res. Hum. Retroviruses* 2001;**17**(6):543–552.

138. Lin, S. J., Roberts, R. L., Ank, B. J., Nguyen, Q. H., Thomas, E. K., Stiehm, E. R. Human immunodeficiency virus (HIV) type-1 GP120-specific cell-mediated cytotoxicity (CMC)

and natural killer (NK) activity in HIV-infected (HIV+) subjects: enhancement with interleukin-2(IL-2), IL-12, and IL-15. *Clin. Immunol. Immunopathol.* 1997;**82**(2):163–173.

139. Geijtenbeek, T. B., Kwon, D. S., Torensma, R. *et al.* DC-SIGN, a dendritic cell-specific HIV-1-binding protein that enhances trans-infection of T cells. *Cell* 2000;**100**(5):587–597.

140. Donaghy, H., Pozniak, A., Gazzard, B. *et al.* Loss of blood CD11c(+) myeloid and CD11c(−) plasmacytoid dendritic cells in patients with HIV-1 infection correlates with HIV-1 RNA virus load. *Blood* 2001;**98**(8):2574–2576.

141. Knight, S. C. Dendritic cells and HIV infection; immunity with viral transmission versus compromised cellular immunity? *Immunobiology* 2001;**204**(5):614–621.

142. Ma, X., Montaner, L. J. Proinflammatory response and IL-12 expression in HIV-1 infection. *J. Leukoc. Biol.* 2000;**68**(3):383–390.

143. Chougnet, C., Thomas, E., Landay, A. L. *et al.* CD40 ligand and IFN-gamma synergistically restore IL-12 production in HIV-infected patients. *Eur. J. Immunol.* 1998;**28**(2): 646–656.

144. McFarland, E. J., Harding, P. A., MaWhinney, S., Schooley, R. T., Kuritzkes, D. R. *In vitro* effects of IL-12 on HIV-1-specific CTL lines from HIV-1-infected children. *J. Immunol.* 1998;**161**(1):513–519.

145. Feldman, S., Stein, D., Amrute, S. *et al.* Decreased interferon-alpha production in HIV-infected patients correlates with numerical and functional deficiencies in circulating type 2 dendritic cell precursors. *Clin. Immunol.* 2001;**101**(2):201–210.

146. Bornemann, M. A., Verhoef, J., Peterson, P. K. Macrophages, cytokines, and HIV. *J. Lab. Clin. Med.* 1997;**129**(1):10–16.

147. Noel, G. J. Host defense abnormalities associated with HIV infection. *Pediatr. Clin. North Am.* 1991;**38**(1):37–43.

148. Mastroianni, C. M., Lichtner, M., Mengoni, F. *et al.* Improvement in neutrophil and monocyte function during highly active antiretroviral treatment of HIV-1-infected patients. *Aids* 1999;**13**(8):883–890.

149. Maloney, M. J., Guill, M. F., Wray, B. B., Lobel, S. A., Ebbeling, W. Pediatric acquired immune deficiency syndrome with panhypogammaglobulinemia. *J. Pediatr.* 1987;**110**(2):266–267.

150. Pahwa, S., Fikrig, S., Menez, R., Pahwa, R. Pediatric acquired immunodeficiency syndrome: demonstration of B lymphocyte defects *in vitro. Diagn. Immunol.* 1986;**4**(1):24–30.

151. de Martino, M., Tovo, P. A., Galli, L. *et al.* Prognostic significance of immunologic changes in 675 infants perinatally exposed to human immunodeficiency virus. The Italian Register for Human Immunodeficiency Virus Infection in Children. *J. Pediatr.* 1991;**119**(5):702–709.

152. Muller, S., Kohler, H. B cell superantigens in HIV-1 infection. *Int. Rev. Immunol.* 1997;**14**(4):339–349.

153. Rutstein, R. M., Rudy, B., Codispoti, C., Watson, B. Response to hepatitis B immunization by infants exposed to HIV. *Aids* 1994;**8**(9):1281–1284.

154. Arpadi, S. M., Markowitz, L. E., Baughman, A. L. *et al.* Measles antibody in vaccinated human immunodeficiency virus type 1-infected children. *Pediatrics* 1996;**97**(5):653–657.

155. Gibb, D., Spoulou, V., Giacomelli, A. *et al.* Antibody responses to *Haemophilus influenzae* type b and *Streptococcus pneumoniae* vaccines in children with human immunodeficiency virus infection. *Pediatr. Infect. Dis. J.* 1995;**14**(2):129–135.

156. Lyall, E. G., Charlett, A., Watkins, P., Zambon, M. Response to influenza virus vaccination in vertical HIV infection. *Arch. Dis. Child.* 1997;**76**(3):215–218.

157. Moir, S., Malaspina, A., Ogwaro, K. M. *et al.* HIV-1 induces phenotypic and functional perturbations of B cells in chronically infected individuals. *Proc. Natl Acad. Sci. USA* 2001;**98**(18):10362–10367.

158. Rodriguez, C., Thomas, J. K., O'Rourke, S., Stiehm, E. R., Plaeger, S. HIV disease in children is associated with a selective decrease in CD23+ and CD62L+ B cells. *Clin. Immunol. Immunopathol.* 1996;**81**(2):191–199.

159. Chirmule, N., Oyaizu, N., Kalyanaraman, V. S., Pahwa, S. Inhibition of normal B-cell function by human immunodeficiency virus envelope glycoprotein, gp120. *Blood* 1992;**79**(5):1245–1254.

160. 1997 revised guidelines for performing CD4+ T-cell determinations in persons infected with human immunodeficiency virus (HIV). Centers for Disease Control and Prevention. *Morb. Mortal. Wkly Rep. Rec. Rep.* 1997;**46**(RR-2):1–29.

161. Mandy, F. F., Nicholson, J. K., McDougal, J. S. Guidelines for performing single-platform absolute CD4+ T-cell determinations with CD45 gating for persons infected with human immunodeficiency virus. Centers for Disease Control and Prevention. *Morb. Mortal. Wkly Rep. Rec. Rep.* 2003;**52**(RR-2):1–13.

162. Malone, J. L., Simms, T. E., Gray, G. C., Wagner, K. F., Burge, J. R., Burke, D. S. Sources of variability in repeated T-helper lymphocyte counts from human immunodeficiency virus type 1-infected patients: total lymphocyte count fluctuations and diurnal cycle are important. *J. Acquir. Immune Defic. Syndr.* 1990;**3**(2):144–151.

163. Hughes, M. D., Stein, D. S., Gundacker, H. M., Valentine, F. T., Phair, J. P., Volberding, P. A. Within-subject variation in CD4 lymphocyte count in asymptomatic human immunodeficiency virus infection: implications for patient monitoring. *J. Infect. Dis.* 1994;**169**(1):28–36.

164. Raszka, W. V., Jr., Meyer, G. A., Waecker, N. J. *et al.* Variability of serial absolute and percent CD4+ lymphocyte counts in healthy children born to human immunodeficiency virus 1-infected parents. Military Pediatric HIV Consortium. *Pediatr. Infect. Dis. J.* 1994;**13**(1):70–72.

165. Shearer, W. T., Rosenblatt, H. M., Schluchter, M. D., Mofenson, L. M., Denny, T. N. Immunologic targets of HIV infection: T cells. NICHD IVIG Clinical Trial Group, and the NHLBI P2C2 Pediatric Pulmonary and Cardiac Complications of HIV Infection Study Group. *Ann. N.Y. Acad. Sci.* 1993;**693**:35–51.

166. Autran, B., Carcelain, G., Debre, P. Immune reconstitution after highly active antiretroviral treatment of HIV infection. *Adv. Exp. Med. Biol.* 2001;**495**:205–212.

167. Sleasman, J. W., Nelson, R. P., Goodenow, M. M. *et al.* Immunoreconstitution after ritonavir therapy in children with human immunodeficiency virus infection involves multiple lymphocyte lineages. *J. Pediatr.* 1999;**134**(5):597–606.

168. Essajee, S. M., Kim, M., Gonzalez, C. *et al.* Immunologic and virologic responses to HAART in severely immunocompromised HIV-1-infected children. *Aids* 1999;**13**(18):2523–2532.

169. Lederman, M. M. Immune restoration and CD4+ T-cell function with antiretroviral therapies. *AIDS* 2001;**15** Suppl **2**:S11–S15.

170. Hainaut, M., Ducarme, M., Schandene, L. *et al*. Age-related immune reconstitution during highly active antiretroviral therapy in human immunodeficiency virus type 1-infected children. *Pediatr. Infect. Dis. J.* 2003;**22**(1):62–69.

171. Gibb, D. M., Newberry, A., Klein, N., de Rossi, A., Grosch-Woerner, I., Babiker, A. Immune repopulation after HAART in previously untreated HIV-1-infected children. Paediatric European Network for Treatment of AIDS (PENTA) Steering Committee. *Lancet* 2000;**355**(9212):1331–1332.

172. Ometto, L., De Forni, D., Patiri, F. *et al*. Immune reconstitution in HIV-1-infected children on antiretroviral therapy: role of thymic output and viral fitness. *AIDS* 2002;**16**(6):839–849.

173. Douek, D. C., Koup, R. A., McFarland, R. D., Sullivan, J. L., Luzuriaga, K. Effect of HIV on thymic function before and after antiretroviral therapy in children. *J. Infect. Dis.* 2000;**181**(4):1479–1482.

174. Vigano, A., Dally, L., Bricalli, D. *et al*. Clinical and immuno-virologic characterization of the efficacy of stavudine, lamivudine, and indinavir in human immunodeficiency virus infection. *J. Pediatr.* 1999;**135**(6):675–682.

175. Havlir, D. V., Schrier, R. D., Torriani, F. J., Chervenak, K., Hwang, J. Y., Boom, W. H. Effect of potent antiretroviral therapy on immune responses to *Mycobacterium avium* in human immunodeficiency virus-infected subjects. *J. Infect. Dis.* 2000;**182**(6):1658–1663.

176. Berkelhamer, S., Borock, E., Elsen, C., Englund, J., Johnson, D. Effect of highly active antiretroviral therapy on the serological response to additional measles vaccinations in human immunodeficiency virus-infected children. *Clin. Infect. Dis.* 2001;**32**(7):1090–1094.

177. Notermans, D. W., de Jong, J. J., Goudsmit, J. *et al*. Potent antiretroviral therapy initiates normalization of hypergammaglobulinemia and a decline in HIV type 1-specific antibody responses. *AIDS Res. Hum. Retroviruses* 2001;**17**(11):1003–1008.

178. Jacobson, M. A., Khayam-Bashi H., Martin, J. N., Black, D., Ng, V. Effect of long-term highly active antiretroviral therapy in restoring HIV-induced abnormal B-lymphocyte function. *J. Acquir. Immune Defic. Syndr.* 2002;**31**(5):472–477.

179. Borkowsky, W., Stanley, K., Douglas, S. D. *et al*. Immunologic response to combination nucleoside analogue plus protease inhibitor therapy in stable antiretroviral therapy-experienced human immunodeficiency virus-infected children. *J. Infect. Dis.* 2000;**182**(1):96–103.

180. Chavan, S., Bennuri, B., Kharbanda, M., Chandrasekaran, A., Bakshi, S., Pahwa, S. Evaluation of T cell receptor gene rearrangement excision circles after antiretroviral therapy in children infected with human immunodeficiency virus. *J. Infect. Dis.* 2001;**183**(10):1445–1454.

181. Jankelevich, S., Mueller, B. U., Mackall, C. L. *et al*. Long-term virologic and immunologic responses in human immunodeficiency virus type 1-infected children treated with indinavir, zidovudine, and lamivudine. *J. Infect. Dis.* 2001;**183**(7):1116–1120.

182. Piketty, C., Weiss, L., Thomas, F., Mohamed, A. S., Belec, L., Kazatchkine, M. D. Long-term clinical outcome of human immunodeficiency virus-infected patients with

discordant immunologic and virologic responses to a protease inhibitor-containing regimen. *J. Infect. Dis.* 2001;**183**(9):1328–1335.

183. Kharbanda, M., Than, S., Chitnis, V. *et al.* Patterns of CD8 T cell clonal dominance in response to change in antiretroviral therapy in HIV-infected children. *AIDS* 2000;**14**(15):2229–2238.

184. Chougnet, C., Jankelevich, S., Fowke, K. *et al.* Long-term protease inhibitor-containing therapy results in limited improvement in T cell function but not restoration of interleukin-12 production in pediatric patients with AIDS. *J. Infect. Dis.* 2001;**184**(2):201–205.

185. Graham, B. S. Clinical trials of HIV vaccines. *Annu. Rev. Med.* 2002;**53**:207–221.

186. Kalyanaraman, V. S., Cabradilla, C. D., Getchell, J. P. *et al.* Antibodies to the core protein of lymphadenopathy-associated virus (LAV) in patients with AIDS. *Science* 1984;**225**(4659):321–323.

187. Sarngadharan, M. G., Popovic, M., Bruch, L., Schupbach, J., Gallo, R. C. Antibodies reactive with human T-lymphotropic retroviruses (HTLV-III) in the serum of patients with AIDS. *Science* 1984;**224**(4648):506–508.

188. Interpretation and use of the western blot assay for serodiagnosis of human immunodeficiency virus type 1 infections. *Morb. Mortal. Wkly Rep.* 1989;**38**(Suppl 7):1–7.

189. Interpretive criteria used to report western blot results for HIV-1-antibody testing–United States. *Morb. Mortal. Wkly. Rep.* 1991;**40**(40):692–695.

190. Constantine, N. T. Serologic tests for the retroviruses: approaching a decade of evolution. *AIDS* 1993;**7**(1):1–13.

191. HIV counseling and testing using rapid tests. *Morb Mortal. Wkly Rep.* 1998;**47**(11):211–215.

192. Stetler, H. C., Granade, T. C., Nunez, C. A. *et al.* Field evaluation of rapid HIV serologic tests for screening and confirming HIV-1 infection in Honduras. *AIDS* 1997;**11**(3):369–375.

193. Nishanian, P., Huskins, K. R., Stehn, S., Detels, R., Fahey, J. L. A simple method for improved assay demonstrates that HIV p24 antigen is present as immune complexes in most sera from HIV-infected individuals. *J. Infect. Dis.* 1990;**162**(1):21–28.

194. Quinn, T. C., Kline, R., Moss, M. W., Livingston, R. A., Hutton, N. Acid dissociation of immune complexes improves diagnostic utility of p24 antigen detection in perinatally acquired human immunodeficiency virus infection. *J. Infect. Dis.* 1993;**167**(5):1193–1196.

195. Schupbach, J., Boni, J., Tomasik, Z., Jendis, J., Seger, R., Kind, C. Sensitive detection and early prognostic significance of p24 antigen in heat-denatured plasma of human immunodeficiency virus type 1-infected infants. Swiss Neonatal HIV Study Group. *J. Infect. Dis.* 1994;**170**(2):318–324.

196. Schupbach, J., Flepp, M., Pontelli, D., Tomasik, Z., Luthy, R., Boni, J. Heat-mediated immune complex dissociation and enzyme-linked immunosorbent assay signal amplification render p24 antigen detection in plasma as sensitive as HIV-1 RNA detection by polymerase chain reaction. *AIDS* 1996;**10**(10):1085–1090.

197. Boni, J., Opravil, M., Tomasik, Z. *et al.* Simple monitoring of antiretroviral therapy with a signal-amplification- boosted HIV-1 p24 antigen assay with heat-denatured plasma. *AIDS* 1997;**11**(6):F47–F52.

198. Jackson, J. B., Drew, J., Lin, H. J. *et al.* Establishment of a quality assurance program for human immunodeficiency virus type 1 DNA polymerase chain reaction assays by the AIDS Clinical Trials Group, ACTG PCR Working Group, and the ACTG PCR Virology Laboratories. *J. Clin. Microbiol.* 1993;**31**(12):3123–3128.

199. Cassol, S., Salas, T., Gill, M. J. *et al.* Stability of dried blood spot specimens for detection of HIV DNA by PCR. *J. Clin. Microbiol.* 1992;**30**:3039–3042.

200. Comeau, A. M., Su, X., Muchinsky, G., Pan, D., Gerstel, J., Grady, G. F. Quality-controlled pooling strategies for nucleic-acid based HIV screening: using PCR as a primary screen on dried blood spot specimens in population studies. In 5th Conference on Retroviruses and Opportunistic Infections; Chicago, IL; 1998.

201. Bremer, J. W., Lew, J. F., Cooper, E., *et al.* Diagnosis of infection with human immunodeficiency virus type 1 by a DNA polymerase chain reaction assay among infants enrolled in the Women and Infants' Transmission Study [see comments]. *J. Pediatr.* 1996;**129**(2):198–207.

202. Owens, D. K., Holodniy, M., McDonald, T. W., Scott, J., Sonnad, S. A meta-analytic evaluation of the polymerase chain reaction for the diagnosis of HIV infection in infants [see comments] [published erratum appears in *J. Am. Med. Assoc.* 1996 Oct 23–30;276(16):1302]. *J Am Med Assoc* 1996;**275**(17):1342–1348.

203. MoH-I. *Guidelines for the Use of Antiretroviral Agents in Pediatric HIV Infection.* 2001.

204. Stanley, S., Ostrowski, M. A., Justement, J. S. *et al.* Effect of immunization with a common recall antigen on viral expression in patients infected with human immunodeficiency virus type 1. *N. Engl. J. Med.* 1996;**334**(19):1222–1230.

205. Staprans, S. I., Hamilton, B. L., Follansbee, S. E. *et al.* Activation of virus replication after vaccination of HIV-1-infected individuals. *J. Exp. Med.* 1995;**182**(6):1727–1737.

206. Brichacek, B., Swindells, S., Janoff, E. N., Pirruccello, S., Stevenson, M. Increased plasma human immunodeficiency virus type 1 burden following antigenic challenge with pneumococcal vaccine. *J. Infect. Dis.* 1996;**174**(6):1191–1199.

207. Ho, D. D., Neumann, A. U., Perelson, A. S., Chen, W., Leonard, J. M., Markowitz, M. Rapid turnover of plasma virions and CD4 lymphocytes in HIV-1 infection. *Nature* 1995;**373**(6510):123–126.

208. Wei, X., Ghosh, S. K., Taylor, M. E. *et al.* Viral dynamics in human immunodeficiency virus type 1 infection. *Nature* 1995;**373**(6510):117–122.

209. Wong, J. K., Hezareh, M., Gunthard, H. F. *et al.* Recovery of replication-competent HIV despite prolonged suppression of plasma viremia. *Science* 1997;**278**:1291–1295.

210. Finzi, D., Hermankova, M., Pierson, T. *et al.* Identification of a reservoir for HIV-1 in patients on highly active antiretroviral therapy. *Science* 1997;**278**:1295–1300.

211. Chun, T., Stuyver, L., Mizell, S. B. *et al.* Presence of an inducible HIV-1 latent reservoir during highly active antiretroviral therapy. *Proc. Natl Acad. Sci. USA* 1997;**94**:13193–13197.

212. Chun, T. W., Carruth, L., Finzi, D. *et al.* Quantification of latent tissue reservoirs and total body viral load in HIV-1 infection [see comments]. *Nature* 1997;**387**(6629):183–188.

213. Persaud, D., Pierson, T., Ruff, C. *et al.* A stable latent reservoir for HIV-1 in resting CD4(+) T lymphocytes in infected children. *J. Clin. Invest.* 2000;**105**(7):995–1003.

214. Palumbo, P. E., Kwok, S., Waters, S. *et al.* Viral measurement by polymerase chain reaction-based assays in human immunodeficiency virus-infected infants. *J. Pediatr.* 1995;**126**(4):592–595.

215. Steketee, R. W., Abrams, E. J., Thea, D. M. *et al.* Early detection of perinatal human immunodeficiency virus (HIV) type 1 infection using HIV RNA amplification and detection. New York City Perinatal HIV Transmission Collaborative Study. *J. Infect. Dis.* 1997;**175**(3):707–711.

216. Delamare, C., Burgard, M., Mayaux, M. J. *et al.* HIV-1 RNA detection in plasma for the diagnosis of infection in neonates. The French Pediatric HIV Infection Study Group. *J. Acquir. Immune. Defic. Syndr. Hum. Retrovirol.* 1997;**15**(2):121–125.

217. Munoz, A., Wang, M. C., Bass, S. *et al.* Acquired immunodeficiency syndrome (AIDS)–free time after human immunodeficiency virus type 1 (HIV-1) seroconversion in homosexual men. Multicenter AIDS Cohort Study Group. *Am. J. Epidemiol.* 1989;**130**(3):530–539.

218. Munoz, A., Kirby, A. J., He, Y. D. *et al.* Long-term survivors with HIV-1 infection: incubation period and longitudinal patterns of CD4+ lymphocytes. *J. Acquir. Immune Defic. Syndr. Hum. Retrovirol.* 1995;**8**(5):496–505.

219. Veugelers, P. J., Kaldor, J. M., Strathdee, S. A. *et al.* Incidence and prognostic significance of symptomatic primary human immunodeficiency virus type 1 infection in homosexual men. *J. Infect. Dis.* 1997;**176**(1):112–117.

220. Lyles, R. H., Munoz, A., Yamashita, T. E. *et al.* Natural history of human immunodeficiency virus type 1 viremia after seroconversion and proximal to AIDS in a large cohort of homosexual men. Multicenter AIDS Cohort Study. *J. Infect. Dis.* 2000;**181**(3):872–880.

221. Vanhems, P., Hirschel, B., Phillips, A. N. *et al.* Incubation time of acute human immunodeficiency virus (HIV) infection and duration of acute HIV infection are independent prognostic factors of progression to AIDS. *J. Infect. Dis.* 2000;**182**(1):334–337.

222. Daar, E. S., Moudgil, T., Meyer, R. D., Ho, D. D. Transient high levels of viremia in patients with primary human immunodeficiency virus type 1 infection. *N. Engl. J. Med.* 1991;**324**(14):961–964.

223. Clark, S. J., Saag, M. S., Decker, W. D. *et al.* High titers of cytopathic virus in plasma of patients with symptomatic primary HIV-1 infection. *N. Engl. J. Med.* 1991;**324**(14):954–960.

224. Rosenberg, E. S., Billingsley, J. M., Caliendo, A. M. *et al.* Vigorous HIV-1-specific CD4+ T cell responses associated with control of viremia. *Science* 1997;**278**(5342):1447–1450.

225. Perelson, A. S., Neumann, A. U., Markowitz, M., Leonard, J. M., Ho, D. D. HIV-1 dynamics *in vivo*: virion clearance rate, infected cell life-span, and viral generation time. *Science* 1996;**271**(5255):1582–1586.

226. Haase, A. T., Henry, K., Zupancic, M. *et al.* Quantitative image analysis of HIV-1 infection in lymphoid tissue. *Science* 1996;**274**(5289):985–989.

227. Cavert, W., Notermans, D. W., Staskus, K. *et al.* Kinetics of response in lymphoid tissues to antiretroviral therapy of HIV-1 infection. *Science* 1997;**276**(5314):960–964.

228. Delwart, E. L., Mullins, J. I., Gupta, P. *et al.* Human immunodeficiency virus type 1 populations in blood and semen. *J. Virol.* 1998;**72**(1):617–623.

229. Poss, M., Rodrigo, A. G., Gosink, J. J. *et al.* Evolution of envelope sequences from the genital tract and peripheral blood of women infected with clade A human immunodeficiency virus type 1. *J. Virol.* 1998;**72**(10):8240–8251.

230. Mellors, J. W., Kingsley, L. A., Rinaldo, C. R., Jr. *et al.* Quantitation of HIV-1 RNA in plasma predicts outcome after seroconversion. *Ann. Intern. Med.* 1995;**122**(8):573–579.

231. Mellors, J. W., Rinaldo, C. R., Jr., Gupta, P., White, R. M., Todd, J. A., Kingsley, L. A. Prognosis in HIV-1 infection predicted by the quantity of virus in plasma. *Science* 1996;**272**(5265):1167–1170.

232. O'Brien, W. A., Hartigan, P. M., Daar, E. S., Simberkoff, M. S., Hamilton, J. D. Changes in plasma HIV RNA levels and CD4+ lymphocyte counts predict both response to antiretroviral therapy and therapeutic failure. VA Cooperative Study Group on AIDS. *Ann. Intern. Med.* 1997;**126**(12):939–945.

233. Hughes, M. D., Johnson, V. A., Hirsch, M. S. *et al.* Monitoring plasma HIV-1 RNA levels in addition to CD4+ lymphocyte count improves assessment of antiretroviral therapeutic response. ACTG 241 Protocol Virology Substudy Team. *Ann. Intern. Med.* 1997;**126**(12):929–938.

234. Finzi, D., Siliciano, R. F. Taking aim at HIV replication. *Nat. Med.* 2000;**6**(7):735–736.

235. Carrington, M., Nelson, G. W., Martin, M. P. *et al.* HLA and HIV-1: heterozygote advantage and B∗35-Cw∗04 disadvantage. *Science* 1999;**283**(5408):1748–1752.

236. Kaslow, R. A., Carrington, M., Apple, R., *et al.* Influence of combinations of human major histocompatibility complex genes on the course of HIV-1 infection. *Nat. Med.* 1996;**2**(4):405–411.

237. O'Brien, S. J., Gao, X., Carrington, M. HLA and AIDS: a cautionary tale. *Trends Mol. Med.* 2001;**7**(9):379–381.

238. Dean, M., Carrington, M., O'Brien, S. J. Balanced polymorphism selected by genetic versus infectious human disease. *Annu. Rev. Genom. Hum. Genet.* 2002;**3**:263–292.

239. Fauci, A. S., Pantaleo, G., Stanley, S., Weissman, D. Immunopathogenic mechanisms of HIV Infection. *Ann. Intern. Med.* 1996;**124**(7):654–663.

240. Bush, C. E., Donovan, R. M., Markowitz, N. P., Kvale, P., Saravolatz, L. D. A study of HIV RNA viral load in AIDS patients with bacterial pneumonia. *J. Acquir. Immune Defic. Syndr. Hum. Retrovirol.* 1996;**13**(1):23–26.

241. Donovan, R. M., Bush, C. E., Markowitz, N. P., Baxa, D. M., Saravolatz, L. D. Changes in virus load markers during AIDS-associated opportunistic diseases in human immunodeficiency virus-infected persons. *J. Infect. Dis.* 1996;**174**(2):401–403.

242. Whalen, C., Horsburgh, C. R., Hom, D., Lahart, C., Simberkoff, M., Ellner, J. Accelerated course of human immunodeficiency virus infection after tuberculosis. *Am. J. Respir. Crit. Care Med.* 1995;**151**(1):129–135.

243. O'Brien, W. A., Grovit-Ferbas K., Namazi, A. *et al.* Human immunodeficiency virus-type 1 replication can be increased in peripheral blood of seropositive patients after influenza vaccination. *Blood* 1995;**86**(3):1082–1089.

244. Fowke, K. R., D'Amico, R., Chernoff, D. N. *et al.* Immunologic and virologic evaluation after influenza vaccination of HIV-1-infected patients. *AIDS* 1997;**11**(8):1013–1021.

245. Premack, B. A., Schall, T. J. Chemokine receptors: gateways to inflammation and infection. *Nat. Med.* 1996;**2**(11):1174–1178.

246. Connor, R. I., Sheridan, K. E., Ceradini, D., Choe, S., Landau, N. R. Change in coreceptor use correlates with disease progression in HIV-1-infected individuals. *J. Exp. Med.* 1997;**185**(4):621–628.

247. Koot, M., van't Wout, A. B., Kootstra, N. A., de Goede, R. E., Tersmette, M., Schuitemaker, H. Relation between changes in cellular load, evolution of viral phenotype, and the

clonal composition of virus populations in the course of human immunodeficiency virus type 1 infection. *J. Infect. Dis.* 1996;**173**(2):349–354.

248. 1994 revised classification system for human immundeficiency virus infection in children less than 13 years. *Morb. Mortal. Wkly Rep.* 1994;**43**:1–19.

249. 1995 revised guidelines for prophylaxis against *Pneumocystis carinii* pneumonia for children infected with or perinatally exposed to human immunodeficiency virus. National Pediatric and Family HIV Resource Center and National Center for Infectious Diseases, Centers for Disease Control and Prevention. *Morb. Mortal. Wkly. Rep.* 1995;**44**(RR-4):1–11.

250. Frederick, T., Mascola, L., Eller, A., O'Neil, L., Byers, B. Progression of human Immunodeficiency virus disease among infants and children infected perinatally with human immunodeficiency virus or through neonatal blood transfusion. Los Angeles County Pediatric AIDS Consortium and the Los Angeles County-University of Southern California Medical Center and the University of Southern California School of Medicine [see comments]. *Pediatr. Infect. Dis. J.* 1994;**13**(12):1091–1097.

251. Jones, D. S., Byers, R. H., Bush, T. J., Oxtoby, M. J., Rogers, M. F. Epidemiology of transfusion-associated acquired immunodeficiency syndrome in children in the United States, 1981 through 1989. *Pediatrics* 1992;**89**(1):123–127.

252. Auger, I., Thomas, P., DeGruttola, V. *et al.* Incubation periods for pedatric AIDS patients. *Nature* 1988;**336**:575–577.

253. Mayaux, M. J., Burgard, M., Teglas, J. P. *et al.* Neonatal characteristics in rapidly progressive perinatally acquired HIV-1 disease. The French Pediatric HIV Infection Study Group. *J. Am. Med. Assoc.* 1996;**275**(8):606–610.

254. Duliege, A. M., Messiah, A., Blanche, S., Tardieu, M., Griscelli, C., Spira, A. Natural history of human immunodeficiency virus type 1 infection in children: prognostic value of laboratory tests on the bimodal progression of the disease. *Pediatr. Infect. Dis. J.* 1992;**11**(8):630–635.

255. Scott, G. B., Hutto, C., Makuch, R. W. *et al.* Survival in children with perinatally acquired human immunodeficiency virus type 1 infection. *N. Engl. J. Med.* 1989;**321**(26):1791–1796.

256. Barnhart, H. X., Caldwell, M. B., Thomas, P. *et al.* Natural history of human immunodeficiency virus disease in perinatally infected children: an analysis from the Pediatric Spectrum of Disease Project. *Pediatrics* 1996;**97**(5):710–716.

257. Blanche, S., Newell, M. L., Mayaux, M. J. *et al.* Morbidity and mortality in European children vertically infected by HIV- 1. The French Pediatric HIV Infection Study Group and European Collaborative Study. *J. Acquir. Immune Defic. Syndr. Hum. Retrovirol.* 1997;**14**(5):442–450.

258. Plaeger-Marshall, S., Isacescu, V., O'Rourke, S., Bertolli, J., Bryson, Y. J., Stiehm, E. R. T-cell activation in pediatric AIDS pathogenesis: three-color immunophenotyping. *Clin. Immunol. Immunopathol.* 1994;**71**(1):19–26.

259. Pollack, H., Zhan, M. X., Ilmet-Moore, T., Ajuang-Simbiri, K., Krasinski, K., Borkowsky, W. Ontogeny of anti-human immunodeficiency virus (HIV) antibody production in HIV-1-infected infants. *Proc. Natl Acad. Sci. USA* 1993;**90**(6):2340–2344.

260. Bryson, Y. J., Luzuriaga, K., Sullivan, J. L., Wara, D. W. Proposed definitions for in utero versus intrapartum transmission of HIV-1. *N. Engl. J. Med.* 1992;**327**(17):1246–1247.

261. Dickover, R. E., Dillon, M., Gillette, S. G. *et al.* Rapid increases in load of human immunodeficiency virus correlate with early disease progression and loss of CD4 cells in vertically infected infants. *J. Infect. Dis.* 1994;**170**(5):1279–1284.

262. De Rossi, A., Masiero, S., Giaquinto, C. *et al.* Dynamics of viral replication in infants with vertically acquired human immunodeficiency virus type 1 infection. *J. Clin. Invest.* 1996;**97**(2):323–330.

263. McIntosh, K., Shevitz, A., Zaknun, D. *et al.* Age- and time-related changes in extracellular viral load in children vertically infected by human immunodeficiency virus. *Pediatr. Infect. Dis. J.* 1996;**15**(12):1087–1091.

264. UNAIDS/WHO. *AIDS Epidemic Update–December 2002.* Geneva: UNAIDS/WHO; 2002.

265. Cohen, J. Is AIDS in Africa a distinct disease? *Science* 2000;**288**(5474):2153–2155.

266. Morgan, D., Whitworth, J. The natural history of HIV-1 infection in Africa. *Nat. Med.* 2001;**7**(2):143–145.

267. Morgan, D., Mahe, C., Mayanja, B., Whitworth, J. A. Progression to symptomatic disease in people infected with HIV-1 in rural Uganda: prospective cohort study. *B. Med. J.* 2002;**324**(7331):193–196.

268. Gortmaker, S. L., Hughes, M., Cervia, J., *et al.* Effect of combination therapy including protease inhibitors on mortality among children and adolescents infected with HIV-1. *N. Engl. J. Med.* 2001;**345**(21):1522–1528.

269. de Martino, M., Tovo, P. A., Balducci, M., *et al.* Reduction in mortality with availability of antiretroviral therapy for children with perinatal HIV-1 infection. Italian Register for HIV Infection in Children and the Italian National AIDS Registry. *J. Am. Med. Assoc.* 2000;**284**(2):190–197.

270. Resino, S., Bellon, J. M., Sanchez-Ramon, S., *et al.* Impact of antiretroviral protocols on dynamics of AIDS progression markers. *Arch. Dis. Child.* 2002;**86**(2):119–124.

271. Holland, C. A., Ma, Y., Moscicki, B., Durako, S. J., Levin, L., Wilson, C. M. Seroprevalence and risk factors of hepatitis B, hepatitis C, and human cytomegalovirus among HIV-infected and high-risk uninfected adolescents: findings of the REACH Study. Adolescent Medicine HIV/AIDS Research Network. *Sex. Transm. Dis.* 2000;**27**(5):296–303.

272. Wilson, C. M., Ellenberg, J. H., Sawyer, M. K. *et al.* Serologic response to hepatitis B vaccine in HIV infected and high-risk HIV uninfected adolescents in the REACH cohort. Reaching for Excellence in Adolescent Care and Health. *J. Adolesc. Health* 2001;**29**(3 Suppl):123–129.

273. Palumbo, P. E., Raskino, C., Fiscus, S. *et al.* Predictive value of quantitative plasma HIV RNA and CD4+ lymphocyte count in HIV-infected infants and children. *J. Am. Med. Assoc.* 1998;**279**(10):756–761.

274. Mofenson, L. M., Korelitz, J., Meyer, W. A., 3rd *et al.* The relationship between serum human immunodeficiency virus type 1 (HIV-1) RNA level, CD4 lymphocyte percent, and long-term mortality risk in HIV-1-infected children. National Institute of Child Health and Human Development Intravenous Immunoglobulin Clinical Trial Study Group. *J. Infect. Dis.* 1997;**175**(5):1029–1038.

275. Abrams, E. J., Weedon, J., Steketee, R. W. *et al.* Association of human immunodeficiency virus (HIV) load early in life with disease progression among HIV-infected infants. New York City Perinatal HIV Transmission Collaborative Study Group. *J. Infect. Dis.* 1998;**178**(1):101–108.

276. Balotta, C., Vigano, A., Riva, C. *et al.* HIV type 1 phenotype correlates with the stage of infection in vertically infected children. *AIDS Res. Hum. Retroviruses* 1996;**12**(13):1247–1253.

277. Spencer, L. T., Ogino, M. T., Dankner, W. M., Spector, S. A. Clinical significance of human immunodeficiency virus type 1 phenotypes in infected children. *J. Infect. Dis.* 1994;**169**(3):491–495.

278. Ometto, L., Zanotto, C., Maccabruni, A. *et al.* Viral phenotype and host-cell suscepti-bility to HIV-1 infection as risk factors for mother-to-child HIV-1 transmission. *AIDS* 1995;**9**(5):427–434.

279. Just, J. J., Casabona, J., Bertran, J., *et al.* MHC class II alleles associated with clinical and immunological manifestations of HIV-1 infection among children in Catalonia, Spain. *Tissue Antigens* 1996;**47**(4):313–318.

280. Kostrikis, L. G., Neumann, A. U., Thomson, B. *et al.* A polymorphism in the regula-tory region of the CC-chemokine receptor 5 gene influences perinatal transmission of human immunodeficiency virus type 1 to African-American infants. *J. Virol.* 1999;**73**(12):10264–10271.

281. Goedert, J. J., Kessler, C. M., Aledort, L. M. *et al.* A prospective study of human immun-odeficiency virus type 1 infection and the development of AIDS in subjects with hemophilia. *N. Engl. J. Med.* 1989;**321**(17):1141–1148.

282. Morris, C. R., Araba-Owoyele L., Spector, S. A., Maldonado, Y. A. Disease patterns and survival after acquired immunodeficiency syndrome diagnosis in human immunode-ficiency virus-infected children. *Pediatr. Infect. Dis. J.* 1996;**15**(4):321–328.

283. Blanche, S., Mayaux, M. J., Rouzioux, C., *et al.* Relation of the course of HIV infection in children to the severity of the disease in their mothers at delivery. *N. Engl. J. Med.* 1994;**330**(5):308–312.

284. Tovo, P. A., de Martino, M., Gabiano, C., *et al.* AIDS appearance in children is associated with the velocity of disease progression in their mothers. *J. Infect. Dis.* 1994;**170**(4):1000–1002.

285. Lambert, G., Thea, D. M., Pliner, V., *et al.* Effect of maternal CD4+ cell count, acquired immunodeficiency syndrome, and viral load on disease progression in infants with perinatally acquired human immunodeficiency virus type 1 infection. New York City Perinatal HIV Transmission Collaborative Study Group. *J. Pediatr.* 1997;**130**(6): 890–897.

286. Krasinski, K., Borkowsky, W., Holzman, R. S. Prognosis of human immunodeficiency virus infection in children and adolescents. *Pediatr. Infect. Dis. J.* 1989;**8**(4):216–220.

287. Bamji, M., Thea, D. M., Weedon, J. *et al.* Prospective study of human immunodeficiency virus 1-related disease among 512 infants born to infected women in New York City. The New York City Perinatal HIV Transmission Collaborative Study Group. *Pediatr. Infect. Dis. J.* 1996;**15**(10):891–898.

288. Blanche, S., Tardieu, M., Duliege, A. *et al.* Longitudinal study of 94 symptomatic infants with perinatally acquired human immunodeficiency virus infection. Evidence for a bimodal expression of clinical and biological symptoms. *Am. J. Dis. Child.* 1990;**144**(11):1210–1215.

289. McKinney, R. E., Jr., Wilfert, C. Growth as a prognostic indicator in children with human immunodeficiency virus infection treated with zidovudine. AIDS Clinical Trials Group Protocol 043 Study Group. *J. Pediatr.* 1994;**125**(5 Pt 1):728–733.

290. Pollack, H., Glasberg, H., Lee, E. *et al.* Impaired early growth of infants perinatally infected with human immunodeficiency virus: correlation with viral load. *J. Pediatr.* 1997;**130**(6):915–922.

291. Nielsen, K., Ammann, A., Bryson, Y. *et al.* A descriptive survey of pediatric HIV-infected long term survivors. In 3rd Conf Retro and Opportun Infect; Jan 28–Feb 1, 1996. p. 150.

292. Bryson, Y. J., Pang, S., Wei, L. S., Dickover, R., Diagne, A., Chen, I. S. Clearance of HIV infection in a perinatally infected infant. *N. Engl. J. Med.* 1995;**332**(13):833–838.

293. Newell, M. L., Dunn, D., De Maria, A., *et al.* Detection of virus in vertically exposed HIV-antibody-negative children. *Lancet* 1996;**347**(8996):213–215.

294. Roques, P. A., Gras, G., Parnet-Mathieu, F. *et al.* Clearance of HIV infection in 12 perinatally infected children: clinical, virological and immunological data. *AIDS* 1995;**9**(12):F19–F26.

295. Bakshi, S. S., Tetali, S., Abrams, E. J., Paul, M. O., Pahwa, S. G. Repeatedly positive human immunodeficiency virus type 1 DNA polymerase chain reaction in human immunodeficiency virus-exposed seroreverting infants. *Pediatr. Infect. Dis. J.* 1995;**14**(8):658–662.

296. Kuhn, L., Meddows-Taylor S., Gray, G., Tiemessen, C. Human immunodeficiency virus (HIV)-specific cellular immune responses in newborns exposed to HIV in utero. *Clin. Infect. Dis.* 2002;**34**(2):267–276.

297. Miller, C. J., Marthas, M., Torten, J. *et al.* Intravaginal inoculation of rhesus macaques with cell-free simian immunodeficiency virus results in persistent or transient viremia. *J. Virol.* 1994;**68**(10):6391–6400.

298. Frenkel, L. M., Mullins, J. I., Learn, G. H. *et al.* Genetic evaluation of suspected cases of transient HIV-1 infection of infants. *Science* 1998;**280**(5366):1073–1077.

299. Stiehm, E. R., Fudenberg, H. H. Serum levels of immune globulins in health and disease: a survey. *Pediatrics* 1966;**37**(5):715–727.

2 The epidemiology of pediatric HIV disease

Mary Lou Lindegren, M.D., Teresa Hammett, M.P.H., and Marc Bulterys, M.D., Ph.D.

Centers for Disease Control and Prevention

Introduction

Worldwide, over 3.2 million children are living with HIV and at least 1700 babies are born each day with HIV infection [1]. Mother-to-child transmission (MTCT) of HIV represents the most common means by which children become infected with HIV. This chapter will review the current epidemiology of HIV infection in children in the USA, and briefly review the growing worldwide impact of HIV on children.

HIV/AIDS among children in the USA

HIV infection and AIDS reporting

Through June 2001, 8994 US children with AIDS were reported to the US Centers for Disease Control and Prevention (CDC) from all 50 states, Puerto Rico, the District of Columbia, and the US Virgin Islands (Table 2.1). Fifty-six percent of all cases were reported from only four states: New York (25%), Florida (16%), New Jersey (8%), and California (7%). The majority of AIDS cases (91%) and virtually all new HIV infections resulted from MTCT. Seven percent of children with AIDS acquired their infection through receipt of contaminated blood or blood products. AIDS also has been reported among children who acquired HIV infection from sexual abuse, mucus membrane exposure to blood, and percutaneous or cutaneous exposures to blood or contaminated needles during home health care [2]. Only 2% of AIDS cases in US children lack an ascribable risk, usually because of incomplete information about the mother [3]. The majority of children with perinatally acquired AIDS were diagnosed at less than 5 years of age (81%), compared to children with hemophilia or transfusion-related AIDS who mostly were diagnosed at 5 years of age or older (95%, 63%, respectively). Black non-Hispanic and Hispanic children are affected disproportionately by the HIV epidemic. AIDS rates reported in 2000 among black, non-Hispanic (1.7 per 100 000) and

Handbook of Pediatric HIV Care, ed. Steven L. Zeichner and Jennifer S. Read.
Published by Cambridge University Press. © Cambridge University Press 2006.

Table 2.1. Cumulative pediatric AIDS cases in the USA, by mode of transmission*

Characteristic no. (%)	Perinatally acquired AIDS (N = 8207)	Hemophilia/coagulation disorder (N = 237)	Transfusion (N = 382)	Pediatric risk not reported or identified (N = 168)	Total (N = 8994)
Age at AIDS					
<1 yr	3237 (39)	0	29 (8)	38 (23)	3301
1–4 years	3462 (42)	11 (5)	112 (29)	39 (23)	3620
5+ years	1508 (18)	226 (95)	241 (63)	91 (54)	2057
Race/ethnicity					
Black, not Hispanic	5058 (62)	34 (14)	88 (23)	103 (61)	5283
Hispanic	1890 (23)	38 (16)	93 (24)	30 (18)	2051
White, not Hispanic	1185 (14)	159 (67)	190 (50)	30 (18)	1564
Asian/ Pacific Islander	34 (<1)	3 (1)	11 (3)	4 (2)	52
American Indian/ Alaska Native	28 (<1)	2 (1)	–	1 (1)	31
Unknown	12 (<1)	1 (<1)	–	–	13
Sex					
Male	4075 (50)	230 (97)	242 (63)	75 (45)	4622
Female	4132 (50)	7 (3)	140 (37)	93 (55)	4372

* Data reported to CDC National AIDS surveillance through June 2001

Hispanic children (0.3 per 100 000) were seventeen and three times higher, respectively, than among white, non-Hispanic children (0.1 per 100 000). The racial/ethnic and age distributions of AIDS and HIV infection among children vary by mode of transmission. For example, cases of AIDS resulting from MTCT of HIV have occurred predominantly among black, non-Hispanic (62%) and Hispanic children (23%), while cases attributed to blood or blood product transfusion are more proportional to the racial/ethnic distribution of the general population.

As of June 2001, HIV infection reporting, using the same methods as for AIDS surveillance, was ongoing in 34 states, the Virgin Islands, and Guam (Table 2.2). As of June 2001, an additional 2206 HIV-infected children have been reported from these areas (Table 2.2) [4]. In many states with HIV reporting, there are over three times as many children living with HIV infection as those living with AIDS (Fig. 2.1).

Modes of acquisition of HIV infection among children
Non-perinatal
Blood/blood products

Since the implementation of heat treatment for clotting factors in 1984, nationwide screening of blood and blood products in 1985, and self-deferral of blood donations from high-risk individuals, incident cases of HIV infection attributable to transmission through blood and blood products have been virtually eliminated in the United States [5]. Transfusion-acquired HIV infection is now extremely rare in the USA.

Sexual transmission

Sexual transmission of HIV infection is the major mode of HIV exposure among adolescents and adults in the United States. A small number of cases of sexual transmission through sexual abuse has been reported among children [6].

Other

There have been rare reports of transmission of HIV in households between siblings where opportunities for skin or mucous membranes exposure to HIV-infected blood were present [7]. One instance of intentional inoculation of a child with HIV-infected blood also has been documented [3]. Because HIV transmission is extremely rare in settings such as homes, schools, and daycare centers, and recommendations have been made to prevent exposure in these settings, no need exists to restrict the placement of HIV-infected children in these settings [8] (see also Chapter 36).

MTCT of HIV
HIV/AIDS among women of childbearing age in the USA

Characteristics of the HIV epidemic in children mirror those of the epidemic in childbearing women. Women account for an increasing proportion of HIV disease in the USA. Of the 784 032 adult and adolescent cases of AIDS reported to the CDC through June 2001 from the USA, Puerto Rico, District of Columbia, and the US Virgin Islands,

Table 2.2. Pediatric HIV infection cases in the USA, by age group, exposure category, race/ethnicity, and gender*

Characteristic no. (%)	Perinatally acquired (N = 1918)	Hemophilia/coagulation disorder (N = 104)	Transfusion (N = 41)	Pediatric risk not reported or identified (N = 143)	Total (N = 2206)
Age at HIV					
<1 yr	934 (49)	2 (2)	0	23 (16)	959
1–4 years	679 (35)	10 (10)	11 (27)	47 (33)	747
5+ years	305 (16)	92 (88)	30 (73)	73 (51)	500
Race/ethnicity					
Black, not Hispanic	1298 (62)	20 (19)	11 (27)	90 (63)	1419
Hispanic	222 (12)	5 (5)	7 (17)	16 (11)	250
White, not Hispanic	373 (19)	76 (73)	22 (54)	22 (15)	493
Asian/ Pacific Islander	8 (<1)	3 (1)	1 (3)	3 (2)	15
American Indian/ Alaska Native	9 (<1)	–	–	2 (1)	11
Unknown	8 (<1)	–	10 (7)	18	
Sex					
Male	908 (47)	102 (98)	17 (41)	70 (49)	1097
Female	1010 (53)	2 (2)	24 (59)	73 (51)	1109

* Data reported to CDC for HIV surveillance through June 2001, from the 36 areas with confidential HIV infection reporting. See also June 2001 CDC HIV/AIDS Surveillance Report.

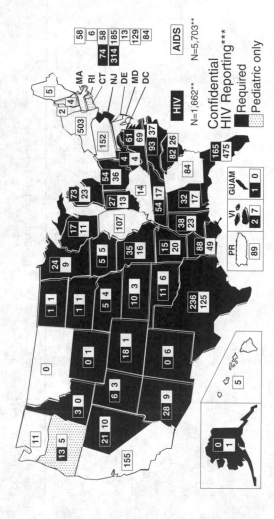

* For areas with confidential HIV infection surveillance reported by patient name. Age based on current age as of December 2000 data reported to CDC.

**Total includes cases missing state of residence data.

Fig. 2.1. Children less than 13 years of age with HIV infection and AID, by state. HIV infection is concentrated in certain states, particularly those with large urban populations and in the South. Many more children are infected with HIV than have AIDS.

134 845 (17%) cases were among women [2]. The proportion of AIDS cases in women has increased from 12.5% in 1988–1992 to 22.6% in 1996–2000 [9]. Of the 145 753 HIV-infected adolescents and adults in the USA, 29% were women; among the 5893 HIV-infected adolescents (aged 13–19 years old), 57% were females, most of whom were infected through heterosexual contact.

Although the HIV/AIDS epidemic in women is concentrated in the Northeast and in the South, recently the greatest increases appear to have been in the South [10]. African-American and Hispanic women are disproportionately affected by the HIV epidemic; in 2000, the highest rates of AIDS were among black, non-Hispanic (46 per 100 000) and Hispanic women (14 per 100 000), compared to white, non-Hispanic women (8 per 100 000). Cumulatively, 40% of AIDS in women is attributable to injection drug use and 41% to heterosexual contact, which surpassed injection drug use in the early 1990s as the predominant mode of transmission among women, particularly among young women [2, 11]. Beginning in the early 1990s, there has been a steady increase in the number of women without a known risk for infection, who are believed to have been infected through heterosexual contact with a partner they did not know to be HIV-infected. Thus, the actual proportion of women infected through heterosexual transmission is likely to be substantially higher than 41%. Among young adults and adolescents, aged 13 to 24 years, 54% of AIDS has been attributable to heterosexual contact. More than 40% of AIDS diagnoses in 1999 were among residents of the poorest counties in the United States [11].

HIV incidence increased among childbearing women through the 1980s, and then stabilized from 1989 to 1995 [12]. Trends varied by region, with declining HIV seroprevalence in the Northeast (4.1 to 3.2/1000 childbearing women) and increasing then stable trends in the South (1.6 to 1.9/1000 childbearing women). Stable HIV seroprevalence may have been a combination of stable HIV incidence among childbearing age women, women aging out of their childbearing years, and reduced fertility among older HIV-infected women due to advanced HIV disease. Particularly high HIV incidence rates (5–6 per 1000 women–years) have been reported from certain institutions that serve an inner-city and high-risk population [13].

The number of persons with AIDS has increased as a result of improved patient survival due to HAART. In 2000, an estimated 338 978 persons were living with AIDS in the USA, including 69 725 women, a 57% increase since 1996. Between 1993 and 2000, the proportion of persons living with AIDS who were women increased from 15% to 21%. Approximately 130 000 women of childbearing age (13–44 years) were living with HIV infection in the USA in 2000, substantially more than the estimated 80 000 HIV-infected women in 1991 [14]. Recent data indicate that pregnancies were less likely to occur among women with advanced HIV disease [15]. Pregnancy rates were higher after the introduction of HAART.

An estimated 40 000 new cases of HIV infection occur each year in the United States and more than 10 000 of these new infections are among women [16]. Recent increases

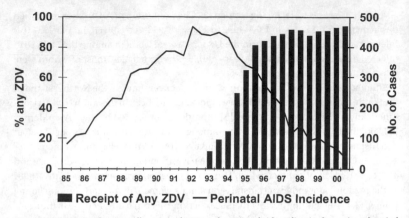

Fig. 2.2. Diagnosis of perinatally acquired AIDS and receipt of zidovudine in the perinatal period as a function of time. Perinatally acquired AIDS diagnoses have declined dramatically since the mid 1990s. At the same time, the rate of zidovudine exposure has increased significantly.

in newly diagnosed HIV infections have created concern that HIV incidence may again be on the rise [17].

Trends in MTCT of HIV

The number of pediatric AIDS cases in the USA increased rapidly in the 1980s, peaked in 1992, and declined 89% from 1992 ($N = 910$) to 2000 ($N = 104$) (35–38) (Fig. 2.2). These declines have been seen in all racial/ethnic groups. Most children who acquired HIV infection through MTCT are non-Hispanic blacks and Hispanics, mirroring the epidemic in women. Declines were seen in all regions of the USA. The earliest and largest declines have occurred among children diagnosed before 1 year of age, reflecting decreased MTCT. Recent declines in AIDS incidence were substantially greater than could be accounted for by declines in births to HIV-infected women [18].

Rapid implementation of US Public Health Service guidelines regarding use of zidovudine (ZDV) prophylaxis to reduce MTCT of HIV and universal, routine HIV counseling and voluntary prenatal HIV testing were associated with the initial decline in the incidence of perinatal HIV infection incidence in the USA. Receipt by mother–infant pairs of all three components of the recommended ZDV prophylaxis regimen was associated with a 68% reduction in perinatal HIV infection rates. Additional data confirmed the effectiveness of ZDV prophylaxis, with MTCT rates of as low as 5–8%. With the introduction of potent combination antiretroviral therapy and cesarean section before labor and ruptured membranes, MTCT rates of less than 2% have been observed [11, 19–21]. However, MTCT continues to occur, especially in populations of women and children who do not receive timely interventions to prevent transmission.

Since an estimated approximately 6000 infants were born to HIV-infected mothers in 2000, if transmission rates were similar to those observed in the late 1980s and early 1990s (about 25%), about 1500 HIV-infected infants would have been born. However, only about 300 infected infants were born [14]. If all infants born to infected mothers were managed optimally, assuming a 2% transmission rate, approximately 120 HIV infected infants would be born each year in the USA. Additional targeted prevention efforts are needed.

The perinatal HIV prevention cascade

Once an HIV-infected woman becomes pregnant, a chain of events must take place to prevent HIV transmission to the child. This chain of events provides a useful framework for considering perinatal HIV prevention interventions and the collection of perinatal surveillance data. This chain includes the following: (a) receipt of early prenatal care; (b) counseling and testing; (c) the acceptance of testing; (d) the acceptance of interventions to prevent transmission, including antiretroviral prophylaxis, cesarean section before labor and ruptured membranes, and avoidance of breastfeeding; (e) adherence to an antiretroviral drug regimen; and (g) follow-up care for both the HIV-infected woman and her infant [22].

Receipt of prenatal care

HIV-infected women are much less likely to receive prenatal care than the general population. Data from 1993 to 1996 indicate that 14% of women received no or minimal prenatal care and 19% initiated prenatal care in the third trimester [24]. This compares to 2% of women in the general population who had late or no prenatal care. As in the general population, prenatal care use among HIV-infected women varied by race and ethnicity, with African-American and Hispanic women likely to have fewer prenatal visits. HIV-infected women who use illicit drugs in pregnancy are much less likely to receive prenatal care, than HIV-infected women who do not use illicit drugs (36% vs. 5%). Reasons drug-using women may not receive prenatal care include social disruption, fear of criminalization, and lack of access to care. HIV-infected women are likely to be subject to many other serious health problems, including a high prevalence of STIs, illegal drug use, and alcohol use, according to a recent report from Michigan, suggesting a need for comprehensive counseling and treatment services to HIV-infected women.

Although many HIV-infected women in the USA receive little or no prenatal care, most deliver in a hospital, providing a crucial opportunity for rapid screening and intervention. The mother infant rapid intervention at delivery (MIRIAD) study is a multicenter project, funded through the CDC, focusing on disadvantaged communities in which many women receive inadequate prenatal care and exhibit relatively high HIV seroprevalence (20). The MIRIAD study aims to evaluate (a) innovative approaches for counseling and voluntary rapid HIV testing program for women in labor presenting with unknown HIV status; (b) the feasibility of obtaining informed consent during labor (or, if not feasible, soon after birth); (c) reasons for lack of prenatal care and/or HIV testing among these women; (d) approaches to antiretroviral prophylaxis administered to the mother and infant; (e) adherence to neonatal therapy; and (f) subsequent receipt of antiretroviral treatment and other services for women identified as HIV-infected. Cost-effectiveness analyses suggest that rapid HIV testing at labor and delivery saves money when HIV prevalence exceeds 0.7 to 1.0% and treatment efficacy exceeds a 5% reduction in perinatal transmission [25], situations that apply in many urban centers in the USA.

Offering and acceptance of HIV counseling and testing

Women receiving prenatal care should be offered testing, but unfortunately many women are not offered it, including mothers in groups that have a high prevalence of HIV infection. The CDC pregnancy risk assessment monitoring system (PRAMS) [26, 27] found that, in 1997, 63% to 87% of mothers received HIV counseling during pregnancy and 58% to 81% were tested for HIV infection, depending on the state. Black mothers, mothers with less than a high school education, young mothers, those with public health care providers, and Medicaid recipients were more likely to receive HIV counseling and testing during pregnancy, which may reflect targeted testing efforts. The highest rates of testing and increases in testing occurred in states with higher HIV seroprevalence.

Updated data from the 1999 PRAMS study indicate a range of prenatal HIV testing from 61% to 81% for states that use an "opt in" approach to testing (i.e., women are provided with pre-HIV test counseling and must consent specifically to an HIV antibody test) [28]. One state, Arkansas, had an "opt-out" testing policy (i.e., women are notified that an HIV test will be included in a standard prenatal battery of tests and that they may refuse testing), which increased prenatal HIV testing rates after the law was implemented, from 57% in 1997 to 71% in 1999. For New York State, prenatal testing rates increased from 69% to 93% after mandatory newborn testing results were made available within 48 hours of delivery. The US Public Revised Guidelines for HIV testing in pregnancy emphasize testing as a routine part of prenatal care and strengthening the recommendation that all pregnant women be tested for HIV [24]. Healthcare facilities serving women at relatively high risk for HIV should also strongly consider implementing a second voluntary universal HIV test during the third trimester of pregnancy, as is done routinely for syphilis. The AAP and the American College of Obstetricians and Gynecologists (ACOG) have issued recommendations in support of the PHS guidelines [29].

Additional data indicate that once women are offered HIV testing, acceptance rates are generally high, over 70% in most settings. However, not all women who are offered testing accept it. CDC's Perinatal Guidelines Evaluation Project evaluated reasons why women were not tested, and the results indicated that some women did not perceive a need for testing because they believed they were not at risk for HIV infection, others knew they had been previously tested for HIV, and because some women had providers who did not strongly recommend testing.

The proportion of pregnant HIV-infected women in whom HIV infection was diagnosed before giving birth is high and increasing. In the seven-state enhanced surveillance project, the proportion of HIV-infected women who were diagnosed before delivery increased from 70% in 1993 to 80% in 1996 [24]. Among women delivering in 1996, approximately half (53%) had their positive HIV test before their pregnancy. Data from 2000 indicate that 93% of HIV-infected women knew their HIV status before delivery [28].

Offering and receipt of antiretroviral drugs

An increasing proportion of HIV-infected mothers and their infants received a component (antepartum, intrapartum, or infant) of the ACTG 076 perinatal transmission prophylaxis regimen; from 37% of children born in 1994 to 90% or more for children born from 1997–2000. The rate of prenatal ZDV receipt increased from almost 30% in 1994 to 71–73% in 1996–1997 and then plateaued. Almost two-thirds of mother–infant pairs in 2000 received all three components of the ZDV regimen. More HIV-infected women are also receiving combination therapy during pregnancy for maternal indications, increasing from 39% in 1998 to 60% in 2000. While the increase in receipt of antiretroviral therapy has resulted in a dramatic decline in perinatally-acquired AIDS incidence in the United States, some women and their infants, including women with substance abuse, who gave birth preterm, or who had less advanced immunosuppression, continue to be at substantial risk of not receiving all three components of the ACTG 076 perinatal transmission prophylaxis regimen [24].

Cesarean Section for the Prevention of MTCT of HIV

Elective cesarean section before onset of labor and rupture of membranes has been shown to decrease the risk of perinatal HIV transmission [30, 31]. The American College of Obstetrician and Gynecologists and the USPHS recommends that HIV-infected pregnant women with HIV RNA of 1000 copies/ml or greater be offered elective cesarean section as an adjunct for prevention of perinatal HIV transmission. Data from the Pediatric Spectrum of HIV Disease Project and pediatric HIV surveillance indicate that the proportion of HIV-infected mothers who had cesarean sections increased from 20% in 1994–1998 to 44% and almost 50% by 2000 [32].

Morbidity and mortality

HIV has been a leading cause of death among children in the USA. Among children aged 1 to 4 years old, annual rates of death per 100 000 persons increased from 1987 to 1995, but then declined dramatically through 1998 (Fig. 2.3). Since 1996, use of potent combination antiretroviral therapy has resulted in substantial reductions in mortality and increased survival of HIV-infected adults and children, as an increasing proportion of HIV-infected children received potent antiretroviral therapy, and reduced proportions

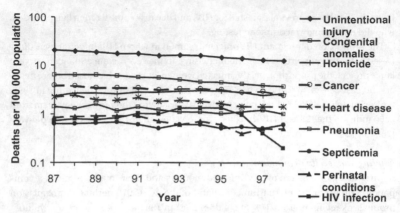

Fig. 2.3. Deaths rates in children for the leading causes of death. Death rates due to HIV infection gradually increased during the late 1980s and early 1990s. Since the mid 1990s death rates in children due to HIV infection have decreased sharply, due to decreased mother-to-child transmission and improved antiretroviral therapy, and prophylaxis and management of opportunistic infections.

of children experience severe immunosuppression [33]. The annual number of children under 13 years of age with HIV infection listed on their death certificate has decreased 81% from 1994 to 1999 [34]. This is likely due to a combination of factors including: prevention of MTCT of HIV, use of potent antiretroviral therapy, and more effective treatment and prevention of opportunistic infections.

The most common AIDS-defining condition in children continues to be *Pneumocystis carinii* pneumonia (PCP) (Table 2.3) (see Chapter 35 [35]). PCP, which occurs predominantly at ages 3 to 6 months, has accounted overall for 33% of all AIDS-defining conditions and 57% of AIDS-defining conditions in infants. PCP prophylaxis guidelines for children were first published in 1991. However, PCP incidence among infants changed little from 1991 through 1993 because HIV infection was not diagnosed early enough for prophylaxis. In 1995, revised guidelines recommended PCP prophylaxis for all perinatally exposed infants at 4 to 6 weeks of age until their infection status is determined. Among infants, rates of PCP and rates of other AIDS conditions declined substantially. Dramatic declines in AIDS incidence in recent years have been attributable primarily to the substantial impact of declining perinatal HIV transmission, although declines in PCP incidence from PCP prevention efforts likely contributed.

Even though fewer HIV-infected children are progressing to AIDS, the relative frequencies of AIDS defining conditions are similar to those observed in previous years of the epidemic [36]. Age-adjusted incidence rates of opportunistic infections were highest for PCP, disseminated MAC disease, esophageal candidiasis, and recurrent bacterial infections, and rates of each declined from 1990 to 1997. Declining

Table 2.3. AIDS-defining conditions diagnosed in US Children with AIDS[*]

	Cumulative no.(%)[*] cases diagnosed with disease $N = 8978$	Number(%) cases diagnosed in 2000 $N = 86$
AIDS-defining conditions		
Pneumocystis carinii pneumonia	2957 (33)	20 (23
Lymphoid interstitial pneumonitis	2084 (23)	10 (12)
Bacterial infection, multiple or recurrent	1834 (20)	13 (15)
HIV wasting syndrome	1613 (18)	14 (16)
HIV encephalopathy	1485 (17)	8 (9)
Candidiasis of esophagus	1408 (16)	9 (10)
Cytomegalovirus disease other than retinitis	723 (8)	6 (7)
Mycobacterium avium complex	727 (8)	2 (2)
Herpes simplex	443 (5)	3 (3)
Candidiasis of bronchi, trachea or lungs	329 (4)	5 (6)
Cryptosporidiosis, chronic intestinal	318 (4)	—
Cytomegalovirus retinitis	167 (2)	3 (3)
Mycobacterial disease, other	118 (1)	2 (2)
Cryptococcosis, extrapulmonary	107 (1)	3 (3)
Toxoplasmosis of brain	76 (1)	2 (2)
M. Tuberculosis, disseminated, or extrapulm	83 (1)	2 (2)
Immunoblastic lymphoma	59 (1)	1 (1)
Burkitt's lymphoma	62 (1)	1 (1)
Progressive multifocal leukoencephalopathy	46 (1)	–
Lymphoma, primary in brain	40 (<1)	1 (1)
Kaposi's sarcoma	31 (<1)	–
Histoplasmosis	24 (<1)	–
Coccidioidomyocosis	12 (<1)	–
Isosporiasis, chronic intestinal	4 (<1)	–

[*] Sum of percentages is greater than 100, because some patients have more than one condition; unadjusted data, Reported to National AIDS surveillance through June 2001

age-adjusted incidence was also observed for cytomegalovirus disease, cryptosporidiosis, and candidiasis [37, 38]. Additional analyses of PSD data showed declines for LIP and wasting. The mean age of HIV-infected children also increased from 4.9 years in 1992 to 8.7 years in 1998. Trends of initial AIDS defining conditions from 1992 to 1999 were analyzed among children reported with perinatally acquired AIDS through June 2000, adjusted for reporting delay and no identified risk, using age-stratified Cochran–Mantel–Haenszel methods (Table 2.4). During this time the median age at AIDS diagnosis had increased from 1 year to 3 years of age. PCP continued to be the most common AIDS defining condition. Significant declines occurred for LIP and MAC, with

Table 2.4. Trends in initial AIDS opportunistic infections among children reported with perinatally acquired AIDS[*]

AIDS defining condition (%)	Year of diagnosis							
	1992	1993	1994	1995	1996	1997	1998	1999
	$n=907$	$n=882$	$n=793$	$n=665$	$n=501$	$n=307$	$n=230$	$n=156$
Pneumocystis carinii pneumonia	24	26	24	23	25	28	25	29
LIP	22	18	18	17	17	11	11	8[*]
Recurrent bact infection	13	15	14	14	16	15	18	19[*]
Encephalopathy	13	13	14	17	17	18	11	14
Wasting	14	13	14	13	13	13	18	12
Candidiasis – esophagus	11	11	12	12	11	8	8	14
Mycobacterium avium complex	4	5	5	4	3	4	3	2[*]

[*] Percentage of children with perinatally acquired AIDS, adjusted for reporting delay, weighted for age; data from national AIDS surveillance for children reported with perinatally acquired AIDS through June 2000, adjusted for reporting delay and no identified risk, using age-stratified Cochran–Mantel–Haenszel methods, [*]$P < 0.05$.

significant increases for recurrent bacterial infections. These trends most likely reflect increasing use of potent combination antiretroviral therapy, improving immune status and use of effective prophylaxis regimens for opportunistic infections [39].

Early treatment with HAART has improved survival and decreased morbidity with more children living longer with HIV infection. With improvements in treatment and survival, increasing numbers of perinatally HIV-infected children are entering adolescence. It has been estimated that there are approximately 10 000 children currently living with perinatally acquired HIV infection in the United States, and that 2200 are currently teenagers. Over the next decade increasing numbers of HIV-infected children will enter adolescence [39, 40]. These HIV-infected teens require a specialized approach (see Chapter 8). The impact of long-term potent antiretroviral treatment on growth and development is not known.

HIV/AIDS among children globally

Throughout the world, the number of HIV infections in children continues to increase. In 2002, an estimated 800 000 children under 15 years of age were newly infected; 3.2 million children were living with HIV infection, and nearly 600 000 died of AIDS [1]. MTCT is the dominant mode of acquisition of HIV among young children worldwide, resulting in at least 1700 new infections each day. Globally, HIV/AIDS is one of

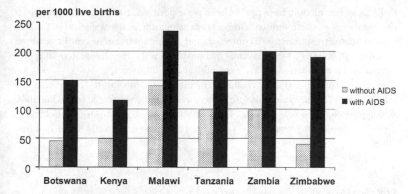

Fig. 2.4. The effect of HIV infection on childhood mortality in six selected sub-Saharan African countries. HIV infection has had a very large negative impact on childhood mortality.

the leading causes of death in children. Figure 2.4 shows the dramatic impact the HIV epidemic is having on under-5 child mortality rates in heavily affected countries in sub-Saharan Africa. In 2002 there were an estimated 14 million children worldwide who have lost one or both parents due to AIDS. Approximately 80% of these children – 11 million – live in sub-Saharan Africa. The severe burden of HIV infection for both infected and uninfected children threatens to dwarf the capacity of families and communities to respond.

Progress has been made towards implementation of MTCT prevention programs in a number of developing countries [41–46]. For instance, Thailand has provided an exemplary model. From October 2000 through July 2001, 93% of 318 721 women who gave birth in 65 provinces were tested for HIV; 69% of HIV-infected women giving birth received zidovudine; and 86% of the infants born to HIV-infected women received zidovudine through the program [47]. Lessons learned from Thailand include the importance of providing regular clinical counseling and management training, and focused monitoring and evaluation data to guide program development, expansion, and improvement.

Increased efforts to interrupt MTCT are being made in several regions with high HIV prevalence, although many barriers remain. In sub-Saharan Africa during 1999–2000, United Nations-sponsored pilot programs were conducted in nine countries with high HIV-1 prevalence; 82 000 women attended antenatal clinics across all sites and HIV prevalence among those tested varied from 13–45%. Of all the women attending antenatal care, only 43% accepted an HIV test. Of the nearly 7000 women who tested positive for HIV infection, 39% received ARV prophylaxis. India has implemented a pilot program among 125 000 pregnant women and has recorded testing and antiretroviral prophylaxis acceptance rates comparable to the African rates. Since early 2000, several private foundations, such as the Elisabeth Glaser Pediatric AIDS Foundation and the

Doris Duke Foundation, have funded large-scale perinatal HIV prevention programs in a number of resource-limited settings. Successful programs to reduce MTCT and to expand treatment options for HIV-infected mothers and their families can be achieved only through improved maternal and child health care services, integrated AIDS prevention and care initiatives, and strong political commitment at all levels.

Additional societal and social challenges further complicate efforts to eliminate HIV infection in children. Sexual abuse of children, mainly girls, and forced sexual initiation also appear common in a number of high HIV prevalence countries in sub-Saharan Africa and Southeast Asia and rape of children is almost universally under-reported [48–50].

Conclusions

Remarkable changes in the epidemiology of pediatric HIV infection in the USA and similar settings have occurred during the last several years, due primarily to successful efforts to prevent MTCT of HIV. Additionally, advances have been made in the diagnosis and treatment of pediatric HIV infection.

However, the global HIV epidemic among infants, children, and adolescents continues in many parts of the world, where there is an ongoing need to implement effective prevention and treatment programs. HIV infection has already caused a precipitous decline in child survival in resource-poor settings. In such settings, prevention of primary HIV infections among women and adolescent girls, particularly adolescent girls who exhibit the highest HIV incidence rates, is critical to the prevention of MTCT of HIV.

REFERENCES

1. UNAIDS. *Report on the Global HIV/AIDS Epidemic.* Geneva: United Nations Progamme on HIV/AIDS (UNAIDS); 2002.
2. Centers for Disease Control and Prevention. *HIV/AIDS Surveillance Report.* Atlanta: Centers for Disease Control and Prevention; 2001. Report No.: 13 (No.1).
3. Centers for Disease Control and Prevention. *HIV/AIDS Surveillance Report.* Atlanta: Centers for Disease Control and Prevention; 2000. Report No.: 12 (No. 1).
4. Hammett, T. A., Bush, T. J., Ciesielski, C. A. Pediatric AIDS cases reported with no identified risk. In American Public Health Association Meeting; San Francisco, CA; 1993.
5. Selik, R. M., Ward, J. W., Buehler, J. W. Trends in transfusion-associated acquired immune deficiency syndrome in the United States, 1982 through 1991. *Transfusion* 1993;**33**(11):890–893.
6. Lindegren, M. L., Hanson, I. C., Hammett, T. A., Beil, J., Fleming, P. L., Ward, J. W. Sexual abuse of children: intersection with the HIV epidemic. *Pediatrics* 1998;**102**(4):E46.
7. American Academy of Pediatrics. Committee of Pediatric AIDS and Committee on Infectious Diseases. Issues related to human immunodeficiency virus transmission in schools,

child care, medical settings, the home, and community. *Pediatrics* 1999;**104**(2 Pt 1): 318–324.

8. American Academy of Pediatrics. Committee on Pediatric AIDS. Education of children with human immunodeficiency virus infection. 2000;**105**(6):58–1360.

9. Centers for Disease Control and Prevention. HIV and AIDS – United States, 1981–2000. *Morb. Mortal. Wkly Rep.* 2001;**50**(21):430–434.

10. Hader, S. L., Smith, D. K., Moore, J. S., Holmberg, S. D. HIV infection in women in the United States: status at the Millennium. *J. Am. Med. Assoc.* 2001;**285**(9):1186–1192.

11. Karon, J. M., Fleming, P. L., Steketee, R. W. *et al.* HIV in the United States at the turn of the century: an epidemic in transition. *Am. J. Pub. Hlth* 2001;**91**(7):1060–1068.

12. Davis, S. F., Rosen, D. H., Steinberg, S., Wortley, P. M., Karon, J. M., Gwinn, M. Trends in HIV prevalence among childbearing women in the United States, 1989–1994. *J. Acquir. Immune Defic. Syndr.* 1998;**19**(2):158–164.

13. Chirgwin, K. D., Feldman, J., Dehovitz, J. A., Minkoff, H., Landesman, S. H. Incidence and risk factors for heterosexually acquired HIV in an inner-city cohort of women: temporal association with pregnancy. *J Acquir. Immune Defic. Syndr. Hum. Retrovirol.* 1999;**20**(3):295–299.

14. Fleming, P. L. M., Byers, R. *et al.* Estimated number of perinatal HIV infections, United States. Presented at the XIV International Conference, Barcelona, Spain; 2002.

15. Blair, J. M., Hanson, C., Jones, J. L. *et al.* Have pregnancy rates among human immunodeficiency virus-infected women changed in the era of effective antiretroviral therapy to prevent perinatal transmission? *Obstet Gynecol* in press.

16. Nakashima, A. K., Fleming, P. L. HIV/AIDS surveillance in the United States, 1981–2001. *J. Acquir. Immune Defic. Syndr.* 2003;32 Suppl 1:S68–S85.

17. Centers for Disease Control and Prevention. Advancing HIV Prevention: New Strategies for a changing epidemic – United States 2003. *Morb. Mortal. Wkly Rep.* 2003;**52**(15):329–332.

18. Lindegren, M. L., Byers, R. H., Jr., Thomas, P. *et al.* Trends in perinatal transmission of HIV/AIDS in the United States. *J. Am. Med. Assoc.* 1999;**282**(6):531–538.

19. Matheson, P. B., Abrams, E. J., Thomas, P. A. *et al.* Efficacy of antenatal zidovudine in reducing perinatal transmission of human immunodeficiency virus type 1. The New York City Perinatal HIV Transmission Collaborative Study Group. *J. Infect. Dis.* 1995;**172**(2):353–358.

20. Simonds, R. J., Steketee, R., Nesheim, S. *et al.* Impact of zidovudine use on risk and risk factors for perinatal transmission of HIV. Perinatal AIDS Collaborative Transmission Studies. *AIDS* 1998;**12**(3):301–308.

21. Cooper, E. R., Nugent, R. P., Diaz, C. *et al.* After AIDS clinical trial 076: the changing pattern of zidovudine use during pregnancy, and the subsequent reduction in the vertical transmission of human immunodeficiency virus in a cohort of infected women and their infants. Women and Infants Transmission Study Group. *J. Infect. Dis.* 1996;**174**(6):1207–1211.

22. Centers for Disease Control and Prevention. US Public Health Service recommendations for human immunodeficiency virus counseling and voluntary testing for pregnant women. *Morb. Mortal. Wkly Rep. Recomm. Rep.* 1995;**44**(RR-7):1–15.

23. Moodley, D., Moodley, J., Coovadia, H. *et al.* A multicenter randomized controlled trial of nevirapine versus a combination of zidovudine and lamivudine to reduce intrapartum and early postpartum mother-to-child transmission of human immunodeficiency virus type 1. *J. Infect. Dis.* 2003;**187**(5):725–735.

24. Public Health Service Task Force. Recommendations for the use of antiretroviral drugs in pregnant HIV-1-infected women for maternal health and interventions to reduce perinatal HIV-1 transmission in the United States. US Public Health Service; 2003.

25. Cooper, E. R., Charurat, M., Mofenson, L. *et al.* Combination antiretroviral strategies for the treatment of pregnant HIV-1-infected women and prevention of perinatal HIV-1 transmission. *J. Acquir. Immune Defic. Syndr.* 2002;**29**(5):484–494.

26. Garcia, P. M., Kalish L. A., Pitt, J. *et al.* Maternal levels of plasma human immunodeficiency virus type 1 RNA and the risk of perinatal transmission. Women and Infants Transmission Study Group. *N. Engl. J. Med.* 1999;**341**(6):394–402.

27. Gilbert, B. C., Shulman, H. B., Fischer, L. A., Rogers, M. M. The Pregnancy Risk Assessment Monitoring System (PRAMS): methods and 1996 response rates from 11 states. *Matern. Child Hlth J.* 1999;**3**(4):199–209.

28. Mofenson, L. M., Lambert, J. S., Stiehm, E. R. *et al.* Risk factors for perinatal transmission of human immunodeficiency virus type 1 in women treated with zidovudine. *Pediatric AIDS Clinical Trials Group Study 185 Team. N. Engl. J. Med.* 1999;**341**(6):385–393.

29. Joint statement of the American Academy of Pediatrics and the American College of Obstetricians and Gynecologists. Human immunodeficiency virus screening. *Pediatrics* 1999;**104**(1 Pt 1):128.

30. The International Perinatal HIV Group. The mode of delivery and the risk of vertical transmission of human immunodeficiency virus type 1– a meta-analysis of 15 prospective cohort studies. *N. Engl. J. Med.* 1999;**340**(13):977–987.

31. The European Mode of Delivery Collaboration. Elective caesarean-section versus vaginal delivery in prevention of vertical HIV-1 transmission: a randomised clinical trial. *Lancet* 1999;**353**(9158):1035–1039.

32. Dominguez, K. L., Lindegren, M. L., D'Almada, P. J. *et al.* Increasing trend of Cesarean deliveries in HIV-infected women in the United States from 1994 to 2000. *J. Acquir. Immune Defic. Syndr.* 2003;**33**(2):232–238.

33. Palella, F. J., Jr., Delaney, K. M., Moorman, A. C. *et al.* Declining morbidity and mortality among patients with advanced human immunodeficiency virus infection. HIV Outpatient Study Investigators. *N. Engl. J. Med.* 1998;**338**(13):853–860.

34. Gortmaker, S. L., Hughes, M., Cervia, J. *et al.* Effect of combination therapy including protease inhibitors on mortality among children and adolescents infected with HIV-1. *N. Engl. J. Med.* 2001;**345**(21):1522–1528.

35. Centers for Disease Control and Prevention. 1995 revised guidelines for prophylaxis against *Pneumocystis carinii* pneumonia for children infected with or perinatally exposed to human immunodeficiency virus. National Pediatric and Family HIV Resource Center and National Center for Infectious Diseases, Centers for Disease Control and Prevention. *Morb. Mortal. Wkly Rep. Recomm.Rep.* 1995;**44**(RR-4):1–11.

36. Fleming, P. L., Ward, J. W., Karon, J. M., Hanson, D. L. Declines in AIDS incidence and deaths in the USA: a signal change in the epidemic. *AIDS* 1998;**12** Suppl A:S55–S61.

37. de Martino, M., Tovo, P. A., Balducci M. *et al.* Reduction in mortality with availability of antiretroviral therapy for children with perinatal HIV-1 infection. Italian Register

for HIV Infection in Children and the Italian National AIDS Registry. *J. Am. Med. Assoc* 2000;**284**(2):190–197.

38. Barnhart, H. X., Caldwell, M. B., Thomas, P. *et al.* Natural history of human immunodeficiency virus disease in perinatally infected children: an analysis from the Pediatric Spectrum of Disease Project. *Pediatrics* 1996;**97**(5):710–716.

39. Frederick, T., Mascola, L., Peters, V. *et al.* Trends in HAART use and immune status among HIV-infected infants and children the in pediatric spectrum of disease project, United States, 1994–2000. XIV International Conference on AIDS; 2002; Barcelona, Spain; 2002.

40. Abrams, E. J., Weedon, J., Bertolli, J. *et al.* Aging cohort of perinatally human immunodeficiency virus-infected children in New York City. New York City Pediatric Surveillance of Disease Consortium. *Pediatr. Infect. Dis. J.* 2001;**20**(5):511–517.

41. Walker, N., Schwartlander, B., Bryce, J. Meeting international goals in child survival and HIV/AIDS. *Lancet* 2002;**360**(9329):284–289.

42. Fowler, M. G., Mercier, E. *et al.* Prevention of mother-to-child HIV transmission in resource-poor countries: translating research into policy and practice. *J. Am. Med. Assoc.* 2000;**283**(9):1175–1182.

43. Lackritz, E. M., Shaffer, N., Luo, C. Prevention of mother-to-child HIV transmission in the context of a comprehensive AIDS agenda in resource-poor countries. *J. Acquir. Immune Defic. Syndr.* 2002;**30**(2):196–199.

44. Nolan, M. L., Greenberg, A. E., Fowler, M. G. A review of clinical trials to prevent mother-to-child HIV-1 transmission in Africa and inform rational intervention strategies. *AIDS* 2002;**16**(15):1991–1999.

45. Laga, M., Schwartlander, B., Pisani, E., Sow, P. S., Carael, M. To stem HIV in Africa, prevent transmission to young women. *AIDS* 2001;**15**(7):931–934.

46. Rollins, N. C., Dedicoat, M., Danaviah, *et al.* Prevalence, incidence, and mother-to-child transmission of HIV-1 in rural South Africa. *Lancet* 2002;**360**(9330):389.

47. Kanshana, S., Simonds, R. J. National program for preventing mother-child HIV transmission in Thailand: successful implementation and lessons learned. *AIDS* 2002;**16**(7):953–959.

48. Buga, G. A., Amoko, D. H., Ncayiyana, D. J. Sexual behaviour, contraceptive practice and reproductive health among school adolescents in rural Transkei. *S. Afr. Med. J.* 1996;**86**(5):523–527.

49. Matasha, E., Ntembelea, T., Mayaud, P. *et al.* Sexual and reproductive health among primary and secondary school pupils in Mwanza, Tanzania: need for intervention. *AIDS Care* 1998;**10**(5):571–582.

50. Watts, C., Zimmerman, C. Violence against women: global scope and magnitude. *Lancet* 2002;**359**(9313):1232–1237.

Part II
General issues in the care of pediatric HIV patients

3 Diagnosis of HIV infection in children

Paul Krogstad, M.D.

Departments of Pediatrics and Molecular and Medical Pharmacology

David Geffen School of Medicine at UCLA, University of California, Los Angeles, CA

Effective management of pediatric HIV-1 infection begins with timely and accurate diagnosis. In infants, early diagnosis is essential. Life-threatening immunodeficiency can develop rapidly and unpredictably, and there are no laboratory or clinical characteristics that accurately predict rapid or slow disease progression [1]. Studies in adults and children have shown that very early treatment can slow the progression of immunodeficiency and preserve HIV-1-specific immune responses. Early detection of HIV-1 infection among pregnant women is necessary to optimize medical care for the HIV-1-infected woman and to prevent mother-to-child transmission of HIV-1. This chapter outlines the use of serology, virus culture, and molecular diagnostic methods to detect HIV-1 infection.

HIV-1 Diagnostic assays

Detection of antibodies to HIV-1

In 1985, enzyme-linked immunosorbent (ELISA) and immunoblot (Western blot) assays were licensed in the United States for detection of HIV-1-specific IgG antibodies in serum. While other tests are now available, they remain the mainstay for serological diagnosis of infection.

ELISA assays detect all antibodies that react with HIV-1 proteins, and are an excellent method for rapid screening. Moreover, minor modifications, such as dilution of the test samples, allow samples with low antibody titers to be identified. This "detuned ELISA" has been successfully used to identify adults with recently acquired HIV-1 infection [2, 3]. In a high-risk population for HIV-1, the positive predictive value of ELISA testing is reported to exceed 99%. However, false-positive reactions still occur (see below), particularly when used in populations at low risk for HIV-1 infection. As a consequence, ELISA results must be confirmed with an assay of greater specificity, usually immunoblot or immunofluorescence assays [4]. The Western blot assay is used

Handbook of Pediatric HIV Care, ed. Steven L. Zeichner and Jennifer S. Read.
Published by Cambridge University Press. © Cambridge University Press 2006.

to identify the presence in a patient's serum of antibodies that are directed against specific structural and enzymatic proteins found in HIV-1 particles. In a Western blot assay, HIV-1 proteins are separated by electrophoresis and transferred to a membrane. Patient serum samples are added to the membrane and allowed to bind to HIV-1 proteins, and after washing, a second reagent is added to detect human IgG antibodies. A pattern of "bands" is created, reflecting the presence of antibodies that bind to viral proteins. Some bands represent reactivity to proteins found in the viral core, each identified by their mass (e.g., the 24-kDa capsid protein is known as p24). Others represent reactivity with the 160-kDa envelope glycoprotein, or its 120-kDa and 41-kDa cleavage products (gp160, gp120, and gp41, respectively) [5]. The Association of State and Territorial Public Health Laboratory Directors' criteria are used in the United States as the definition of a positive immunoblot (Western blot) [6]. By these guidelines, a positive Western blot assay reveals the presence of antibodies to any two of the following proteins: p24, gp41, or gp120/gp160. A negative assay shows no reactivity against any HIV-1 proteins. An indeterminate Western blot assay indicates the presence of the patient's antibodies against one or more HIV-1 proteins, but not those required for a positive assay. Most indeterminate assays have bands representing antibodies to p17, p24, p55, or a combination of these proteins. Patients with indeterminate Western blot assays require additional testing to exclude or confirm HIV-1 infection. Generally, the Western blot is repeated soon thereafter, and one or more virological tests are performed as well.

The serological methods described above are complex tests that must be performed by skilled personnel in a medical laboratory. Rapid serological methods to detect IgG antibodies to HIV-1 in blood, oral fluid, and urine have been developed, and are commercially available [4]. These tests permit HIV-1 antibodies to be detected in as little as 10 to 20 minutes, without the use of sophisticated equipment, but confirmation by other methods is recommended [7]. Rapid serological tests could potentially play an important role in efforts to prevent perinatal transmission of HIV-1, by identifying pregnant women and their exposed infants [8,9]. Studies are under way to test the utility of rapid testing methods in this setting.

All results from serologic tests for HIV-1 infection mandate careful clinical interpretation. False negative reactions are found among patients who have not begun to produce antibody (acute antiretroviral syndrome), or, rarely, among those in whom antibodies are no longer being produced (late stages of HIV-1 infection with resulting hypogammaglobulinemia). Rare cases have been described in which HIV-1 infected individuals with disrupted immunoglobulin production are serologically negative; infection was demonstrated by virological assays (see below). False-positive ELISA reactions have been reported among patients with acute DNA viral infections, those with autoimmune disorders, and among multiparous or multiply transfused individuals. Moreover, the shortcomings of serological assays must be born in mind when evaluating infants and young children. The transplacental transfer of maternal IgG antibody during gestation causes all children born to HIV-1-infected women to be seropositive at birth; only a fraction are truly infected [1].

HIV-1 RNA and DNA detection methods

Because HIV-1 is a retrovirus, its genome exists both as an RNA form in virions and as a DNA form in infected cells (see Chapter 1). HIV-1 DNA polymerase chain reaction (PCR) analysis of blood leukocyte DNA is an extremely sensitive assay, and 30% to 50% of infections in infants can be detected at birth [9–11]. False-negative results occur in the first several weeks of age because many infants acquire HIV-1 infection in the immediate peripartum period. However, by 1 month of age, nearly all perinatally-acquired infections can be detected (see below).

The amount of virion-packaged HIV-1 RNA in the peripheral blood ("viral load") is an important measure of disease activity and of the effectiveness of antiretroviral therapy. This genomic viral RNA can be measured using reverse transcriptase PCR (RT-PCR) or other RNA quantification techniques such as branched DNA (bDNA) or nucleic acid sequence-based amplification (NASBA). Provided that samples of blood are promptly processed, HIV-1 RNA detection assays are highly sensitive and specific for the diagnosis of HIV-1 infection [12, 13].

PCR assays to detect DNA and RNA are extremely sensitive, and problems can arise if rigorous attention to cross-contamination is not provided. False-positive reactions may also occur owing to sample mix-up and laboratory errors, principally cross-contamination [13, 14].

Other virological assays
Viral p24 antigen detection

ELISA detection of the presence of the p24 antigen of HIV-1 in serum is an alternative method for diagnosis of HIV-1 infection. In general terms, sera to be tested are allowed to bind to p24-specific antibody that is either bound to a well of a microtiter plate or to the surface of polystyrene beads. After appropriate incubation and washing steps, the well or beads are incubated with a goat or rabbit antibody that reacts with any p24 antigen captured by the first step. Finally, an anti-goat or anti-rabbit antibody is added, which is coupled to an enzyme that produces a colorimetric reaction in the presence of a chemical substrate. ELISA measurements of the HIV-1 capsid protein (p24), have been used to diagnose HIV-1 infection in all age groups, but have low (30%–70%) sensitivity among infants less than three months of age [9, 15]. The inability to detect p24 antigen is largely the result of the presence of HIV-1 specific antibodies that in an infant are the result of transplacental transfer. Dissociation of antibody from p24 antigen in serum specimens greatly enhances the sensitivity of the p24 ELISA. In the ICD (immune complex dissociated) p24 assay, serum or plasma samples are treated briefly with acid, which dissociates HIV-1 antibodies from their bound antigens. Following neutralization of the sample, the ELISA is run as described above. However, ICD-p24 antigen testing should not be used for the diagnosis of infection in infants less than a month of age because of an unacceptably high number of false-positive results [9, 15]. Other investigators have used heat denaturation of plasma samples to release viral antigen (HD-Ag testing), prior to ELISA. HD-Ag testing appears to be very sensitive for the detection of viremia (16), but a small number of false-positive results occur, compared to PCR testing of the same specimen [17]. Antigen detection methods remain a potentially useful alternative approach to the diagnosis of perinatal HIV infection, with recognition of the need for confirmation of these results.

Culture

Since the initial isolation of HIV-1 in the early 1980s, cultures have been used to detect HIV-1 and to measure the number of HIV-1 infected peripheral blood lymphocytes. In general terms, patient peripheral blood mononuclear cells (PBMCs) are incubated with PBMCs from an HIV-1-seronegative (i.e., uninfected) donor, and cultured for up to 6 weeks in media containing interleukin 2 (IL-2, originally known as T-cell growth factor) which activates the PBMCs and facilitates high levels of viral replication within the cells. The growth of HIV-1 in the cells is determined by assaying for capsid protein (p24) by ELISA performed on culture fluid medium. Cultures are designated as positive when significant p24 antigen is detected (usually ≥ 30 pg/ml) [18].

Although cumbersome, time-consuming, and costly to perform, HIV-1 cultures have high specificity and sensitivity. False-positive test results are rare and generally result from laboratory errors such as specimen mislabeling. In the absence of antiretroviral treatment, falsely negative cultures are unusual among adult patients, but may exist in early infancy because of small specimen volumes and low amounts of virus soon after perinatal infection. Nonetheless, under optimal conditions, the sensitivity of culture and HIV-1 DNA PCR are equal for detection of HIV-1 infection in infants [19].

Diagnosing HIV-1 infection in infants and children

Using virological assays, HIV-1 infection can be detected in most infants by 1 month of age, and in nearly all by 6 months of age. HIV-1 DNA PCR is currently the diagnostic method of choice for perinatally exposed children under 18 months of age (Table 3.1). Umbilical cord specimens must not be used because contamination of the specimen by maternal blood can occur. Approximately 40% of infants will test positive in the first 24 hours of life. The sensitivity of HIV-1 DNA PCR rises rapidly, and most infants with perinatally-acquired infection who test negative at birth will have positive PCR test results by 2 weeks of age. In a meta-analysis of several published studies, the sensitivity of HIV-1 DNA PCR was 93% at 2 weeks of age (95% confidence interval: 76% to 97%) [10]. The small number of infants who do not have detectable HIV-1 DNA by this time will generally test positive by the end of the second month of life [19]. Early diagnosis of HIV-1 infection is desirable, to allow antiretroviral therapy to be instituted or modified.

Table 3.1. Detection of HIV-1 infection in infants and children

---

HIV-1-infected

   a. Child <18 mo known to be seropositive or born to an HIV-1-infected mother with:

      1. Positive results on two separate determinations (excluding cord blood) from one of the following detection assays:

         HIV-1 DNA PCR or HIV-1 RNA detection assays

         HIV-1 culture

         HIV-1 p24 antigen (Only used in infants above one month of age);

         or

      2. Meets the clinical criteria for AIDS diagnosis based on the 1987 AIDS surveillance case definition.

   b. Child ≥18 mo with:

      1. Positive HIV-1 antibody detection tests (e.g., repeatedly positive ELISA and confirmatory test (Western blot or immunofluorescence assay));

         or

      2. Meets any criteria outlined in (a)

HIV-1-uninfected (seroreverter)

   Child born to an HIV-1-infected mother, who has:

      1. Negative HIV-1 antibody tests (2 or more negative ELISA tests performed one month apart, both after 6 months of age);[a]

         or

      2. No other laboratory evidence of HIV-1 infection (has not had two positive viral detection tests, if performed);

         and

         No evidence of an AIDS-defining condition.

---

[a] In the absence of hypogammaglobulinemia.

Adapted from [20]. (Updates available at www.hivatis.org/guidelines/Pediatric/Dec12_01/peddec.pdf)

Testing should be performed within 48 hours of birth, at 1 to 2 months of age, and again at 4 to 6 months of age. Any positive tests should be verified as quickly as possible by a second virologic test [20].

HIV-1 infection can be excluded with high accuracy when an asymptomatic child has had two or more negative virologic tests, using blood samples drawn at or after 1 month of age, with at least one drawn after 4 months of age. HIV-1 infection also can be excluded when HIV-1 antibodies are not detected in two or more antibody tests (spaced one month apart) performed at or after 6 months of age, in a child who has no signs or symptoms of HIV-1 infection. Finally, HIV-1 infection can be ruled out when antibody tests (ELISA or Western blot) are negative, in the absence of hypogammaglobulinemia, in a child at least 18 months of age who lacks any clinical evidence of HIV-1 infection.

HIV-1 infection is diagnosed when two positive HIV-1 virological tests are obtained (HIV-1 RNA or DNA PCR, p24 antigen (for children above one month of age), or culture). Separate blood specimens should be used for these tests. There have been rare reports of infants with positive virological tests, and subsequent negative tests. Although transient HIV-1 infection has been proposed to explain this finding, nearly all such cases are false positive tests resulting from sample mix-up and laboratory error, including PCR contamination [14]. A diagnosis of HIV-1 can be made by serological methods in children 18 months of age or older who have antibodies to HIV-1 detected by ELISA and confirmed by Western blot or immunofluorescence methods.

Diagnosis of non-subtype B HIV-1 infection

The two human immunodeficiency viruses, HIV-1 and HIV-2, exhibit tremendous genetic heterogeneity, which may complicate PCR-based diagnosis [21]. HIV-1 variants are currently classified into three groups: M (main), O (outlier), and N (non-M/non-O). Within group M, clusters (clades) of related strains have been further classified into subtypes A–D, F-H, J, and K. In addition, inter-subtype recombinants have been identified in several regions of the world [21, 22]. A similar classification of HIV-2 subtypes exists.

All of the ELISAs that are currently licensed for use in the USA will detect HIV-1 specific antibodies, but only a subset will detect antibodies to HIV-2. None of these ELISA or confirmatory tests will reliably detect HIV-1 subtype O, and none of the confirmatory tests available will consistently detect HIV-2 antibodies [4]. Fortunately, infections with HIV-1 subtype O and HIV-2 are still rare outside of countries in west central Africa (e.g., Cameroon, Ivory Coast), and commercially available serological tests can be used to detect most infections worldwide.

The genetic diversity of HIV-1 particularly complicates PCR detection of the virus in infants. Subtype B is the most common subtype in the USA and Western Europe, and the commercially available Amplicor HIV-1 DNA detection kit (Roche) employs oligonucleotide primers that detect it and the most closely related subtypes (e.g., subtypes D and G) [9, 12, 23]. However, the majority of HIV-1 infections in the world are caused by the other subtypes, which may not be detected (e.g., subtypes A and C) [21, 23, 24]. Alternatives to the use of the Amplicor HIV-1 DNA PCR in these cases include the use of commercial HIV-1 RNA detection methods that include primers with broader specificity (Amplicor HIV-1 Monitor 1.5, NASBA, and bDNA). These alternative methods should be considered when the maternal history suggests the possibility of infection by an unusual subtype, or when an infant has signs or symptoms of HIV-1 infection, despite negative initial testing. Changes in the worldwide epidemiology of HIV-1 will likely necessitate repeated reevaluation of methods to detect viral DNA and RNA detection to ensure detection of HIV-1 in all individuals in a given geographic area.

Summary

Many assays are commercially available to detect HIV-1 infection in children. In children who are 18 or more months of age, and in adolescents and adults, serologic assays (e.g., ELISA, Western blot) constitute the most cost-effective diagnostic assay for HIV-1 infection. For children younger than 18 months, HIV-1 DNA PCR is the preferred method for early HIV-1 detection. These assays provide clinicians the opportunity to make a prompt diagnosis of HIV-1 infection, and to initiate antiretroviral therapy as well as prophylaxis against opportunistic infections.

Acknowledgments

The author is an Elizabeth Glaser Scientist sponsored by the Pediatric AIDS Foundation. Elizabeth Glaser is remembered with great admiration for her courage and her work on behalf of all families affected by HIV.

REFERENCES

1. King, S. M. and The American Academy of Pediatrics Committee on pediatric AIDS. Evaluation and treatment of the human immuno-deficiency virus-1-exposed infant. *Pediatrics* 2004;**114**:497–505.

2. Janssen, R. S., Satten, G. A., Stramer, S. L. *et al.* New testing strategy to detect early HIV-1 infection for use in incidence estimates and for clinical and prevention purposes. *J. Am. Med. Assoc.* 1998;**280**:42–48.

3. Machado, D. M., Delwart, E. L., Diaz, R. S. *et al.* Use of the sensitive/less-sensitive (detuned) EIA strategy for targeting genetic analysis of HIV-1 to recently infected blood donors. *AIDS* 2002;**16**:113–119.

4. CDC. Revised Guidelines for HIV Counseling, Testing, and Referral Technical Expert Panel Review of CDC HIV Counseling, Testing and Referral Guidelines. *Morb. Mortal. Wkly. Rep.* 2001;**50**:1–58.

5. Bylund, D. J., Ziegner, U. H., Hooper, D. G. Review of testing for human immunodeficiency virus. *Clin. Lab. Med.* 1992;**12**;12:305–333.

6. CDC. Interpretation and use of the Western blot assay for serodiagnosis of human immunodeficiency virus type 1 infections. *Morb. Mortal. Wkly. Rep.* 1989;**38**:1–7.

7. CDC. Revised Guidelines for HIV Counseling, Testing and Referral. *Morb. Mortal. Wkly Rep.* 2001; 50 (RR19):1–58.

8. Minkoff, H., O'Sullivan, M. J. The case for rapid HIV testing during labor. *J. AM. Med. Assoc.* 1998;**279**:1743–1744.

9. Nielsen, K., Bryson Y. J. Diagnosis of HIV infection in children. *Pediatr. Clin. North. Am.* 2000;**47**:39–63.

10. Dunn, D. T., Brandt, C. D., Krivine, A. *et al.* The sensitivity of HIV-1 DNA polymerase chain reaction in the neonatal period and the relative contributions of intra-uterine and intra-partum transmission. *AIDS* 1995;**9**:F7–F11.

11. Shearer, W. T., Quinn, T. C., LaRussa, P. *et al*. Viral load and disease progression in infants infected with human immunodeficiency virus type 1. Women and Infants Transmission Study Group. *N. Engl. J. Med.* 1997;**336**:1337–1342.

12. Delamare, C., Burgard, M., Mayaux, M. J. *et al*. HIV-1 RNA detection in plasma for the diagnosis of infection in neonates. The French Pediatric HIV Infection Study Group. *J. Acquir. Immune. Defic. Syndr. Hum. Retrovirol.* 1997;**15**:121–125.

13. Simonds, R. J., Brown, T. M., Thea, D. M. *et al*. Sensitivity and specificity of a qualitative RNA detection assay to diagnose HIV infection in young infants. Perinatal AIDS Collaborative Transmission Study. *AIDS* 1998;**12**:1545–1549.

14. Frenkel, L. M., Mullins, J. I., Learn, G. H. *et al*. Genetic evaluation of suspected cases of transient HIV-1 infection of infants. *Science* 1998;**280**:1073–1077.

15. Miles, S. A., Balden, E., Magpantay, L. *et al*. Rapid serologic testing with immune-complex-dissociated HIV p24 antigen for early detection of HIV infection in neonates. Southern California Pediatric AIDS Consortium. *N. Engl. J. Med.* 1993;**328**:297–302.

16. Schupbach, F. M., Pontelli, D., Tomasik, Z., Luty, R., Boni, J. Heat-mediated immune complex dissociation and enzyme-linked immunosorbent assay signal amplification render p24 antigen detection in plasma as sensitive as HIV-1 RNA detection by polymerase chain reaction. *AIDS* 1996;**10**:1085–1090.

17. Schupbach, B. J., Tomasik, Z., Jendis, J., Seger, R., Kind, C. Sensitive detection and early prognostic significance of p24 antigen in heat-denatured plasma of human immunodeficiency virus type 1-infected infants. Swiss Neonatal HIV Study Group. *J. Infect. Dis.* 1994;**170**:318–324.

18. Hollinger, F. B., Bremer, J. W., Myers, L. E., Gold, J. W., McQuay, L. Standardization of sensitive human immunodeficiency virus coculture procedures and establishment of a multicenter quality assurance program for the AIDS Clinical Trials Group. The NIH/NIAID/DAIDS/ACTG Virology Laboratories. *J. Clin. Microbiol.* 1992;**30**:1787–1794.

19. Owens, D. K., Holodniy, M., McDonald, T. W., Scott, J., Sonnad, S. A meta-analytic evaluation of the polymerase chain reaction for the diagnosis of HIV infection in infants. *J. Am. Med. Assoc.* 1996;**275**:1342–1348.

20. CDC. Recommendations of the U.S. Public Health Service Task Force on the use of zidovudine to reduce perinatal transmission of human immunodeficiency virus. *Morb. Mortal. Wkly. Rep.* 1995;**44**:1–20.

21. McCutchan, F. Global diversity in HIV. In Crandall, K., ed. *Evolution of HIV*. Baltimore, MD: The John Hopkins University Press, 1999.

22. Robertson, D. L., Anderson, J. P., Bradac, J. A. *et al*. HIV-1 nomenclature proposal. *Science* 2000;**288**:55–56.

23. Bogh, M., Machuca, R., Gerstoft, J. *et al*. Subtype-specific problems with qualitative Amplicor HIV-1 DNA PCR test. *J. Clin. Virol.* 2001;**20**:149–153.

24. Rouet, F., Montcho, C., Rouzioux, C. *et al*. Early diagnosis of paediatric HIV-1 infection among African breast-fed children using a quantitative plasma HIV RNA assay. *AIDS* 2001;**15**:1849–1856.

4 Prevention of mother-to-child transmission of HIV

Jennifer S. Read, M.D., M.S., M.P.H., D.T.M.&H.

Pediatric, Adolescent, and Maternal AIDS (PAMA) Branch, NICHD, NIH, Bethesda, MD

Introduction

Over the past several years, major successes have been achieved in prevention of mother-to-child transmission (MTCT) of human immunodeficiency virus type 1 (HIV). However, these successes have occurred primarily in those countries with the greatest resources and the lowest burden of HIV infection among women and children. Significant challenges remain, particularly in those countries with more limited resources and a greater population burden of HIV infection. Each day an estimated 2000 infants become infected with HIV, virtually all residing in resource-poor settings [1]. MTCT of HIV can occur during pregnancy, at the time of labor and delivery, and postnatally (through breastfeeding) [2]. Rates of MTCT of HIV have been calculated in studies conducted around the world in the absence of interventions to decrease transmission [3]. Overall, most studies reported a transmission rate in the range of 25%–30% and higher transmission rates were observed in resource-poor settings (13%–42%) than in resource-rich settings (14%–25%). In this chapter, risk factors for MTCT of HIV will be reviewed briefly. In addition, interventions for the prevention of MTCT of HIV will be discussed, both those already shown to be efficacious and those under study. Finally, strategies to prevent MTCT of HIV will be addressed.

Risk factors for, and interventions to prevent, mother-to-child transmission of HIV

Numerous risk factors for MTCT of HIV have been identified or are under investigation [4]. General categories of risk factors include: the amount of virus to which the child is exposed, the duration of such exposure, factors facilitating the transfer of virus from mother to child, characteristics of the virus, and the child's susceptibility to infection. Table 4.1 summarizes selected known or potential risk factors for MTCT of HIV, and the

Handbook of Pediatric HIV Care, ed. Steven L. Zeichner and Jennifer S. Read.
Published by Cambridge University Press. © Cambridge University Press 2006.

Table 4.1. Selected known or potential risk factors for, and associated interventions to prevent, MTCT of HIV

Category	Factor	Intervention
Amount of virus	Higher maternal viral load	• Decrease maternal viral load and/or provide pre-/post-exposure prophylaxis to the infant
	• In peripheral blood	• Administer antiretroviral drug(s) to the mother
	• In cervicovaginal fluid	• Administer antiretroviral drug(s) to the mother
		• Administer viricidal agent(s) to the mother (cervicovaginal cleansing) and/or to the newborn
	• In breast milk	• Administer antiretroviral drug(s) to the mother
		• Administer antiretroviral prophylaxis to the infant
		• Treat breast milk with heat or chemicals
Duration of exposure	Mode of delivery (vaginal delivery or cesarean section after labor and/or after ruptured membranes)	• Cesarean section before labor and before ruptured membranes
	Breastfeeding	• Avoid breastfeeding (if safe, affordable, and feasible)
		• If breastfeeding unavoidable, early weaning (if possible)
Factors facilitating transfer of the virus from mother to child	Vitamin A deficiency	• Administer vitamin A supplementation to the mother and/or infant
	Chorioamnionitis	• Administer antibiotics to the mother
	Mixed breastfeeding	• Exclusive breastfeeding

associated interventions (already identified under investigation) for preventing such transmission.

Amount of virus to which the child is exposed

The amount of virus the infant is exposed to represents a major risk factor for MTCT of HIV. A higher maternal HIV RNA concentration (viral load) in the peripheral bloodstream is associated with a higher risk of MTCT of HIV [5]. Although the risk of transmission of HIV from mothers with peripheral blood viral loads below the lower limit of detection is very low, no threshold of peripheral blood viral load below which transmission does not occur has been identified. Although the association between maternal peripheral blood viral load and MTCT remains even among women who received zidovudine prophylaxis [6], receipt of antiretroviral therapy (ART) attenuates the relationship between maternal viral load and transmission [5]. Women receiving highly active antiretroviral therapy (HAART) [7, 8] have very low rates of MTCT.

Antiretroviral interventions for the prevention of MTCT of HIV began with the success of the AIDS Clinical Trials Group (ACTG) Protocol 076, published in 1994 [9] (Table 4.2). Subsequently, the efficacy of other antiretroviral prophylaxis regimens has been demonstrated in different countries around the world [10–19] (Table 4.2). The efficacy of antiretroviral prophylaxis is diminished (or eradicated [16]) in breastfeeding populations, due to continued breastfeeding transmission after prophylactic drug administration has been discontinued. Simplification of the ACTG 076 regimen (oral intrapartum zidovudine, shorter maternal or infant administration) can still result in reductions in vertical transmission rates similar to those observed with ACTG 076, although longer antepartum courses of zidovudine are associated with lower transmission rates [14]. Not all of the protective effect of antiretroviral drugs is explained by lowering of maternal peripheral blood viral load, and pre- and postexposure prophylaxis of the infant is also important [20,21]. Finally, the combination of two antiretroviral drugs (zidovudine with nevirapine) substantially reduces transmission compared to a single drug (zidovudine) [19]. More and more HIV-infected women in the resource-rich settings are receiving combination ART, including HAART, for their own health. Receipt of more potent ART regimens is associated with rates of MTCT of HIV of less than 2 [7,8].

Analysis of transmission rates among HIV-infected women and their infants who received one or more components (antepartum, intrapartum, and/or postnatal) of the ACTG 076 zidovudine prophylaxis regimen suggested there are reductions in the rates of MTCT of HIV even if abbreviated regimens of zidovudine are received [22, 23]. The observed transmission rates (according to when zidovudine prophylaxis was initiated) were: antepartum: 6.1%; intrapartum: 10.0%; within 48 hours after birth: 9.3% (5.9% if within 12 hours after birth and 25% if within 12–24 hours after birth); three days or more after birth: 18.4%; and none: 26.6%.

In addition to peripheral blood viral load, a higher genital tract viral load is independently associated with a higher risk of MTCT of HIV [24, 25]. The utility of cervicovaginal cleansing, with or without immediate surface decontamination of the infant, with virucidal agents such as benzalkonium chloride and chlorhexidine has been evaluated in several studies in sub-Saharan Africa [26–29].

A higher breast milk viral load is associated with a higher risk of MTCT of HIV [30, 31]. If breastfeeding is unavoidable, then it is possible that one or more of the following interventions to decrease the viral load of the breast milk could prevent transmission:

Table 4.2. Randomized clinical trials: antiretroviral prophylaxis

Drug(s) evaluated	Trial	Location	Breastfeeding	Randomization	Transmission rates	Efficacy
Zidovudine (ZDV)	Connor 1994 [9]	USA, France	No	Mother: ZDV 100 mg po 5 times per day beginning at 14–34 weeks gestation, 2 mg/kg IV over a one hour period, then 1 mg/kg per hour until delivery Infant: 2 mg/kg po q 6 hours for 6 weeks, beginning 8–12 hours after birth	7.9% (95%CI: 4.1, 11.7)	71%
				Placebo	27.7% (95%CI: 21.2, 34.1)	
	Shaffer 1999 [10]	Thailand	No	Mother: ZDV 300 mg po BID from 36 weeks gestation, q 3 hours from onset of labor until delivery Infant: No ZDV	9.4% (95%CI: 5.2, 13.5)	50%
				Placebo	18.9% (95%CI: 13.2, 24.2)	
	Wiktor 1999 [11]	Cote d'Ivoire	Yes (most)	Mother: ZDV 300 mg po BID from 36 weeks gestation, q 3 hours from onset of labor until delivery Infant: No ZDV	12.2% (1 month) 15.7% (3 months)	44% (1 month) 37% (3 months)
				Placebo	21.7% (1 month) 24.9% (3 months)	
	Dabis 1999 [12]	Cote d'Ivoire	Yes (most)	Mother: ZDV 300 mg po BID from 36–38 weeks gestation until labor,	18.0% (6 months)	38%

Study	Country		Intervention	Transmission rate	Results/comments
Leray 2002 [13]	Burkina Faso	No	600 mg at beginning of labor, 300 mg po BID × 7 days Infant: No ZDV Placebo	27.5%	No statistically significant differences in three arms (long-long, long-short, short-long)
Lallemant 2000 [14]	Thailand		All participants: • Mother: ZDV 300 mg po BID until labor, then 300 mg po q 3 hours until delivery • Infant: ZDV 2 mg/kg po q 6 hours with randomization to one of four arms: Long-long: maternal ZDV from 28 weeks, infant ZDV for 6 weeks Short-short: maternal ZDV from 35 weeks, infant ZDV for 3 days Long-short: maternal ZDV from 28 weeks, infant ZDV for 3 days Short-long: maternal ZDV from 35 weeks, infant ZDV for 6 weeks	6.5% (4.1, 8.9) (final analysis) 10.5% (interim analysis; enrolment into this arm discontinued) 4.7% (2.4, 7.0) (final analysis) 8.6% (5.6, 11.6) (final analysis)	Transmission rate among those randomized to arms with longer (from 28 weeks) antepartum ZDV: 1.6% (0.7, 2.6) Transmission rate among those randomized to arms with shorter (from 36 weeks) antepartum ZDV: 5.1% (3.2, 7.0)

(cont.)

Table 4.2. *(cont.)*

Drug(s) evaluated	Trial	Location	Breastfeeding	Randomization	Transmission rates	Efficacy
ZDV vs. nevirapine (NVP)	Jackson 2003 [15]	Uganda	Yes (most)	NVP 200 mg po at onset of labor (infant NVP 2 mg/kg within 72 hours of birth)	11.8% by 6–8 weeks 13.5% by 14–16 weeks 15.7% by 18 months	41% by 18 months
				ZDV 600 mg po at onset of labor and 300 mg q 3 hours until delivery (infant ZDV 4 mg/kg po BID for 7 days after birth)	20.0% by 6–8 weeks 22.1% by 14–16 weeks 25.8% by 18 months	
ZDV with lamivudine (3TC)	PETRA 2002 [16]	South Africa, Tanzania, Uganda	Yes (some)	Antepartum ZDV 300 mg po BID with lamivudine (3TC) 150 mg po BID from 36 weeks gestation		No statistically significant differences in transmission rates at 18 months
				Intrapartum ZDV 300 mg × 1, then 300 mg po q 3 hrs with 3TC 150 mg × 1, then 150 mg q 12 hours Postpartum (Mother): ZDV 300 mg po BID with 3TC 150 mg po BID for one week Postnatal (Infant): ZDV 4 mg/kg with 3TC 2 mg/kg po BID for one week		
				Arm A: Antepartum, intrapartum, and postpartum/postnatal	5.7% at 6 weeks 15% (9–23) at 18 months	
				Arm B: Intrapartum and postpartum/postnatal only	8.9% at 6 weeks 18% (12–26) at 18 months	
				Arm C: Postpartum/postnatal only	14.2% at 6 weeks 20% (13–30) at 18	

	Location	Breastfeeding	Control	Regimen	Transmission rate	Notes
			Placebo		15.3% at 6 weeks 22% (16–30) at 18 months	
Moodley 2003	South Africa	Yes (some)	Placebo	Mother: ZDV 600 mg po × 1, then 300 mg po q 3 hours until delivery and 300 mg po BID for 1 week after delivery. 3TC 150 mg po × 1, then 150 mg po q12 hours until delivery and 150 mg po BID for 1 week. Infant: ZDV 12 mg po BID for 1 week and 3TC 6 mg po BID for 1 week (if birth weight <2 kg, then ZDV 4 mg/kg and 3TC 2 mg/kg)	9.3% (7.0, 11.6)	No statistically significant differences in transmission rates
				Mother: NVP 200 mg po at labor onset, and another dose 48 hours later if still in labor, followed by 200 mg 24–48 hours postpartum. Infant: NVP 6 mg at 24–48 hours after birth (if birth within 2 hours of the maternal labor dose, another 6-mg dose within 6 hours after delivery)	12.3% (9.7, 15.0)	
NVP Dorenbaum 2002[a]	USA, Brazil, Europe, Bahamas	No		Mother: NVP 200 mg po after onset of labor. Infant: NVP 2 mg/kg at 48–72 hours after birth	1.4% (0.6, 2.7)	No statistically significant difference in transmission rates
				Placebo	1.6% (0.8, 2.9)	

(cont.)

Table 4.2. (*cont.*)

Drug(s) evaluated	Trial	Location	Breastfeeding	Randomization	Transmission rates	Efficacy
	Lallemant 2002[b] [19]	Thailand	No	Mother: NVP 200 mg po × 1 at the onset of labor Infant: NVP 6 mg po × 1 within 48–72 hours after birth Arm 1: NVP to mother and NVP to infant Arm 2: NVP to mother and Placebo to infant Arm 3: Placebo to mother and Placebo to infant	1.9% (0.9, 3.0) 2.8% (1.5, 4.1) 6.5% enrolment into this arm stopped because transmission significantly higher than in Arm 1	No statistically significant difference in transmission rates between ARM 1 and ARM 2

[a] All women received at least zidovudine perinatal transmission prophylaxis according to the ACTG 076 protocol, and most received combination antiretroviral therapy

[b] All women received zidovudine prophylaxis (300 mg po BID) beginning at 28 weeks gestation or as soon as possible thereafter (at least 2 weeks), and 300 mg po q 3 hours from the onset of labor until delivery. Infants received zidovudine prophylaxis for one week (or for 4–6 weeks if mothers received less than four weeks of zidovudine during pregnancy).

administration of antiretroviral drugs to the mother while breastfeeding, antiretroviral prophylaxis administered to the infant, and treatment of breast milk with heat or chemical agents.

Before considering specific interventions to prevent breastfeeding transmission of HIV, it is important to consider the potential effects of breastfeeding on the HIV-infected woman herself. One such potential effect is increased mortality among breastfeeding HIV-infected women. The results of two studies evaluating the risk of mortality among HIV-infected women according to infant feeding modality (breastfeeding compared with formula feeding) have been conflicting [32, 33]. A third study, the Breastfeeding and HIV International Transmission Study, found that mother's mortality during the 18-month period after delivery did not differ significantly according to children's feeding modality [34].

It is possible that HIV transmission through breastfeeding could be decreased with antiretroviral drugs administered either to the mother or to the infant while breastfeeding. The efficacy of continued administration of antiretroviral prophylaxis to breastfeeding infants is being investigated in studies in India and in different parts of Africa. These studies are evaluating administration of different antiretroviral drugs to the infant for varying lengths of time (1 week to 6 months). Observational studies and randomized clinical trials involving administration of combinations of antiretroviral drugs to breastfeeding, HIV-infected women in sub-Saharan Africa are being initiated to evaluate the effectiveness and efficacy of maternal combination ART to prevent MTCT of HIV during breastfeeding. Drugs being evaluated include zidovudine, lamirudine, and didanosine [35].

Treatment of breast milk with either chemical agents or heat to inactivate HIV has been investigated in several studies [36–39]. Obviously, utilization of all of these methodologies would not be feasible in many settings. Additionally, while lowering breast milk viral load, these methodologies are unlikely to eliminate HIV from the milk completely. Finally, with any treatment to inactivate HIV, the extent to which the treatment diminishes the protective or nutritional components of breast milk must be carefully assessed.

Duration of exposure to the virus
Intrapartum
A longer duration of ruptured membranes is associated with a greater risk of MTCT of HIV. The risk of MTCT of HIV increases approximately 2% with each increase of one hour in the duration of ruptured membranes [40]. Incorporating data from North America and Europe, an individual patient data meta-analysis [41] suggested a lower risk of MTCT of HIV with cesarean section before labor and before ruptured membranes (ECS). The transmission rates with ECS without ART was 10.4%, as compared with a rate of 19.0% with other modes of delivery without ART. The respective rates with ART during the antepartum, intrapartum, and postnatal periods were 2.0% and 7.3%. Simultaneously, a randomized clinical trial of mode of delivery among HIV-infected

Table 4.3. Randomized clinical trials: mode of delivery and infant feeding modality.

Trial	Location	Randomization	Transmission rates	Efficacy
European mode of delivery Collaboration 1999 [42]	Europe	Cesarean section Vaginal delivery	1.8% 10.5%	83%
Nduati 2000 [44]	Kenya	Formula feeding Breastfeeding	20.5% (14.0–27.0) 36.7% (29.4–44.0)	44%

women in Europe documented the efficacy of cesarean section in preventing MTCT [42]: 1.8% transmission among those randomized to cesarean delivery versus 10.5% among those randomized to vaginal delivery (Table 4.3).

Postnatally (through breastfeeding)

A longer duration of breastfeeding is associated with an increased risk of HIV transmission [43]. A randomized clinical trial of breastfeeding versus formula feeding among HIV-infected women in Kenya [44] demonstrated HIV transmission through breastfeeding and prevention of such transmission with formula feeding (Table 4.3). If complete avoidance of breast milk is not possible, early weaning from breast milk (e.g., at 6 months of age), if feasible, would limit exposure to HIV-infected breast milk while allowing the child to experience the benefits of breastfeeding. Early weaning from breast milk is being evaluated in trials in Zambia [45] and elsewhere.

Factors facilitating transfer of the virus from mother to child

Several factors potentially facilitate transfer of the virus from mother to child, including vitamin A deficiency, chorioamnionitis, mixed breastfeeding, and maternal breast pathology and infant thrush. Modification of these factors in order to decrease the likelihood of MTCT has been or is being evaluated.

Maternal vitamin A deficiency has been associated with an increased risk of MTCT of HIV [46]. However, results from three completed vitamin A supplementation trials indicated no benefit of supplementation with regard to prevention of MTCT of HIV [47–49]. Enrolment in a fourth vitamin A supplementation trial in Zimbabwe has been completed.

Placental membrane inflammation (chorioamnionitis and funisitis) has been associated with an increased risk of MTCT of HIV [50–52]. Therefore, a clinical trial of antibiotic treatment to reduce chorioamnionitis in HIV-infected women was initiated. However, the trial was discontinued after interim analyses no effect indicated [53].

In South Africa, data from a randomized clinical trial of vitamin A supplementation to prevent MTCT of HIV [48] were reanalyzed to evaluate a possible association between feeding patterns among infants of breastfeeding, HIV-infected mothers and the risk of MTCT [54]. In this study, breastfeeding was categorized as exclusive or mixed, i.e., without or with water, other fluids, and food. Women who chose to breastfeed were counseled to consider exclusive breastfeeding. Follow-up visits after birth, during which an infant feeding history was obtained, occurred at 1 week, 6 weeks, and 3 months of age, and every 3 months thereafter. By 15 months of age, children who ever breast-fed were more likely to have become HIV-infected (31.6%) than those children who never breastfed (19.4%), $P = 0.007$. Of children who ever breastfed, those with exclusive breastfeeding until at least 3 months of age but no longer than 6 months of age had a lower estimated transmission point estimate than those with mixed feeding, but the confidence limits for these point estimates overlap (exclusive: 24.7% [95%CI: 16.0–34.4%]; mixed: 35.9% [95%CI: 26.7–45.1%]). The authors proposed that the mechanism of their findings was that contaminated fluids and foods given to infants with mixed breastfeeding damaged the bowel and facilitated the entry of HIV into tissues. The results of this hypothesis-generating study prompted several investigators to pursue new studies of exclusive breastfeeding to assess more carefully the risk of HIV transmission according to feeding modality. For example, data from Zimbabwe suggest mixed breastfeeding is associated with a higher risk of MTCT of HIV and death [55]. However, exclusive breastfeeding is not the norm in Africa and other parts of the world. Despite this, programs to promote exclusive breastfeeding have had some success. For example, the prevalence of exclusive breastfeeding at 5 months of age increased from 6% to 70% with home-based counseling by peer counselors (mothers from the local community with training for ten days) in Bangladesh [56].

Both maternal breast pathology (e.g., breast abscesses [25, 57, 58], mastitis [25, 30, 59], and nipple lesions [58]) and oral candidiasis of the infant [59] are associated with late postnatal transmission of HIV. One program under way in Zimbabwe involved education of women who choose to breastfeed following individual counseling regarding exclusive breastfeeding until the infant is four to six months of age followed by rapid weaning. Education and counseling also are provided regarding proper positioning during breastfeeding, prompt seeking of medical care if breast problems arise or if the infant develops oral candidiasis or other lesions, avoiding breastfeeding from the affected breast, and safe sex practices while breastfeeding [60].

Summary of studies of interventions to prevent MTCT

Although many different interventions to prevent MTCT of HIV have been and are being investigating, efficacy has been demonstrated to date for only the following:
- antiretroviral prophylaxis;
- cesarean section before labor and before ruptured membranes; and
- complete avoidance of breastfeeding.

In addition to these interventions, observational data strongly suggest that combination ART, including HAART, is associated with very low rates of transmission.

Table 4.4. Interventions for the prevention of MTCT of HIV

Intervention	Resource-rich settings	Resource-poor settings
Voluntary counseling and testing (VCT)	Yes	Yes
Antiretroviral prophylaxis/therapy	Yes	Yes (but therapy generally not widely available)
Cesarean section before labor and before ruptured membranes	Yes	Generally no
Complete avoidance of breastfeeding	Yes	Generally no

Strategies for the prevention of mother-to-child transmission of HIV

Although prevention of MTCT of HIV is often conceptualized as only beginning once an HIV-infected woman is pregnant, prevention of MTCT optimally begins before pregnancy and before acquisition of HIV infection, i.e., through prevention of acquisition of HIV infection by adolescent girls and by women of reproductive age. In the absence of primary prevention, then prevention of unwanted pregnancies is important. Assuming an HIV-infected adolescent girl or a woman has become pregnant, then prevention of MTCT of HIV in the USA and other resource-rich settings, where the seroprevalence of HIV among adults is below 1% [61], has incorporated the following interventions: voluntary HIV counseling and testing, complete avoidance of breastfeeding, cesarean section before labor and before ruptured membranes, and antiretroviral drugs (from zidovudine prophylaxis, at a minimum, to combination ART) (Table 4.4). However, in resource-poor settings, where the seroprevalence of HIV among adults is often over 20% [61] and the burden of HIV disease is much greater than in resource-rich settings, complete avoidance of breastfeeding is generally not possible or acceptable, and cesarean delivery for the prevention of MTCT of HIV is generally not feasible due to lack of clinical infrastructure and staffing (Table 4.4). In these settings, efforts to find new, or adapt old, interventions so that they are feasible and affordable to implement remains an urgent priority. Concomitantly there is a growing realization that, if the real goal is to increase the likelihood of children's HIV-free survival (and not just to decrease MTCT rates), it is best for many reasons to work towards optimizing the health of the HIV-infected woman herself since one of the best predictors of children's deaths is their mothers' own deaths. Obviously, provision of treatment for HIV-infected pregnant women is an important goal in and of itself, aside from secondary benefits in terms of lower MTCT rates.

Voluntary HIV counseling and testing

Voluntary HIV counseling and testing has represented an essential component of prevention efforts in the USA [62] and other resource-rich settings, since the greatest effectiveness of current preventive interventions (such as cesarean delivery and antiretroviral prophylaxis) is predicated upon a pregnant woman knowing her HIV infection status before becoming pregnant or else as early as possible during pregnancy. The US Public Health Service recommended in 1995 that HIV counseling and testing be offered to all pregnant women [63]. The proportion of mothers of HIV-exposed or -infected children in the USA whose HIV infection was diagnosed before their child's birth increased from 70% in 1993 (before the original US Public Health Service guidelines were issued in 1995) to 94% in 1997 [64]. However, while a decreasing proportion of the overall population of pregnant women in the USA have delayed or no prenatal care (25% in 1989 but 18% in 1997) [65], such may not be the case among HIV-infected women. Additionally, receipt of prenatal care does not guarantee HIV counseling and testing will occur. Data from several studies have indicated missed opportunities for antenatal HIV counseling and testing [66, 67]. Such data prompted the US Institute of Medicine to recommend universal, routine testing of pregnant women with patient notification [68]. The US Public Health Service subsequently made similar recommendations [69].

In many resource-poor settings, however, where few or no treatment or prophylactic interventions for HIV-infected individuals exist, acceptance of voluntary HIV counseling and testing (including return to receive results of HIV diagnostic testing) may not be high. For example, only 78% of women receiving antenatal care in Cote d'Ivoire consented to HIV testing and, of these, only 58.4% returned to receive the results [70]. With the use of rapid diagnostic tests (such that results can be made available to the individual being testing on the same day, as opposed to requiring a return visit to the clinic), and with increasing availability of both therapeutic and prevention interventions, it is anticipated that acceptance of voluntary HIV counseling and testing will increase.

Complete avoidance of breastfeeding

Complete avoidance of breastfeeding (e.g., by using infant formula) is an intervention of obvious utility in settings where it is feasible (i.e., where clean water is available), affordable, and culturally acceptable. In resource-rich settings such as the USA, complete avoidance of breastfeeding by HIV-infected women has been advised for several years [71, 73]. Breastfeeding among HIV-infected women is uncommon in the US. Estimates of the proportion of HIV-infected women in the USA have ranged from 1%–3% before 1994 [74], and less than 1% in 1994 or later [75]. HIV-infected mothers are significantly less likely to breastfeed their children if they are aware of their infection status before delivery, highlighting the need for access to prenatal care and HIV counseling and testing [74].

However, complete avoidance of breastfeeding is not feasible in many resource-poor settings, for reasons including the cost associated with procurement of replacement feeding, the stigma associated with not breastfeeding, and the potential morbidity and mortality associated with replacement feeding. Even in the Nairobi clinical trial of breastfeeding versus formula feeding [44], in which one of the enrollment criteria was access to municipal-treated water, the two groups of children (those whose mothers were randomized to breastfeeding and those whose mothers were randomized to formula feeding) experienced similar rates of mortality during the first 2 years of life [76]. Assessment of the feasibility of complete avoidance of breastfeeding or of early weaning involves consideration of an individual woman's situation and local circumstances. The World Health Organization recommends that HIV-infected women who decide to not breastfeed their children, or who decide to wean their children from breast milk early, should receive specific guidance and support during at least the first 2 years of their children's lives to assure adequate replacement feeding [77].

Since complete avoidance of breastfeeding or early weaning may not be possible in many settings, it is extremely important to develop and implement culturally appropriate interventions to prevent breast milk transmission of HIV in resource-poor settings [77]. Further, in light of the evidence of the association of maternal breast pathologies and breastfeeding transmission, the WHO recommends that HIV-infected women who breastfeed should receive education and counseling to assure good breastfeeding technique to decrease the risk of development of such conditions, and if such conditions arise, they should be treated as quickly and completely as possible [77]. Similarly, oral candidiasis in children should be treated promptly.

Cesarean section before labor and ruptured membranes

Subsequent to the publication of studies demonstrating the efficacy of cesarean section before labor and delivery for the prevention of MTCT [42], and indicating an association between mode of delivery and transmission remained among HIV-infected women receiving antiretroviral therapy (ART) (most likely zidovudine prophylaxis) [41], the American College of Obstetricians and Gynecologists [78] and the US Public Health Service [79] issued recommendations that cesarean section, as an intervention to prevent transmission, should be discussed and recommended for women with peripheral blood viral loads greater than 1000 copies/ml irrespective of receipt of ART. Cesarean delivery for the prevention of MTCT of HIV has been performed with increasing frequency in clinical centers in the USA over the past several years [80]. As noted previously, cesarean delivery as an intervention to prevent MTCT of HIV is generally not feasible in resource-poor settings because of the lack of a skilled attendant during labor and other reasons.

In settings where adequate staffing and infrastructure exist, issues that have been raised regarding use of cesarean section as an intervention to prevent transmission include concerns regarding its effectiveness among women with low viral loads or who are receiving potent ART, potentially increased maternal and infant morbidity associated with surgical delivery in populations of HIV-infected women, and the risk of health care worker infection associated with surgical delivery. Despite the conservative wording of US recommendations [78, 79], more recent data suggest a persistent effect of cesarean section delivery even among those HIV-infected pregnant women with viral loads of less than 1000 copies/ml [21, 81–84]. It has been estimated that the rate of

MTCT of HIV would have to be extremely low before cesarean section would no longer be cost effective in the USA and similar settings [85].

The potential benefit of cesarean section before labor and ruptured membranes for prevention of MTCT of HIV must be weighed against possible deleterious effects of surgical delivery for the mother, for the infant, and for the obstetrician [86–88]. Cesarean delivery may be associated with a slightly increased risk of postpartum morbidity among HIV-infected women compared to uninfected women, but assessment of currently available data suggest postpartum morbidity rates among HIV-infected women are not sufficiently frequent or severe to outweigh the potential benefit of cesarean section for the prevention of MTCT of HIV [79]. There are no published data regarding the risk of neonatal morbidity according to HIV-infected women's mode of delivery. Finally, although we know the risk must be extremely small, there are essentially no data regarding the relative risk of accidental acquisition of HIV infection by obstetricians or other health care workers according to mode of delivery [88].

Antiretroviral transmission prophylaxis and antiretroviral treatment of HIV-infected pregnant women

Shortly after the release of the results of ACTG 076 [9], the US Public Health Service issued guidelines regarding the use of zidovudine for perinatal HIV transmission prophylaxis [89]. Zidovudine prophylaxis has played a central role in the prevention of MTCT in resource-rich settings for the past several years [64].

More recently, an increasing number of HIV-infected women are receiving combination ART, including HAART, for their own health, including women in North America [8]. Guidelines for initiation of ART in adults and adolescents have been developed by several groups, including the US Public Health Service [90]. Criteria for initiation of ART according to these guidelines include: symptomatic HIV disease, CD4+ lymphocyte count of 350 cells/mm^3 or less, plasma HIV RNA levels over 55 000 copies/ml. In addition, guidelines more specifically focused on the use of antiretroviral drugs in pregnant women have been developed by the US Public Health Service [79], the British HIV Association [91], and the European Consensus Panel [92]. These guidelines provide generally similar recommendations, although cesarean section before labor and ruptured membranes is emphasized to a greater extent in the British and European guidelines as compared to the US guidelines.

The US Public Health Service guidelines [79] address different groups of HIV-infected women and their infants (Table 4.5). Specifically, the groups addressed are those women who have not received prior ART, those women who are already receiving ART during the current pregnancy, those women in labor who have not received therapy previously, and infants born to mothers who have received no ART during the antepartum or intrapartum periods.

Guidelines for initiation of ART in adults and adolescents also have been developed by the World Health Organization [93]. These guidelines address initiation of therapy if CD4+ lymphocyte testing is or is not available: if CD4 testing is available, initiation

Table 4.5. Recommendations for antiretroviral prophylaxis to prevent MTCT of HIV: according to timing of maternal presentation

Time period at presentation	Previous antiretroviral therapy	Recommendation	Comment/alternatives
Antepartum	No	Women should receive at least the three-part ACTG 076 regimen: Mother: ZDV 100 mg po 5 times per day beginning at 14–34 weeks gestation, 2 mg/kg IV over a one hour period, then 1 mg/kg per hour until delivery Infant: ZDV 2 mg/kg po q 6 hours for 6 weeks, beginning 8–12 hours after birth	• Acceptable alternatives to the maternal regimen in the clinical trial (100 mg orally five times daily) are oral zidovudine administered as 200 mg three times daily or 300 mg twice daily. Combining this zidovudine prophylactic regimen with additional antiretroviral drugs for treatment of the mother's HIV infection is recommended for women whose clinical, immunologic, or virologic status requires treatment or who have peripheral blood viral loads of over 1000 copies/mL. • Alternatives to the ACTG 076 prophylactic regimen (prophylactic regimen initiated during the antepartum period) are listed in Table 4.2: ○ Mother: ZDV 300 mg po BID from 36 weeks gestation, q 3 hours from onset of labor until delivery [10, 11] ○ Mother: ZDV 300 mg po BID from 36–38 weeks gestation, 600 mg × 1 at onset of labor, 300 mg po BID for 7 days after delivery [12] ○ Mother: ZDV 300 mg po BID until onset of labor, then 300 mg po q 3 hours until delivery beginning at 28 weeks gestation; Infant 2 mg/kg po q 6 hours for 3 days (6 weeks of infant ZDV if maternal ZDV initiated at/after 35 weeks) [14]

| Antepartum | Yes | Women should continue therapy if the pregnancy is identified after the first trimester. ZDV should be a component of the antepartum regimen after the first trimester if possible. Irrespective of the antepartum regimen, intrapartum and infant ZDV as per the ACTG 076 regimen is recommended. [Mother: ZDV 2 mg/kg IV over a 1-hour period, then 1 mg/kg per hour until delivery Infant: ZDV 2 mg/kg po q 6 hours for 6 weeks, beginning 8–12 hours after birth | ○ Mother: ZDV/3TC 300 mg/150 mg po BID from 36 weeks gestation; ZDV 300 mg × 1 after onset of labor, then 300 mg po q 3 hours until delivery; 3TC 150 mg × 1 at onset of labor, then 150 mg po q 12 hours until delivery; ZDV/3TC 300/150 mg po BID for 1 week; Infant: ZDV 4 mg/kg with 3TC 2 mg/kg po BID for week [PETRA 2002, Arm A]

○ Mother: ZDV po BID beginning at 28 weeks gestation, ZDV 300 mg po q 3 hours from onset of labor until delivery, with or without NVP 200 mg po × 1 at the onset of labor; infant: ZDV 2 mg/kg po q 6 hours for 1 week, with or without NVP 6 mg po × 1 within 48–72 hours after birth

• See below for alternative intrapartum and postnatal regimens. |

(cont.)

Table 4.5. (*cont.*)

Time period at presentation	Previous antiretroviral therapy	Recommendation	Comment/alternatives
Intrapartum	No	Women/infants should receive at least the intrapartum/postnatal components of the ACTG 076 regimen: Mother: ZDV 2 mg/kg IV over a 1-hour period, then 1 mg/kg per hour until delivery Infant: ZDV 2 mg/kg po q 6 hours for 6 weeks, beginning 8–12 hours after birth	• Mother: NVP 200 mg po × 1 at onset of labor; Infant: NVP 2 mg/kg within 48–72 hours of birth [102] • Mother: ZDV 300 mg × 1 after onset of labor, then 300 mg po q 3 hours until delivery; 3TC 150 mg × 1 at onset of labor, then 150 mg po q 12 hours until delivery; ZDV/3TC 300/150 mg po BID for 1 week; Infant: ZDV 4 mg/kg with 3TC 2 mg/kg po BID for one week [16, Arm B] • Intrapartum ZDV administered intravenously, followed by 6 weeks of oral ZDV to the infant, combined with one dose of ZVP at the onset of the labor and one dose of –ZVP to the infant at 48–72 hours after birth (intrapartum and infant components of the ACTG 076 regimen, combined with the HIVNET 012 regimen) [14]
Postnatal	No (infant born to mother who did not receive any antiretroviral therapy during the antepartum or intrapartum periods)	Postnatal component of the ACTG 076 regimen: Infant: ZDV 2 mg/kg po q 6 hours for 6 weeks, beginning 8–12 hours after birth	The efficacy of administering a combination of antiretroviral drugs to the infant for prevention of transmission is under study, and the efficacy is not known at this time.

of ART is recommended for those with WHO Stage IV disease; those with WHO stage III disease and a CD4+ cell count below 350/mm³; and those with Stage I and II disease and a CD4+ cell count below 200/mm³. If CD4 testing is unavailable, initiation of ART is recommended for those with WHO Stage III or IV disease and those with WHO Stage II or III disease, if the total lymphocyte count is below 1200/mm³. The use of antiretroviral drugs for treatment of HIV-infected pregnant women and for perinatal transmission prophylaxis in resource-poor settings is currently quite limited in terms of the overall, global need. Hopefully, with increasing availability of drugs, as well as the infrastructure and staffing for the management of HIV-infected individuals, including pregnant women, this will change.

Important issues to address regarding the use of antiretroviral drugs in general, and their use among pregnant women and infants especially, are the drugs' known toxicities and potential adverse effects, which can affect patients' adherence to the drugs. In turn, poor adherence can facilitate the emergence of antiretroviral drug resistance. Both the known or potential adverse effects of antiretroviral drug use among pregnant women and their infants, and antiretroviral drug resistance as it relates to prevention of MTCT of HIV, have been reviewed in detail [94, 95]. Data from Thailand suggested women who receive intrapartum NVP may be less likely to achieve virologic suppression with subsequent treatment regimens containing NVP [96]. However, more recent data indicate receipt of single-dose NVP does not affect subsequent treatment success if treatment is initiated 6 months or more after delivery [97]. Additional studies are planned or under way.

Potential safety problems related to antiretroviral prophylaxis for prevention of MTCT can be categorized as follows [94]: fetal toxicity, resulting in adverse pregnancy outcomes such as low birth weight, preterm delivery, congenital anomalies, and fetal/neonatal death; short-term adverse effects on the mother and on the infant, including laboratory abnormalities (e.g., hematologic abnormalities or other laboratory abnormalities suggesting liver or other organ dysfunction) and clinical abnormalities (e.g., rash or other morbidity, mortality); long-term adverse consequences for the child, including mitochondrial toxicity resulting in organ damage or death and development of cancer; and long-term adverse effects on the mother and on the child who becomes infected despite interventions to prevent MTCT, such as more rapid disease progression or development of resistance subsequent to receipt of perinatal transmission prophylaxis with antiretroviral drug(s). Although follow-up of exposed mothers and children should be performed to detect short- and long-term consequences of such exposure, the available data suggest that adverse effects of exposure to antiretroviral drugs for prevention of MTCT are minimal.

Limited data exist regarding antiretroviral prophylaxis regimens and the development of resistance. The US Public Health Service guidelines [79] recommend resistance testing for the same indications in pregnant women as for non-pregnant adults, i.e., acute infection, viral failure or suboptimal viral Supresion or a high likelihood of having resistant. However, other groups recommend resistance testing for all pregnant women with detectable HIV RNA levels, irrespective of previous receipt of antiretroviral drug(s), in order to maximize the response to ART [98, 99]. Although MTCT virus resistant HIV has been reported [100], it is unknown whether the presence of HIV resistance mutations increases the risk of MTCT. Therefore, it remains controversial whether pregnancy represents a specific indication for resistance testing.

Conclusions

The field of prevention of MTCT is changing rapidly. For those countries with greater resources and a lower disease burden, utilization of currently available interventions and combination ART to decrease maternal viral load and to provide pre- and post exposure prophylaxis, has resulted in low transmission rates. However, there are ongoing needs. These needs are: to make interventions and therapy more widely available, to address potential problems with existing interventions (e.g., drug toxicity, antiretroviral resistance, postpartum and neonatal morbidity related to surgical delivery), to develop new and better interventions (e.g., passive and active immunization against HIV [101, 102], and to emphasize primary prevention. However, the great majority of mothers and children affected by HIV in the world reside in those countries with fewer resources with which to fight the disease. In these settings, there is an urgent need to implement known efficacious interventions, to incorporate prevention of MTCT into overall maternal–child health programs, to develop new and better (and simpler, cheaper, and more feasible) interventions, especially with regard to transmission through breastfeeding, and to emphasize primary prevention. Therefore, despite successes in the prevention of MTCT of HIV over the past several years, significant clinical and public health challenges exist.

REFERENCES
1. UNAIDS. AIDS Epidemic Update: December 2003 (Available at www.unaids.org).
2. Kourtis, A. P., Bulterys, M., Nesheim, S. R., Lee, F. K. Understanding the timing of HIV transmission from mother to infant. *J. Am. Med. Assoc.* 2001;**285**:709–712.
3. Working Group on Mother-to-Child Transmission of HIV. Rates of mother-to-child transmission of HIV-1 in Africa, America, and Europe: results from 13 perinatal studies. *J. Acquir. Immune Defic. Syndr. Hum. Retrovirol.* 1995;**8**:506–510.
4. Fowler, M. G., Simonds, R. J., Roongpisuthipong, A. Update on perinatal HIV transmission. *Pediatr. Clin. North Am.* 2000;**47**:21–38.
5. Contopoulos-Ioannidis, D. G., Ioannidis, J.P.A. Maternal cell-free viremia in the natural history of perinatal HIV-1 transmission. *J. Acquir. Immune Defic. Syndr.* 1998;**18**: 126–135.
6. Mofenson, L. M., Lambert, J. S., Stiehm, E. R. *et al.* Risk factors for perinatal transmission of human immunodeficiency virus type 1 in women treated with zidovudine. Pediatric AIDS Clinical Trials Group Study 185 Team. *N. Engl. J. Med.* 1999;**341**:385–393.

7. Cooper, E. R., Charurat, M., Mofenson, L. *et al.* Combination antiretroviral strategies for the treatment of pregnant HIV-1-infected women and prevention of perinatal HIV-1 transmission. *J. Acquir. Immune Defic. Syndr.* 2002;**29**:484–494.

8. Shapiro, D., Tuomala, R., Pollack, H. *et al.* Mother-to-child HIV transmission risk according to antiretroviral therapy, mode of delivery, and viral load in 2895 U.S. women (PACTG 367). Eleventh Conference on Retroviruses and Opportunistic Infections (February 2004; San Francisco, CA.), Program and Abstracts. (Abstract S-80).

9. Connor, E. M., Sperling, R. S., Gelber, R. *et al.* Reduction of maternal–infant transmission of human immunodeficiency virus type 1 with zidovudine treatment. *N. Engl. J. Med.* 1994;**331**:1173–1180.

10. Shaffer, N., Chuachoowong, R., Mock, P. A. *et al.* Short-course zidovudine for perinatal HIV-1 transmission in Bangkok, Thailand: a randomised controlled trial. *Lancet* 1999;**353**:773–780.

11. Wiktor, S. Z., Ekpini, E., Karon, J. M. *et al.* Short-course zidovudine for prevention of mother-to-child transmission of HIV-1 in Abidjan, Cote d'Ivoire: a randomised trial. *Lancet* 1999;**353**:781–785.

12. Dabis, F., Msellati, P., Meda, N. *et al.* 6-month efficacy, tolerance and acceptability of a short regimen of oral zidovudine to reduce vertical transmission of HIV in breastfed children in Cote d'Ivoire and Burkina Faso: a double-blind placebo-controlled multicentre trial. *Lancet* 1999;**353**:786–792.

13. Leroy, V., Karon, J. M., Alioum, A. *et al.* Twenty-four month efficacy of a maternal short-course zidovudine regimen to prevent mother-to-child transmission of HIV-1 in West Africa. *AIDS* 2002;**16**:631–641.

14. Lallemant, M., Jourdain, G., Le Coeur, S., *et al.* A trial of shortened zidovudine regimens to prevent mother-to-child transmission of human immunodeficiency virus type 1. *N. Engl. J. Med.* 2000;**353**:982–991.

15. Jackson, J.B., Musoke, P., Fleming, T. *et al.* Intrapartum and neonatal single-dose nevirapine compared with zidovudine for prevention of mother-to-child transmission of HIV-1 in Kampala, Uganda: 18-month follow-up of the HIVNET 012 randomised trial. *Lancet* 2003;**362**:859–863.

16. The Petra study team. Efficacy of three short-course regimens of zidovudine and lamivudine in preventing early and late transmission of HIV-1 from mother to child in Tanzania, South Africa, and Uganda (Petra study): a randomized, double-blind, placebo-controlled trial. *Lancet* 2002;**359**:1178–1186.

17. Moodley, D., Moodley, J., Coovadia, H. *et al.*, for the South African Intrapartum Nevirapine Trial (SAINT) Investigators. A multicenter randomized controlled trial of nevirapine versus a combination of zidovudine and lamivudine to reduce intrapartum and early postpartum mother-to-child transmission of human immunodeficiency virus type 1. *J. Infect. Dis.* 2003;**187**:725–735.

18. Dorenbaum, A., Cunningham, C. K., Gelber, R. D. *et al.* Two-dose intrapartum/newborn nevirapine and standard antiretroviral therapy to reduce perinatal HIV transmission: a randomized trial. *J. Am. Med. Assoc.* 2002;**288**:189–198.

19. Lallemant, M., Jourdain, G., Le Coeur, S., *et al.* Single-dose perinatal nevirapine plus standard zidovudine to prevent mother-to-child transmission of HIV-1 in Thailand. *N. Engl. J. Med.* 2004;**351**:217–228.

20. Sperling, R. S., Shapiro, D. E., Coombs, R. W. *et al.* Maternal viral load, zidovudine treatment, and the risk of transmission of human immunodeficiency virus type 1 from mother to infant. *N. Engl. J. Med.* 1996;**335**:1621–1629.

21. Ioannidis, J. P. A., Abrams, E. J., Ammann, A. *et al.* Perinatal transmission of human immunodeficiency virus type 1 by pregnant women with RNA virus loads <1000 copies/ml. *J. Infect. Dis.* 2001;**183**:539–545.

22. Wade, N. A., Birkhead, G. S., Warren, B. L. *et al.* Abbreviated regimens of zidovudine prophylaxis and perinatal transmission of the human immunodeficiency virus. *N. Engl. J. Med.* 1998;**339**:1409–1414.

23. Wade, N. A., Birkhead, G. S., French, P. T. Short courses of zidovudine and perinatal transmission of HIV [letter] *N. Engl. J. Med.* 1999;**340**:1042–1043.

24. Chuachoowong, R., Shaffer, N., Siriwasin, W. *et al.* Short-course antenatal zidovudine reduces both cervicovaginal human immunodeficiency virus type 1 RNA levels and risk of perinatal transmission. *J. Infect. Dis.* 2000;**181**:99–106.

25. John, G. C., Nduati, R. W., Mbori-Ngacha, D. A. *et al.* Correlates of mother-to-child human immunodeficiency virus type 1 (HIV-1) transmission: association with maternal plasma HIV-1 RNA load, genital HIV-1 DNA shedding, and breast infections. *J. Infect. Dis.* 2001;**182**;206–212.

26. Mandelbrot, L., Msellati, P., Meda, N. *et al.* 15 month follow up of African children following vaginal cleansing with benzalkonium chloride of their HIV infected mothers during late pregnancy and delivery. *Sex. Transm. Infect.* 2002;**78**:267–270.

27. Biggar, R. J., Miotti, P. G., Taha, T. E. *et al.* Perinatal intervention trial in Africa: effect of a birth canal cleansing intervention to prevent HIV transmission. *Lancet* 1996;**347**:1647–1650.

28. Gaillard, P., Mwanyumba, F., Verhofstede, C. *et al.* Vaginal lavage with chlorhexidine during labor to reduce mother to child HIV transmission: clinical trial in Mombasa, Kenya. *AIDS* 2001;**15**:389–396.

29. Wilson, C., Gray, G., Read, J. S. *et al.* Tolerance and safety of different concentrations of chlorhexidine for peripartum vaginal and infant washes: HIVNET 025. *J. Acquir. Immune Defic. Syndr* 2004;**35**:138–143.

30. Semba, R. D., Kumwenda, N., Hoover, D. R. *et al.* Human immunodeficiency virus load in breast milk, mastitis, and mother-to-child transmission of human immunodeficiency virus type 1. *J. Infect. Dis.* 1999;**180**:93–98.

31. Richardson, B., Stewart-John, G. C., Hughes, J. P. *et al.* Breast-milk infectivity in human immunodeficiency virus type 1-infected mothers. *J. Infect. Dis.* 2003;**187**: 736–740.

32. Nduati, R., Richardson, B. A., John, G. *et al.* Effect of breastfeeding on mortality among HIV-1 infected women: a randomised trial. *Lancet* 2001;**357**:1651–1655.

33. Coutsoudis, A., Coovadia, H., Pillay, K., Kuhn, L. Are HIV-infected women who breastfeed at increased risk of mortality? *AIDS* 2001;**15**:653–655.

34. The Breastfeeding and, International HIV Transmission Study (BHITS) Group. Mortality according to infant feeding modality among HIV-infected, breastfeeding women in sub-Saharan Africa. *J. Acquir. Immune Defic. Syndr.* 2005;**39**:430–438..

35. Gaillard, P., Fowler, M. G., Dabis, F. *et al.* Use of antiretroviral drugs to prevent HIV-1 transmission through breast-feeding: from animal studies to randomized clinical trials. *J. Acquir. Immune Defic. Syndr*. 2004; **35:** 178–187.

36. Krebs, F. C., Miller, S. R., Malamud, D., Howett, M. K., & Wigdahl, B. Inactivation of human immunodeficiency virus type 1 by nonoxynol-9, C31G, of an alkyl sulfate, sodium dodecyl sulfate. *Antiviral Res.* 1999;**43**:157–173.

37. Chantry, C. J., Morrison, P., Panchula, J. *et al*. Effects of lipolysis or heat treatment on HIV-1 provirus in breast milk. *J. Acquir. Immune. Defic. Syndr.* 2000; **24**:325–329.

38. Orloff, S. L., Wallingford, J. C., McDougal, J. S. Inactivation of human immunodeficiency virus type 1 in human milk: effects of intrinsic factors in human milk and of pasteuriza- tion. *J. Hum. Lact.* 1993;**9**:13–17.

39. Jeffery, B. S., Webber, L., Mokhondo, K. R., Erasmus, D. Determination of the effective- ness of inactivation of human immunodeficiency virus by Pretoria pasteurization. *J. Trop. Pediatr.* 2001;**47**:345–349.

40. The International Perinatal HIV Group. Duration of ruptured membranes and vertical transmission of HIV-1: a meta-analysis from fifteen prospective cohort studies. *AIDS* 2001;**15**:357–368.

41. The International Perinatal HIV Group. The mode of delivery and the risk of vertical transmission of human immunodeficiency virus type 1: a meta-analysis of 15 prospec- tive cohort studies. *N. Engl. J. Med.* 1999;**340**:977–987.

42. The European Mode of Delivery Collaboration. Elective caesarean section versus vaginal delivery in preventing vertical HIV-1 transmission: a randomised clinical trial. *Lancet* 1999;**353**:1035–1037.

43. The Breastfeeding and HIV International Transmission Study Group. Late postnatal transmission of HIV-1 in breast-fed childern: an individual patient data meta-analysis. *J. Infect. Dis.* 2004; **189**: 2154–2166.

44. Nduati, R., John, G., Mbori-Ngacha, D. *et al*. Effect of breastfeeding and formula feeding on transmission of HIV-1: a randomized clinical trial. *J. Am. Med. Assoc.* 2000; **283**:1167– 1174.

45. Piwoz, E.G., Kasonde, P., Vwalika, C. *et al*. The feasibility of early rapid breastfeeding cessation to reduce postnatal transmission of HIV in Lusaka, Zambia. 14th International Conference on AIDS (Barcelona, Spain; July 7–12, 2002), Program and Abstracts, abstract TuPeF5393.

46. Semba, R. D., Miotti, P. G., Chiphangwi, J. D. *et al*. Maternal vitamin A deficiency and mother-to-child transmission of HIV-1. *Lancet* 1994;**343**:1593–1597.

47. Kumwenda, N., Miotti, P. G., Taha, T. E. *et al*. Antenatal vitamin A supplementation increases birthweight and decreases anemia, but does not prevent HIV transmission or decrease mortality in infants born to HIV-infected women in Malawi. *Clin. Infect. Dis.* 2002;**35**:618–624.

48. Coutsoudis, A., Pillay, K., Spooner, E. *et al*. Randomized trial testing the effect of vitamin A supplementation on pregnancy outcomes and early mother-to-child HIV-1 transmis- sion in Durban, South Africa. *AIDS* 1999;**13**:1517–1524.

49. Fawzi, W. W., Msamanga, G. I., Hunter, D. *et al*. Randomized trial of vitamin supplements in relation to transmission of HIV-1 through breastfeeding and early child mortality. *AIDS* 2002;**16**:1935–1944.

50. St. Louis, M., Kamenga, M., Brown, C. *et al*. Risk of perinatal HIV-1 transmission according to maternal immunologic, virologic, and placental factors. *J. Am. Med. Assoc.* 1993;**269**:2853–2859.

51. Temmerman, M., O'Nyong's, A., Bwayo J. *et al.* Risk factors for mother-to-child transmission of human immunodeficiency virus-1 infection. *Am. J. Obstet. Gynecol.* 1995;**172**:700–705.

52. Wabwire-Mangen, F., Gray, R. H., Mmiro, F. A. *et al.* Placental membrane inflammation and risks of maternal-to-child transmission of HIV-1 in Uganda. *AIDS* 1999;**22**:379–385.

53. Kafulafula, G., Martinson, F., Msamanga, G., Sinkala, M., and the HIVNET 024 Team Phase III Trial of Antibiotics to Reduce Chorioamnionitis-Associated MTCT of HIV. *XV International AIDS Conference (Bangkok, Thailand; July 11–16, 2004) Program and Abstracts* (abstract ThOrC1418).

54. Coutsoudis, A., Pillay, K., Kuhn, L., Spooner, E., Tsai, W. Y., Coovadia, H. M. Method of feeding and transmission of HIV-1 from mothers to children by 15 months of age: prospective cohort study from Durban, South Africa. *AIDS* 2001;**15**:379–387.

55. Iliff, P. J., Piwoz, E. G., Tavengwa, N. V. *et al.* Early exclusive breastfeeding reduces the risk of postnatal HIV-1 transmission and increases HIV-free survival. AIDS. 2005; **19**(7):699–708.

56. Haider, R., Ashworth, A., Kabir, I., Huttly, S. R. Effect of community-based peer counsellors on exclusive breastfeeding practices in Dhaka, Bangladesh: a randomised controlled trial. *Lancet* 2000;**356**:1643–1647.

57. Van de Perre, P., Hitimana, D. G., Simonon, A. *et al.* Postnatal transmission of HIV-1 associated with breast abscess. *Lancet* 1992;**339**:1490–1491.

58. Ekpini, E. R., Wiktor, S. Z., Satten, G. A. *et al.* Late postnatal mother-to-child transmission of HIV-1 in Abidjan, Côte d'Ivoire. *Lancet* 1997;**349**:1054–1059.

59. Embree, J. E., Njenga, S., Datta, P. *et al.* Risk factors for postnatal mother-child transmission of HIV-1. *AIDS* 2000;**14**:2535–2541.

60. Tavengwa, N., Piwoz, E., Gavin, L., Zunguza, C., Iliff, P., Humphrey, J. Development, implementation, and evaluation of a program to counsel women about infant feeding in the context of HIV. *14th International Conference on AIDS* (Barcelona, Spain; July 7–12, 2002), Program and Abstracts, abstract MoPeF3881.

61. UNAIDS. 2004 Report on the Global AIDS epidemic. (http://www.unaids.org)

62. Read, J. S. Preventing mother-to-child transmission of HIV: the USA experience. *Prenat. Neonat. Med.* 1999;**4**:391–397.

63. Centers for Disease Control and Prevention. U.S. Public Health Service recommendations for human immunodeficiency virus counseling and voluntary testing for pregnant women. *Morb. Mortal. Wkly Rep.* 1995;**44** (RR-7):1–15.

64. Lindegren, M. L., Byers, R. H. Jr, Thomas, P. *et al.* Trends in perinatal transmission of HIV/AIDS in the United States. *J. Am. Med. Assoc.* 1999;282:531–538.

65. Centers for Disease Control and Prevention. Entry into prenatal care – United States, 1989–1997. *Morb. Mortal. Wkly Rep.* 2000;**49** (18):393–398.

66. Mills, W. A., Martin, D. L., Bertrand, J. R., Belongia, E. A. Physicians' practices and opinions regarding prenatal screening for human immunodeficiency virus and other sexually transmitted diseases. *Sex. Transm. Dis.* 1998;**25**:169–175.

67. Phillips KA, Morrison KR, Sonnad SS, Bleecker T. HIV counseling and testing of pregnant women and women of childbearing age by primary care providers: self-reported beliefs and practices. *Acquir. Immune Defic. Hum. Retrovirol.* 1997;**14**:174–178.

68. Institute of Medicine (IOM). (1998) *Reducing the Odds: Preventing Perinatal Transmission of* HIV *in the United States.* Washington, DC: National Academy Press.

69. Centers for Disease Control and Prevention. Advancing HIV prevention: new strategies for a changing epidemic – United States, 2003. *Morb. Mortal. Wkly Rep.* 2003;**52** (15):329–332.

70. Cartoux, M., Msellati, P., Meda, N. *et al.* Attitude of pregnant women toward HIV testing in Abidjan, Cote d'Ivoire and Bobo-Dioulasso, Burkina Faso. *AIDS* 1998;**12**:2337–2344.

71. Centers for Disease Control. Current recommendations for assisting in the prevention of perinatal transmission of human T-lymphotropic virus type III/lymphadenopathy-associated virus and acquired immunodeficiency syndrome. *Morb. Mortal. Wkly Rep.* 1985;**34**:721–726.

72. American Academy of Pediatrics, Committee on Pediatric AIDS. Human milk, breast-feeding, and transmission of human immunodeficiency virus in the United States. *Pediatrics.* 1995;**96**:977–979.

73. Read, J. S., and the Committee on Pediatric AIDS, American Academy of Pediatrics. Human milk, breastfeeding, and transmission of human immunodeficiency virus in the United States. *Pediatrics* 2003;**112**:1196–1205.

74. Bertolli, J. M., Hsu, H., Frederick, T. *et al.* Breastfeeding among HIV-infected women, Los Angeles and Massachusetts, 1988–1993. *11th World AIDS Conference*, Vancouver, 1996. Abstract We.C.3583.

75. Simonds, R. J., Steketee, R., Nesheim, S. *et al.* Impact of zidovudine use on risk and risk factors for perinatal transmission of HIV. *AIDS* 1998;**12**:301–308.

76. Mbori-Ngacha, D., Nduati, R., John, G. *et al.* Morbidity and mortality in breastfed and formula-fed infants of HIV-1-infected women: a randomized clinical trial. *J. Am. Med. Assoc.* 2001;**286**:2413–2420.

77. World Health Organization. Report of the WHO Technical Consultation on Behalf of the UNFPA/UNICEF/WHO/UNAIDS Inter-Agency Task Team on Mother-to-Child Transmission of HIV, October 11–13, 2000. New data on the prevention of mother-to-child transmission of HIV and their policy implications. Geneva, Switzerland: WHO; January 15, 2001. (Available at www.unaids.org/publications/documents/mtct/index.html).

78. American College of Obstetricians and Gynecologists. Scheduled cesarean delivery and the prevention of vertical transmission of HIV infection. ACOG Committee Opinion Number 234. Washington, D.C.: ACOG, May 2000.

79. Centers for Disease Control and Prevention. US Public Health Service Task Force recommendations for the use of antiretroviral drugs in pregnant women infected with HIV-1 for maternal health and for reducing perinatal HIV-1 transmission in the United States. MMWR 1998;47 (No. RR-2): 1–30. (Most recent revision of the guidelines available at http://AIDS Info.nih.gov.).

80. Dominguez, K. L., Lindegren, M. L., D'Almada, P. J. *et al.* Increasing trend of Cesarean deliveries in HIV-infected women in the United States from 1994 to 2000. *J. Acquir. Immune Defic. Syndr.* 2003;**33**:232–238.

81. Shaffer, N., Roongpisuthipong, A., Siriwasin, W. *et al.* Maternal viral load and perinatal HIV-1 subtype E transmission, Thailand. *J. Infect. Dis.* 1999;**179**:590–599.

82. The European Collaborative Study. Maternal viral load and vertical transmission of HIV-1: an important factor but not the only one. *AIDS* 1999;**13**:1377–1385.

83. Fiscus, S., Adimora, A, Schoenbach *et al*. Elective c-section may provide additional benefit in conjunction with maternal combination antiretroviral therapy to reduce perinatal HIV transmission. *XIII World AIDS Conference* (July 2000, Durban, South Africa), Abstract WePpC1388.

84. European Collaborative Study. Mother-to-child transmission of HIV infection: the era of highly active antiretroviral therapy. *Clin. Infect. Dis.* 2005;**40**:458–465.

85. Mrus, J. M., Goldie, S. J., Weinstein, M. C., Tsevat, J. The cost-effectiveness of elective Cesarean delivery for HIV-infected women with detectable HIV RNA during pregnancy. *AIDS* 2000;**14**:2543–2552.

86. Read, J. S., Cesarean section delivery to prevent vertical transmission of human immunodeficiency virus type 1: associated risks and other considerations. *Ann. NY Acad. Sci.* 2000;**918**:115–121.

87. Read, J. S. Preventing mother to child transmission of HIV: the role of caesarean section. *Sex. Transm. Infect.* 2000;**76**:231–232.

88. Ippolito, G., Puro, V., Heptonstall, J., Jagger, J., De Carli, G., Petrosillo, N. Occupational human immunodeficiency virus infection in health care workers: worldwide cases through September 1997. *Clin. Infect. Dis.* 1999;**28**:365–383.

89. Center for Disease Control and Prevention. Recommendations of the US Public Health Service Task Force on the use of zidovudine to reduce perinatal transmission of human immunodeficiency virus. *Morb. Mortal Wkly Rep.* 1994;**43** (RR11):1–20.

90. Centers for Disease Control and Prevention. Guidelines for the use of antiretroviral agents in HIV-infected adults and adolescents. *MMWR* 1998;**47**: 47 (No. RR-5) 43–82 (updates available at http://AIDSInfo.nih.gov).

91. Lyall, E.G.H., Blott, M., de Ruiter, A. *et al*. Guidelines for the management of HIV infection in pregnant women and the prevention of mother-to-child transmission. *HIV Med.* 2001;**2**:314–334.

92. Newell, M.-L., Rogers, M. Pregnancy and HIV infection: a European Consensus on management. *AIDS* 2002;**16** (Suppl. 2):S1–S18.

93. World Health Organization. Scaling up antiretroviral therapy in resource-limited settings: treatment guidelines for a public health approach (2003 revision). (http://www.who.int/3by5/publications/documents/arv˙guidelines/en).

94. Mofenson, L. M., Munderi, P. Safety of antiretroviral prophylaxis of perinatal transmission for HIV-infected pregnant women and their infants. *AIDS* 2002;**30**:200–215.

95. Nolan, M., Fowler, M. G., Mofenson, L. M. Antiretroviral prophylaxis of perinatal HIV-1 transmission and the potential impact of antiretroviral resistance. *AIDS* 2002;**30**:216–229.

96. Jourdain, G., Ngo-Giang-Huong, N., Le Coeur, S., *et al*. Intrapartum exposure to neivrapine and subsequent maternal responses to nevirapine-base antiretroviral therapy. *N. Engl. J. Med.* 2004;**351**:229–240.

97. Lockman, S., Smeaton, L. M., Shapiro, R. L. *et al*. Maternal and infant response to nevirapine (NVP)-based antiretroviral treatment (ART) following peripartum single-does NVP or placebo (Plc.) Program and Abstracts of the 43rd Annual Meeting of IDSA (San Francisco; October 6–9, 2005); abstract LB-5.

98. Hirsch, M. S., Brun-Vézinet, F., Clotet, B. *et al*. Antiretroviral drug resistance testing in adults infected with human immunodeficiency virus type 1: 2003 recommendations of an International AIDS Society-USA panel. *Clin. Infect. Dis.* 2003;**37**:113–128.

99. The EuroGuidelines Group for HIV Resistance. Clinical and laboratory guidelines for the use of HIV-1 drug resistance testing as part of treatment management: recommendations for the European setting. *AIDS* 2001;**15**:309–320.

100. Johnson, V. A., Petropoulos, C. J., Woods, C. R. *et al.* Vertical transmission of multi-drug resistance human immunodeficiency virus type 1 (HIV-1) and continued evolution of drug resistance in an HIV-1-infected infant. *J. Infect. Dis.* 2001;**183**:1688–1693.

101. Guay, L. A., Musoke, P., Hom, D. L. *et al.* Phase I/II trial of HIV-1 hyperimmune globulin for the prevention of HIV-1 vertical transmission in Uganda. *AIDS* 2002;**16**:1391–1400.

102. Biberfeld, G., Buonaguro, F., Lindberg, A., de The, G., Yi, Z., Zetterstrom, R. Prospects of vaccination as a means of preventing mother-to-child transmission of HIV-1. *Acta Paediatr.* 2002;**91**:241–242.

5 Routine pediatric care

[1] **Elaine Abrams, MD,** [2] **Rachel Y. Moon, MD,**
[3] **Lisa-Gaye Robinson, MD,** [4] **Russell B. Van Dyke, MD**

[1] Department of Pediatrics, Harlem Hospital Center and College of Physicians and Surgeons,
Columbia University, New York, NY

[2] Division of General Pediatrics and Community Health, Children's National Medical Center,
Washington, DC

[3] Department of Pediatrics, Harlem Hospital Center and College of Physicians and Swgeons,
Columbia University, New York, NY

[4] Department of Pediatrics, Tulane University Health Sciences Center, New Orleans, LA

Introduction

HIV infection is a chronic illness with diverse clinical manifestations and psychosocial challenges. The routine care of HIV-infected children demands a dedicated multidisciplinary approach from a variety of health care professionals including medical sub-specialists, nurses, psychiatrists, psychologists, dentists, social workers and case managers. The HIV primary care provider, while ensuring health maintenance and preventing disease, must serve as the coordinator of an array of services crucial to the management of these children in the context of the family. Important management considerations attend the care of both HIV-exposed children and those children ultimately identified as HIV-infected.

Care of the HIV-exposed infant

Routine care for the infant born to an HIV-infected mother should begin well before the infant's birth. Clinicians should collaborate with the mother's primary care providers to minimize the risk of HIV transmission. Care of the infant after birth includes continued interventions to reduce the risk of HIV infection, as well as HIV diagnostic evaluations and routine infant care (Table 5.1). Care of the HIV-exposed newborn in the hospital begins with a thorough maternal history, including HIV disease status [HIV RNA concentration (viral load), CD4+ lymphocyte count, and HIV-related complications), receipt of interventions to prevent mother-to-child transmission (e.g.,

Handbook of Pediatric HIV Care, ed. Steven L. Zeichner and Jennifer S. Read.
Published by Cambridge University Press. © Cambridge University Press 2006.

antiretroviral prophylaxis, cesarean delivery before labor and before ruptured membranes), and history of other infections (e.g., syphilis, herpes simplex virus, hepatitis B and C, cytomegalovirus, toxoplasmosis, gonorrhea, or tuberculosis (TB)). Psychosocial issues that could affect the child (e.g., substance abuse, homelessness, mental illness, immigration status) should be identified in order to provide any necessary additional services.

Antiretroviral perinatal transmission prophylaxis

Antiretroviral prophylaxis, cesarean delivery before labor and before ruptured membranes, and avoidance of breastfeeding reduce the risk of mother-to-child transmission (MTCT) of HIV (see Chapter 4). In the USA, a 6-week course of oral zidovudine (ZDV) for infants of HIV-infected mothers is recommended [1], irrespective of the medical and surgical management of the mother during the antepartum and intrapartum periods. Therefore, all infants born to HIV-infected women should begin ZDV (2 mg/kg every 6 hours) prophylactic therapy as close to the time of birth as possible (preferably within 12 hours) [2, 3]. ZDV should be continued through the end of the sixth week of life unless the infant is identified as being infected, at which time it should be immediately discontinued (and the infant should be fully evaluated, see below) [4]. Mild reversible anemia is associated with ZDV prophylaxis in the newborn. Therefore, clinicians should check a hemogram at birth and at 2–4 weeks of age to monitor for anemia. The primary care provider should consider potential complications of antiretroviral exposure as an etiology for unexplained presenting signs and symptoms, especially those with characteristics of mitochrondrial dysfunction (see Chapter 13). Furthermore, the long-term side effects of in utero exposure to antiretroviral therapies have not been delineated. Therefore, it is important that the history of antiretroviral exposure remain in the child's medical record and that families understand the importance of this information. Long-term follow-up and surveillance studies continue to investigate whether there are long-term toxicities related to interventions to prevent MTCT of HIV.

HIV diagnostic evaluations

All infants born to HIV-infected women, or women whose HIV infection status is unknown, should be tested for HIV infection beginning at birth. Such diagnostic testing should be performed using a DNA polymerase chain reaction (PCR) assay. HIV RNA assays also can be used for diagnosis of HIV infection, though some studies have demonstrated that a low copy number may yield a false positive test during the early months of life [5, 6]. If the PCR test result at birth is negative, it should be repeated at two weeks and again at one month of age. If the one month result is negative, a final test should be repeated after four months of life. The infant can be considered definitively HIV-uninfected if there are at least two negative HIV virologic detection tests, with one test obtained at or after one month of age and the second test obtained at or after 4 months of age. It is unknown if and how routine maternal highly active

Table 5.1. Care of the HIV-exposed infant

Age	PHC[§]	Immunizations[¶]	Laboratory assays	ZDV prophylaxis[b]	TMP-SMZ prophylaxis
Birth	§	Hepatitis B (Hep B) #1	HIV DNA PCR[a]	Begin within 12 hours of birth	
2 weeks	§		HIV DNA PCR[a]		
4 weeks	§	Hep B # 2	HIV DNA PCR[a]		
6 weeks	§			↓	Begin[d]
2 months	§	DPT, HIB, IPV, Pneumococcal #1		Stop[c]	↓
4 months	§	DPT, HIB, IPV, Pneumococcal #2	HIV DNA PCR[a]		Stop[e]
6 months	§	DPT, HIB, Hep B, Pneumococcal #3 (*Influenza*)			
9 months	§				
12 months	§	MMR, varicella	Hemogram[f] Lead HIV ELISA[h]		
	TST[g]				

§ PHC = preventive health care. This includes all the elements of a comprehensive preventive care program recommended by the American Academy of Pediatrics (AAP) for all pediatric patients. All evaluations should include an interval history, assessment of growth and development, anticipatory guidance and recommended immunizations.

¶ The immunizations recommended in this table are for HIV-exposed infants who are immunologically normal.

[a] A positive test should be repeated immediately. In addition, a hemogram and lymphocyte subsets should be obtained at that time. Infants suspected of being exposed to a non-subtype-B HIV-1 virus (African or Asian origin) may require alternative testing (see text).

[b] Zidovudine (ZDV) prophylaxis should be started within 12 hours of birth irrespective of the medical and surgical management of the mother during the antepartum and intrapartum periods. Addition of supplementary antiretrovirals should only be done in conjunction with an expert in pediatric HIV.

[c] ZDV prophylaxis should be discontinued prior to 6 weeks if the infant has laboratory confirmation of HIV infection.

[d] Trimethoprim-sulfamethoxazole (TMP-SMZ) should be started prior to 6 weeks of life if the infant has laboratory confirmation of HIV infection and is older than 4 weeks of age.

[e] TMP-SMZ prophylaxis should only be discontinued when there is laboratory confirmation that the infant in not infected and is without clinical signs of HIV infection.

[f] A hemogram is recommended by the AAP for all children at 12 months of age.

[g] Tuberculin skin test.

[h] Median age at the time of loss of maternal HIV antibody is at 10 months of life. Documentation of two negative ELISAs to confirm an uninfected status remains a recommendation of the AAP. However, with the low transmission rates in the USA and some other countries, and the extremely low probability of infection with multiple negative PCR tests, this recommendation may no longer be warranted in the USA and similar settings.

antiretroviral therapy during pregnancy may affect the timing of detection of infant HIV infection.

The American Academy of Pediatrics currently recommends that all patients have HIV antibody tests to confirm absence of infection. The median age at the time of loss of maternal antibody is 10 months. An uninfected infant should no longer have detectable IgG antibody to HIV by 18 months of age. Given the low rate of mother-to-child transmission of HIV in North America, and the extremely low probability of HIV infection in a clinically well infant with negative PCR assay results, documentation of loss of maternal antibody may not be warranted [7]. However, parents may request that the test be done and some child welfare and foster care agencies continue to require follow-up antibody testing.

A positive HIV DNA PCR result in any infant should be repeated immediately. Positive results on two separate specimens, not including cord blood, represent definitive laboratory criteria for HIV infection. More than 95% of all HIV-infected infants test positive by 1 month of age [8]. It is important to note that infection with a non-B HIV subtype (e.g., in Africa and Asia) may not be recognized by the commercial HIV DNA PCR assays routinely available in the US. Infants born to HIV-infected mothers who could be infected with a non-B subtype may require testing using an alternative test, e.g., the branched-chain DNA (bDNA) test capable of detecting multiple subtypes (see Chapter 3). This testing should be done in consultation with an expert in pediatric HIV.

Routine infant care

Anticipatory guidance for the primary caretaker is an important component of the care of an HIV-exposed infant. The caretaker must be advised that it may take several months before the child can be determined to either be uninfected or infected. This often creates significant anxiety. Informing the child's caregiver of the rationale for perinatal HIV transmission prophylaxis with ZDV, as well as for immunizations and opportunistic infection prophylaxis, can be important in optimizing adherence to these necessary regimens. Caretaker also should be repeatedly educated about other aspects of HIV disease, including diagnosis, treatment, prognosis, and about signs of infection and symptoms that should cause them to seek immediate medical attention for the infant.

Immunizations

In the USA, routine pediatric immunizations should be given to all HIV-exposed children according to the schedule recommended by the Advisory Committee on Immunization Practices (ACIP) and the American Academy of Pediatrics (AAP) (Table 5.2) (9, 10). HIV-exposed children should not receive live virus or live bacteria vaccines, with the exception of measles-mumps-rubella (MMR) vaccine and varicella vaccine. The inactivated polio vaccine (IPV) should be given instead of the live oral polio vaccine (OPV) (Table 5.3).

Table 5.2. Recommended childhood and adolescent immunization schedule: United States, 2005

Vaccine ▼ / Age ▶	Birth	1 month	2 months	4 months	6 months	12 months	15 months	18 months	24 months	4–6 years	11–12 years	13–18 years
Hepatitis B[1]	HepB #1	HepB #2			HepB #3						HepB Series	
Diphtheria, Tetanus, Pertussis[2]			DTaP	DTaP	DTaP		DTaP	DTaP		DTaP	Td	Td
Haemophilus influenzae type b[3]			Hib	Hib	Hib	Hib						
Inactivated Poliovirus			IPV	IPV		IPV				IPV		
Measles, Mumps, Rubella[4]						MMR #1				MMR #2	MMR #2	MMR #2
Varicella[5]							Varicella			Varicella	Varicella	
Pneumococcal Conjugate[6]			PCV	PCV	PCV	PCV	PCV		PCV	PPV	PPV	
Influenza[7]						Influenza (Yearly)				Influenza (Yearly)	Influenza (Yearly)	
Hepatitis A[8]										Hepatitis A Series		

Vaccines below this line are for selected populations

■ Range of recommended ages
■ Preadolescent assessment
▨ Only if mother HBsAg(–)
■ Catch-up immunization

This schedule indicates the recommended ages for routine administration of currently licensed childhood vaccines, as of December 1, 2004, for children through age 18 years. Any dose not administered at the recommended age should be administered at any subsequent visit when indicated and feasible. ■ Indicates age groups that warrant special effort to administer these vaccines not previously administered. Additional vaccines may be licensed and recommended during the year. Licensed combination vaccines may be used whenever any components of the combination are indicated and other components of the vaccine

are not contraindicated. Providers should consult the manufacturers' package inserts for detailed recommendations. Clinically significant adverse events that follow immunization should be reported to the Vaccine Adverse Event Reporting System (VAERS). Guidance about how to obtain and complete a VAERS form is available at **www.vaers.org** or by telephone, **800-822-7967**.

The Childhood and Adolescent Immunization Schedule is approved by:
Advisory Committee on Immunization Practices www.cdc.gov/nip/acip
American Academy of Pediatrics www.aap.org
American Academy of Family Physicians www.aafp.org

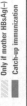

DEPARTMENT OF HEALTH AND HUMAN SERVICES
CENTERS FOR DISEASE CONTROL AND PREVENTION

Table 5.2. (*cont.*)

[1] **Hepatitis B (HepB) vaccine.** All infants should receive the first dose of HepB vaccine soon after birth and before hospital discharge; the first dose may also be administered by age 2 months if the mother is hepatitis B surface antigen (HBsAg) negative. Only monovalent HepB may be used for the birth dose. Monovalent or combination vaccine containing HepB may be used to complete the series. Four doses of vaccine may be administered when a birth dose is given. The second dose should be administered at least 4 weeks after the first dose, except for combination vaccines which cannot be administered before age 6 weeks. The third dose should be given at least 16 weeks after the first dose and at least 8 weeks after the second dose. The last dose in the vaccination series (third or fourth dose) should not be administered before age 24 weeks.

Infants born to HBsAg-positive mothers should receive HepB and 0.5 mL of hepatitis B immune globulin (HBIG) at separate sites within 12 hours of birth. The second dose is recommended at age 1–2 months. The final dose in the immunization series should not be administered before age 24 weeks. These infants should be tested for HBsAg and antibody to HBsAg (anti-HBs) at age 9–15 months.

Infants born to mothers whose HBsAg status is unknown should receive the first dose of the HepB series within 12 hours of birth. Maternal blood should be drawn as soon as possible to determine the mother's HBsAg status; if the HBsAg test is positive, the infant should receive HBIG as soon as possible (no later than age 1 week). The second dose is recommended at age 1–2 months. The last dose in the immunization series should not be administered before age 24 weeks.

[2] **Diphtheria and tetanus toxoids and acellular pertussis (DTaP) vaccine.** The fourth dose of DTaP may be administered as early as age 12 months, provided 6 months have elapsed since the third dose and the child is unlikely to return at age 15–18 months. The final dose in the series should be given at age ≥4 years. **Tetanus and diphtheria toxoids (Td)** is recommended at age 11–12 years if at least 5 years have elapsed since the last dose of tetanus and diphtheria toxoid-containing vaccine. Subsequent routine Td boosters are recommended every 10 years.

[3] **Haemophilus influenzae type b (Hib) conjugate vaccine.** Three Hib conjugate vaccines are licensed for infant use. If PRP-OMP (PedvaxHIB® or ComVax® [Merck]) is administered at ages 2 and 4 months, a dose at age 6 months is not required. DTaP/Hib combination products should not be used for primary immunization in infants at ages 2, 4 or 6 months but can be used as boosters after any Hib vaccine. The final close in the series should be administered at age ≥ 12 months.

4 **Measles, mumps, and rubella vaccine (MMR).** The second dose of MMR is recommended routinely at age 4–6 years but may be administered during any visit, provided at least 4 weeks have elapsed since the first dose and both doses are administered beginning at or after age 12 months. Those who have not previously received the second dose should complete the schedule by age 11–12 years.

5 **Varicella vaccine.** Varicella vaccine is recommended at any visit at or after age 12 months for susceptible children (i.e., those who lack a reliable history of chickenpox). Susceptible persons aged ≥13 years should receive 2 doses administered at least 4 weeks apart.

6 **Pneumococcal vaccine.** The heptavalent **pneumococcal conjugate vaccine (PCV)** is recommended for all children aged 2–23 months and for certain children aged 24–59 months. The final dose in the series should be given at age ≥12 months. **Pneumococcal polysaccharide vaccine (PPV)** is recommended in addition to PCV for certain high-risk groups. see *MMWR* 2000;49(No. RR-9):1–35.

7 **Influenza vaccine.** Influenza vaccine is recommended annually for children aged ≥6 months with certain risk factors (including, but not limited to, asthma, cardiac disease, sickle cell disease, human immunodeficiency virus [HIV], and diabetes), healthcare workers, and other persons (including household members) in close contact with persons in groups at high risk (see *MMWR* 2004;53;[RR-6];1–40). In addition, healthy children aged 6–23 months and dose contacts of healthy children aged 0–23 months are recommended to receive influenza vaccine because children in this age group are at substantially increased risk for influenza-related hospitalizations. For healthy persons aged 5–49 years, the intranasally administered live, attenuated influenza vaccine (LAIV) is an acceptable alternative to the intramuscular trivalent inactivated influenza vaccine (TIV). See *MMWR* 2003;52[RR-6]:1–40. Children receiving TIV should be administered a dosage appropriate for their age (0.25 mL if aged 6–35 months or 0.5 mL if ≥3 years). Children aged ≤8 years who are receiving influenza vaccine for the first time should receive 2 doses (separated by at least 4 weeks for TIV and at least 6 weeks for LAIV).

8 **Hepatitis A vaccine.** Hepatitis A vaccine is recommended for children and adolescents in selected states and regions and for certain high-risk groups; Consult your local public health authority. Children and adolescents in these states, regions, and high-risk groups who have not been immunized against hepatitis A can begin the hepatitis A immunization series during any visit. The 2 doses in the series should be administered at least 6 months apart. See *MMWR* 1999;48(RR-12):1–37.

Table 5.3. Guidelines for active and passive immunization in HIV-exposed and -infected children (and their contacts)

Vaccine	HIV-exposed (infection status indeterminate)	HIV-infected, asymptomatic	HIV-infected, symptomatic	Close contact of HIV-infected individual	Schedule
Hepatitis B[a]	Yes	Yes	Yes	Yes	Birth, 1 month, 6 months
DTaP/DTP[b]	Yes	Yes	Yes	Yes	2 months, 4 months, 6 months, 12–18 months, 4–6 yrs; Td or Tdap recommended at 11–12 years
HIB	Yes	Yes	Yes	Yes	2 months, 4 months, 6 months, 12–18 months
Polio, inactivated[c]	Yes	Yes	Yes	Yes	2 months, 4 months, 12–18 months, 4–6 years
Polio, oral[d]	**No**	**No**	**No**	**No**	
MMR[e]	Yes	Yes	Yes	Yes	12 months, 1 month after first dose
Varicella[f]	Yes	Yes	**No**	Yes	At 12 months or older. HIV-infected children receive a second dose 3 months after first dose
Pneumococcal Conjugate, 7-valent (PCV-7)[g]	Yes	Yes	Yes	Yes	2 months, 4 months, 6 months, 12–15 months
Pneumococcal 23-valent (PPV-23)[g]	N/A	Yes	Yes	**No**	≥ 2 years old and ≥ 2 months after last dose of PCV7; 3–5 years after first dose
Hepatitis A[h]	If risk factors	If risk factors	If risk factors	If risk factors	Not recommended unless other risk factors (see below)
Influenza[i]	Yes	Yes	Yes	Yes	Each autumn after 6 months of age; repeat annually
BCG[j]	**No**	**No**	**No**	**No**	Not recommended in the USA and in areas of low prevalence of tuberculosis; consider in asymptomatic infants in high prevalence areas.
Meningococca conjugate, 4-valent (MCV-4)	**Yes**	**Yes**	**Yes**	**Yes**	11–12 years old

Borrelia burgdorferi (Lyme)[k]	No	No	No	No	No	Only recommended for persons over 15 years of age who are at high risk of exposure
Plague[l]	No	No	No	No	No	Not recommended for persons less than 18 years old; only for those at high risk of exposure
Rabies[m]	Postexposure	Postexposure	Postexposure	Postexposure	Postexposure	Only for postexposure prophylaxis; days 1, 3, 7, 14, and 28
Rotavirus[n]	No	No	No	No	No	
Typhoid[o]	If travelling to endemic area	If travelling to endemic area	If travelling to endemic area	If travelling to endemic area	If travelling to endemic area	May be considered if travelling to endemic area. Live, attenuated vaccine should not be given
Yellow fever[p]	No	No	No	No	Yes	May be considered in asymptomatic persons travelling to endemic areas

[a] **Hepatitis B:** Hepatitis B immunoglobulin (HBIG) should be given to HIV-exposed and infected children according to the recommended pediatric immunization schedule [10]. Infants with perinatal exposure to Hepatitis B should receive 0.5 ml HBIG within 12 hours of birth concurrently with the first hepatitis B vaccine. Sexual partners of persons with acute HBV infection should receive 0.06 ml/kg HBIG and begin the Hepatitis B vaccine series. HBIG and hepatitis B vaccination should also be considered when there is direct exposure to blood products that potentially could contain Hepatitis B surface antigen [11].

[b] **Tetanus:** As in immunocompetent persons, tetanus immunoglobulin (TIG) should be administered if the patient sustains a tetanus-prone wound (e.g., wounds contaminated with dirt, feces, saliva; puncture wounds; wounds where there is devitalized tissue, such as crush injury, frostbite, or necrosis; bite wounds) [10]. The wound should be thoroughly cleaned and debrided. A dose of 250 units of TIG should be given.

[c] **Polio, inactivated (IPV):** Uninfected siblings should be immunized with IPV to decrease the risk of possible vaccine-associated paralytic polio in the HIV-infected child.

[d] **Polio, oral (OPV):** OPV is contraindicated in HIV-infected children in the USA [12]. In addition, because of prolonged fecal shedding of virus and the possibility of vaccine-associated paralytic polio in immunocompromised patients, contacts of HIV-infected individuals should not receive OPV. If OPV is inadvertently administered to a household or close contact, care must be taken to minimize contact with the HIV-infected child for four to six weeks after vaccination. The World Health Organization recommends use of OPV routinely for all infants [13]. In many developing

Notes to Table 5.3 (cont.)

countries, where polio is endemic and thus the relative importance of vaccine-associated paralytic polio is decreased, OPV has several advantages over IPV: lower cost, inducement of intestinal immunity, and capability for herd immunity.

[e] **Measles-Mumps-Rubella (MMR):** MMR vaccine is currently contraindicated in HIV-infected children with severe immunosuppression (CDC Immunologic Category 3) (Table 5.4) [14–16]. However, although it is a live vaccine, MMR should be administered to HIV-infected children who are not severely immunocompromised because of the increased risk of morbidity with measles infection. As measles is not transmitted to contacts of patients immunized with measles vaccine, it can and should be given to household and other close contacts of HIV-infected children. To increase the likelihood of an adequate immunologic response, the first dose of MMR should be administered at 12 months of age (before further decline in immune status), and the second dose given as early as 4 weeks after the first dose. If there is increased risk of exposure to measles (i.e., an outbreak), the MMR can be given as early as 6 months of age, with an additional dose given at 12 months of age [16]. If an HIV-infected child is regularly receiving intravenous immunoglobulin, the presence of passively acquired antibodies may prevent response to the MMR vaccine. However, because of the potential benefits of the MMR, vaccination should be considered two weeks before the next immunoglobulin dose. A second dose should be repeated in 4 weeks unless otherwise contraindicated [14]. There is presently no consensus regarding the utility of checking antibody titers in patients receiving immunoglobulin.

Measles: Immunoglobulin (IG) should be given within 6 days of exposure. IG should also be given to any measles-susceptible household contacts with asymptomatic HIV infection, especially if they are less than 1 year of age [14]. If the patient has received IVIG within three weeks of exposure, IG is not necessary. The dose of IG is 0.5 ml/kg (maximum 15 ml) for symptomatic HIV-infected children, and 0.25 ml/kg (maximum 15 ml) for HIV-exposed children or asymptomatic, HIV-infected children.

[f] **Varicella:** Varicella vaccine should be considered at 12 months of age in asymptomatic or mildly symptomatic children in CDC Immunologic Category 1 (Table 5.4) [17]. Children should receive two doses of varicella vaccine, three months apart. Because vaccinees with impaired cellular immunity may be at increased risk for severe adverse effects from the vaccine, patients should be re-evaluated if they develop a post-vaccination varicella-like rash. Varicella vaccine can and should be given to susceptible contacts of HIV-infected children [18]. No precautions are needed if the vaccinated contact does not develop a rash. If the vaccinated contact develops a rash, direct contact with susceptible immunocompromised persons should be avoided while the rash is present. However, varicella zoster Immunoglobulin (VZIG) is not indicated in the case of contact with a recent vaccinee. Any adult in the household who lacks a history of varicella should have serologic testing for VZV and should receive the vaccine if seronegative. There is no contraindication to administering the vaccine to family members of HIV-infected children. Susceptible HIV-infected children should avoid exposure to persons with varicella or shingles (herpes zoster).

Varicella Immunoglobulin (VZIG): VZIG should be administered within 96 hours of exposure [10]. VZIG is not necessary if the patient has received IVIG or VZIG within three weeks of exposure. The dose of VZIG to be given is one vial (125 units, approximately 1.25 ml)/10 kg, with a minimum 125 units (one vial) and a maximum 625 units (five vials). Patients receiving VZIG are potentially infectious for a period extending from day 8 to day 28 after exposure to infection. As noted above, if an HIV-infected child who is not known to be immune to VZV is exposed to varicella or zoster, he she should receive an injection of VZIG as soon as possible but within 96 hours of the exposure [17]. The use of oral acyclovir for postexposure prophylaxis following exposure to VZV is not recommended and should not replace VZIG for the immunosuppressed host. In the healthy HIV-uninfected child who is susceptible to varicella, the live attenuated varicella vaccine can be administered following exposure to VZV to prevent or modify disease. However, in the HIV-infected child, VZIG should be given. The varicella vaccine should not be given with VZIG, since antibody may interfere with the activity of the live virus vaccine.

g **Pneumococcus:** Because *Streptococcus pneumoniae* is a common bacterial pathogen in young children, and because of increasing resistance to antibiotics, pneumococcal vaccination is critical. There are two pneumococcal vaccines available: the heptavalent pneumococcal conjugate vaccine (PCV7) and the 23-valent pneumococcal vaccine (PPV23). The PPV23, which contains the purified capsular polysaccharide antigens of 23 serotypes, provides protection against many more serotypes of pneumococcus, but is ineffective in children less than 2 years of age. Therefore, the two different vaccines are given sequentially in HIV-infected children [19]. The PCV7, which is a multivalent protein conjugate vaccine, should be given to all HIV-infected children in the USA beginning at 2 months of age according to the schedule for routine pediatric immunizations [19]. If a child between the ages of 24 and 59 months has not received the PCV7, two doses administered 2 months apart should be given. In two studies of HIV-infected children, a single dose of PCV7 was found to be more immunogenic than a dose of PPV23; however, children receiving PCV7 subsequently mounted a booster antibody response with PPV23 [20–21]. The PPV23 should be given at 2 years of age, at least 2 months after the last PCV7 dose. A second dose of PPV23 should be given 3 to 5 years after the first dose. If a child is diagnosed with HIV between 24 and 59 months of age, the first PCV7 should be given at the time of diagnosis. If the diagnosis is made after 5 years of age, PPV23 should be given.

h **Hepatitis A:** Hepatitis A vaccine consists of inactivated viral antigen. It is not routinely recommended for HIV-exposed or HIV-infected children. It is unknown whether the vaccine is immunogenic in immunocompromised children. However, some studies suggest that HIV-infected adults develop lower antibody levels after immunization with hepatitis A vaccine [22]. Hepatitis A vaccine should be given to individuals who are 2 years of age or older if there are risk factors for hepatitis A, such as: (1) travel to countries with endemic HAV infection (in general, these countries include those other than Australia, Canada, Japan, New Zealand, Western Europe, and Scandinavia), (2) residence in a community with high endemic rates and/or periodic outbreaks of HAV (e.g., Native Americans, Alaskan natives), (3) chronic liver disease, (4) clotting factor disorders, (5) homosexual/bisexual men, (6) illicit or injection drug use, or (7) occupational risk for hepatitis A. If hepatitis A vaccine is indicated in a child with HIV infection, it should be given according to the recommended pediatric immunization schedule [23]. Persons who have not been previously immunized with hepatitis A vaccine should be given intramuscular immunoglobulin (IG) if there is recent (less than 2 weeks) exposure to hepatitis A. Such exposures include:

Notes to Table 5.3 (*cont.*)

(1) household and sexual contacts of patients with serologically confirmed hepatitis A, (2) sharing illicit drugs with someone with serologically confirmed hepatitis A infection, (3) staff and attendees of childcare centers/family childcare homes if at least one child, one employee, and/or two household contacts of attendees are infected, (4) food handlers working in the same establishment as a hepatitis A-infected food handler [22]. One intramuscular dose of IG (0.02ml/kg) should be given as soon as possible after exposure but not more than 2 weeks after the last exposure. Hepatitis A vaccine can be administered simultaneously with IG.

[i] **Influenza:** Influenza vaccine consists of inactivated whole virus (whole-virus vaccine) or viral components (split-virus vaccine). Influenza vaccine should be administered annually in the autumn to HIV-infected children at least 6 months of age and their close contacts [23]. For children less than 9 years of age, two doses administered 1 month apart are required when the vaccine is given for the first time. Thereafter, one dose annually is adequate. Children aged 12 years or less should receive split-virus vaccine only; children over the age of 12 years can receive split or whole virus vaccine. Children less than 3 years of age should receive half of the usual dose. The efficacy of the influenza vaccine in children less than 6 months of age is not known.

There are studies that have demonstrated a transient (6- to 8-week) increase in HIV viral load in some HIV-infected patients after influenza immunization [24–26]. This has raised concerns that introducing new antigens through immunization could stimulate macrophages and lymphocytes that could harbor HIV and thereby accelerate progression of disease. Studies in adult and pediatric patients have not shown clinical or immunologic deterioration in relation to this transient increase in viral load [27–28]. Because influenza can cause serious disease with complications in HIV-infected children and because immunization may offer some protection, it is currently recommended that all HIV-infected children receive influenza vaccine.

An intranasally administered, live attenuated influenza vaccine is now available in the USA. Although it is unknown whether this vaccine will be approved for use in HIV-infected children, inadvertent exposure to the vaccine is unlikely to result in serious side effects [29–30].

[j] **Bacille Calmette–Guerin (BCG):** BCG is a live attenuated vaccine that is used to prevent disseminated tuberculosis. Complications or dissemination of BCG occur, and symptomatic HIV-infected persons may be at higher risk for complications. Therefore, in the USA and in other areas with low prevalence of tuberculosis, BCG is not recommended [31–32]. However, in countries with high prevalence of tuberculosis, the World Health Organization recommends BCG in asymptomatic HIV-infected children. The WHO does not recommend BCG for HIV-exposed or-infected children who live in areas with low prevalence of tuberculosis or who are at otherwise low risk for tuberculosis infection [33–34]. The World Health Organization recommends BCG for HIV-infected children in countries with high prevalence of tuberculosis [33–34].

[k] *Borrelia burgdorferi* (**Lyme disease**): This vaccine is a recombinant outer surface protein (rOspA) vaccine. It is not approved for children less than 15 years of age [35].

l **Plague:** A formalin-activated vaccine is no longer available in the USA. It is only indicated for persons between 18 and 61 years of age with high risk for exposure: laboratory personnel who are routinely in contact with *Yersinia pestis*, and persons with regular contact with wild rodents or their fleas in areas where *Y. pestis* is endemic [36].

m **Rabies:** Human rabies vaccine can be given to HIV-infected children according to the recommendations for healthy children who are exposed to rabies [37]. It should not be given as pre-exposure prophylaxis. There are three vaccines available in the USA, and five doses (1.0 ml each) are required on days 1, 3, 7, 14, and 28. As antibody response may not be adequate in immunocompromised persons, it is recommended that antibody titers be obtained to assure an appropriate response. As in immunocompetent persons, human rabies immune globulin (HRIG) should be used concurrently with the first rabies vaccine dose [37]. The recommended dose of HRIG is 20 IU/kg; as much as possible should be used to infiltrate the wound area. The remainder of the dose should be administered intramuscularly using a separate needle and syringe.

n **Rotavirus:** The original rotavirus vaccine, a live virus vaccine, is contraindicated in HIV-exposed and -infected children in the USA [38]. It is no longer available.

o **Typhoid:** Routine typhoid vaccination is not recommended in the USA. If an HIV-infected child is travelling to an area where *Salmonella typhi* is endemic, vaccination with the Vi capsular polysaccharide vaccine or the inactivated vaccine may be given. The Vi capsular polysaccharide vaccine consists of one dose (0.5ml) given intramuscularly, and it should not be given to children less than 2 years old. The inactivated vaccine must be given in two intramuscular doses separated by at least 4 weeks, and should not be given to those less than 6 months of age. Live, attenuated TY21a vaccine is contraindicated in HIV-exposed infants and HIV-infected children [39].

p **Yellow fever:** While yellow fever vaccine, a live virus vaccine, is not contraindicated in HIV-infected children, there is a theoretical risk of encephalitis in immunosuppressed individuals. If travelling to an endemic area cannot be avoided, patients should be given instructions on avoiding mosquitoes, and asymptomatic HIV-infected persons could be given the option of vaccination [40]. The vaccine is contraindicated for infants under 4 months of age, and ideally vaccination should be postponed until 9 to 12 months of age.

Table 5.4. CDC immunologic classification of HIV infection in children less than 13 years of age

Immunologic categories	CD4+ lymphocyte count (cells/μl) and CD4%		
	< 12 mo	1–5 yrs	6–12 yrs
1. No evidence of suppression	≥ 1500 or ≥ 25%	≥ 1000 or ≥ 25%	≥500 or ≥ 25%
2. Moderate suppression	750–1499 or 15–24%	500–999 or 15–24%	200–499 or 15–24%
3. Severe suppression	< 750 or < 15%	< 500 or < 15%	< 200 or < 15%

From [15].

Opportunistic infection prophylaxis

All infants born to HIV-infected mothers should receive prophylaxis for *Pneumocystis jiroveci* pneumonia (PJ). Because PJ rarely occurs before 2 months of age, initiation of PJ prophylaxis in HIV-exposed infants can be safely delayed until 6 weeks of age, following discontinuation of ZDV prophylaxis. This will help to avoid neutropenia which can result from concomitant administration of ZDV and trimethoprim-sulfamethoxazole (TMP-SMZ). Prophylaxis for PJ can be discontinued if the child is confirmed to be HIV-uninfected (usually by four to six months).

Care of the HIV-infected child

The overall goals of routine care of the HIV-infected child are the same as those for all children: health maintenance and disease prevention. Important aspects of routine care of the HIV-infected child include comprehensive general medical care, HIV disease progression monitoring, treatment of HIV infection, opportunistic infection prophylaxis, mental health evaluation and treatment, and education of and support for both the patient and the family.

Comprehensive general medical care

Routine health maintenance – including assessment of growth, nutrition, development, and mental health; immunizations; evaluation and management of intercurrent illnesses; anticipatory guidance for the prevention of injury and disease; dental referrals; and screening for hearing and vision – should be provided for all children. Some HIV-infected children receive all of their care directly from a team that manages the medical, social and mental health issues associated with HIV. Alternatively, a general pediatrician provides the bulk of routine care in close consultation with an HIV specialist. The specialist may see a child whose condition is stable two to three times per year, with the general pediatrician providing the remainder of the care. Availability of services and parent preference generally determine the choice of care model. In either model, it is imperative that the child be managed by someone expert in the field.

Assessment of growth and development

Sequential assessment of growth and physical development is of particular importance. Growth failure or failure-to-thrive was described as a common finding in children with HIV infection early in the epidemic [41]. A small number are born with low birth weight, but most infected infants grow normally in utero and cannot be distinguished from uninfected infants by size at birth [41, 42]. During the first year of life, some infected infants, particularly those with a more rapid disease course, deviate from their previous growth pattern, and their growth velocity slows significantly [43]. While often associated with disease progression, the etiology of failure-to-thrive is multifactorial, including genetic predisposition, intrauterine environment (drug and alcohol exposure), and medication side effects [43]. The introduction of combination antiretroviral therapy has decreased the prevalence of failure-to-thrive among HIV-infected children, but other growth abnormalities have emerged. Paradoxically, obesity has been noted among some HIV-infected children. Delayed puberty also has been reported [44]. Long-term treatment with combination antiretroviral therapy also appears to put some children at risk for the development of lipodystrophy, a syndrome of abnormal fat distribution and serum lipid elevation [45, 46] (see Chapter 13). All children should have sequential measurements of their growth, and growth charts should be maintained to monitor their patterns and velocity of growth. Special attention should be paid to the timing of pubertal changes and to the distribution of body fat, particularly among children receiving combination antiretroviral therapy. Patients should have serial assessments of neurological and developmental status. Early in the epidemic, developmental abnormalities were reported in a large proportion of infants and young children [47]. Neurological disorders appear as developmental delays in younger children and as cognitive deficits, behavioral problems, psychiatric manifestations, and school failure in older children and young teens [48]. Children with abnormalities on screening should undergo neuropsychological and/or educational testing (see Chapter 10).

Active and passive immunization

HIV-infected children in the USA generally should receive routine pediatric immunizations according to the schedule recommended by the Advisory Committee on Immunization Practices (ACIP) and the American Academy of Pediatrics (AAP) (Table 5.2), with specific caveats (Table 5.3) [9, 10]. Children with symptomatic HIV infection generally tend to have poor immunologic responses to vaccines, with decreasing responses as the infection progresses. There is evidence that HIV-infected children have dysfunctional humoral immune responses to antigen challenges, and such dysfunctional responses occur as early as the first year of life in those children who acquire HIV perinatally. Thus, antibody production in response to vaccine administration may be compromised. In addition, as the disease progresses, cellular immune function also declines. Therefore, if the patient is directly exposed to a vaccine-preventable disease, he/she should be considered susceptible, regardless of immunization status, and should receive the appropriate passive immunization. Presently, there is no evidence to support increased doses or booster doses of immunizations to augment the immune response. While some clinicians obtain post-vaccination antibody titers, there is no consensus regarding their utility. Since immunocompromised individuals can develop disease from vaccine strains of organisms (found in live vaccines), HIV-infected children generally should not receive live virus or live bacteria vaccines, with the exception of measles-mumps-rubella (MMR) vaccine and varicella vaccine [14, 17], and IPV should be given instead of the live OPV (Table 5.3). However, testing for HIV infection in asymptomatic children without risk factors for HIV is not indicated before administering live virus vaccines.

HIV disease progression monitoring
Initial evaluation of the HIV-infected child
The initial evaluation of the HIV-infected child should include a comprehensive history, a physical examination, an assessment of the patient's developmental, behavioral, and mental health, and baseline laboratory tests as outlined in Table 5.5. A comprehensive evaluation allows the clinician to stage the child clinically, immunologically and virologically and to determine the need for therapeutic and/or prophylactic interventions.

The initial evaluation also should include an assessment of the family's adjustment to the diagnosis as well as knowledge and understanding of HIV infection. The initial evaluation marks the beginning of a dialogue with the child and family about a wide range of social and psychological matters integral to HIV care.

A detailed medical history, including the mother's pregnancy, labor and delivery, and the child's medical, growth and developmental history, will enable the provider to assess the clinical stage of disease. However, historical data may be incomplete. Tanner staging and menstrual history should be included for preteens and adolescents. A comprehensive family history should include the HIV infection status of other family members, especially siblings. Parents should be encouraged to have the HIV infection status of all the children in the family determined. The initial history also should aim to assess the coping skills and mental health needs of the caregiver and child. A comprehensive social history should be obtained and a family profile developed to determine appropriate assistance and support services. A complete evaluation may not be accomplished during a single visit and may require a number of meetings with different members of the multidisciplinary team. Over time, disclosure of HIV status within the family and community, and to the child, should be explored. Finally, providers should make themselves aware of any cultural and religious beliefs that could influence care and treatment.

Table 5.5. Initial evaluation of the HIV-infected pediatric patient

	Assessment
History	
Mother's medical history	HIV disease stage
	• CD4+ lymphocyte count
	• Viral load (HIV RNA assay)
	• Clinical stage, complications
	Receipt of antiretroviral drugs
	Antiretroviral resistance testing
	HIV subtype (clade)
	Drug and alcohol use
	Labor and delivery history (mode of delivery, duration of ruptured membranes, complications)
Child's medical history	Gestational age
	Birth weight
	Receipt of antiretroviral drugs
	Neonatal medical problems
	Breastfeeding history
	Recurrent symptoms
	Serious illnesses
	Age of puberty, menstruation
	Hospitalizations
	Chronic medications, allergies
	Immunizations
	Growth history
	Developmental history
	School history (grade, achievement)
	Behavioral and mental health history
	Sexual history
Family history	Primary caretaker
	Family history of illness including HIV, TB
	Source of care for other family members with HIV
	Family members taking antiretroviral therapy
	Foster care and adoption history, as appropriate
	Relationship with biologic family members for children in alternative care settings (foster, adoptive, group homes)
Social history	Primary language in household
	Disclosure to child and family members
	Religious and cultural beliefs
	Legal issues related to guardianship
	Source of household income
	Insurance coverage
	Other caretakers who assist in care
Physical examination	A complete comprehensive physical examination including a developmental evaluation

Table 5.5. (cont.)

	Assessment
Laboratory	HIV ELISA and Western blot (if not already done)
	CBC with differential[a]
	CO4+ lymphocyte count
	Viral load (HIV RNA assay)[a]
	Blood urea nitrogen, creatinine
	Liver function tests
	Cholesterol, triglyceride
	Urinalysis
	Hepatitis B and C serologies
	Cytomegalovirus (CMV), toxoplasmosis, syphilis and varicella serologies[b]
	Tuberculin skin test (TST)
	Chest radiograph
	Brain CT or MRI (if clinically indicated)
	Electrocardiogram/Echocardiogram[c]

[a] The initial results should be repeated within 4 weeks to confirm the results prior to initiating any therapy.

[b] If the child is <12 months old, positive serologies should be repeated after 12 months of age to document seroreversion.

[c] Some centers advocate baseline electrocardiogram and echocardiogram on all children at the initial evaluation. Insurance funding may not be available to cover these costs.

The physical examination should include careful determination of the child's height, weight and, from birth through 2 years of age, head circumference. A comprehensive examination looking for specific organ system involvement is important. Patients should have a thorough neurological examination and neuropsychological assessment (see Chapter 10). In some settings, the primary provider may prefer to use a simplified screening tool to assess developmental status and refer only those children with abnormalities on screening for specialized assessments. Similarly, the mental health status and, when appropriate, educational achievement of the child should be assessed, again either by the primary provider or by a specially trained mental health professional.

The diagnostic tests that are suggested for the first evaluation allow the clinician to obtain baseline immunologic and virologic data (CD4+ lymphocyte counts, plasma HIV RNA concentration), to assess organ system involvement (complete blood count with differential, serum chemistries, liver and renal function tests, lipid profile, urinalysis, and a chest radiograph), and to determine exposure to vertically acquired infections and potential opportunistic pathogens (CMV, *Toxoplasma gondii*, syphilis, varicella, hepatitis B and C serologies). If clinically indicated, neuroimaging (brain CT or MRI) or a cardiac evaluation should be obtained. A tuberculin skin test should be placed on all children over the age of 1 year and all those with a known exposure to an adult with active TB.

Follow-up evaluations of the HIV-infected child

A complete evaluation of the disease status of an HIV-infected infant, child, or adolescent must include immunologic, virologic, and clinical evaluations. The most useful assays for the evaluation of immune function in HIV-infected children are determination of the absolute number and percentage of CD4+ and CD8+ T lymphocytes. CD4+ lymphocyte count is independently predictive of the likelihood of disease progression [49]. Interpretation of CD4+ T cell counts should take into consideration the age of the child since the normal number of cells declines with age over the first 6 years of life (see Chapter 1). Routine monitoring should be performed every 3 months in an otherwise stable child (Table 5.6). However, precipitous decreases in the CD4+ lymphocyte absolute count or percentage, changes in plasma HIV RNA concentration, changes in clinical status, or initiation of a new treatment regimen may dictate more frequent measurements.

The plasma HIV RNA concentration (viral load) provides information regarding the child's response to therapy and the child's risk of disease progression [49–52]. It should be monitored every 3 to 4 months in a stable child (Table 5.6), but more frequently for the following groups of children: those with significant increases in viral load measurements, those with significant deteriorations in clinical or immune status, and those whose antiretroviral therapy regimen has changed. There are several different methods available for quantifying HIV RNA, each with different levels of sensitivity (see Chapter 1). It is therefore important to use the same assay repeatedly for a given patient as the results of the different assays may be significantly disparate.

All children should be assessed for organ system disease at regular intervals with a thorough history and a complete physical examination. For some organ systems, specific tests may reveal evidence of disease before symptoms develop. Helpful screening assessments (outlined in Table 5.6) include:

- central nervous system – yearly developmental assessment after 2 years of age, yearly neurologic examination;
- cardiovascular – chest radiograph, electrocardiogram and echocardiogram every 3 to 5 years;
- pulmonary – yearly tuberculin skin test, chest radiograph every 3 to 5 years;
- gastrointestinal – liver function testing every 3 months;
- renal – yearly urinalysis; and
- hematologic – complete blood count with differential.

Most of the latter tests should be carried out at the suggested intervals in asymptomatic children or at any time when a child presents with a history or symptoms suggestive of disease related to a specific organ system. Patients with advanced disease may require more frequent evaluations dictated by their clinical status. In addition,

Table 5.6. Schedule for follow-up laboratory and diagnostic evaluations for the HIV-infected pediatric patient

Frequency	Assessment
Every 3 months[a]	Complete blood count with differential
	CD4+ lymphocyte count
	Plasma HIV RNA concentration (viral load)
	Laboratory tests for assessment of toxicities of antiviral and concomitant treatments[b]
Every 6 months	Developmental evaluations to 2 years of age
	Ophthalmologic examination for children with positive CMV or toxoplasmosis serology and CD4+ lymphocyte counts placing them at risk for retinitis[c]
Every 12 months	Urinalysis
	CMV and toxoplasma serologies (if previously negative)
	Tuberculin skin test (TST)
	Developmental evaluation after 2 years of age
	Dental referral after 1 year of age
	Vision and hearing screen
Every 3–5 years	Chest radiograph
	Electrocardiogram/Echocardiogram[d]

[a] More often if medically indicated.

[b] Laboratory tests that are performed depend on potential toxicities of the specific drugs given. Baseline studies prior to initiation of therapy are warranted. Routine lipid studies to assess for toxicity are recommended every 6 months.

[c] If the child is <12 months old, positive serologies should be repeated after 12 months of age to document seroreversion.

[d] Some centers advocate baseline electrocardiogram and echocardiogram on all children at the initial evaluation. Insurance funding may not be available to cover these costs.

children receiving antiretroviral therapy will need routine monitoring for toxicities (e.g., complete blood count with differential, liver aminotransferases, pancreatic enzymes and lipid profiles) associated with specific treatments. A schedule for obtaining these tests is provided in Table 5.6. Follow-up visits should serve to deliver routine pediatric care; to monitor the child's disease status, medication adherence, complications of treatment, and mental health status; and to provide support and education for the child and family. The schedule for follow-up medical visits will largely depend upon the severity of the child's disease and the complexity and toxicity of the treatment regimen. Children with advanced disease require frequent visits, as often as every 4 to 6 weeks, while those with more stable disease can be seen quarterly (Table 5.6). For newly diagnosed patients, consideration should be given to shorter intervals between visits during the first 6 to 9 months after diagnosis. This allows the caregiver time to become familiar with the staff and the concept of attending to the medical needs of a child with a chronic illness. Children beginning new treatment regimens may require weekly visits to reinforce adherence and to closely monitor virologic and immunologic response. Clinically stable children who are not taking antiretroviral medications require less frequent monitoring, every 3 to 4 months. On the other hand, those with advanced disease who are not receiving antiretroviral medications, generally because of adherence difficulties, should be monitored as often as every 1 to 2 months.

The interim history should attempt to elicit signs and symptoms of specific organ dysfunction, medication adherence, intolerance and toxicity, and new mental health or behavioral problems. The physical examination should be comprehensive. The laboratory tests that should be obtained are outlined in Table 5.6. More frequent testing may be in order for patients with decreasing CD4+ cell counts, increasing HIV RNA copy number, and/or deterioration in clinical status. Additionally, antiviral resistance testing (genotypic and/or phenotypic) would be recommended for a patient on antiretroviral therapy with virologic failure who may have developed viral resistance to specific agents.

Involving the child in the treatment plan as much as possible with age-appropriate education and acknowledgment of the complexities of their medical regimens and social issues will lay a foundation for future ongoing participation in their long-term healthcare. It is important to keep in mind that, due the nature of the illness, most children will remain in care for the duration of their lives.

Treatment of HIV infection

Pediatric antiretroviral therapy continues to evolve. Those prescribing antiretroviral therapy should be thoroughly familiar with the drugs and how to use them, potential drug toxicities, and drug interactions. Clinicians caring for HIV-infected children should routinely monitor children's response to antiretroviral therapy, as well as adherence to such drug therapy (see Chapters 11–16).

In addition to clinical and laboratory (viral load and CD4+ T cell counts and percentages) evaluations prior to the initiation of antiretroviral therapy, the family's readiness should be assessed thoroughly. Children sometimes need advance training to ensure that they will adhere adequately to the prescribed regimen and may need pill swallowing training if no liquid formulation. After initiation of a new antiretroviral regimen, viral load assays and CD4+ T cell counts should be monitored monthly. If viral suppression is achieved, virologic and immunologic evaluations, and laboratory monitoring for toxicity (including complete blood count, liver function tests, lipid profile), can be performed every 3 months. A deterioration in the clinical status may prompt more frequent assessment. Starting and changing antiretroviral therapy is addressed in Chapter 15). Adherence to antiretroviral therapy is crucial for long-term success of antiretroviral therapy (see Chapter 7).

Opportunistic infection prophylaxis

HIV-infected individuals are at risk of acquiring opportunistic infections, and the routine care of HIV-infected children should include prevention of such infections. For most HIV-associated opportunistic infections, the risk of infection is correlated with the patient's degree of immunosuppression. Thus, guidelines for initiating prophylaxis are generally based upon the number of circulating CD4+ lymphocytes in the peripheral blood. The normal CD4+ lymphocyte count is substantially higher in infants than in older children and adults, with normal values decreasing over the first few years of life. However, the normal percentage of CD4+ lymphocyte is relatively independent of age (Table 5.4) [15]. Infants have a less effective cellular immune response than do older children (see Chapter 1).

Highly active antiretroviral therapy (HAART) often results in a dramatic increase in the CD4+ lymphocyte count and a decrease in the risk of opportunistic infections. This has led to a dramatic fall in the mortality from AIDS in the USA [53]. Thus, the most effective means of preventing opportunistic infections is to aggressively treat the underlying HIV infection in order to maintain a normal CD4+ lymphocyte count. However, viral resistance or poor adherence to therapy can result in a failure of HAART, leading to a fall in the CD4+ lymphocyte count over time. Also, certain infections, such as pneumonia, sinusitis, and herpes zoster, occur in HIV-infected children who are not severely immunosuppressed and these are likely to remain common despite HAART.

A number of studies in adults have demonstrated that prophylaxis against PCP, toxoplasmosis, and *Mycobacterium avium* complex (MAC) can be safely discontinued once a patient responds to HAART with a sustained increase in their CD4+ lymphocyte count [54]. There are limited data on the safety of discontinuing prophylaxis in children at this time, and many authorities have extrapolated the adult data to children. Currently, a number of studies in adults and children are attempting to characterize the immune reconstitution that results from HAART. Questions such as the need for re-immunization with the childhood vaccines following immune reconstitution remain to be answered.

In addition to PCP and MAC, other common opportunistic infections in HIV-infected children children include chronic and recurrent mucosal and esophageal candidiasis, cytomegalovirus infections, *Cryptosporidium* enteritis, herpes zoster, and mucocutaneous herpes simplex virus [55] (Table 5.7). HIV-infected children are also at increased risk of common childhood infections such as otitis media, sinusitis, viral respiratory infections, bacterial pneumonia, bacteremia, gastroenteritis, and meningitis.

Even when it is not possible to completely suppress HIV replication and maintain a normal CD4+ lymphocyte count, careful attention to opportunistic infection prophylaxis in HIV-infected children can significantly reduce morbidity and mortality. Comprehensive guidelines for the prevention of opportunistic infections in children and adults are published, as are guidelines for the treatment of opportunistic infections in children [4, 32]. These are available on the internet (http://AIDSInfo.nih.gov)

Table 5.7. Incidence of opportunistic infections in HIV-infected children in the pre-HAART era (1988–1998)

	Event rate (per 1000 patient–years)
Serious bacterial infections	151
Herpes zoster	29
Disseminated MAC	18
Pneumocystis jiroveci pneumonia (PJ)	13
Candidiasis	12
Cryptosporidiosis	6
CMV retinitis	5
Tuberculosis	4
CMV, other than retinitis	2
Fungal, other than *Candida*	1
Toxoplasmosis	0.6
Progressive multifocal leukoencephalopathy	0.6

From [55]. Used with permission.

and are updated on a regular basis. They should be consulted for the most up-to-date information.

Prophylaxis strongly recommended as standard of care

Pneumocystis jiroveci (formerly *Pneumocystis carinii*) pneumonia (PCP)

Although there are no known effective measures to prevent exposure to the organism, antimicrobial prophylaxis is very effective in preventing PCP. As noted above, all infants born to HIV-infected women should receive PCP prophylaxis, with such prophylaxis being discontinued once HIV infection has been definitively excluded. HIV-infected children over 1 year of age should continue to receive PCP prophylaxis if indicated by their CD4+ values (Table 5.8). The decision to continue prophylaxis in an infected child over the age of 1 year who no longer meets criteria for prophylaxis should be made on an individual basis. PCP prophylaxis should also be considered for any HIV-infected child with a rapidly falling CD4+ lymphocyte count.

The drug of choice for PCP prophylaxis is TMP-SMZ (Table 5.8). For children who are co-infected with *T. gondii*, TMP-SMZ is also effective in preventing toxoplasmosis. However, as many as 15% of children are intolerant to TMP-SMZ; adverse reactions include rash, fever, neutropenia, anemia, and, rarely, the Stevens–Johnson syndrome. Neutropenia is particularly troublesome in children receiving both TMP-SMZ and ZDV. In adults, the gradual introduction of TMP-SMZ in an escalating dose over the first 14 days of therapy reduces the rate of initial adverse reactions [56]. If an adverse reaction is not life-threatening, rechallenge with TMP-SMZ is successful in 57%–75% of adults.

Table 5.8. Prophylaxis to prevent first episode of opportunistic disease among infants and children infected with human immunodeficiency virus

Pathogen	Indication	Preventive regimen	
		First choice	Alternative
Strongly recommended as standard of care			
Pneumocystis carinii[a]	HIV-infected, or HIV indeterminate, infants aged 1–12 mos; HIV-infected children aged 1–5 yrs with CD4$^+$ count of <500/µl or CD4$^+$ percentages of <15%; HIV-infected children aged 6–12 yrs with CD4$^+$ count of <200/µl or CD4+ percentages of <15%	Trimethoprim-sulfamethoxazole (TMP-SMZ), 150/750 mg/m^2 per day in two divided doses by mouth three times weekly on consecutive days (AII); acceptable alternative dosage schedules: (AII) single dose by mouth three times weekly on consecutive days; two divided doses by mouth daily; or two divided doses by mouth three times weekly on alternate days	Dapsone (children aged ≥1 mos), 2 mg/kg body weight (max 100 mg) by mouth daily or 4 mg/kg body weight (max 200 mg) by mouth weekly (CII); aerosolized pentamidine (children aged ≥5 yrs), 300 mg every month via Respirgard II (manufactured by Marquest, Englewood, Colorado) nebulizer (CIII); atovaquone (children aged 1–3 mos and >24 mos, 30 mg/kg body weight by mouth daily; children aged 4–24 mos, 45 mg/kg body weight by mouth daily) (CII)
Mycobacterium tuberculosis			
Isoniazid-sensitive	Tuberculin skin test (TST) reaction, ≥5 mm or prior positive TST result without treatment; or contact with any person with active tuberculosis, regardless of TST result	Isoniazid, 10–15 mg/kg body weight (max 300 mg) by mouth daily for 9 mos (AII); or 20–30 mg/kg body weight (max 900 mg) by mouth twice weekly for 9 months (BII)	Rifampicin, 10–20 mg/kg body weight (max 600 mg) by mouth daily for 4–6 mos (BIII)
Isoniazid-resistant	Same as previous pathogen; increased probability of exposure to isoniazid-resistant tuberculosis	Rifampin, 10–20 mg/kg body weight (max 600 mg) by mouth daily for 4–6 mos (BIII)	Uncertain
Multidrug-resistant (isoniazid and rifampin)	Same as previous pathogen; increased probability of exposure	Choice of drugs requires consultation with public health	—

			to multidrug-resistant tuberculosis	authorities and depends on susceptibility of isolate from source patient	
Mycobacterium avium complex[b]	For children aged ≥6 yrs with CD4+ count of <50/μl; aged 2–6 yrs with CD4+ count of <75/μl; aged 1–2 yrs with CD4+ count of <500/μl; aged <1 yr with CD4+ count of <750/μl	Clarithromycin, 7.5 mg/kg body weight (max 500 mg) by mouth twice daily (AII), or azithromycin, 20 mg/kg body weight (max 1200 mg) by mouth weekly (AII)	Azithromycin, 5 mg/kg body weight (max 250 mg) by mouth daily (AII); children aged ≥6 yrs, rifabutin, 300 mg by mouth daily (BI)
Varicellazoster virus[c]	Substantial exposure to varicella or shingles with no history of chickenpox or shingles	Varicella zoster immunoglobulin (VZIG), 1 vial (1.25 ml)/10 kg body weight (max 5 vials) intramuscularly, administered ≤96 hrs after exposure, ideally in ≤48 hrs (AII)	—
Vaccine-preventable pathogens[d]	HIV exposure/infection	Routine immunizations (see text)	—
Usually recommended			
Toxoplasma gondii[e]	Immunoglobulin G (IgG) antibody to *Toxoplasma* and severe immunosuppression	TMP-SMZ, 150/750 mg/m² per day in two divided doses by mouth daily (BIII)	Dapsone (children aged ≥1 mos), 2 mg/kg body weight or 15 mg/m² (max 25 mg) by mouth daily plus pyrimethamine, 1 mg/ kg body weight by mouth daily plus leucovorin, 5 mg by mouth every 3 days (BIII); atovaquone, children aged 1–3 mos and >24 mos, 30 mg/kg body weight by mouth daily; children aged 14–24 mos, 45 mg/kg body weight by mouth daily (CIII)
Varicella zoster virus	HIV-infected children who are asymptomatic and not immunosuppressed	Varicella zoster vaccine (see vaccine-preventable pathogens section of this table)	Varicella zoster vaccine (see vaccine-preventable pathogens section of this table) (BII)
			—

(cont.)

Table 5.8. (*cont.*)

Pathogen	Indication	Preventive regimen First choice	Preventive regimen Alternative
Influenza virus	All patients, annually, before influenza season	Inactivated split trivalent influenza vaccine (see vaccine preventable section of this table) (BIII)	Oseltamivir (during outbreaks of influenza A or B) for children aged ≥13 years, 75 mg by mouth daily (CIII); rimantadine or amantadine (during outbreaks of influenza A), children aged 1–9 yrs, 5 mg/kg body weight in 2 divided doses (max 150 mg/day) by mouth daily; children aged ≥10 yrs, use adult doses (CIII)

Not recommended for the majority of children; indicated for use only in unusual circumstances

Pathogen	Indication	Preventive regimen First choice	Preventive regimen Alternative
Invasive bacterial infections[f]	Hypogammaglobulinemia (i.e., IgG <400 mg/dl)	Intravenous immunoglobulin (400 mg/kg body weight every 2–4 weeks) (AI)	—
Cryptococcus neoformans	Severe immunosuppression	Fluconazole, 3–6 mg/kg body weight by mouth daily (CII)	Itraconazole, 2–5 mg/kg body weight by mouth every 12–24 hrs (CII)
Histoplasma capsulatum	Severe immunosuppression, endemic geographic area	Itraconazole, 2–5 mg/kg body weight by mouth every 12–24 hrs (CIII)	—
Cytomegalovirus (CMV)[g]	CMV antibody positivity and severe immunosuppression	Oral ganciclovir, 30 mg/kg body weight by mouth three times daily (CIII)	—

Notes: Information included in these guidelines might not represent Food and Drug Administration (FDA) approval or approved labeling for products or indications. Specifically, the terms *safe* and *effective* might not be synonymous with the FDA-defined legal standards for product approval. Letters and Roman numerals in parentheses after regimens indicate the strength of the recommendation and the quality of the evidence

[a] Daily TMP-SMZ reduces the frequency of certain bacterial infections. Apparently, TMP-SMZ, dapsone-pyrimethamine, and possibly atovaquone (with or without pyrimethamine) protect against toxoplasmosis, although data have not been prospectively collected. When compared with weekly dapsone, daily dapsone is associated with lower incidence of *Pneumocystis carinii* pneumonia (PCP) but higher hematologic toxicity and mortality (**Source:** McIntosh K, Cooper E, Xu J *et al.* Toxicity and efficacy of daily vs. weekly dapsone for prevention of *Pneumocystis carinii* pneumonia in children infected with human immunodeficiency virus. ACTG 179 Study Team. AIDS Clinical Trials Group. *Pediatr. Infect. Dis. J.* 1999;18:432–9). The efficacy of parenteral pentamidine (e.g., 4 mg/kg body weight every 2–4 weeks) is controversial. Patients receiving therapy for toxoplasmosis with sulfadiazine-pyrimethamine are protected against PCP and do not need TMP-SMZ.

[b] Substantial drug interactions can occur between rifamycins (i.e., rifampin and rifabutin) and protease inhibitors and non-nucleoside reverse transcriptase inhibitors. A specialist should be consulted.

[c] Children routinely being administered intravenous immunoglobulin (IVIG) should receive VZIG if the last dose of IVIG was administered >21 days before exposure.

[d] HIV-infected and -exposed children should be immunized according to the childhood immunization schedule (see Ref. [32] and text), which has been adapted from the January–December 2001 schedule recommended for immunocompetent children by the Advisory Committee on Immunization Practices, the American Academy of Pediatrics, and the American Academy of Family Physicians. This schedule differs from that for immunocompetent children in that both the conjugate pneumococcal vaccine (PCV-7) and the pneumococcal polysaccharide vaccine (PPV-23) are recommended (BII) and vaccination against influenza (BIII) should be offered. Measles, mumps, and rubella should not be administered to severely immunocompromised children (DIII). Vaccination against varicella is indicated only for asymptomatic non-immunosuppressed children (BII). After an HIV-exposed child is determined not to be HIV-infected, the schedule for immunocompetent children applies.

[e] Protection against toxoplasmosis is provided by the preferred antipneumocystis regimens and possibly by atovaquone. Atovaquone can be used with or without pyrimethamine. Pyrimethamine alone probably provides limited, if any, protection (for definition of severe immunosuppression, see Table 5.4).

[f] Respiratory syncytial virus (RSV) IVIG (750 mg/kg body weight), not monoclonal RSV antibody, can be substituted for IVIG during the RSV season to provide broad anti-infective protection, if this product is available.

[g] Oral ganciclovir and perhaps valganciclovir results in reduced CMV shedding among CMV-infected children. Acyclovir is not protective against CMV.

Gradual reintroduction over one to two weeks is more likely to be successful than direct rechallenge with the full dose [57]. Successful gradual reintroduction has been reported in a small number of children [58]. If a child develops an adverse reaction to TMP-SMZ, the medication should be discontinued. Once the symptoms resolve, if the reaction was not life threatening, TMP-SMZ can be gradually reintroduced (sometimes termed "oral desensitization"). The concomitant use of an antihistamine is recommended. Addition of a non-steroidal anti-inflammatory agent or corticosterioids may be considered during the reintroduction and for any reactions which develop during ongoing treatment. Alternatives for PCP prophylaxis in children who cannot tolerate TMP-SMZ include dapsone, pentamidine, and atovaquone (Table 5.8).

Adults who have responded to HAART with an increase in their CD4+ lymphocyte count to greater than 200 cells/μl can safely stop PCP prophylaxis [59, 60]. It is recommended that patients' CD4+ lymphocyte counts be maintained above 200 cells/μl for at least three months and that patients have at least partial suppression of their HIV viral load before PCP prophylaxis is discontinued. If the CD4+ lymphocyte count subsequently falls to below 200 cells/μL, then prophylaxis should be restarted. Although the safety of discontinuing PCP prophylaxis in children has not been established, many authorities will discontinue prophylaxis if a child responds to HAART therapy with a sustained suppression in HIV viral load and an increase in CD4+ lymphocytes to CDC Immunologic Category 1 or 2 for at least 3 to 6 months.

Tuberculosis (TB)

All children born to HIV-infected mothers and all children living in a household with HIV should have a tuberculin skin test (TST, 5-TU PPD) at or before 9 to 12 months of age, which should be repeated at least annually. In addition, all newly diagnosed HIV-infected children and adolescents should have annual testing. In this setting, 10 mm or more of induration is considered a positive TST. If the child is HIV-infected, has a known TB exposure, or has clinical or radiographic findings compatible with TB, induration of 5 mm or more is considered a positive test. If the TST is positive, the child should be evaluated for active TB, including chest radiography. If no evidence of active disease is found, the child should be treated for latent TB. Children living in a household with a TST-positive person should be evaluated for TB. Children exposed to a person with active TB should be treated for latent TB once active disease has been excluded, regardless of the result of their own TST. In HIV-infected children, nine to 12 months of isoniazid is recommended for treatment of latent TB unless the child is suspected to be infected with a resistant organism (Table 5.8). Directly observed therapy should be utilized if available (see Chapter 31).

Disseminated *Mycobacterium avium* complex (MAC)

Although there are no known effective measures to prevent exposure to environmental mycobacteria (mostly MAC) (see Chapter 32), antimicrobial prophylaxis is effective in preventing MAC infections. MAC is rare in the first year of life but becomes more common with increasing age and decreasing CD4+ lymphocyte count. Therefore, prophylaxis of disseminated MAC is recommended for children with advanced HIV disease, based upon CD4+ criteria (Table 5.8). Clarithromycin or azithromycin are the preferred agents, and rifabutin is an alternative agent (although, because of drug interactions, its use should be avoided unless a macrolide cannot be used). The combination of clarithromycin and rifabutin should be avoided since it is no more effective than clarithromycin alone and has a higher rate of adverse events that either drug alone [61].

The safety of discontinuing MAC prophylaxis with immunologic reconstitution following HAART has been demonstrated in adults [32]. Although the safety of discontinuing prophylaxis has not been demonstrated in children, many authorities will stop prophylaxis once a child has a sustained increase in the CD4+ lymphocyte count to CDC Immunologic Category 1 or 2.

Varicella and other vaccine-preventable diseases
Prevention of these diseases is addressed above under "Immunizations" and in Table 5.3.

Prophylaxis usually recommended as standard of care: toxoplasmosis

Congenital toxoplasmosis is uncommon in the USA, as is encephalitis caused by *T. gondii* among HIV-infected children. Appropriate management of HIV-infected women, with serologic testing for *T. gondii* and with prophylaxis and therapy as appropriate, will prevent congenital toxoplasmosis. TMP-SMZ can be safely administered during pregnancy and is active in preventing reactivation of *T. gondii*. HIV-infected women with a primary *T. gondii* infection or active reactivation disease during pregnancy should receive treatment, in consultation with a specialist in treating toxoplasmosis during pregnancy. Infants born to women infected with both HIV and *T. gondii* should be evaluated for congenital toxoplasmosis.

Older children and adults acquire toxoplasmosis by ingesting cysts in poorly cooked meat, ingesting sporulated oocysts in contaminated food or water, or from contact with infected cats and their feces (e.g., in litter boxes). HIV-infected individuals should avoid eating undercooked meat; meat should be cooked until it is no longer pink inside. Hands should be washed after handling raw meat and after gardening; raw fruits and vegetables should be well washed before eaten raw. Domestic cats are commonly infected with *Toxoplasma*. If the family owns a cat, the litter box should be changed daily, before excreted oocysts have had time to sporulate. Hand washing is essential, and it is best for HIV-infected persons and all pregnant women to avoid changing a litter box. Families need not part with their cat or have the cat tested for *T. gondii*, but should be aware of the risk of cat ownership.

HIV-infected children who are severely immunosuppressed (CDC Immunologic Category 3) and infected with *T. gondii* should receive prophylaxis against both toxoplasmosis and PCP. TMP-SMZ, when administered for PCP prophylaxis, also provides prophylaxis against toxoplasmosis. Atovaquone might also provide protection against toxoplasmosis. The child who does not meet criteria for PCP prophylaxis is at low risk for toxoplasmosis and prophylaxis is not necessary. HIV-infected children who meet criteria for PCP prophylaxis, but who are receiving an agent other than TMP-SMZ or atovaquone, are not receiving adequate prophylaxis against toxoplasmosis. Therefore, they should have serologic testing for *T. gondii* performed on an annual basis, starting at 12 months of age, to determine if they are infected with *T. gondii*. If seropositive for *T. gondii*, they should receive prophylaxis for both PCP and toxoplasmosis. If the child cannot tolerate TMP-SMZ, then atovaquone or dapsone/pyrimethamine/leukovorin are recommended (Table 5.8).

Prophylaxis not recommended for the majority of children; indicated for use only in unusual circumstances

Invasive bacterial infections (bacterial pneumonia, bacteremia, and other invasive bacterial infections)

HIV-infected children are at increased risk for common childhood infections such as otitis media and sinusitis. Recurrent sinusitis can be problematic in some children. In addition, HIV-infected children have frequent invasive bacterial infections, including pneumonia, bacteremia, and meningitis (Table 5.7). The organisms causing these infections are generally the same as for normal children, with *Streptococcus pneumoniae* the predominant pathogen [62, 63]. These organisms are common in the community and there is no effective way to limit exposure to them. As noted previously, all HIV-infected children should be vaccinated against *Haemophilus influenzae* type b and against *Streptococcus pneumoniae* (Table 5.3) [32].

The use of TMP-SMZ for PCP prophylaxis results in a reduction in the risk of bacterial infections. There may be an advantage to using daily dosing ($150/750$ mg/m^2 per day in two divided doses) in children with recurrent infections. TMP-SMZ prophylaxis will not prevent all pneumococcal infections, since the majority of penicillin-resistant strains are also resistant to TMP-SMZ. Other antibiotics may be considered for prophylaxis in individual cases, recognizing the risk of promoting drug resistance with antibiotic prophylaxis.

Monthly infusions of intravenous immunoglobulin (IVIG) (400 mg/kg per dose q month) are effective in preventing recurrent bacterial infections in selected children (Table 5.8) (62, 63). HIV-infected children have functional hypogammaglobulinemia, despite having elevated immunoglobulin levels. Because of the cost, risk of complications, and discomfort associated with IVIG infusions, the use of IVIG is generally limited to the following indications [4].

1. Children who experience recurrent bacterial infections despite appropriate antimicrobial prophylaxis and therapy. In children with hypogammaglobulinemia, it may be reasonable to initiate IVIG infusions without attempting antimicrobial prophylaxis. IVIG may not provide additional benefit to children receiving daily TMP-SMZ prophylaxis (63).

2. Children living in a region with a high prevalence of measles, without detectable antibody to measles despite receiving two measles immunizations.
3. HIV-associated thrombocytopenia (platelet count < 20 000/mm^3 while receiving antiretroviral therapy) (see Chapter 25).
4. HIV-infected children with chronic bronchiectasis who fail to respond to antibiotics and pulmonary care may respond to high-dose IVIG (600 mg/kg per month).

Cryptococcosis, histoplasmosis, and coccidioidomycosis

Invasive fungal infections are less common in HIV-infected children than in adults, presumably because of less frequent exposure to these pathogens (see Chapter 33). These organisms are present in the environment and are acquired by inhalation of airborne organisms in contaminated soil. Dissemination may occur in those with severe immunosuppression. Histoplasmosis and coccidioidomycosis each have a distinct geographic distribution, and infection is common among persons living in endemic regions. Severely immunosuppressed persons living in or visiting a region endemic for *Histoplasma* should avoid activities known to cause exposure, such as creating dust from soil, cleaning chicken coops, disturbing soil beneath bird roosting sites, remodeling or demolishing old buildings, and exploring caves. Likewise, for *Coccidioides*, severely immunosuppressed persons should avoid exposure to disturbed native soil such as at excavation sites or during dust storms.

Routine skin testing of persons living in endemic regions for *Histoplasma* and *Coccidioides* is not recommended since the results do not predict disease. Fluconazole and itraconazole prophylaxis reduce the frequency of cryptococcal disease among patients with advanced HIV infection (Table 5.8). However, routine antifungal prophylaxis is not recommended because no survival benefit has been shown, infection is uncommon, and therapy is costly, may promote drug resistance, and is associated with drug interactions. Prophylaxis with itraconazole will reduce the frequency of histoplasmosis among patients with advanced HIV disease living in an endemic region but no improvement in survival has been shown [64]. Primary prophylaxis for coccidioidomycosis has not been shown to be effective. Because these invasive fungal infections are uncommon in children, primary prophylaxis is not recommended.

Cytomegalovirus

Cytomegalovirus infections are common in HIV-infected children (see Chapter 34). However, infection is often asymptomatic and it is difficult to determine the extent to which CMV contributes to disease [65]. CMV disease in children often results from a primary infection rather than from reactivation of a past infection, the more common situation in adults. CMV co-infection is likely to accelerate the course of HIV disease in children infected with both viruses [66]. Thus, there may be a benefit to identifying those HIV-infected children who are also CMV-infected.

Most HIV-infected women are co-infected with CMV and both in utero and intrapartum transmission of CMV to the infant can occur. The infant also can acquire CMV through breastfeeding. Intrapartum transmission of CMV, but not in utero infection, may be more common in women co-infected with HIV and CMV than in those infected with CMV alone [67, 68]. The most common route of transmission of CMV during childhood is horizontal spread through contact with saliva or urine. Sexual contact and blood transfusion are less common routes of transmission in childhood. HIV-infected children who are CMV-uninfected or of unknown CMV status and who require a transfusion should receive CMV-seronegative or leukocyte-depleted blood products.

It may be useful to identify which HIV-infected children are co-infected with CMV by doing yearly serologic testing starting at 12 months of age. This will allow a CMV-infected child who is severely immunosuppressed (CDC Immunologic Category 3) to be evaluated by an experienced ophthalmologist on a regular basis (every 4 to 6 months) in order to detect early retinitis. Alternatively, children can be screened for CMV once they are severely immunosuppressed. Older children should be taught to recognize "floaters" and changes in visual acuity which could represent retinitis.

Prophylaxis with oral ganciclovir can be considered for CMV-infected children who are severely immunosuppressed, such as those with a CD4+ lymphocyte count <50 cells/μl [32, 69] (Table 5.8). However, disadvantages of ganciclovir prophylaxis include cost, the toxicity of oral ganciclovir (anemia and neutropenia), limited efficacy data, and the risk of developing resistant virus. A liquid preparation of ganciclovir for use in children can be prepared from the parenteral preparation; the dose is 30 mg/kg per dose PO TID. Valganciclovir, an oral pro-drug of ganciclovir with much greater bioavailability, is not available in a liquid formulation. It is approved for the treatment of CMV retinitis in adults but is not approved for the prophylaxis of CMV disease in either adults or children.

Other organisms

Cryptosporidium and microsporidiosis

Cryptosporidium parvum, a protozoan, is a common cause of self-limited watery diarrhea in normal infants and children. Transmission is by fecal–oral spread, and outbreaks of *C. parvum* infection are frequent in the day care setting [70]. Large outbreaks in metropolitan areas have resulted from contaminated drinking water and several outbreaks have been associated with public swimming pools. Other sources of infection include contact with infected adults and children, lake and river water, contaminated foods, and young household pets. In children with advanced HIV disease, cryptosporidiosis is characterized by severe and protracted diarrhea with abdominal pain and anorexia. The infection may result in substantial weight loss and even death. The stools are watery in consistency and may contain mucus but lack blood or inflammatory cells. Patients with advanced immunosuppression have protracted infections which rarely clear without immune reconstitution [71]. *C. parvum* has been implicated as a cause of sclerosing cholangitis in HIV-infected persons [72].

Children with severe immunodeficiency should avoid exposure to potential sources of *C. parvum*. Hand washing is recommended following possible exposure. Families may choose to avoid having their child drink tap water; boiling water for 1 minute will reduce the risk of infection. Drinking bottled water and the use of a submicron personal-use water filter also can reduce the risk of infection; effective filtering of commercial bottled water should be confirmed. Filters should remove particles of one micrometer in diameter in order to remove oocysts. (For detailed information on bottled water and water filters, consult the USPHS/IDSA guidelines [32].)

The most effective means to prevent cryptosporidiosis is to avoid immunosuppression with effective antiretroviral therapy. Chemoprophylaxis for *C. parvum* infection is not recommended. Clarithromycin and rifabutin, when used for MAC prophylaxis, may prevent the development of cryptosporidiosis [73]. This benefit is not seen with azithromycin. However, there are insufficient data to recommend use of these drugs solely to prevent cryptosporidiosis.

Microsporidia are a group of protozoa that cause acute and chronic diarrhea in HIV-infected persons. Infections in humans are zoonotic or waterborne. The incidence of microsporidiosis has declined dramatically with effective antiretroviral therapy. Hand washing and other personal hygiene measures are the only effective means to prevent exposure. Chemoprophylaxis is not available.

Bartonellosis

Bartonella henselae is the cause of cat-scratch disease. Severely immunosuppressed HIV-infected persons are at high risk for developing disease caused by infection with *Bartonella*, including bacillary angiomatosis. Cats are the reservoir for human disease, with cats less than 1 year of age most likely to transmit infection. Cat scratches and saliva are believed to be the principal sources of infection. Fleas transmit the organism between cats and may occasionally transmit infection to humans. *Bartonella* infection is very common in cats and serologic testing of cats is not recommended.

HIV-infected children who are severely immunosuppressed should avoid exposure to cats, particularly cats less than 1 year of age. Families should be aware of the risk of cat ownership. Declawing is not advised, but children should avoid rough play with cats, which could result in a bite or scratch. Cats should not be allowed to lick open wounds, and cat-associated wounds should be washed promptly. Families should practice good flea control of cats. Chemoprophylaxis is not recommended.

Candidiasis

Candida organisms commonly colonize the skin, mucous membranes, and gastro-intestinal tract, and infants acquire the organism early in life. Oral candidiasis is the most common mucocutaneous disease of HIV-infected children. Chronic and recurrent infections of skin and mucous membranes are frequently the presenting infection in HIV-infected children. Judicious use of antibiotics will prevent overgrowth of *Candida* and limit clinical disease. Indwelling venous catheters should be managed with care to avoid contamination and subsequent infection. Fluconazole prophylaxis will prevent mucosal candidiasis but is not generally recommended since treatment is effective and because of concerns about developing resistance, adverse reactions, drug interactions, and cost. However, in selected individuals with severe or frequent recurrent candidiasis, a course of prophylactic fluconazole may be considered (see Chapter 33).

Herpes simplex virus (HSV)

Neonatal herpes simplex virus infection is usually acquired during delivery from a mother with an active genital HSV (see Chapter 34). It can result in devastating disseminated infection or encephalitis in the newborn. In older infants and children, HSV is acquired by contact. Sexual acquisition is common once an adolescent is sexually active. Recommendations for the prevention of neonatal HSV include delivery by cesarean section if the membranes have not been ruptured for more than 4–6 hours. Oral acyclovir prophylaxis during late pregnancy for women with recurrent genital HSV is a controversial strategy that is recommended by some experts to prevent neonatal HSV. For pregnant women with frequent recurrences of HSV, prophylactic acyclovir might be considered. No fetal toxicity has been reported with acyclovir exposure during pregnancy [74]. HIV-infected children should avoid direct contact with individuals with active HSV infections. Use of latex condoms during all acts of sexual intercourse will reduce the risk of exposure to HSV as well as other sexually transmitted diseases (see Chapter 8).

Human herpesvirus 8 (HHV-8)

Persons co-infected with HIV and HHV-8 are at risk for developing Kaposi's sarcoma (KS). HHV-8 is transmitted by oral secretions, semen, and the sharing of needles. In regions of the world where HHV-8 is endemic, mother-to-child transmission of HHV-8 is reported, as is horizontal transmission between children [75]. KS is rare in children in developed countries, but is much more common in some regions, particularly sub-Saharan Africa. It is reasonable to recommend that HIV-infected children avoid contact with the oral secretions of an individual with KS. Serologic testing for HHV-8 is not recommended to prevent exposure and no recommendations are available to prevent child-to-child transmission. Use of latex condoms should be effective in reducing the risk of sexual transmission.

Human papillomavirus (HPV)

Cutaneous HPV infections are commonly acquired during childhood by person-to-person contact. Warts can be very extensive in HIV-infected individuals. Laryngeal papillomatosis is a rare condition which results from an infant aspirating infectious genital tract secretions during birth. It is not known if this is more likely to occur in a child born to an HIV-infected mother. Anogenital warts are generally acquired through sexual contact but may occasionally result from exposure during birth. HPV genital infections are extremely common in sexually active adolescents, frequently leading to cervical dysplasia and the risk of carcinoma. Latex condoms should be used during sexual intercourse, although they are unlikely to completely prevent the transmission of genital HPV, which also can occur as the result of manual inoculation. Sexually active adolescents should be evaluated for genital HPV infection on a regular basis (see Chapter 8). HPV vaccines targeting high-risk genotypes are in development.

Hepatitis B virus and hepatitis C virus

The principal route of acquisition of hepatitis B virus (HBV) in childhood is mother-to-child, with most transmission occurring at the time of delivery. It is not known if HIV co-infection increases the rate of HBV transmission. All pregnant women should be evaluated for HBV infection. All infants born to HIV/HBV co-infected women should receive prophylaxis with hepatitis B immunoglobulin (HBIG) and the hepatitis B vaccine. In older children and adolescents, transmission is by person-to-person exchange of blood and through sexual contact.

Mother-to-child transmission is also the principal route of acquisition of hepatitis C (HCV) in childhood. Maternal risk factors for transmission of HCV to the infant include co-infection with HIV, a higher HCV viral load, and intravenous drug use. The overall rate of transmission from a co-infected mother is 15%–22% with rates ranging from 5%–36% in different studies. The mode of delivery (vaginal vs. cesarean section) and breastfeeding do not influence the rate of transmission [76]. Thus, a cesarean section should not be performed solely to prevent transmission of hepatitis C. All children born to mothers co-infected with HIV and HCV should be evaluated for HCV infection. Since maternal HCV antibody can persist in a child for up to 18 months, serologic testing is not useful in children less than 18 months of age. In this age group, reverse transcriptase-PCR for HCV RNA should be performed to identify virus in the blood. Children infected with HCV, if susceptible, should be vaccinated against hepatitis A virus and hepatitis B virus since infection with a second hepatitis virus can result in fulminant hepatitis. In adolescents and adults, injection drug use is the primary route of HCV transmission; the rate of sexual transmission of HCV is low. Adolescents should avoid injection drug use, body-piercing, and unprotected sexual intercourse.

Mental health evaluation and monitoring

A wide variety of mental health needs have been described for HIV-infected children, including emotional, cognitive, learning, and behavioral problems [48, 77]. These children have to grapple with the experience of living with a stigmatizing chronic illness while experiencing the normal developmental milestones of puberty, autonomy, peer relationships, and sexuality. Furthermore, many children and youth with HIV infection are primarily from ethnic minority, socioeconomically disadvantaged families with high rates of substance abuse, psychiatric disorders, chronic stress, and psychological impairment. The complexities of HIV infection in conjunction with extraordinary social inadequacies contribute to the wide variety of diagnoses among HIV-infected children, including developmental delay, school failure, attention deficit disorder, depression, antisocial behavior, and post-traumatic stress syndrome. Increased sensitivity and attention to these issues by the primary provider is essential, and frequent assessments (e.g., at each medical visit) for possible problems should be conducted. The inclusion of mental health professionals within the multidisciplinary team facilitates evaluation and treatment of this set of problems. Counseling and/or pharmacologic intervention may be appropriate as well as imperative for the medical and psychological well-being of the child and their family. Adolescents with HIV infection represent a particularly challenging population of patients (see Chapter 8).

Education of, and support for, the patient and family
Support and education for HIV-infected children

As HIV-infected children become older, it is important to involve them in their own medical/psychosocial management, including an ongoing dialogue about how HIV infection affects their health and why interventions are instituted. Involvement of the child in the decision-making processes regarding drug regimens will likely enhance adherence. Families should be encouraged to disclose infection status to the child when the child becomes developmentally capable of understanding the information. Many families may be unwilling or unprepared to address issues of disclosure and require ongoing support as they move towards open discussions with their child [78]. As the child approaches adolescence, the issue of disclosure must be resolved to prevent secondary transmission (see Chapter 8).

Family assessment, support and education

HIV affects multiple family members and reaches out into the local community. All family members are profoundly affected by caring for a child with a chronic illness, especially one with complex medical management, daily medications, and significant social stigma. It is imperative to acknowledge and address the psychological and social needs of all family members to enable them to seek maximal medical and emotional well-being. Young mothers identified as HIV-infected through perinatal testing must face the challenges of caring for a newborn while coping with the stress of learning their infection status. Depression and other psychiatric disorders, limited parenting experience, poor coping skills, and substance abuse may interfere with these mothers' abilities to meet their children's, as well as their own, needs. Parents of older children may require care for their own disease and often continue to struggle with the high risk behaviors, such as alcohol and drug use, which lead to HIV infection. Foster and adoptive parents, who willingly and lovingly took home young infants with HIV, may find themselves overwhelmed by the growing emotional and psychological needs of these children as they enter adolescence. The multidisciplinary HIV team should be able to assess and address these complex issues and provide appropriate care, case management, and/or referrals to other providers.

The family and child should be engaged in a partnership with the multidisciplinary team in the management of the child's disease and treatment decisions. Routine care of the child and youth with HIV infection should include ongoing education about the disease: the natural history, clinical signs and symptoms, and laboratory evaluations for HIV infection, the risks and benefits of antiretroviral therapy and opportunistic infection prophylaxis, and information about intercurrent illnesses. The need for strict adherence and the identification of barriers to adherence must be discussed frequently. The provider should assess the family's comfort with treatment as well as their personal beliefs and commitment to strict adherence to chronic therapeutic regimens with multiple daily doses. School and daycare attendance offer special challenges for HIV-infected children (see Chapter 36).

Summary

Routine pediatric care of the HIV-exposed and -infected child must be delivered by a primary care provider who is knowledgeable in this chronic disease. Coordination of medical subspecialities and psychosocial services is needed to deliver optimal routine care. The HIV-exposed infant who is identified as uninfected will require less demanding medical interventions but may continue to require attention to his or her psychosocial needs by virtue of the nature of this chronic infection within the family unit. The infected child and family will be faced with challenging acute needs and the demands of a chronic and ultimately fatal disease. However, employing a sophisticated multidisciplinary approach, providing new effective treatment regimens and actively engaging the child and caretaker in the medical/psychosocial care plan will likely enable many HIV-infected children to enter adulthood.

REFERENCES
1. Connor, E. M., Sperling, R. S., Gelber, R. *et al*. Reduction of maternal-infant transmission of human immunodeficiency virus type 1 with zidovudine treatment. *N. Engl. J. Med.* 1994;**331**(18):1173–1180.
2. Wade, N. A., Birkhead, G. S., Warren, B. L. *et al*. Abbreviated regimens of zidovudine prophylaxis and perinatal transmission of the human immunodeficiency virus. *N. Engl. J. Med.* 1998;**339**(20):1409–1414.
3. Wade, N., Birkhead, G., French, P. T. Short courses of zidovudine and perinatal transmission of HIV. *N. Engl. J. Med.* 1999;**340**:1042–1043.
4. Working group on antiretroviral therapy and medical management of infants, children and adolescents with HIV infection. Antiretroviral therapy and medical management of the HIV-infected child. *Pediatrics* 1998;**102**(4):1005–1062. (Most recent revision of the guidelines available at AIDSinfo.nih.gov. Accessibility verified October 29, 2005.)
5. Cunningham, C. K., Charbonneau, T. T., Song, K. *et al*. Comparison of human immunodeficiency virus 1 DNA polymerase chain reaction and qualitative and quantitative RNA polymerase chain reaction in human immunodeficiency virus 1-exposed infants. *Pediatr. Infect. Dis. J.*, 1999;**18**:30–35.

6. Delamare, C., Burgard, M., Mayaux, M. J. *et al.* HIV-1 RNA detection in plasma for the diagnosis of infection in neonates. The French Pediatric HIV Infection Study Group. *J. Acquir. Immune Defic. Syndr. Hum. Retrovirol.* 1997;**15**(2):121–125.

7. Benjamin, D. K., Miller, W. C., Fiscus, S. A. *et al.* Rational testing of the HIV-exposed infant. *Pediatrics* 2001;**108**(1):E3.

8. Dunn, D. T., Brandt, C. D., Krivine, A. *et al.* The sensitivity of HIV-1 DNA polymerase chain reaction in the neonatal period and the relative contributions of intra-uterine and intra-partum transmission. *AIDS* 1995;**9**:F7–F11.

9. Centers for Disease Control and Prevention. Recommended childhood immunization schedule – United States, 2002. *Morb. Mortal. Wkly. Rep.* 2002;**51**(2):31–33.

10. Centers for Disease Control and Prevention. Recommendations of the Advisory Committee on Immunization Practices: use of vaccines and immune globulins in persons with altered immunocompetence. *Morb. Mortal. Wkly Rep.* 1993;**42** (No RR-4).

11. Centers for Disease Control and Prevention. Hepatitis B virus: a comprehensive strategy for eliminating transmission in the United States through universal childhood vaccination: recommendations of the Advisory Committee on Immunization Practices (ACIP). *Morb. Mortal. Wkly Rep.* 1991;**40**.

12. Centers for Disease Control and Prevention. Poliomyelitis prevention in the United States – updated recommendations of the Advisory Committee on Immunization Practices (ACIP). *Morb. Mortal. Wkly Rep.* 2000;**49**(No. RR-5).

13. Technical Consultative Group to the World Health Organization on the Global Eradication of Poliomyelitis. "Endgame" issues for the global poliomyelitis eradication initiative. *Clin. Infect. Dis.* 2002;**34**:72–77.

14. Centers for Disease Control and Prevention. Measles, mumps, and rubella – vaccine use and strategies for elimination of measles, rubella, and congenital rubella syndrome and control of mumps: recommendations of the Advisory Committee on Immunization Practices (ACIP). *Morb. Mortal. Wkly Rep.* 1998;**47**(No. RR-8).

15. Centers for Disease Control. 1994 classification system for human immunodeficiency virus infection in children less than 13 years of age. *Morb. Mortal. Wkly Rep.* 1994;**43** (No. RR-12): 1–10.

16. Committee on Infectious Diseases and Committee on Pediatric AIDS, American Academy of Pediatrics. Measles immunization in HIV-infected children. *Pediatrics* 1999;**103**:1057–1060.

17. Centers for Disease Control and Prevention. Prevention of varicella – updated recommendations of the Advisory Committee on Immunization Practices (ACIP). *Morb. Mortal. Wkly Rep.* 1999;**48** (No. RR-6).

18. Centers for Disease Control and Prevention. Update: vaccine side effects, adverse reactions, contraindications, and precautions – recommendations of the Advisory Committee on Immunization Practices (ACIP). *Morb. Mortal. Wkly Rep.* 1996;**45** (No. RR-12).

19. Centers for Disease Control and Prevention. Preventing pneumococcal disease among infants and young children – recommendations of the Advisory Committee on Immunization Practices (ACIP). *Morb. Mortal. Wkly Rep.* 2000;**49** (No. RR-9).

20. King, J. C., Vink, P. E., Farley, J. J., Smilie, M., Parks, M., Lichenstein, R. Safety and immunogenicity of three doses of a five-valent pneumococcal conjugate vaccine in children

younger than 2 years with and without human immunodeficiency virus infection. *Pediatrics* 1997;**99**:575–580.

21. King, J. C., Vink, P. E., Farley, J. J. Comparison of the safety and immunogenicity of a pneumococcal conjugate with a licensed polysaccharide vaccine in human immunodeficiency virus and non-human immunodeficiency virus-infected children. *Pediatr. Infect. Dis. J.* 1996;**15**:192–196.

22. Centers for Disease Control and Prevention. Prevention of Hepatitis A through active or passive immunization – recommendations of the Advisory Committee on Immunization Practices (ACIP). *Morb. Mortal. Wkly Rep.* 1999;**48**: (No. RR-12).

23. Advisory Committee on Immunization Practices. Prevention and control of influenza – recommendations of the Advisory Committee on Immunization Practices (ACIP). *Morb. Mortal. Wkly Rep.* 2001;**50** (RR-4).

24. O'Brien, W. A., Grovit-Ferbas, K., Namazi A. *et al.* Human immunodeficiency virus type 1 replication can be increased in peripheral blood of seropositive patients after influenza vaccination. *Blood* 1995; **86**:1082–1089.

25. Ramilo, O., Hicks, P. J., Borvak, J. *et al.* T cell activation and human immunodeficiency virus replication after influenza immunization of infected children. *Pediatr. Infect. Dis. J.* 1996;**15**:197–203.

26. Staprans, S. K., Hamilton, B. L., Follansbee, S. E. *et al.* Activation of virus replication after vaccination of HIV-1 infected individuals. *J. Exp. Med.* 1995;**182**:1727–1737.

27. Sullivan, P. S., Hanson, D. L., Dworkin, M. S. *et al.* Effect of influenza vaccination on disease progression among HIV-infected persons. *AIDS* 2000;**14**:2781–2785.

28. Kroon, F., van Dissel, J., de Jong, J., Zwinderman, K., van Furth, R. Antibody response after influenza vaccination in HIV-infected individuals: a consecutive 3-year study. *Vaccine* 2000; **18**:3040–3049.

29. King, J. J., Fast, P., Zangwill, K. *et al.* Safety, vaccine virus shedding and immunogenicity of trivalent, cold-adapted, live attenuated influenza vaccine administered to human immunodeficiency virus-infected and noninfected children. *Pediatr. Infect. Dis. J.* 2001;**20**:1124–1131.

30. King, J. J., Treanor, J., Fast, P. *et al.* Comparison of the safety, vaccine virus shedding, and immunogenicity of influenza virus vaccine, trivalent, types A and B, live cold-adapted, administered to human immunodeficiency virus (HIV)-infected and non-HIV-infected adults. *J. Infect. Dis.* 2000;**181**:725–728.

31. Centers for Disease Control and Prevention. The role of BCG vaccine in the prevention and control of tuberculosis in the United States – a joint statement by the Advisory Council for the Elimination of Tuberculosis and the Advisory Committee on Immunization Practices (ACIP). *Morb. Mortal. Wkly Rep.* 1996;**45** (No. RR-4).

32. Centers for Disease Control and Prevention. Guidelines for the prevention of opportunistic infections among HIV-infected persons – 2002 recommendations of the U.S. Public Health Service and the Infectious Diseases Society of America. *Morb. Mortal. Wkly Rep.* 2002; **51** (No. RR-8): 1–52.

33. Harries, A. D., Maher D., *TB/HIV: A Clinical Manual.* Geneva, Switzerland: World Health Organization, 1996.

34. World Health Organization. Special Programme on AIDS and expanded programme on immunizations: joint statement – consultation on human immunodeficiency

virus (HIV) and routine childhood immunizations. *Wkly Epidemiol. Rec.* 1987;**62**:297–299.

35. Centers for Disease Control and Prevention. Recommendations for the use of Lyme disease vaccine – recommendations of the Advisory Committee on Immunization Practices (ACIP). *Morb. Mortal. Wkly Rep.* 1999;**48** (No. RR-7).

36. Centers for Disease Control and Prevention. Prevention of plague – recommendations of the Advisory Committee on Immunization Practices (ACIP). *Morb. Mortal. Wkly, Rep.* 1996;**45** (No. RR-14).

37. Centers for Disease Control and Prevention. Human rabies prevention – United States, 1999 – recommendations of the Advisory Committee on Immunization Practices (ACIP). *Morb. Mortal. Wkly Rep.* 1999;**48** (No. RR-1).

38. Centers for Disease Control and Prevention. Rotavirus vaccine for the prevention of rotavirus gastroenteritis among children – recommendations of the Advisory Committee on Immunization Practices (ACIP). *Morb. Mortal. Wkly Rep.* 1999;**48** (No. RR-2).

39. Centers for Disease Control and Prevention. Typhoid immunization – recommendations of the Advisory Committee on Immunization Practices (ACIP). *Morb. Mortal. Wkly Rep.* 1994;**43** (No. RR-14).

40. Centers for Disease Control and Prevention. *Health information for international travelers 2001–2002*. Atlanta: US Department of Health and Human Services, Public Health Service, 2001.

41. McKinney, R. E., Robertson, J. W. Effect of human immunodeficiency virus infection on the growth of young children. Duke Pediatric AIDS Clinical Trials Unit. *J. Pediatr.* 1993;**123**(4):579–582.

42. Abrams, E. J., Matheson, P. B., Thomas, P. A. *et al.* Neonatal predictors of infection status and early death among 332 infants at risk of HIV-1 infection monitored prospectively from birth. *Pediatrics* 1995;**96**:451–458.

43. Moye, J., Rich, K. C., Kalish, L. A. *et al.* Natural history of somatic growth in infants born to women infected by human immunodeficiency virus. *J. Pediatr* 1996;**128**:58–69.

44. DeMartino, M., Tovo, P. A., Galli, L. *et al.* Puberty in perinatal HIV-1 infection: a multi-center longitudinal study of 212 children. *AIDS* 2001;**15**(12):1527–1534.

45. Arpadi, S. M., Cuff, P. A., Horlick, M., Wang J., Kotler, D. P. Lipodystrophy in HIV-infected children is associated with high viral load and low CD4+ -lymphocyte count and CD4+ -lymphocyte percentage at baseline and use of protease inhibitors and stavudine. *J. Acquir. Immune Defic. Syndr.* 2001;**27**(1):30–34.

46. Melvin, A. J., Lennon, S., Mohan, K. M., Purnell, J. Q. Metabolic abnormalities in HIV type 1-infected children treated and not treated with protease inhibitors. *AIDS Res. Hum. Retroviruses* 2001;**17**(12):1117–1123.

47. Diamond, G. W. Developmental problems in children with HIV infection. *Ment. Retard.* 1989;**27**(4):213–217.

48. Brown, L. K., Lourie, K. J., Pao, M. Children and adolescents living with HIV and AIDS: a review. *J. Child Psychol. Psychiatry* 2000;**41**(1):81–96.

49. Mofenson, L. M., Korelitz, J., Meyer, W. A. *et al.* The relationship between serum human immunodeficiency virus type 1 (HIV-1) RNA level, CD4 lymphocyte percent, and long-term mortality risk in HIV-1 infected children. National Institute of Child Health and Human Development Intravenous Immunoglobulin Clinical Trial Study Group. *J. Infect. Dis.* 1997;**175**:1029–1038.

50. Abrams, E. J., Weedon, J., Steketee, R. W. *et al.* Association of HIV viral load early in life with disease progression among HIV-infected infants. *J. Infect. Dis.* 1998;**178**:101–108.

51. Shearer, W. T., Quinn, T. C., LaRussa, P. *et al.* Viral load and disease progression in infants infected with human immunodeficiency virus type 1. *N. Engl. J. Med.* 1997;**336**:1337–1342.

52. Palumbo, P. E., Raskino, C., Fiscus, S. *et al.* Predictive value of quantitative plasma HIV RNA and CD4+ lymphocyte count in HIV-infected infants and children. *J. Am. Med. Assoc.* 1998;**279**(10):756–761.

53. Palella, F. J., Delaney, K. M., Moorman, A. C. *et al.* Declining morbidity and mortality among patients with advanced human immunodeficiency virus infection. *N. Engl. J Med.* 1998;**338**:853–861.

54. Mussini, C., Pezzotti, P., Govoni, A. *et al.* Discontinuation of primary prophylaxis for *Pneumocystis carinii* pneumonia and toxoplasmic encephalitis in human immunodeficiency virus type-I-infected patients: the changes in opportunistic prophylaxis study. *J. Infect. Dis.* 2000;**181**:1635–1642.

55. Dankner, W. M., Lindsey, J. C., Levin, M. J. Correlates of opportunistic infections in children infected with the human immunodeficiency virus managed before highly active antiretroviral therapy. *Pediatr. Infect. Dis. J.* 2001;**20**:40–48.

56. Para, M. F., Finkelstein, D., Becker, S., Dohn, M., Walawander, A., Black, J. R. Reduced toxicity with gradual initiation of trimethoprim-sulfamethoxazole as primary prophylaxis for *Pneumocystis carinii* pneumonia: AIDS Clinical Trials Group 268. *J. Acquir. Immune Defic. Syndr.* 2000;**24**:337–343.

57. Leoung, G. S., Stanford, J. F., Giordano, M. F. *et al.* Trimethoprim-sulfamethoxazole (TMP-SMZ) dose escalation versus direct rechallenge for *Pneumocystis carinii* pneumonia prophylaxis in human immunodeficiency virus-infected patients with previous adverse reaction to TMP-SMZ. *J. Infect. Dis.* 2001;**184**:992–997.

58. Kletzel, M., Beck, S., Elser, J., Shock, N., Burks, W. Trimethoprim sulfamethoxazole oral desensitization in hemophiliacs infected with human immunodeficiency virus with a history of hypersensitivity reactions. *Am. J. Dis. Child* 1991;**145**:1428–1429.

59. Schneider, M.M.E., Borleffs, J.C.C., Stolk R. P. *et al.* Discontinuation of prophylaxis for *Pneumocystis carinii* pneumonia in HIV-1-infected patients treated with highly active antiretroviral therapy. *Lancet* 1999; **353**:201–203.

60. Lopez Bernaldo de Quiros, J. C., Miro, J. M., Pena, J. M. *et al.* Randomized trial of the discontinuation of primary and secondary prophylaxis against *Pneumocystis carinii* pneumonia after highly active antiretroviral therapy in patients with HIV infection. *N. Engl. J. Med.* 2001;**344**:159–167.

61. Havlir, D. V., Dube, M. P., Sattler, F. R. *et al.* Prophylaxis against disseminated *Mycobacterium avium* complex with weekly azithromycin, daily rifabutin, or both. *N. Engl. J. Med.* 1996;**335**:392–398.

62. NICHD IVIG Study Group. Intravenous immune globulin for the prevention of bacterial infection in children with symptomatic human immunodeficiency virus infection. *N. Engl. J. Med.* 1991;**325**:73–80.

63. Spector, S. A., Gelber, R. D., McGrath, N. *et al.* A Controlled trial of intravenous immune globulin for the prevention of serious bacterial infections in children receiving zidovudine for advanced human immunodeficiency virus infection. *N. Engl. J. Med.* 1994;**331**:1181–1187.

64. McKinsey, D. S., Wheat, L. F., Cloud, G. A. *et al.* Itraconazole prophylaxis for fungal infections in patients with advanced human immunodeficiency virus infection: randomized, placebo-controlled, double-blind study. *Clin. Infect. Dis.* 1999;**28**:1049–1056.

65. Frenkel, L. D., Gaur, S., Tsolia, M. *et al.* Cytomegalovirus infection in children with AIDS. *Rev. Infect. Dis.* 1990;**12** (Suppl 7): S820–S826.

66. Nigro, G., Krzystofiak, A., Gattinara, G. *et al.* Rapid progression of HIV diseases in children with CMV DNAemia. *AIDS* 1996;**10**:1127–1133.

67. Mussi-Pinhata, M. M., Yamamoto, Y., Figueiredo, L. T. M. *et al.* Congenital and perinatal cytomegalovirus infection in infants born to mothers infected with human immunodeficiency virus. *J. Pediatr.* 1998;**132**:285–290.

68. Kovacs, A., Schlucter, M., Easley, K. *et al.* Cytomegalovirus infection and HIV-1 disease progression in infants born to HIV-1-infected women. *N. Engl. J. Med.* 1999; **341**: 77–84.

69. Spector, S. A., McKinley, G. F., Lalezari, J. P. *et al.* Oral ganciclovir for the prevention of cytomegalovirus disease in persons with AIDS. *N. Engl. J. Med.* 1996;**334**:1491–1497.

70. Cordell, R. L., Addiss, D. G. Cryptosporidiosis in child care settings: a review of the literature and recommendations for prevention and control. *Pediatr. Infect. Dis. J.* 1994;**13**:310–317.

71. Flanigan, T., Whalen, C., Turner, J. *et al. Cryptosporidium* infection and CD4 counts. *Ann. Intern. Med.* 1992;**116**:840–842.

72. Cello, J. P., Acquired immunodeficiency syndrome cholangiopathy: spectrum of disease. *Am. J. Med.* 1989;**86**:539–546.

73. Holmberg, S. D., Moorman, A. C., Von Bargen, J. C. *et al.* Possible effectiveness of clarithromycin and rifabutin for cryptosporidiosis chemoprophylaxis in HIV disease. *J. Am. Med. Assoc.* 1998;**279**:384–386.

74. Centers for Disease Control and Prevention. Pregnancy outcomes following systemic prenatal acyclovir exposure: June 1, 1984–June 30, 1993. *Morb. Mortal. Wkly Rep.* 1993;**42**:806–809.

75. Plancoulaine, S., Abel, L., van Beveren, M. *et al.* Human herpesvirus 8 transmission from mother to child and between siblings in an endemic population. *Lancet* 2000;**356**:1062–1065.

76. Yeung LTF, King SM, Roberts EA. Mother-to-infant transmission of hepatitis C virus. *Hepatology* 2001;**34**:223–229.

77. Havens, J.F., Mellins, C.A., Hunter, J. Psychiatric Aspects of HIV/AIDS in childhood and adolescence. In Rutter, M., Taylor, E. eds *Child and Adolescent Psychiatry: Modern Approaches*, 4th edn. Oxford, UK: Blackwell, 2001:828–841.

78. Mellins, C. A., Brackis-Cott, E., Dolezal, C., Richards, A., Nicholas, S., Abrams, E. J. Patterns of HIV status disclosure to perinatally infected HIV-positive children and subsequent mental health outcomes. *Clin. Child Psychol. Psychiatry*. 2001;**7**:101–114.

6 Emergency evaluation and care

James M. Callahan, MD

Department of Emergency Medicine, SUNY – Upstate Medical University
Syracuse, NY

Any clinician who sees sick children in an acute care setting may treat children with HIV and should be familiar with the atypical and sometimes life-threatening diseases that affect HIV-infected children. HIV-infected children are frequently seen in the emergency department (ED) [1]. HIV–infected children present to the ED with different complaints, are more likely to have diagnostic or therapeutic procedures performed and are more likely to be admitted to the hospital than uninfected children [2]. HIV status may not be known at the time of an ED visit. Manifestations of HIV infection may not be recognized [3, 4].

Even with the wide variety of antiretroviral therapies currently available, the quick recognition and aggressive treatment of the infectious complications of HIV infection in children may be life saving. Initial diagnosis of HIV infection may be made when a child presents with an acute and possibly life-threatening illness. Physicians must know the right questions to ask and the signs to look for. They must also be familiar with the appropriate evaluation and treatment options available to these children.

Emergency department presentation

History

HIV-infected children, whose diagnosis is unknown, may first present to the ED. Physicians must be familiar with historical factors that may put a parent or child at risk for HIV infection (Table 6.1). Today, almost all pediatric patients with HIV infection have perinatally acquired infections.

Pediatric patients with HIV infection present in many ways. Poor growth or delayed development may be seen. Multiple hospital admissions for invasive bacterial illnesses (e.g., meningitis, cellulitis, sinusitis, and/or pneumonia) [4] and oral thrush unresponsive to treatment or occurring after the first year of life may suggest HIV disease. A history of otherwise common pediatric problems resistant to usual therapy (e.g., severe

Handbook of Pediatric HIV Care, ed. Steven L. Zeichner and Jennifer S. Read.
Published by Cambridge University Press. © Cambridge University Press 2006.

Table 6.1. Possible indications of HIV infection from the history

Parental history

History of HIV infection

IV drug abuse

Other substance abuse or addiction

Sexual contact with IV drug user(s)

Multiple sexual partners

Prostitution

Absence of parents (death or inability to care for child may be due to parental HIV infection)

Patient history

Unexplained small-for-gestational age birth

Unexplained failure to thrive

Multiple serious (invasive) bacterial infections

Unexpectedly severe consequences of common viral infections

Recurrent thrush or oral thrush after 12 months of age

Unexplained developmental delay; loss of milestones

Persistent or recurrent diarrhea

Sexually transmitted diseases

---

eczematous or seborrheic rashes) may also be a sign of HIV disease [5–7]. Patients with sexually transmitted diseases, especially adolescents with recurrent pelvic inflammatory disease, should be counseled that they are at risk for HIV infection and should be screened.

In some children, the diagnosis may not be made until the child is 6 to 8 years of age or older. The ED physician must remain open to the possibility that an older child's symptoms or presentation may be due to HIV infection. Children may present with early onset of symptoms, opportunistic infections (especially *Pneumocystis carinii* pneumonia (PCP), rapid progression and early death [5, 6]. In contrast, they may have a more indolent course with signs of lymphadenopathy, hepatosplenomegaly, parotid swelling, and recurrent episodes of bacterial illnesses. These latter children are more likely to have lymphoid interstitial pneumonitis (LIP) and slowly progressive neurologic symptoms. These two types of presentation are not mutually exclusive. Children with a slower progression of illness may develop the acute onset of severe symptoms including opportunistic infections.

Physical examination

Table 6.2 lists physical examination findings suggestive of pediatric HIV infection. Many of these findings are non-specific. Certainly, a combination of several of these findings should prompt an evaluation for HIV infection.

Table 6.2. Physical findings associated with pediatric HIV infection

General
Failure to thrive; severe wasting
Extensive and/or persistent lymphadenopathy
Hepatosplenomegaly

Pulmonary
Unexplained digital clubbing
Persistent respiratory distress (especially if hypoxic or associated with a reticulonodular pattern or a chronic interstitial pneumonia on X-ray)
Hypoxia out of proportion to respiratory distress

Head and neck
Oral thrush unresponsive to therapy or in children > 12 months of age
Persistent or recurrent parotid swelling
Severe or recalcitrant otitis media or sinusitis
Unexplained microcephaly
Severe stomatitis secondary to herpes simplex virus

Skin
Unusually severe manifestations of viral illnesses (rubeola, varicella)
Extensive molluscum contagiosum
Recurrent folliculitis
Severe or recurrent ulcers due to herpes simplex virus
Severe eczematous or seborrheic dermatitis
Purpura or petechial rashes

Neurologic
Unexplained developmental delay or loss of milestones
Unexplained spasticity

Laboratory and radiologic abnormalities

Certain abnormalities (Table 6.3) found on diagnostic testing done in the ED should prompt consideration of HIV as an underlying diagnosis. If these are found in a patient with other signs or symptoms of HIV disease, this diagnosis should be entertained. Unexplained hematuria or proteinuria or both can be due to HIV-mediated renal disease. Patients who have an elevated serum total protein with a normal or low serum albumin may have an increased globulin fraction owing to the increased production of IgG, particularly in the setting of lymphadenopathy and hepatosplenomegaly.

Presentation of children with known HIV infection

Patients with known HIV infection may present to the ED for related or unrelated complaints. The approach to these patients may have to be modified (e.g., additional diagnostic tests may need to be performed and disposition and treatment decisions

Table 6.3. Non-specific laboratory and radiologic abnormalities potentially suggestive of HIV infection

Laboratory
Anemia
Neutropenia
Thrombocytopenia
Increased globulin fraction
Hematuria, proteinuria

Radiologic
Chronic, interstitial pneumonitis
Hilar lymphadenopathy
Reticulonodular pattern on chest X-ray

Table 6.4. Important history in patients with known HIV infection

CDC classification
HIV RNA level
CD4+ count
Antiretroviral therapy
Prophylaxis for opportunistic infections; particularly *Pneumocystis carinii* pneumonia
Past opportunistic infections

may need to be altered). In the ED, HIV-exposed children with indeterminate infection should be treated as if they are HIV-infected [6].

In obtaining a history in patients with known HIV infection, some key information should be elicited (Table 6.4). Patients with evidence of severe immunocompromise or previous episodes of opportunistic infections, especially PCP, are at a much higher risk of developing a new, potentially life-threatening, opportunistic infection. The absence of these factors does not mean that a patient does not have PCP or another opportunistic infection.

A key component of caring for patients with HIV infection is ensuring good follow-up care. The primary care physician must be informed of the ED visit, what was done, and when the patient needs to follow up before the patient is discharged.

HIV testing in the emergency department

When a patient presents to the ED with signs or symptoms of possible HIV infection, he or she should be tested for HIV. If HIV testing is to be done in the ED, appropriate pre- and post-test counseling must be available. It must be ensured that the patient can be contacted if he or she does not return for follow-up. Ideally, the same healthcare provider or providers should see the patient on both visits. There should be adequate time for discussion of test results and their ramifications. In a busy ED where personnel work variable shifts this may be difficult to do. ED social workers may be very helpful in counseling patients or arranging follow-up. If good follow-up, counseling, and patient confidentiality can be ensured, then testing can be done in the ED. Many families may not have regular healthcare providers and may go to the ED for all medical care. Not testing these patients may mean that they won't get tested.

If testing in the ED is not feasible, the patient must be referred for appropriate testing. The parents or caretakers should be informed why there is a concern about the patient. A referral should be made to the primary care physician or another resource where testing can be done. Contact must be made with that provider to inform them as to why the patient is being referred. An appointment is ideally made for the patient and given to the caretaker before discharge from the ED.

In any case, treatment for potentially life-threatening complications and manifestations of HIV infection should not be delayed pending a definitive diagnosis. Children with potentially life-threatening presentations should be treated presumptively as being HIV-infected. For example, an infant with respiratory distress, failure to thrive, lymphadenopathy and organomegaly on physical examination should be presumptively treated for PCP, even if no definitive HIV testing is available.

Postexposure testing and prophylaxis

A special case when HIV testing is desirable in the ED is when a patient is to undergo postexposure prophylaxis (PEP) following accidental needlestick injuries or an episode of sexual assault. There are very few data about the use of PEP in pediatric and adolescent patients. One recent report documented the experience at one pediatric ED [8]. If PEP is to be instituted, baseline HIV testing should be done in the ED. In some states, it is currently required that physicians offer the option of PEP to victims of sexual assault. This requires a set plan for when PEP and testing should be offered, how medications will be obtained and paid for, and who will counsel the patient and family. Appropriate follow-up including informing the patient and family of test results must be arranged before ED discharge. This may be coordinated with the patient's primary care physician or another hospital-based service (e.g., adolescent medicine, child abuse referral team, or pediatric infectious diseases).

Life-threatening presentations

Children with HIV infection may present with life-threatening complications (Table 6.5). A common acute presentation is a child with respiratory distress, fever, and cough. This can be due to a variety of etiologies including PCP, bacterial, and viral pneumonias. PCP pneumonitis can be rapidly progressive and fatal; PCP may be the initial presentation of HIV infection in young infants. The clinician must maintain a high degree of suspicion. Hypoxia, usually more severe than expected from the degree of respiratory distress, is a common finding [5]. The chest X-ray may be normal, especially early in the course of the illness or may show a diffuse alveolar and/or interstitial

Table 6.5. Life-threatening symptomatology in patients with HIV infection

---

Sepsis
  Increased incidence of invasive bacterial disease
  Fever or hypothermia with decreased perfusion

Respiratory distress
  Respiratory distress with marked hypoxia
  Consider and begin therapy for *Pneumocystis carinii* pneumonia
  Cytomegalovirus (CMV) pneumonitis may also be rapidly progressive

Gastrointestinal bleeding
  Bacterial, viral, and parasitic gastroenteritides
  CMV enteritis can cause severe
      gastrointestinal bleeding; experimental therapy ganciclovir may be helpful

Seizure and/or abrupt change in mental status
  Consider meningitis (bacterial, viral, and opportunistic pathogens)
  Stroke is a rare but reported complication
  Metabolic and toxic etiologies, not directly related to HIV disease

---

pattern [6]. If PCP is suspected, therapy with intravenous trimethoprim-sulfamethoxazole (TMP-SMX) should be initiated immediately (see Chapter 35). Diagnostic tests may be performed after the patient is stabilized.

Pediatric patients with HIV infection are at increased risk of invasive bacterial illnesses. Fever may be the only sign of these illnesses. Patients may present with sepsis and shock (see Chapter 30 and the text that follows).

Most children with HIV infection have neurologic involvement at some time in their illness. However, this involvement is usually a slow, progressive process. Seizures or an acute change in mental status are rare [5]. Neurologic presentations should prompt an investigation to rule out meningitis due to routine or opportunistic organisms, central nervous system (CNS) malignancies or stroke, particularly in patients with thrombocytopenia (see Chapter 19).

Gastrointestinal bleeding can be seen as a manifestation of disseminated CMV infection with CMV enteritis. Submucosal bleeding in this disease can produce lead points, which lead to intussusception, a rare presentation. Disseminated CMV infection may be treated with ganciclovir, but the prognosis is grave regardless of therapy (see Chapters 26 and 34).

Fever

Fever is the single, most common chief complaint among HIV-infected children who present to the ED [9]. Many of these children are well-appearing or have minimal symptoms. Invasive bacterial illnesses are common [10] (see Chapters 3, 5, and 32).

Causes

Fever in an HIV-infected child may result from invasive bacterial infections or opportunistic infections. Children with HIV infection experience increased rates of bacteremia, bacterial pneumonia, sinusitis (including chronic infections), urinary tract infections, osteomyelitis, meningitis, oral candidiasis and abscesses of internal organs [5, 10–13] (see Chapter 30).

PCP is the most common and potentially the most serious opportunistic infection [10]. Affected patients usually present with abrupt onset of fever and cough, respiratory distress and hypoxia. Hypoxia is often more severe than one would expect from the amount of respiratory distress. Other opportunistic infections, including cryptococcosis, toxoplasmosis, and *M. avium–intracellulare* complex (MAC) may be seen. These infections are more often seen in children with advanced disease; such children frequently present with chronic fevers. Chronic, almost daily fevers can also be seen in children as a manifestation of their HIV infection, especially in advanced stages.

Viral infections can also cause fevers in children with HIV infection. Asymptomatic children may handle routine infections without much difficulty [11, 13]. However, children with HIV infection may have severe or disseminated infections with agents such as respiratory syncytial virus (RSV), varicella, and rubella. Children with these and other usually well-tolerated viral infections should be approached in a cautious manner. Good supportive care, close observation and follow-up, and specific antiviral agents when available (e.g., acyclovir for varicella) all are indicated.

Evaluation and treatment of the well-appearing febrile child

Well-appearing children who have never had a serious bacterial or opportunistic infection should have a minimal outpatient evaluation (Table 6.6) [6, 11]. A complete blood count (CBC) is usually obtained. However, in one study the white blood count (WBC) was not useful in identifying patients with bacteremia or serious infections [9]. Even with episodes of invasive pneumococcal disease, the WBC and other laboratory tests are neither sensitive nor specific in identifying patients with invasive disease [14–16]. However, children with a high WBC, especially if accompanied by a bandemia, should be admitted for parenteral antibiotics. Children receiving zidovudine (AZT) or lamivudine may have neutropenia as a side effect of therapy [6]. The two agents together may accentuate this effect.

Invasive pneumococcal infections (IPI) are the most common serious bacterial infection in HIV-infected children [14–16]. Rates of IPI are significantly higher than in uninfected children [14]. Patients with HIV disease are less likely to have leukocytosis or other laboratory abnormalities than uninfected children [14–16] and more likely to have pneumococcal isolates that are penicillin resistant [15]. In one study, patients with occult pneumococcal bacteremia tended to do well and did not develop meningitis or other complications or sequelae when treated as outpatients [16]. Empiric antibiotics significantly decreased the rate of persistent bacteremia at their return visit. Patients who were afebrile and well-appearing at revisit were safely treated as outpatients [16].

Table 6.6. Evaluation of the febrile child

Well-appearing

Thorough history and physical examination

CBC with differential

Blood culture

Pulse oximetry

Chest X-ray if signs of respiratory illness

Urinalysis and urine culture in children who are not toilet-trained or older children
    with urinary symptoms

Stool for WBCs and culture if there is a history of diarrhea

Ill-appearing

Thorough history and physical examination

Close monitoring of vital signs

CBC with differential

Platelet count

Coagulation studies (PT, PTT, fibrin degradation products, fibrinogen; especially if
    platelet count is low or there is evidence of bleeding)

Blood culture for bacteria (consider mycobacteria and fungi)

Chest X-ray

Pulse oximetry (arterial blood gases if marked respiratory distress, decreased
    perfusion or unexplained tachypnea)

Urinalysis and urine culture

Cerebrospinal fluid for cell count and differential, Gram's stain, glucose, protein and
    bacterial culture, if indicated; consider special studies for opportunistic infections

---

Neutropenic patients with fever should be admitted for parenteral antibiotics pending culture results. Children with indeterminate HIV infection status should be given the "benefit of the doubt" and treated as if they are HIV-infected [6]. Children with a history of fever who are afebrile on presentation should be treated the same way.

If no infection, or only a presumed viral infection (e.g., an upper respiratory infection), is found, the patient may be managed as an outpatient without antibiotics. If a localized bacterial infection is found (e.g., otitis media or sinusitis) in a patient who appears well, appropriate oral antibiotics can be given and the child managed as an outpatient with close follow-up. Children with HIV infection have frequent episodes of otitis media and these infections seem to be more resistant and recurrent in nature than in healthy children [17, 18] (see Chapter 22). Treatment with the usual oral antibiotics (amoxicillin) is appropriate. As these children have an increased rate of infection with resistant organisms, high-dose amoxicillin (80–90 mg/kg per day) should be used. If the patient does not respond rapidly, agents with a broader spectrum (amoxicillin-clauvulanate, cefuroxime, or axetil) or other agents (erythromycin-sulfisoxazole, clarithromycin or azithromycin) may be considered. All children with fever who are managed as outpatients should have follow-up within 24 to 48 hours.

Table 6.7. Indications for hospital admission in febrile children

---

Toxic appearance (lethargy, unexplained tachycardia or tachypnea, hypotension)

Neutropenia

Presence of indwelling venous devices (some centers treat well-appearing patients with antibiotics and follow closely as outpatients)

Increased WBCs or bandemia

Previous episodes of serious invasive bacterial disease or opportunistic infections

---

Families should return for a recheck if their condition worsens. It is important to know how the family can be contacted. The family's address, multiple phone numbers, and even cellular phone and radiopager numbers should be obtained and noted on the chart. Communication with the patient's primary care provider to arrange a follow-up appointment is very important before the patient leaves the ED. The parent or caretaker must know exactly what to look for if the child is becoming more ill and what symptoms should prompt an immediate recheck.

Children with previous episodes of serious bacterial infections (e.g., sepsis or meningitis), a previous history of opportunistic infections, or a history of low CD4 counts should be treated more conservatively. There should be a very low threshold for admitting these patients when they present with fever, even if they look well [11]. Patients receiving periodic treatments with intravenous immunoglobulin (IVIG) are not completely protected against bacterial infections. IVIG has no effect on the incidence of opportunistic infections.

Patients with in-dwelling central venous catheters who present with fevers may be admitted for intravenous antibiotics pending blood cultures. If well-appearing, these patients may be given a single dose of intravenous antibiotics with close follow-up as outpatients. Indications for admission of febrile children with HIV infection are listed in Table 6.7.

Fever control for children with HIV infection can be accomplished with acetaminophen or ibuprofen as long as no other contraindications to the use of these medicines exist. Patients with thrombocytopenia or renal disease should not use ibuprofen or other non-steroidal anti-inflammatory drugs (NSAIDs).

Evaluation and treatment of the ill-appearing febrile child

All HIV-infected children with fever who are ill-appearing should have an immediate evaluation (see Table 6.6) and begin broad-spectrum parenteral antibiotics. These children all should be hospitalized. *Streptococcus pneumoniae* is the most common cause of invasive bacterial infections [15, 19]. Other organisms, including *Haemophilus influenzae* type b, *Salmonella* sp., and other gram-negative enteric organisms, may also cause invasive disease [5, 9–11, 19]. Children who present in shock, especially those with indwelling central venous devices and those colonized with *Pseudomonas* sp. may have infections due to *Pseudomonas*. Fungal sepsis, disseminated viral infections, and PCP may cause children to have fever and appear ill. Any child with fever and respiratory distress should be treated for PCP until a diagnosis is made (see Chapters 30, 33, 35 and the following text).

The history and physical examination may give clues to the cause of the patient's deterioration. Vital signs should be watched closely. In children, hypotension is a late and ominous sign. Tachycardia, prolonged capillary refill, anxiety or depressed mental status for age are signs of compensated shock and should prompt immediate action. Fluid therapy with boluses of isotonic fluids and vasopressor support, if needed, are just as important as giving the appropriate antibiotics.

A chest X-ray should be obtained. Bacterial pneumonia can occur suddenly in children. PCP can present with fever, cough, respiratory distress, and hypoxia. Patients with sepsis syndrome may develop pulmonary edema and the acute respiratory distress syndrome (ARDS). Pulse oximetry and arterial blood gas values should be followed closely.

Patients who present with fever accompanied by seizures, irritability, marked lethargy, a change in mental status, or other signs of meningitis should have a lumbar puncture. Bacterial meningitis is the primary concern. Opportunistic infections may also be present, although not so frequently.

Treatment of ill-appearing febrile children with HIV infection demands meticulous monitoring and supportive care (fluid resuscitation and therapy; vasopressor agents, oxygen, ventilatory support, and blood product support as needed). Early administration of broad spectrum, parenteral antibiotics is imperative. A third generation cephalosporin is often an appropriate choice. Cefotaxime or ceftriaxone provide good coverage for both gram-positive and gram-negative organisms as well as adequate penetration of the CSF. Ill-appearing children with in-dwelling catheters should receive broader coverage. A reasonable choice would include the addition of an antistaphylococcal penicillin (e.g., nafcillin or oxacillin). Patients with previous episodes of disease secondary to *Pseudomonas* sp. and those in shock should be treated for possible infection with these organisms [11]. Ceftazidime and an aminoglycoside would be appropriate.

Studies have shown high rates of resistance to penicillin and cephalosporins among *S. pneumoniae* isolates in patients with HIV infection [15, 19]. Patients with meningitis usually appear ill at presentation [16]. In patients with meningitis or those for whom there is a high suspicion of pneumococcal illness, broader coverage, such as the addition of vancomycin or rifampin, should be given. If corticosteroids are to be given in patients with meningitis, rifampin is the preferred additional agent. Antibiotic therapy should be refined when culture and sensitivity results are available.

Evaluation of the child with persistent fevers

Many HIV-infected children have persistent or recurrent fevers as part of their primary illness. Often, extensive workups have already been performed. These children should

Table 6.8. Major causes of respiratory distress

Bacterial pneumonia
   Streptococcus pneumoniae, Haemophilus influenzae type b, group A streptococci,
   Staphylococcus aureus, Mycoplasma pneumoniae, Branhamella catarrhalis,
   Pseudomonas aeruginosa and other gram-negative organisms
Common viral pathogens (e.g., respiratory syncytial virus, influenza, adenovirus)
Pneumocystis carinii pneumonia
Lymphoid interstitial pneumonitis
Underlying reactive airway disease
Other opportunistic infections (MAC, tuberculosis, aspergillosis, *Legionella*)
Cytomegalovirus pneumonitis
Cardiac disease

---

be evaluated thoroughly. Any change in clinical status should prompt a renewed evaluation. This includes any change in the frequency or character of the patient's febrile episodes. The clinician best able to make these judgments is the patient's primary care physician. If this physician is unable to see the patient, the ED clinician should at least contact the primary care physician to discuss the patient's clinical presentation and prior workup. The primary concern in evaluating these patients in the ED is to be confident (based upon clinical evaluation and, if necessary ancillary studies) that a new, acute process is not present.

Respiratory distress

Respiratory distress can be an ominous sign in HIV-infected children. PCP is still the most common opportunistic infection in these children and a major cause of morbidity [20]. Respiratory infections are the most common cause of mortality in HIV-infected children [21]. Many other causes – both infectious and non-infectious – may be responsible for producing respiratory distress. Respiratory distress in an HIV-infected child should prompt an immediate evaluation and quick treatment.

Causes

The major causes of respiratory distress in children with HIV infections are listed in Table 6.8. Some of these causes are relatively rare (e.g., opportunistic infections other than PCP and CMV infection). Bacterial pneumonias are common. Children may also suffer from infections with common viral pathogens.

PCP is the most worrisome cause of respiratory distress. LIP is a common finding in children with HIV infection. It causes a slow but progressive decrease in pulmonary function. Children with HIV infection may have underlying reactive airway disease as well [22] (see Chapter 24). The impact of HIV infection on other organ systems including the effects of cardiomyopathy may cause respiratory distress. Children may also have

Table 6.9. Emergency evaluation of children with respiratory distress

---

Complete history and physical examination
Chest radiograph
CBC and differential
Pulse oximetry
Induced sputum or BAL to rule out PCP (unless another diagnosis is definitive)

If indicated:
    Arterial blood gas
    Lactate dehydrogenase (LDH) level
    Blood culture
    Viral studies
    PPD and anergy testing

---

respiratory distress due to other opportunistic infections, including MAC, tuberculosis, aspergillosis, and *Legionella* infection.

Evaluation

Table 6.9 outlines the usual evaluation of children with HIV infection and respiratory distress. Prior history of opportunistic infections (especially PCP) or a bacterial pneumonia should be determined. The PPD status of the patient, family, and contacts should be ascertained [23]. Tuberculosis, although relatively rare, requires aggressive therapy. A prior history of reactive airway disease or LIP can guide therapy and evaluation.

Children with known reactive airway disease who present with mild, diffuse wheezing, are afebrile and look relatively well may be given a trial of beta-agonists. If they improve with minimal treatment, are not hypoxic, and continue to look well, no further evaluation needs to be done [22]. Ipratropium may be added as it has been shown to decrease admission rates in children without HIV infection that are having moderate to severe attacks. Oral corticosteroids should be prescribed for a brief course. These children should have close follow-up to be sure that they do not have deterioration in their status. Their primary care physician must be informed and follow-up scheduled in 1 to 2 days.

In all other children, a chest X-ray and CBC should be done in addition to pulse oximetry. Children with bacterial pneumonias present with fever, cough, tachypnea, and varying degrees of respiratory distress [20, 22, 23]. Hypoxemia may be present. Many pneumonias in children result from hematogenous seeding of the lung during episodes of occult bacteremia. Respiratory symptoms may be minimal. Chest X-rays usually show lobar or segmental infiltrates [22–24]. In patients with pleural effusions, pleurocentesis may provide relief of symptoms and identify an etiologic agent. The WBC is usually elevated, and there is usually a left shift in the differential.

Children with HIV infection may also have infections with common respiratory pathogens. When infected with respiratory syncytial virus, children with HIV infection are less likely to have wheezing and more likely to present with pneumonia [20, 25]. HIV-infected children have prolonged viral shedding. Measles infection may lead to severe pneumonia in children with AIDS [20]. Diagnosis may be made with nasal washings for rapid viral diagnostic tests. If children have severe symptoms or are not improving as would be expected, simultaneous infection with bacterial pathogens, PCP, or other pathogens may be present.

Pneumocystis carinii pneumonia

PCP can manifest at any age, but 50% of reported cases in children with HIV infection occur in the first six months of life [26]. PCP may be the first manifestation of HIV-related disease. Consideration of PCP should trigger the initiation of therapy. Usually, children have acute onset of tachypnea, dyspnea, and cough [6, 20]. However, they may also present with a cough of days to weeks in duration with only slowly progressive tachypnea [22, 23]. Physical examination shows tachypnea, dyspnea, rhonchi, and wheezes. Rales may be present but are rare [22]. There is usually hypoxia, which is more marked than would be expected from the patient's symptoms. Chest X-rays typically show a diffuse, interstitial pattern, although clear radiographs (especially early in the disease process), hyperinflation, lobar infiltrates, or even severe changes consistent with ARDS have been reported [20, 22]. Lactate dehydrogenase (LDH) levels are usually markedly elevated (>500 IU), and the alveolar–arterial oxygen gradient is usually high (>30 mm Hg) [20, 22, 27]. Definitive diagnosis is made on specimens obtained by induced sputum or bronchoalveolar lavage (see Chapter 24 for a detailed discussion of diagnosis and therapy of PCP). Therapy should not wait until a definitive diagnosis is made.

Lymphoid interstitial pneumonitis

LIP is a slowly progressive finding in many children with HIV infection and is the most common respiratory complication in these children [23]. Usually, children present after 1 year of age [28]. Patients may have a cough but often present only with mild tachypnea [22]. Digital clubbing is often present. Hypoxia is usually mild but chronic. Often, children with LIP have associated lymphadenopathy, hepatosplenomegaly, and parotid enlargement. They frequently have clear breath sounds, but wheezing and other signs of bronchospasm may be present. Chest X-rays show a diffuse, interstitial process often with a reticulonodular pattern [20, 22, 23, 27, 28]. LIP can progress to respiratory failure if not recognized and treated [24]. LDH is mildly elevated (usually 250–500 IU) [22]. There may be some overlap of LDH values with children with PCP (see Chapter 24).

Cytomegalovirus

Patients with HIV infection and prior infection with CMV may have reactivation of their CMV with immune dysfunction or immunosuppressed patients may have acute infections. Pneumonia may be one manifestation. Retinitis, hepatitis, and colitis may

Table 6.10. Treatment of children with respiratory symptoms

Condition	Treatment
Reactive airway disease	Bronchodilators (including ipratropium), corticosteroids
Bacterial pneumonia	Amoxicillin, amoxicillin-clavulanate, or cefuroxime PO or cefuroxime IV (if severely ill or accompanied by sepsis, use broader antibiotic coverage)
Bacterial pneumonia in recently hospitalized patients	Ceftriaxone and antistaphylococcal penicillin IV (consider coverage for *Pseudomonas*, e.g., ceftazidime and an aminoglycoside)
Pneumocystis carinii pneumonia	Trimethoprim-sulfamethoxazole or pentamidine IV
Lymphoid interstitial pneumonitis – pulmonary lymphoid hyperplasia	Corticosteroids PO (may give IV if critically ill)
Viral processes	Supportive care (consider ribavirin for respiratory syncytial virus, amantadine for influenza, ganciclovir for cytomegalovirus, acyclovir for varicella)

All children should receive supportive care including oxygen, bronchodilator therapy, ventilatory support, and IV fluids as indicated.

also be seen [22]. Pneumonia accompanied by one of these findings is very suggestive of CMV disease. Pneumonia due to CMV often looks like PCP on chest X-rays. CMV may cause co-infection with PCP and may contribute to a lack of improvement with conventional therapy for PCP [30]. Lung biopsy may be required to definitively diagnose the cause of the patient's respiratory compromise (see Chapter 24).

Therapy

A summary of treatments for specific respiratory conditions in children with HIV infection can be found in Table 6.10. Supportive care, including oxygen therapy, ventilatory support, bronchodilator therapy, and intravenous fluids, should be provided as needed. Patients who may be developing respiratory failure should be kept nothing by mouth (NPO) in anticipation of possible endotracheal intubation. PCP can rapidly be fatal. If PCP is considered, therapy should be begun immediately [5, 20, 22, 23]. Corticosteroids have been shown to be helpful in pediatric patients with PCP and are usually also begun [21, 29–31]. (Therapy for PCP is covered in detail in Chapter 24).

Afebrile children who present with diffuse wheezing and respiratory distress may be given a trial of bronchodilator therapy. Patients with moderate to severe symptoms often benefit from the addition of ipratropium to beta-agonists. Ipratropium is not used as chronic therapy. If they improve rapidly and show no signs of a coexisting infection, they may be discharged to continue bronchodilator therapy at home. Corticosteroids, 1 to 2 mg/kg per day of prednisone or prednisolone, should be given for 4 to 5 days. Hypoxia, moderate to severe distress or rapidly recurring symptoms are indications for hospital admission just as they are for patients with reactive airway disease without HIV infection (therapy for reactive airway disease in the HIV-infected child is discussed in Chapter 24). Fever, a first episode of wheezing, severe distress, hypoxia, or failure to improve with usual therapy are indications to obtain a chest radiograph. Febrile children with wheezing who have rales, abnormal chest X-rays, or leukocytosis should receive antibiotics as well [22].

Patients with lobar or segmental infiltrates should be treated for bacterial pneumonia. If the diagnosis is not clear or if the patient is ill appearing, treatment may be initiated simultaneously for both bacterial infections and PCP pending definitive diagnosis. Patients who are only mildly symptomatic, not dehydrated, not hypoxic, and able to tolerate oral medications may be given a trial of oral antibiotics with close follow-up. If transportation back to the hospital is not readily available, or if the family is unable to adequately monitor the child's progress, the child should be admitted.

Amoxicillin, amoxicillin-clavulanate, and cefuroxime may be good choices for oral therapy, depending on local patterns of antibiotic resistance. Doubling the usual dose of the antibiotic has been recommended, especially in areas where there is a significant incidence of pneumococci with intermediate sensitivities to beta-lactams [22]. Remember that when this is done with amoxicillin-clavulanate, the clinician must be careful not to be giving too high a dose of clavulanate so as to cause gastrointestinal irritation and diarrhea (see Chapter 26). TMP-SMX should be reserved for patients with presumed PCP. Patients should be re-examined within 24 hours. Patients whose clinical status worsens at any time should be admitted for parenteral antibiotics. Patients on oral antibiotics who fail to improve within 24 to 48 hours should also be admitted for parenteral antibiotics. Failure to improve should also prompt a serious reconsideration of the underlying diagnosis.

Cefuroxime 100–150 mg/kg per day, divided into three doses is an excellent choice for otherwise uncomplicated cases requiring parenteral therapy. Patients who have recently been hospitalized should receive coverage to include therapy for *S. aureus* and gram-negative organisms. Ceftriaxone and an antistaphylococcal penicillin is a good alternative. If *Pseudomonas* sp. is suspected, ceftazidime and an aminoglycoside are appropriate. Seriously ill patients should also receive broader coverage.

Patients must be monitored closely. Deterioration or failure to improve should prompt reconsideration of the diagnosis, broadening the antibiotic coverage, and additional diagnostic testing. Although rare, patients with PCP may have lobar or segmental infiltrates on chest X-ray. The addition of TMP-SMX or pentamidine may be considered.

In children with hypoxia and findings consistent with LIP, treatment with corticosteroids may be helpful. Prednisone or prednisolone (if a liquid preparation is needed) at 1 to 2 mg/kg per day is given for several weeks [20, 22, 23]. Chapter 35 discusses therapy for LIP in more detail. Dosages are then slowly tapered as tolerated. Tuberculosis and pulmonary disease with MAC may look similar to LIP. If the patient has a history of fevers, these should be excluded before the patient is begun on corticosteroid therapy [22].

Most viral respiratory infections require only good supportive care. Critically ill children may be treated with specific antiviral agents (e.g., ribavirin for respiratory syncytial virus, acyclovir for varicella, ganciclovir for CMV pneumonitis, and amantadine for influenza) if a diagnosis is made.

Gastrointestinal emergencies

Diarrhea

Diarrhea, both acute and chronic, is a common problem in HIV-infected children. Acute diarrhea can cause dehydration, especially if accompanied by vomiting or fever. Chronic diarrhea and wasting may make an HIV-infected child more prone to dehydration from an intercurrent illness. Dehydration should be treated aggressively with fluids, which may be given intravenously, if necessary. Determining a causative agent may permit specific therapy and more rapid resolution of symptoms. Gastrointestinal disorders are discussed more completely in Chapter 26.

Differential diagnosis

Common causes of diarrhea in HIV-infected children are listed in Table 6.11. Patients who experience an abrupt onset of diarrhea without preceding vomiting are more likely to have a bacterial infection [32]. Bloody stools are more often seen in children with bacterial gastroenteritis. The finding of more than five stool leukocytes per high-power field is suggestive of bacterial infection.

Patients with emesis of several hours' duration followed by the onset of watery or occasionally mucoid diarrhea frequently have viral gastroenteritis [32]. Children with HIV infection experience infections with routine viral pathogens. However, these agents often cause prolonged symptoms [32, 33]. HIV-infected children may also experience gastroenteritis due to CMV and other uncommon causes.

Opportunistic infections including parasitic diseases and MAC may produce diarrhea in children – often of a chronic nature. Cryptosporidiosis has been reported to cause episodes of severe diarrhea, especially in patients with advanced symptoms [34]. Children with prolonged symptoms should be evaluated for these illnesses and treated as outlined in Chapter 26.

Evaluation

The evaluation of diarrhea in HIV-infected children is outlined in Table 6.12. The clinician should look for signs of dehydration or cardiovascular compromise and attempt to identify a causative agent. History of exposure to infectious agents can be helpful. Vomiting often precedes diarrhea with viral infections [32]. Bloody stools are common

Table 6.11. Common causes of diarrhea

Bacteria
  Salmonella sp.
  Shigella sp.
  Campylobacter sp.
  Yersinia enterocolitica
  Escherichia coli
  Clostridium difficile

Viruses
  Rotavirus
  Enteroviruses
  Adenovirus
  Cytomegalovirus

Opportunistic infections.
  Mycobacterium avium–intracellulare
  Giardia lamblia
  Cryptosporidium
  Entamoeba histolytica
  Microsporidia
  Isopora belli
  Cyclospora

in bacterial gastroenteritis. *Clostridium difficile*, CMV, and *Entamoeba histolytica* can also cause bloody stools. Tenesmus is common with *Shigella* and *E. histolytica*.

Caretakers should be asked about the patient's oral intake, activity level, and urine output. On physical examination, lethargy may indicate severe dehydration requiring prompt fluid resuscitation. Signs of dehydration or poor perfusion should also be looked for. Tachycardia, dry mucous membranes, cool extremities, and prolonged capillary refill all are worrisome signs. Decreased activity level may also indicate dehydration. Hypotension is a late sign signaling decompensated shock. Children who progress to this are near collapse and resuscitation may be difficult. It is imperative to intervene early before this occurs.

The presence of fecal leukocytes makes the diagnosis of bacterial gastroenteritis more likely. Sheets of leukocytes are often seen with *Shigella* infections. However, the absence of fecal leukocytes does not exclude bacterial sources. Children with HIV infection have a higher risk of developing invasive disease due to *Salmonella* sp. and other enteric organisms [32]. Gastroenteritis due to *Salmonella* should be treated with oral or parenteral antibiotics. Any signs of systemic illness (fever, rigors, poor perfusion) should raise the concern that the patient is bacteremic. Intravenous antibiotics should be administered in addition to rapid fluid resuscitation. Blood cultures should be obtained before antibiotics are given.

Table 6.12. Evaluation of HIV-infected children with diarrhea

History
    Possible exposure to infectious agents
    Presence and time course of vomiting
    Nature of diarrhea
    Presence of abdominal pain
    Presence of tenesmus
    Activity level
    Urine output

Physical examination
    Temperature
    Close attention to vital signs
    Signs of dehydration or poor perfusion
    Abdominal tenderness

Laboratory tests
    CBC with differential
    Serum electrolytes and glucose (glucose testing should be done at bedside)
    Blood culture for bacterial pathogens
    Stool examination for leukocytes
    Stool culture for bacterial pathogens
    Stool culture for viral pathogens
    Stool for *Clostridium difficile* toxins
    Stool examination for ova and parasites

A CBC may show leukocytosis with a left shift, especially if bacteremia is present. Patients with *Shigella* often have low or normal total WBCs but a marked bandemia in which band forms often exceed the number of mature neutrophils. Atypical lymphocytes may be seen in children with viral gastroenteritis. Serum electrolytes and glucose should be checked. Marked acidosis may call for bicarbonate replacement. Patients with a history of wasting and decreased body stores may be especially prone to hypoglycemia. In patients with prolonged diarrhea who have negative bacterial cultures and viral antigen tests, stools should be tested for *C. difficile* toxin and examined for ova and parasites and mycobacteria. Enteric cryptosporidiosis can cause severe diarrhea in patients with advanced HIV infection [34].

Therapy

The main goal of therapy in the patient with diarrhea is to ensure adequate hydration and end-organ perfusion. Children with mild diarrhea who can tolerate oral fluids may be able to be managed with oral electrolyte solutions or other dietary manipulations. Children who appear more than mildly dehydrated, who have diarrhea accompanied by marked emesis, or who have signs or symptoms of systemic disease that might be consistent with bacteremia should be rapidly rehydrated with intravenous fluids.

Initial fluid therapy consists of 20 ml/kg boluses of isotonic fluid (0.9% normal saline solution (NSS) or Ringer's lactate). Boluses are repeated until signs of decreased perfusion resolve. Urine output should be monitored. In children with signs of decompensated shock (i.e., hypotension), rapid fluid administration is still the first line of therapy. Vasopressor agents should be started if there is no response after 60–80 ml/kg of crystalloid fluids. Intraosseous needles may be used if intravenous access cannot be obtained. The anterior tibial plateau is the preferred site for intraosseous access in young children. The distal, anterior femur may also be used in young infants. In children over 3 years of age and especially in patients greater than 6 years of age, the distal tibia just cephalad to the medial malleolus is the preferred site. Any fluid or medication (including blood products), which would be administered through a standard intravenous line, may be given intraosseously.

Administration of glucose should be guided by serum glucose testing. Boluses of large volumes of glucose-containing fluids should be avoided. Bedside testing allows for rapid determination of the serum glucose. If low, glucose should be administered at a dose of 0.25–0.50 g/kg (2.5–5 ml/kg of 10% dextrose [D_{10}], 1–2 ml/kg of D_{25}, or 0.5–1 ml/kg of D_{50}). Lower concentrations (e.g., D_{10}) are less likely to cause phlebitis or venous irritation leading to a loss of intravenous access.

After fluid resuscitation and treatment of hypoglycemia have been completed, children should be begun on dextrose-containing fluids with saline to slowly replace fluid and electrolyte deficits (e.g., D_5, 0.45% NSS at 1.5 times maintenance). Deficits should be replaced over a period of 24 to 48 hours (48 to 72 hours in patients who are hypernatremic).

If a bacterial infection is suspected, antibiotics should be started (Table 6.13). Signs of toxicity, dehydration, poor perfusion, or inability to tolerate oral medications should prompt the institution of intravenous regimens. Cultures should be obtained before antibiotic therapy is begun. After results are available, sensitivity profiles should be used to guide antibiotic therapy.

Most viral pathogens are not amenable to specific therapy. CMV enteritis, when biopsy confirmed, may be treated with ganciclovir or foscarnet [32, 33]. When found, various parasitic and opportunistic infections may be treatable.

Abdominal pain
Differential diagnosis
Children with gastroenteritis may have abdominal pain as part of their constellation of symptoms. Diarrhea or vomiting or both may accompany the pain or follow soon after. *Y. enterocolitica* or MAC infection may cause mesenteric adenitis (inflammation of the mesenteric lymph nodes), which can lead to symptoms of severe abdominal pain, fever, and vomiting. It may be difficult to distinguish these symptoms from appendicitis or other acute abdominal processes.

Table 6.13. Antibiotics for bacterial gastroenteritis

Suspected agent	Oral antibiotics	Parenteral antibiotics
Salmonella sp.	Amoxicillin	Ampicillin
	TMP–SMX	TMP–SMX, Ceftriaxone
Shigella sp.	TMP–SMX, Amoxicillin (high rates of resistance in some areas), Tetracycline (in patients > 8 years of age)	TMP–SMX, Ampicillin Ceftriaxone Chloramphenicol
Campylobacter sp.	Erythromycin, Tetracycline (in patients > 8 years of age)	Aminoglycosides
Yersinia enterocolitica	TMP–SMX	TMP–SMX Chloramphenicol
Escherichia coli (there are no studies supporting the effectiveness of antibiotics in the treatment of *E. coli* enterocolitis) [36]	TMP–SMX	TMP–SMX
Clostridium difficile	Vancomycin, Metronidazole	

TMP-SMX, trimethoprim-sulfamethoxazole.
Once available, sensitivity testing should guide antibiotic choice.

Patients with HIV infection may have appendicitis. One adult study showed that HIV-infected individuals presented to the ED relatively late in their course and had a higher appendiceal perforation rate than non-infected controls [35]. None of the individuals with appendicitis had an elevated WBC. Patients with classic signs of appendicitis should have prompt surgical evaluation. Equivocal findings may be evaluated with abdominal and pelvic CT scans.

Patients with intussusception can present with abdominal pain, vomiting, and varying degrees of lethargy. Intussusception may result from lead points due to various disease processes (e.g., submucosal bleeding in patients with CMV enteritis). Other common causes of abdominal pain such as urinary tract infection and constipation may be seen in HIV-infected children as well. Pneumonia, especially involving the lower lobes may also present with abdominal pain (and may be accompanied by vomiting). HIV-infected children are also at risk for less common causes of abdominal pain.

Esophagitis due to *Candida* infections may be seen. Usually, pain is retrosternal or epigastric in location and occurs especially with swallowing [32, 33]. Esophagitis may or may not be accompanied by oral thrush. *Herpes simplex* virus (HSV) may lead to esophagitis with similar symptoms. Usually, oral ulcers accompany HSV esophagitis [32]. Young children may refuse to drink or have drooling as presenting signs.

HIV-infected children develop pancreatitis at increased rates [36]. In this group of patients, pancreatitis was associated with the use of pentamidine, especially in patients with very low CD4 counts. PCP, CMV, cryptosporidium, and MAC were all associated with pancreatitis. Patients with pancreatitis virtually all have abdominal pain and vomiting. Didanosine (ddI), lamivudine (3TC), stavudine (d4T), and zalcitibine (ddC) are also associated with pancreatitis [21, 37].

Splenic abscesses [38] and hydrops-like cholecystitis due to cryptosporidial endocholecystitis [39] are rare causes of recurrent or persistent abdominal pain that have been reported. Extrapulmonary *Pneumocystis carinii* infections can also involve abdominal organs.

Evaluation

Evaluation begins with a thorough history and physical examination. Fever may accompany gastroenteritis. Fever is also seen with urinary tract infections, lower lobe pneumonias, and acute abdominal processes such as appendicitis. Many patients with pancreatitis have fever as well. Absence of fever makes infections or suppurative causes of abdominal pain less common but does not exclude them completely.

A medication history may reveal the use of pentamidine, ddI, 3TC, d4T, ddC, or steroids. All of these agents have been associated with pancreatitis. A past history of pancreatitis, urinary tract infections, or recurrent problems with constipation may make one of these processes the most likely diagnosis. Emesis that is not followed by diarrhea within 12 to 24 hours makes gastroenteritis a less likely cause of abdominal pain. Pancreatitis, intussusception, or acute abdominal processes leading to an ileus or obstruction should be considered. Bilious emesis may be seen with an ileus but should raise the concern of a mechanical obstruction. All children with bilious emesis should have abdominal X-rays with multiple views to rule out an obstruction.

Peritoneal signs should prompt surgical consultation. Right lower quadrant pain and tenderness, rebound tenderness, and guarding are seen with appendicitis. Remember, the WBC may not be elevated. Abdominal and pelvic CT scans may be helpful. Right upper quadrant tenderness and possibly a mass may be seen with cholecystitis. Periumbilical, epigastric, and flank pain can be seen in pancreatitis. Often, the physical signs in children with pancreatitis seem to be less than would be expected from the child's symptoms. Severe pain and emesis are the most common symptoms seen. Intermittent, cramping, severe pain, which may be relieved by episodes of emesis, is more typical of intussusception. A mass may be felt in children with intussusception, usually in the right side of the abdomen. Bloody stools (currant-jelly stools) are a late sign of intussusception indicating mucosal ischemia and compromise. The goal should be to make this diagnosis before this occurs.

Unless the history and physical clearly point to a benign cause of abdominal pain (e.g., constipation) or gastroenteritis, HIV-infected children with abdominal pain should have some screening laboratory and radiologic studies performed. At least two radiologic views of the abdomen should be obtained. A CBC with differential, urinalysis, urine gram stain and culture should be obtained. Serum transaminases, bilirubin, lipase, and amylase determinations are helpful in the evaluation. In patients with pancreatitis, serum calcium, glucose, and electrolytes should be followed closely.

Esophagrams or esophagoscopy may be required to diagnose *Candida* or HSV esophagitis. Ultrasonography may be used to diagnose cholecystitis or monitor patients with pancreatitis for pseudocyst formation. It may also be useful in the diagnosis of appendicitis and some cases of intussusception. Air-contrast or barium enema remains the diagnostic tool of choice as well as the initial treatment for intussusception. Hepatic and splenic abscesses may be found with ultrasound or abdominal computed tomography (CT) scans.

Therapy

The main goal of therapy is to provide good supportive care until the underlying cause can be found. Hydration status should be monitored closely. Intravenous fluids and glucose and electrolytes should be given, if needed. Delaying the administration of analgesics while diagnostic studies are performed is not necessary. After a diagnosis is made, definitive therapy may be begun.

Children with esophagitis due to *Candida* may be treated with ketoconazole and mycostatin orally [32]. Failure to respond to this therapy in a few days should prompt the institution of parenteral therapy. Amphotericin B or fluconazole are possible alternatives [32] (see Chapter 33).

Treatment of pancreatitis is supportive in nature. Patients should be made NPO and have a nasogastric tube placed and put to low, intermittent suction to effect complete bowel rest. Intravenous fluids and parenteral hyperalimentation should be begun. Nasogastric losses should be replaced. Analgesia with opioids should be provided. Respiratory status, serum calcium, electrolytes, and glucose should be monitored carefully. Serial ultrasound or abdominal CT scans should be performed to monitor for the development of pancreatic pseudocysts, abscesses, or hemorrhagic complications. Medications that could have caused pancreatitis should be discontinued. Corticosteroids are not indicated and antibiotics should only be given for specific suppurative complications.

Parenchymal abscesses may be treated with antibiotics or antifungal agents if a causative organism is known. However, most parenchymal lesions require surgical drainage at some point [38]. Common causes of abdominal pain should be managed as they would in children without HIV infection (see Chapter 26).

Neurologic emergencies

Most HIV-infected children have neurologic involvement at some point [5, 7], usually an encephalopathy due to primary infection of the CNS [5–7]. Emergency presentations of this encephalopathy are rare. The acute onset of seizures or a change in mental status warrants emergency investigation and treatment. Chapters 10 and 19 contain more

Table 6.14. Differential diagnosis of seizures

Bacterial meningitis
Streptococcus pneumonia
Haemophilus influenzae type b
Escherichia coli
Salmonella sp.
Other bacteria

Opportunistic infections
Toxoplasma gondii
Cryptococcus neoformans
Candida albicans
Mycobacterium tuberculosis
Atypical mycobacteria

Viral infections
Cytomegalovirus
Herpes simplex virus

CNS malignancy

CNS hemorrhage or infarction

Rapidly progressive HIV encephalopathy

---

detailed discussions of the neurologic and neuropsychologic disorders associated with HIV infection.

Seizures

Differential diagnosis

HIV encephalopathy usually is not associated with seizures except when it is rapidly progressive [5, 7]. Other causes must be ruled out. The differential diagnosis of seizures in HIV-infected children is found in Table 6.14. CNS infections are a major cause of morbidity. Opportunistic infections of the CNS are less common than bacterial meningitis [7]. Pneumococcal and HiB disease may be seen even in patients with complete immunizations. Children may present with fever, headache, lethargy or irritability, nuchal rigidity, and possibly focal deficits. Seizures with fever may be seen.

Opportunistic infections caused by *Toxoplasma gondii*, *Cryptococcus neoformans*, *Candida albicans*, *Mycobacterium tuberculosis*, and atypical mycobacteria may cause focal or generalized seizures in patients with HIV infection. Meningeal signs and signs of increased intracranial pressure may be seen. Viral infections with CMV and HSV as well as common viruses such as enteroviruses may cause meningitis or encephalitis and seizures.

CNS malignancies, usually lymphoma, and hemorrhage or infarction may cause seizures, focal deficits, or an abrupt change in mental status [6, 7, 40, 41]. A small number

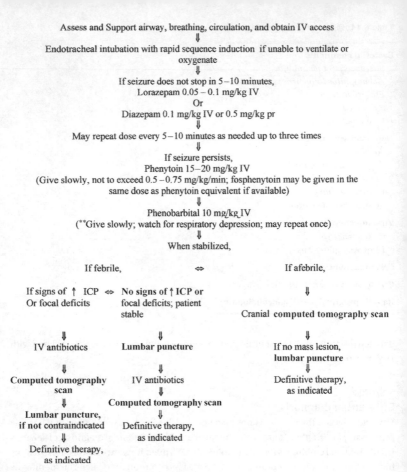

Assess and Support airway, breathing, circulation, and obtain IV access

⇓

Endotracheal intubation with rapid sequence induction if unable to ventilate or oxygenate

⇓

If seizure does not stop in 5–10 minutes,
Lorazepam 0.05 – 0.1 mg/kg IV

Or

Diazepam 0.1 mg/kg IV or 0.5 mg/kg pr

⇓

May repeat dose every 5–10 minutes as needed up to three times

⇓

If seizure persists,
Phenytoin 15–20 mg/kg IV
(Give slowly, not to exceed 0.5 – 0.75 mg/kg/min; fosphenytoin may be given in the same dose as phenytoin equivalent if available)

⇓

Phenobarbital 10 mg/kg IV
(**Give slowly; watch for respiratory depression; may repeat once)

⇓

When stabilized,

| If febrile, | ⇔ | | If afebrile, |

| If signs of ↑ ICP ⇔ Or focal deficits | No signs of ↑ ICP or focal deficits; patient stable | | ⇓ Cranial computed tomography scan |

| ⇓ IV antibiotics | ⇓ Lumbar puncture | | ⇓ If no mass lesion, lumbar puncture |

| ⇓ Computed tomography scan | ⇓ IV antibiotics | | ⇓ Definitive therapy, as indicated |

| ⇓ Lumbar puncture, if not contraindicated | ⇓ Computed tomography scan | | |

| ⇓ Definitive therapy, as indicated | ⇓ Definitive therapy, as indicated | | |

Fig. 6.1. Evaluation and treatment of seizures.

of pediatric HIV patients have developed CNS aneurysms (42). Infarctions have been reported in children with HIV encephalopathy and may account for their initial presentation [7, 40]. HIV-infected children may also have seizures due to the same causes seen in other children, including trauma, ingestions, and metabolic derangements.

Evaluation and treatment

Emergency evaluation and management of HIV-infected children with seizures proceed hand in hand (Fig. 6.1). The airway should be supported and the patient ventilated, if necessary. Bag–valve–mask ventilation is usually sufficient. If ventilation is not effective, or if prolonged hypoventilation occurs with the use of anticonvulsant medications, endotracheal intubation is indicated. In patients with uncontrolled status epilepticus or signs of increased intracranial pressure, rapid sequence intubation should be considered for cerebral protection. If the clinician is unable to obtain intravenous access, intraosseous needles may be used or diazepam may be given per rectum.

Seizures that continue for more than a few minutes should be treated with benzodiazepines. If seizures do not abate, phenytoin may be added. Phenytoin does not cause respiratory depression. Phenytoin should be given slowly (no more than 0.5 to 0.75 mg/kg per min) or hypotension and cardiovascular collapse may occur. Fosphenytoin does not seem to have this untoward side effect. Phenobarbital may also be added. Its respiratory depressive effects are additive to those of the benzodiazepines.

After stabilization, the cause of the seizure must be determined. Emergent neuroradiologic imaging with close monitoring should be performed. A prospective, ED study among HIV-infected adolescents and adults showed that new seizures, depressed or altered orientation, or headaches, different in quality from a usual headache for the patient were all highly associated with the presence of focal lesions on non-contrast head CT [43].

Patients with signs of impending herniation should undergo rapid sequence intubation and hyperventilation and receive mannitol. If bacterial meningitis is suspected (e.g., the patient is febrile), antibiotic therapy should be begun. In this situation, antibiotic therapy should not be delayed until CSF is obtained. In febrile patients without signs of increased intracranial pressure or focality, a lumbar puncture can be obtained before CT and then antibiotics can be administered. Vancomycin in addition to cefotaxime or ceftriaxone is an appropriate empiric regimen (see discussion of treatment of bacterial meningitis in Chapters 19 and 30).

CSF should be obtained even in the absence of fever. However, cranial CT scans should be performed first in these cases. CSF cell count and differential, glucose and total protein, and Gram's stain and bacterial culture and sensitivity should be ordered. CSF should also be sent for viral culture, India ink stain or cryptococcal antigen, and fungal cultures. Serum glucose, electrolytes, and calcium levels should be checked. Laboratory and radiologic findings in patients with various causes of seizures are outlined in Table 6.15. After the cause of the seizure has been determined, specific therapy may be begun. Malignancies may be amenable to therapy. Supportive care and possible neurosurgical intervention are indicated for cerebrovascular accidents.

Altered mental status

Children with CNS infections, malignancies, or cerebrovascular accidents may present with an acute alteration in their mental status. The differential diagnosis is similar to that for seizures. Neuroradiologic imaging should be performed. CT scans are usually more appropriate in an acute setting than magnetic resonance imaging (MRI). A CT scan will reveal major problems (e.g., new mass lesion, acute hemorrhage, etc.) and

Table 6.15. Laboratory and radiologic findings for specific causes of seizures

Cause	Laboratory or radiologic findings
Bacterial meningitis	Cerebrospinal fluid (CSF) pleocytosis, low glucose, elevated protein, and positive Gram stain and culture.
Toxoplasmosis	Single- or multiple-ring-enhancing mass lesions on cranial CT with contrast
Cryptococcal meningitis	Positive India ink stain or cryptococcal antigen in CSF
Viral meningitis/encephalitis	CSF pleocytosis and elevated protein, Herpes simplex virus may give ring-enhancing lesions on cranial CT with contrast
Mycobacterial meningitis	CSF lymphocytic pleocytosis with markedly elevated protein and low glucose; mass lesions may be seen on CT
CNS malignancy	Mass lesion on CT
CNS hemorrhage	Fresh blood on CT
CNS infarction	CT showing edema initially followed by increased lucency over several days
CNS aneurysms	Aneurysms on CT or MRI [42]

guide initial management. MRI may be done when the patient is more stable. Patients with fever should have a lumbar puncture to exclude CNS infection as a cause of their deterioration. Opportunistic infections and some viral encephalitides may present without classic signs of meningitis. Altered mental status with or without fever may be the only presenting sign. For patients without fever, imaging studies should precede the lumbar puncture.

Summary

Children with HIV infection may present with an acute change in status for a variety of reasons. Sepsis, pulmonary, gastrointestinal, and neurologic emergencies all are major causes of morbidity and mortality. Recognizing the causes of these emergencies and knowing how to treat them are important for any clinician working in the acute care setting. In addition, physicians who work in the emergency department setting must recognize the ways in which HIV infection manifests itself in children. Identifying infected children and referring them for appropriate care can lead to a prolonged survival and an improved quality of life.

REFERENCES
1. Hsia, D. C., Fleishman, J. A., East, J. A., Hellinger, F. J. Pediatric human immunodeficiency virus infection: recent evidence on the utilization and costs of health services. *Arch. Pediatr. Adolesc. Med.* 1995;**149**:496–498.

2. Friedland, L. R., Bell, L. M., Rutstein, R. Utilization and clinical manifestations of human immunodeficiency virus type 1-infected children to a pediatric emergency department. *Pediatr. Emerg. Care* 1991;**7**:72–75.

3. Schweich, P. J., Fosarelli, P. D., Duggan, A. K., Quinn, T. C., Baker, J. L. Prevalence of human immunodeficiency virus seropositivity in pediatric emergency room patients undergoing phlebotomy. *Pediatrics* 1990;**86**:660–665.

4. Fein, J. A., Friedland, L. R., Rutstein, R., Bell, L. M. Children with unrecognized human immunodeficiency virus infection: an emergency department perspective. *Am. J. Dis. Child.* 1993;**147**:1104–1108.

5. Crain, E. F., Bernstein, L. J. Pediatric HIV infection for the emergency physician: epidemiology and overview. *Pediatr. Emerg. Care* 1990;6214–6218.

6. Walker, A. R., HIV infections in children. *Emerg. Med. Clin. North Am.* 1995;**13**:147–162.

7. Zuckerman, G., Metrou, M., Bernstein, C. J., Crain, E. F. Neurologic disorders and dermatologic manifestations in HIV-infected children. *Pediatr. Emerg. Care* 1991;**7**:99–105.

8. Babl, F., Cooper, E. R., Damon, B. *et al.* HIV postexposure prophylaxis for children and adolescents. *Am. J. Emerg. Med.* 2000;**18**:282–287.

9. Pinkert, H., Harper, M. D., Cooper, T., Fleisher, G. R. HIV-infected children in the pediatric emergency department. *Pediatr. Emerg. Care* 1993;**9**:265–269.

10. Nicholas, S. W., The opportunistic and bacterial infections associated with pediatric human immunodeficiency virus disease. *Acta Pediatr.* Suppl 1994;**400**:46–50.

11. Nicholas, S. W., Management of the HIV-positive child with fever. *J. Pediatr.* 1991;**119**:S21–S24.

12. Larson, T., Bechtel, L. Managing the child infected with HIV. *Primary Care* 1995;**22**:23–50.

13. Principi, N., Marchisio, P., Tornaghi, R. *et al.* Occurrence of infection in children infected with human immunodeficiency virus. *Pediatr. Infect. Dis. J.* 1991;**10**:190–193.

14. Farley, J. J., King, J. C., Jr., Nair, P. *et al.* Invasive pneumococcal disease among infected and uninfected children of mothers with human immunodeficiency virus infection. *J. Pediatr.* 1994;**124**:853–858.

15. Mao, C., Harper, M., McIntosh, K. *et al.* Invasive pneumococcal infections in human immunodeficiency virus-infected children. *J. Infect. Dis.* 1996;**173**:870–876.

16. Dayan, P. S., Chamberlain, J. M., Arpadi, S. M. *et al.* Streptococcus pneumoniae bacteremia in children infected with HIV: presentation, course, and outcome. *Pediatr. Emerg. Care* 1998;**14**:194–197.

17. Principi, N., Marchisio, P., Tornaghi, R. *et al.* Acute otitis media in human immunodeficiency virus-infected children. *Pediatrics* 1991;**88**:566–571.

18. Barnett, E. D., Klein, J. O., Pelton, S. I., Luginbuhl, L. M. Otitis media in children born to human immunodeficiency virus-infected mothers. *Pediatr. Infect. Dis. J.* 1992;**11**:360–364.

19. Andiman, W. A., Mezger, J., Shapiro, E. Invasive bacterial infections in children born to women infected with human immunodeficiency virus type 1. *J. Pediatr.* 1994;**124**:846–852.

20. Bye, M. R. HIV in children. *Clin. Chest Med.* 1996;**17**:787–796.

21. Harper, M. B. Human immunodeficiency virus infection. In Fleisher, G. R., Ludwig, S., eds. *Textbook of Pediatric Emergency Medicine*, 4th ed. Philadelphia: Lippincott, Williams and Wilkins, 2000:795–809.

22. Cunningham, S. J., Crain, E. F., Bernstein, L. J. Evaluating the HIV-infected child with pulmonary signs and symptoms. *Pediatr. Emerg. Care* 1991;**7**:32–37.

23. Hauger, S. B., Approach to the pediatric patient with HIV infection and pulmonary symptoms. *J. Pediatr.* 1991;**119**:S25–S33.

24. Cowan, M. J., Shelhamer, J. H., Levine, S. J. Acute respiratory failure in the HIV-seropositive patient. *Crit. Care Clin.* 1997;**13**:523–552.

25. King, J. C., Burke, A. R., Clemens, J. D. *et al.* Respiratory syncytial virus illnesses in human immunodeficiency virus- and non-infected children. *Pediatr. Infect. Dis. J.* 1993;**12**:733–739.

26. Simonds, R. J., Oxtoby, M. J., Caldwell, B. *et al. Pneumocystis carinii* pneumonia among US children with perinatally acquired HIV infection. *J. Am. Med. Assoc.* 1991;**265**:1963–1967.

27. Connor, E., Bagarazzi, M., McSherry, G. *et al.* Clinical and laboratory correlates of *Pneumocystis carinii* pneumonia in children infected with HIV. *J. Am. Med. Assoc.* 1991;**265**:1963–1967.

28. Schneider, R. F. Lymphoid interstitial pneumonitis and nonspecific interstitial pneumonitis. *Clin. Chest Med.* 1996;**17**:763–766.

29. Sheikh, S., Bakshi, S. S., Pahwa, S. G. Outcome and survival in HIV-infected infants with *Pneumocystis carinii* pneumonia and respiratory failure. *Pediatr. AIDS HIV Infec.* 1996;**7**:155–163.

30. Williams, A. J., Duong, T., McNally, L. M. *et al. Pneumocystis carinii* pneumonia and cytomegalovirus infection in children with vertically acquired HIV infection. *AIDS* 2001;**15**:335–339.

31. Sleasman, J. W., Hemenway, C., Klein, A. S., Barrett, D. J. Corticosteroids improve survival of children with AIDS and *Pneumocystis carinii* pneumonia. *Am. J. Dis. Child.* 1993;**147**:30–34.

32. Powell, K. R. Approach to gastrointestinal manifestations in infants and children with HIV infection. *J. Pediatr.* 1991;**119**:S34–S40.

33. Lewis, J. D., Winter, H. S. Intestinal and hepatobiliary diseases in HIV-infected children. *Gastroenterol. Clin. N. Am.* 1995;**24**:119–132.

34. Guarino, A., Castaldo, A., Russo, S. *et al.* Enteric cryptosporidiosis in pediatric HIV infection. *J. Pediatr. Gastroenterol. Nutr.* 1997;**25**:182–187.

35. Bova, R., Meagher, A. Appendicitis in HIV-positive patients. *Aust. N. Z. J. Surg.* 1998;**68**:337–339.

36. Miller, T. L., Winter, H. S., Luginbuhl, L. M. *et al.* Pancreatitis in pediatric human immunodeficiency virus infection. *J. Pediatr.* 1992;**120**:223–227.

37. Love, J. T., Shearer, W. T. Prevention, diagnosis and treatment of pediatric HIV infection. *Comprehen. Ther.* 1996;**22**:719–726.

38. Smith, M. D., Nio, M., Cawel, J. E. *et al.* Management of splenic abscess in immunocompromised children. *J. Pediatr. Surg.* 1993;**28**:823–826.

39. Boige, N., Bellaiche, M., Carnet, D. *et al.* Hydrops-like cholecystitis due to cryptosporidiosis in an HIV-infected child. *J. Pediatr. Gastroenterol. Nutr.* 1998;**26**:219–221.

40. Visudtibhan, A., Visudhiphan, P., Chiemchanya, S. Stroke and seizures as the presenting signs of pediatric HIV infection. *Pediatr. Neurol.* 1999;**20**:53–56.

41. Butler, C., Hittelman, J., Hauger, S. B. Approach to neurodevelopmental and neurologic complications in pediatric HIV infection. *J. Pediatr.* 1991;**119**:S41–S46.

42. Husson, R. N., Saini, R., Lewis, L. L. *et al.* Cerebral artery aneurysms in children infected with human immunodeficiency virus. *J. Pediatr.* 1992;**121**:927–930.

43. Rothman, R. E., Keyl, P. M., McArthur, J. C. *et al.* A decision guideline for emergency department utilization of noncontrast head computed tomography in HIV-infected patients. *Acad. Emerg. Med.* 1999;**6**:1010–1019.

7 Adherence to antiretroviral therapy in children and youth

John Farley, MD, MPH

University of Maryland School of Medicine, MD

Improved health outcomes for HIV-infected children and youth will not be achieved without maximal viral suppression. Highly active antiretroviral therapy (HAART) represents a major breakthrough in HIV management, but not all patients respond optimally to HAART. Non-adherence is well established as a major cause of clinical failure, and intermittent non-adherence is a particular problem. Studies in adults have demonstrated that $\geq$95% adherence to HAART is necessary for durable suppression of viral load [1–3]. In the presence of selective pressure by antiretroviral agents, high rates of viral replication and viral mutation lead to the development of drug resistance. Mutations conferring resistance against one antiretroviral agent often confer cross-resistance to other agents; poor adherence can render a whole class of antiretroviral drug ineffective.

Although a crucial component of good clinical care, assessment of adherence to HAART in HIV-infected children and youth is challenging and labor intensive. Patient and parent (or other caregiver) characteristics associated with optimal adherence are not well characterized. Studies evaluating interventions to improve adherence in this group are encouraging but few.

HIV as a chronic illness

Pediatric HIV infection is now referred to as the "newest chronic illness in childhood" [4, 5]. Chronic illness alters a person's life by creating permanent changes in daily living. Adherence is a major problem in management of patients with any chronic illness. Non-adherence occurs with half of all medical recommendations made to chronically ill patients [6]. Chronic illness in children presents many unique adherence challenges. Caregivers are responsible for the adherence of children and so have a profound impact on adherence. Children living in families in which the adult caregiver is ill, is subject to significant stress, lacks effective organizational skills, lacks social support, or

Handbook of Pediatric HIV Care, ed. Steven L. Zeichner and Jennifer S. Read.
Published by Cambridge University Press. © Cambridge University Press 2006.

is not motivated to administer medications, will be at high risk for non-adherence. Depression and ongoing substance abuse are associated with poor adherence among HIV-infected adults, and one would expect a similar association among caregivers of HIV-infected children [2, 7, 8]. Use of outreach staff to provide additional support for families with such challenges may enhance adherence.

Adherence of children to complex medical regimens is influenced by the parent or caregiver's knowledge of the illness, understanding of treatment recommendations, and duration of treatment [9]. Previous studies of pediatric chronic illnesses have found a relationship between poor adherence and the caregiver's understanding of the prescribed regimen and the complexity of the regimen [10]. Difficulties with adherence are observed with other chronic diseases, such as diabetes. The complexity and numerous demands associated with diabetes treatment often lead to significant declines in adherence over the course of treatment. Periodic non-adherence is often viewed as the rule, rather than the exception [11]. Thus, providers need to emphasize caregiver education, and realize that adherence will likely decrease over time without intervention.

Children's understanding of, and reactions to, illness change during development through a series of systematic stages that correspond to cognitive abilities [12]. The child's level of cognitive, motor, social, emotional, and psychological functioning affects the course and management of the disease. Their ability to perceive their own illness, approach medical treatment, and respond to interventions is influenced by their developmental level. It is important for care providers to be certain that a child's understanding of his or her illness is periodically updated to keep pace with cognitive and emotional development. Older children can assume increasing responsibility for their own care and are influenced by peers and their social setting [10]. Providers need to assess the influence of developmental factors on adherence periodically and adjust interventions to improve adherence as the child matures.

For newly diagnosed adolescents and older perinatally infected youth, the initiation of HAART and the necessary adherence to HAART is a significant behavioral change. The process of behavior change is complex and is described by the Stages of Change Model. Based on a comparative analysis of major therapy systems [13, 14], the model describes a cyclical pattern of movement through five specific stages [15]. Individuals are: (a) unaware or unwilling to do anything about the problem, (b) consider the possibility of change, (c) become determined and prepared to make the change, (d) take action, and (e) sustain the change over time [16]. The stages are designated: precontemplation, contemplation, preparation, action, and maintenance. It is important to note that the precontemplation stage is quite diverse, that an individual frequently recycles or "relapses" several times through different stages, and that an individual may not progress linearly through the stages. The major clinical implications of the model are that providers must carefully assess an individual's readiness for action (i.e., adherence) before prescribing HAART, and that periodic relapse (i.e., non-adherence) is to be expected, necessitating a plan to minimize the clinical impact of non-adherence. For example, caregivers should be taught to stop all antiretrovirals rather than just some.

Assessment of adherence

A number of methods have been used to assess adherence in clinical practice and in research studies. Each method has distinctive benefits and drawbacks. The methods include caregiver interviews, pill counts, pharmacy refill records, electronic monitoring, drug level monitoring, monitoring response to therapy, and utilizing records of other health behaviors such as appointment keeping. While it is clear that close to 100% adherence is necessary for sustained viral suppression, the cutoff for an adequate level of adherence does vary somewhat depending upon the assessment method used. The adherence cutoff value may also vary with different antiretroviral therapies. For example, since a single point mutation resulting in a single amino acid change leads to high level resistance to all of the available non-nucleoside reverse transcriptase inhibitors (NNRTIs), regimens including NNRTIs may be less forgiving of adherence lapses than other regimens. A summary of adherence assessment modalities studied in HIV-infected children is shown in Table 7.1.

Caregiver self-report

Caregiver interview or self-report is considered especially subject to bias, as parents may inflate their adherence report to satisfy clinicians. However, it can be used to identify some poor adherers [17], and these poor adherers can respond to interventions [18]. While useful as a reinforcement tool, parent self-monitoring (i.e., using a calendar to record doses given) is subject to the same bias as caregiver interviews or other approaches to self-report when used as a measurement tool. Caregiver self-report to assess adherence among perinatally HIV-infected children has been utilized with useful but imperfect results. The best-known instrument is the Pediatric AIDS Clinical Trial Group (PACTG) Pediatric Adherence Questionnaire Modules 1 and 2 (http://www.fstrf.org/qol/peds/pedadhere.html). Module 1 of the PACTG Adherence Questionnaire begins with identification of antiretroviral medications and then asks the subject about doses missed during the prior 3 days. Module 2 presents a number of potential problems with adherence and asks the caregiver if any of these potential problems have occurred in the past 14 days.

Good adherence as assessed by self-report instruments is associated with good clinical outcomes. A study using the PACTG instrument in HIV-infected children enrolled in a clinical trial involving a HAART regimen (PACTG protocol 377) found a correlation between the child's virologic outcome and caregiver self-reported adherence during the 3 days prior to interview [19]. Another larger study ($n = 90$) using a similar but not identical self-report questionnaire found that children whose caregivers reported no missed doses in the previous week were more likely to have a HIV viral load <400 copies/ml [20]. Even though the self-report instruments can predict clinical outcomes, the data obtained using these instruments may not be entirely accurate. Two studies showed that a caregiver self-report questionnaire dramatically overestimated adherence compared with pill count and/or electronic monitoring [21, 22]. It may be possible

Table 7.1. Adherence assessment modalities studied in HIV-infected children

[Reference] Assessment modality and adherence definition	Number adherent (%)	Number non-adherent (%)	Association with viral load <400 copies/ml.
[34] (4–6 months follow-up)			
Prescription refill (≥75% all antiretrovirals)	42 (58%)	30 (42%)	P = 0.001
[21] (3 months follow-up)			
Self-report (<20% missed doses in prior 3 days)	29 (96.7%)	1 (3.3%)	NS
Pill Count (≥80% all antiretrovirals)	18 (69.2%)	8 (30.8%)	NS
MEMS Track Cap™ (≥80% all antiretrovirals)	2 (25%)	6 (75%)	NS
[20] (cross-sectional)			
Self-report (no missed doses in prior week)	50 (57%)	39 (43%)	P = 0.04
[19] (clinical trial, 6–12 months follow-up)			
Self-report (no missed doses in prior 3 days)	88 (70%)	37 (30%)	P = 0.02
[22] (6 months follow-up)			
MEMS Track Cap™ (≥80% one antiretroviral)	17 (65%)	11 (35%)	P < 0.001
Prescription refill (≥80% all antiretrovirals)	19 (73%)	8 (27%)	P = 0.002
Self-report (no missed doses in prior 3 days)	20 (100%)	0 (0%)	NS
Physician assessment (≥80% all antiretrovirals)	14 (74%)	5 (26%)	P < 0.001
No missed clinic appointments	18 (69%)	8 (31%)	P = 0.009

to improve self-report questionnaires to enhance their accuracy. In one study, participants were more likely to self-report adherence difficulty when questions focused on problems rather than missed doses [22], suggesting a possible strategy for design of alternative self-report instruments and an approach for care providers during patient care visits. Several variations of self-report instruments have been developed. The pills identification test (PIT) uses a display board with two similar pills for each antiretroviral prescribed and asks patients to identify which pill they are taking. Correct PIT scores have been shown to be associated with adherence in HIV-infected adults [23], suggesting a potential adjunct to self-report for pediatric providers. Audio computer-assisted self-interviewing has been shown to encourage more honest answers from patients on sensitive topics than face to face interviews [24]. The evidence concerning the reliability of self-report, particularly outside of the clinical trial setting, is mixed. Care providers should recognize that self-report generally overestimates adherence, and strongly consider incorporating an alternative adherence assessment strategy as part of patient care.

Provider assessment

Physician estimate or clinical judgment of adherence has been studied in adults with chronic illness. Several studies concluded that clinicians do no better than chance when judging whether or not an adult patient is adherent [25–27]. In a study of HIV-infected adults, physician adherence assessment was found to correlate poorly with pill counts [28]. Pediatricians appear to be just as inaccurate as physicians caring for adults when estimating patient adherence [29, 30]. One small study demonstrated an unexpectedly high reliability for provider assessment in HIV-infected children. In this study, physicians relied heavily on pharmacy refill records and virologic response [22], suggesting a useful strategy for clinical practice.

Pill counts

The pill count method to estimate adherence involves a comparison between the amount of medication remaining in the child's bottle and the amount that should be remaining based on the amount and dosage of the initial prescription and the length of time since the patient began using the bottle. This method provides a measure of adherence over time, but is subject to bias due to "pill dumping" (i.e., the parent may not leave all unused pills in the bottle in an effort to falsely increase the apparent level of adherence and please the clinician), and determining the date when the patient commenced using the current bottle can be a challenge. The PACTG Adherence to Therapy Subcommittee has developed a pill count case report form (CRF). The PACTG Pill Count Form, example cases, and an Excel spreadsheet model to easily perform the calculations are available on the public domain portion of the PACTG website (http://www.fstrf.org/qol/peds/pedadhere.html). Although labor intensive, pill counts are likely the most practical and readily available non-self-report adherence assessment tool. Disappointingly, the one published study to date in HIV-infected children found a poor correlation for pill counts with both electronic monitoring and virologic response. However, sample sizes were small ($n = 8$ for electronic monitoring, $n = 30$ for virologic response) [21]. The utility of this tool in the clinical setting needs to be more widely assessed.

Pharmacy refill records

The chances of pill dumping bias or reporting bias are minimized by using pharmacy medication refill records (i.e., comparing refill data from the pharmacy with the estimated refill requirement if all doses were administered). This method has been utilized in HIV-infected adults [7, 31, 32] and found to correlate with virologic response [31, 33]. Pharmacy refill records were utilized in a study of 72 children receiving HAART. Only 42 (58%) were considered adherent (defined as refilling $\geq 75\%$ of protease inhibitors and $\geq 75\%$ of all antiretrovirals in a 6-month interval). Of the 42 children classified as adherent, 22 (52%) achieved and maintained an undetectable viral load [34]. This method is less labor intensive than pill counts, but it does require pharmacist collaboration or access to health insurance claims data. The method generally overestimates adherence, since the availability of medication in the home does not necessarily mean the medication was actually administered. However, this method utilized over several months will usually identify adherence problems. Combining this method with periodic pill counts may enhance sensitivity.

Electronic monitoring

Pharmacy refill records and pill counts provide a general assessment of the number of doses taken, but fail to yield any information regarding patterns of poor adherence. Electronic monitoring of adherence offers a more detailed assessment, demonstrating problems with dosing intervals in addition to missed doses. The medication event monitoring system (MEMS, Aprex/Aardex Corp., Menlo Park, CA) uses a microprocessor in the medication container cap to record the date and time of each vial opening. Studies in HIV-infected adults have demonstrated that electronic monitoring of adherence was the method of adherence assessment which correlated most robustly with virologic suppression [3, 35–37]. Several groups are utilizing this methodology in ongoing studies of HIV-infected children [21, 22]. A study of 26 perinatally HIV-infected children demonstrated similar findings to the adult studies, with electronic monitoring more robustly associated with virologic response than pharmacy refill records or caregiver self-report [22]. Improved technology is now available so this monitoring approach can be used for bottles containing liquids or powders. Caregivers or youth who lay out pills in advance or use a pill box storage device are currently excluded, but new technology utilizing electronic monitoring for tablet/capsule "blister packs" is under development. Placement of the MEMS™ bottle cap requires caregiver cooperation and/or pharmacist collaboration and caps may become defective or lost, occasionally resulting in incomplete data. The approximate cost of monitoring is US$100 per patient per year for a single drug. The company has developed a SmartCap™ option, which provides patients with a reminder beep when doses are due and an information "window" telling them when was the last time they opened the bottle. This is attractive as a combined monitor and intervention for older children.

Drug level monitoring

Therapeutic drug monitoring for individual patients is under study in adults and proposed in children with the goal of maintaining levels sufficient to suppress viral load and prevent viral mutation and resistance. Therapeutic drug monitoring is discussed in more detail in Chapter 16. As pediatric therapeutic drug monitoring protocols are developed, it will be important to assess the utility of trough drug levels as an adherence assessment tool. This strategy has been employed in HIV-infected adults [38–40] and has been described in children [41, 42]. Evaluation will require incorporation of other adherence measures for comparison within protocols utilizing therapeutic drug monitoring. An anticipated limitation of drug levels as an adherence assessment tool is that the level will only reflect adherence behavior during a period of time (variable depending on drug metabolism) immediately prior to obtaining the level. Utility in the clinical care setting is limited at this time.

Appointment keeping

In a study of 26 perinatally HIV-infected children over a 6-month period, no missed appointment in the interval was associated with virologic response, but agreement with the adherence rate assessed by electronic monitoring was limited [22]. Further study of the association between adherence and appointment keeping behavior in a larger population seems warranted, as appointment records are commonly available to providers.

Improving adherence

There is clear evidence based on caregiver self-report that poor palatability and unpleasant or inconvenient formulations remain major barriers to excellent adherence in children. In the PACTG 377 study discussed previously, caregivers cited "taste" and "child refuses" as common adherence problems for the ritonavir liquid formulation and "taste" and "scheduling interferes with lifestyle" for nelfinavir (dosed three times a day in this study) [19]. In the study by Reddington et al., the top two desired interventions caregivers cited as potentially very helpful were: "better tasting medications" (81%) and "take meds fewer times each day" (72%) [20]. Antiretroviral therapy regimens requiring less frequent administration have been associated with better adherence in HIV-infected adults. In a study of 244 patients with adherence assessed by self-report, $\geq$80% adherence to pre-HAART antiretrovirals was associated with once or twice a day dosing on multivariate analysis [43] and this was confirmed in a later HAART study [37]. Thus, it is resoundingly clear that care providers should choose the least complex and most palatable regimen possible. As an alternative to liquid formulations, some of which are notorious for palatability problems, a procedure for teaching young children to swallow pills was first described in 1984, and is now commonly employed by pediatric HIV care providers [44]. If palatability problems are anticipated, delaying initiation of the regimen while pill-swallowing training is attempted should be considered. If palatability issues are otherwise insurmountable, physicians have occasionally resorted to the placement of gastrostomy tubes for HIV-infected children to improve adherence with excellent outcomes in one case series [45].

In addition to addressing regimen complexity issues and ongoing education, clinicians need not only to provide caregivers and patients with adherence aids, but should also work with patients to plan how adherence will be incorporated in the daily "routine" [46]. Before initiating a regimen, patients and their families should be interviewed about the details of their daily routine and adjustments to the treatment regimen (such as timing of dosing) made to accommodate the routine. Weekends may need to be discussed separately from weekdays. Whenever possible, medication dosing should be "cued" to another regular event such as mealtimes or washing up at bedtime. Medication should be available where the routine event dosing is "cued" to takes place (i.e., kitchen or bathroom). Adherence aids such as pill boxes with a compartment for doses for each day and time, or an alarm device should be encouraged. The effectiveness of different adherence aids will vary from family to family, and will depend upon the details of the family's routine and the patient's specific drug regimen.

While a falling viral load is a powerful positive reinforcement for caregivers and patients, many providers also utilize a "token economy" as an adherence intervention (i.e., a reward for good adherence is given on a regular basis and then eventually withdrawn with the hope that good adherence will be maintained). This intervention has not been formally evaluated in this setting, but a "token economy" is commonly used to address other pediatric behavioral issues with demonstrated efficacy [47]. For example, a caregiver may give a child with behavior problems interfering with medication administration a reward when the child behaves well. However, many adherence problems are more complex, necessitating targeting both caregiver and child behaviors, and requiring a more complex intervention. In addition, eventual withdrawal of the reward must be done carefully to maximize the chance that the desired behavior (i.e., good adherence) will be maintained. Planning and conducting a "token economy" intervention is more complicated than one would assume, and mental health supervision should be considered.

There remains a paucity of data identifying characteristics associated with poor adherence that would facilitate the design and implementation of adherence interventions likely to be efficacious. Nonetheless, a prospective randomized trial of an intensive home-based nursing intervention showed that the nursing intervention was associated with improved adherence to HAART and virologic outcome [48]. This suggests that interventions to enhance caregiver knowledge and self-efficacy can overcome child-related barriers to adherence, and provide social support for some caregivers.

An implication of the Stages of Change Model for health behavior among youth primarily responsible for their own medication adherence is that individuals starting therapy prematurely or without adequate preparation may nonetheless benefit from failure, learning lessons that could advance the probability of success on the next attempt. However, this may have serious adverse consequences in the case of HAART therapy. The Treatment Regimens Enhancing Adherence in Teens (TREAT) Program was developed as an adolescent-focused, multi-faceted program, based on the Stages of Change Model, to promote optimal long-term adherence to HAART [49]. The TREAT program was designed primarily for treatment-naïve HIV-infected youth, and was developed and piloted as part of the Reaching for Excellence in Adolescent Care and Health (REACH) study for youth infected through sexual activity and injection drug use sponsored by the US National Institutes of Health at multiple sites in the USA. A striking finding of the TREAT Program pilot study was that 39% of the youth currently prescribed HAART were staged in a manner discordant with their treatment status, i.e., they were prescribed HAART but were staged as precontemplation, contemplation, or preparation [49] and were non-adherent, suggesting care providers need to take more care to assess patient readiness prior to initiating HAART. The pilot did suggest that the TREAT intervention was successful in facilitating movement through stages, with 78% of the small number of subjects who completed the full program moving forward [49].

Development of new antiretroviral formulations has facilitated the testing of once daily directly observed therapy (DOT), in which a health care provider observes the patient taking medication. A clinical trial utilizing DOT for youth newly initiating HAART is under development. Although highly successful for the treatment of tuberculosis, this expensive and labor intensive intervention has been utilized in one study among HIV-infected adults, with disappointing findings concerning efficacy [50].

Conclusion

While each adherence assessment method has advantages and disadvantages, incorporation of adherence assessment and strategies to optimize adherence into the clinical care of HIV-infected children and youth is essential. A summary of recommendations for clinical practice is shown in Table 7.2. Measuring and improving adherence for children and youth will be even more challenging in the future. In developed countries, an increasing proportion of perinatally HIV-infected children are reaching adolescence, and increasing numbers of adolescents are infected through risky behaviors. A majority of patients cared for by pediatric HIV specialists in developed country settings will soon be adolescents. In a study of HIV-infected pregnant women, being an adolescent was the most important factor associated with poor adherence to antiretroviral

Table 7.2. Approaches to improving treatment adherence

Prior to prescribing HAART
- Assess stage of readiness to be adherent and/or explore Health Belief Model determinants and other potential determinants such as substance abuse or depression
- Identify and address potential barriers to adherence such as palatability issues, disclosure, or alternate caregivers
- Consider the patient's daily life routine when choosing a regimen and minimize dosing frequency to no more than twice a day if possible
- Educate the patient and/or caregiver concerning the importance of adherence, special administration requirements, and possible side effects
- Cue dosing to regular life events and offer adherence aids, such as a pill box, if possible

After initiating HAART
- Follow-up frequently during the initial months of therapy
- When evaluating adherence, supplement self-report with a second adherence assessment method
- Provide positive reinforcement and frequent education boosters
- Identify adherence problems early and consider prescribed drug holiday while addressing adherence problems

---

therapy [7], underscoring the adherence difficulties for this age group. In developing countries, potential adherence barriers unique to this setting will need to be identified and addressed. While challenging, attention to adherence can significantly improve clinical outcomes, leading to longer, healthier lives for our patients.

REFERENCES

1. Miller, L. D., Hays, R. D. Adherence to combination antiretroviral therapy: synthesis of the literature and clinical implications. *AIDS Reader* 2000;**10**:177–185.
2. Gifford, A. L., Bormann, J. E., Shively, M. J., Wright, B. C., Richman, D. D., Bozzette, S. A. Predictors of self-reported adherence and plasma HIV concentrations in patients on multi-drug antiretroviral regimens. *J. Acquir. Immune Defic. Syndr.* 2000;**23**:386–395.
3. Arnsten, J. H., Demas, P. A., Farzadegan, H. *et al.* Antiretroviral therapy adherence and viral suppression in HIV-infected drug users: comparison of self-report and electronic monitoring. *Clin. Infect. Dis.* 2001;**33**:1417–1423.
4. Lipson, M., What do you say to a child with AIDS? *Hastings Center Rep.* 1993;**23**:6–12.
5. Maieron, M. J., Roberts, M. C., Prentice-Dunn, S. Children's perception of peers with AIDS. Assessing the impact of contagion information, perceived similarity, and illness conceptualization. *J. Pediatr. Psychol.* 1996;**21**:321–334.
6. Cameron, K., Gregor, F. Chronic illness and compliance. *J. Adv. Nursing* 1987;**12**:671–676.

7. Laine, C., Newschaffer, C. J., Zhang, D., Cosler, L., Hauck, W. W., Turner, B. J. Adherence to antiretroviral therapy by pregnant women infected with human immunodeficiency virus: a pharmacy claims-based analysis. *Obstet. Gynecol.* 2000;**95**:167–173.

8. Gordillo, V., del Amo, J., Soriano, V., Gonzalez-Lahoz, J. Sociodemographic and psychologic variables influencing adherence to antiretroviral therapy. *AIDS* 1999;**13**:1763–1769.

9. Parrish, J. Parent compliance with medical and behavioral recommendations. In Krasnegor, N., Arasteh, J., Cataldo, M., eds. *Child Health Behavior*. New York: Wiley; 1986; 453–501.

10. Thompson, R. J., Gustafson, K. E., *Adaption to Chronic Childhood Illness*. Washington DC: American Psychological Association; 1996.

11. LaGreca, A., Schuman, W. B. Adherence to prescribed medical regimens. In Roberts, M. C., ed. *Handbook of Pediatric Psychology*. 2nd edn. New York: Guilford Press; 1995: 55–83.

12. Peterson, L., Coping by children undergoing stressful medical procedures: some conceptual, methodological, and therapeutic issues. *J. Cons. Clin. Psychol.* 1989;**57**:380–387.

13. Prochaska, J. O., *Systems of Psychotherapy: A Transtheoretical Analysis*. Homewood IL: Dorsey Press; 1979.

14. Prochaska, J. O., DiClemente, C. C. Stages and processes of self-change of smoking: toward an integrative model of change. *J. Cons. Clin. Psychol.* 1983;**51**:390–395.

15. Prochaska, J. O., DiClemente, C. C., Norcross, J. C. In search of how people change: Applications to addictive behaviors. *Am. Psychol.* 1992;**47**:1102–1114.

16. DiClemente, C. C. Motivational interviewing and the stage of change. In Miller, W. R., Rollnick, S., eds. *Motivational Interviewing: Preparing People for Change*. New York: Guilford Press; 1991.

17. Gordis, L., Markowitz, M., Lilienfield, A. M. The inaccuracy in using interview to estimate patient reliability in taking medications at home. *Med. Care* 1969;**17**:49–54.

18. Haynes, R. B., Taylor, D. W., Sackett, D. L., Gibson, E. S., Bernholz, C. D., Mukherjee, J. Can simple clinical measurements detect patient noncompliance? *Hypertension* 1980;**2**: 757–764.

19. Van Dyke, R. B., Lee, S., Johnson, G. M. *et al.* Reported adherence as a determinant of response to highly active antiretroviral therapy in HIV-infected children. *Pediatrics* 2002;**109**:e61.

20. Reddington, C., Cohen, J., Raldillo, A. *et al.* Adherence to medication regimens among children with human immunodeficiency virus infection. *Pediatr. Infect. Dis. J.* 2000;**19**:1148–1153.

21. Steele, R. G., Anderson, B., Rindel, B. *et al.* Adherence to antiretroviral therapy among HIV-positive children: examination of the role of caregiver health beliefs. *AIDS Care* 2001;**13**:617–629.

22. Farley, J. J., Hines, S. E., Musk, A. E., Ferrus, S., Tepper, V. E. Assessment of adherence to antiviral therapy in HIV-infected children using the medication event monitoring system (MEMS) compared with pharmacy refill, provider assessment, and caregiver self-report. *J. Acquir. Immune Defic. Syndr.* 2003;**33**:211–218.

23. Parienti, J. J., Verdon, R., Bazin, C., Bouvet, E., Massari, V., Larouze, B. The pills identification test: a tool to assess adherence to antiretroviral therapy [letter]. *J. Am. Med. Assoc.* 2001;**285**:412.

24. Metzger, D. S., Koblin, B., Turner, C. *et al*. Randomized controlled trial of audio computer-assisted self-interviewing: utility and acceptability in longitudinal studies. HIVNET Vaccine Preparedness Study Protocol Team. *Am. J. Epidemiol.* 2000;**152**:99–106.

25. Caron, H. S., Roth, H. P. Patient's cooperation with a medical regimen. *J. Am. Med. Assoc.* 1968;**203**:922–926.

26. Davis, M. S. Variations in patients' compliance with doctors' orders: Analysis of congruence between survey responses and results of empirical investigations. *J. Medi. Educat.* 1966;**41**:1037–1048.

27. Mushlin, A. I., Appel, F. A. Diagnosing potential noncompliance: Physician's ability in a behavioral dimension of medical care. *Arch. Intern. Medi.* 1977;**137**:318–321.

28. Bangsberg, D. R., Hecht, F. M., Clague, H. *et al*. Provider assessment of adherence to HIV antiretroviral therapy. *J. Acquir. Immune Defic. Syndr.* 2001;**26**:435–442.

29. Charney, E., Bynum, R., Eldredge, D. *et al*. How well do patients take oral penicillin? A collaborative study in private practice. *Pediatrics* 1967;**40**:188–195.

30. Wood, H. F., Feinstein, A. R., Taranta, A. *et al*. Rheumatic fever in children and adolescents: a long-term epidemiologic study of subsequent prophylaxis, streptococcal infections, and clinical sequelae. *Ann. Intern. Medi.* 1964;**60** suppl.:31–46.

31. Maher, K., Klimas, N., Fletcher, M. A. *et al*. Disease progression, adherence, and response to protease inhibitor therapy for HIV infection in an urban Veteran's Affairs medical center. *J. Acquir. Immune Defici. Syndr.* 1999;**22**:358–363.

32. Turner, B. J., Newschaffer, C. J., Zhang, D., Cosler, L., Houch, W. W. Antiretroviral use and pharmacy-based measurement of adherence in post-partum HIV-infected women. *Med. Care* 2000;**38**:911–925.

33. Low-Beer, S., Yip, B., O'Shaughnessy, M. V., Hogg, R. S., Montaner, J. S. G. Adherence to triple therapy and viral load response [letter]. *J. Acquir. Immune Defic. Syndr.* 2000;**23**:360–361.

34. Watson, D. C., Farley, J. J. Efficacy of and adherence to highly active antiretroviral therapy in children infected with human immunodeficiency virus type 1. *Pediatr. Infect. Dis. J.* 1999;**18**:682–689.

35. Liu, H., Golin, C. E., Miller, L. G. *et al*. A comparison study of multiple measures of adherence to HIV protease inhibitors. *Ann. Intern. Med.* 2001;**134**:968–977.

36. Bangsberg, D. R., Hecht, F. M., Charlebois, E. D. *et al*. Adherence to protease inhibitors, HIV-1 viral load, and development of drug resistance in an indigent population. *AIDS* 2000;**14**:357–366.

37. Paterson, D. L., Swindells, S., Mohr, J. *et al*. Adherence to protease inhibitor therapy and outcomes in patients with HIV infection. *Ann. Intern. Med.* 2000;**133**:21–30.

38. Tuldra, A., Ferrer, M. J., Fumaz, C. R. Monitoring adherence to HIV therapy [letter]. *Arch. Intern. Med.* 1999;**159**:1376–1377.

39. Samet, J. H., Libman, H., Steger, K. A. Compliance with zidovudine in patients infected with human immunodeficiency virus, type 1: a cross-sectional study in a municipal hospital clinic. *Am. J. Med.* 1992;**92**:495–502.

40. Murri, R., Ammassari, A., Gallicano, K. *et al*. Patient reported nonadherence to HAART is related to protease inhibitor levels. *J. Acquir. Immune Defic. Syndr.* 2000;**24**:123–128.

41. Albano, F., Spagnuolo, M. I., Berni Canani, R., Guarino, A. Adherence to antiretroviral therapy in HIV-infected children in Italy. *AIDS Care* 1999;**11**:711–714.

42. Kastrissios, H., Suarez, JR, Hammer, S. *et al.* The extent of non-adherence in a large AIDS clinical trial using plasma dideoxynucleoside concentrations as a marker. *AIDS* 1998;**12**:2305–2311.

43. Eldred, L. J., Wu, A. W., Chaisson, R. E., Moore RD. Adherence to antiretroviral and pneumocystis prophylaxis in HIV disease. *J. Acquir. Immune Defic. Syndr.* 1998;**18**:117–125.

44. Dahlquist, L. M., Blount, R. L. Teach a six-year-old girl to swallow pills. *J. Behav. Ther. Exp. Psychiatry* 1984;**15**:171–173.

45. Shingadia, D., Viani, R. M., Yogev, R. *et al.* Gastrostomy tube insertion for improvement of adherence to highly active antiretroviral therapy in pediatric patients with human immunodeficiency virus. *Pediatrics* 2000;**105**:e80.

46. Chesney, M. A. Factors affecting adherence to antiretroviral therapy. *Clin. Infect. Dis.* 2000;**30**(Suppl2):S171–S176.

47. Carney, R. M., Schechter, K., Davis, T. Improving adherence to blood glucose testing in insulin-dependent diabetic children. *Behav. Ther.* 1983;**14**:247–254.

48. Berrien, V. M., Salazar, J. C., Reynolds, E., Mckay, K. Adherence to antiretroviral therapy in HIV-infected pediatric patients improves with home-based intensive nursing intervention. *AIDS Patient Care STDs* 2004;**18**:355–363.

49. Rogers, A. S., Miller, S., Murphy, D. A., Tanney, M., Fortune, T. The TREAT (therapeutic regimens enhancing adherence in teens) program: theory and preliminary results. *J. Adolesc. Hlth* 1991;**292S**:30–38.

50. Altice, F. L. Trust and the acceptance of and adherence to antiretroviral therapy. *J. Acquir. Immune Defic. Syndr.* 2001;**28**:47–58.

8 Adolescents and HIV

Ligia Peralta, MD

University of Maryland School of Medicine, Department of Pediatrics, Baltimore, MD

Bret J. Rudy, MD

Children's Hospital of Philadelphia, The University of Pennsylvania School of Medicine, PA

Introduction

HIV-infected adolescents represent an important part of the global AIDS epidemic. In this chapter, the epidemiology of HIV infection in adolescents will be addressed, as well as adolescent development, HIV counseling and testing, and prevention of acquisition of HIV infection by adolescents. Finally, management of HIV-infected adolescents, including reproductive health and gynecologic care, will be addressed. It is not the intent of this chapter to review all aspects of management of HIV-infected adolescents, but rather to address issues that are unique to adolescents. This chapter emphasizes adolescent HIV infection as seen in the USA, but many of the principles are applicable to adolescents in other settings.

Epidemiology

The epidemiology of HIV infection among adolescents in the USA generally mirrors the epidemiology of HIV infection among adolescents in other resource-rich countries. In resource-poor countries, the epidemiology of HIV infection among adolescents is somewhat different in that HIV infection disproportionately affects young women, who generally become infected through heterosexual contact, often with older men.

By the end of 2001, the Centers for Disease Control and Prevention (CDC) estimated that adolescents aged 13 to 19 years made up less than 1% (4428 cases), and young adults aged 20–24 years represented 3.5% (28 665 cases), of all reported individuals with AIDS in the USA [1]. It is estimated that over 100 000 adolescents are living with HIV in the USA, although most are unaware of their infection [2]. Statistical modeling suggests that one in four new HIV infections in the USA occurs in persons under the age of 22 years [3]. The number of HIV infections is increasing in young women, with acquisition of infection through heterosexual transmission, and in young men, through

Handbook of Pediatric HIV Care, ed. Steven L. Zeichner and Jennifer S. Read.
Published by Cambridge University Press. © Cambridge University Press 2006.

male-to-male sexual transmission. Globally, more than half of new infections occur in individuals under 25 years of age.

Male-to-male sexual transmission represents the most common mode of acquisition of HIV infection among young men in the USA For example, in 2001, 35% of AIDS diagnoses in young men from 13 to 19 years of age were attributable to male-to-male sexual transmission [1]. This proportion increased to 61% in young men from 20 to 24 years of age. In the Young Men's Survey, the prevalence of HIV infection among 3492 men aged 15 to 22 years who had sex with men (MSM) was 7.2% [4]. The prevalence was highest among African-American and Latino men. Importantly, only 18% of the 249 HIV-infected men were aware of their infection.

The most common mode of acquisition of HIV infection for those aged 13–19 years old (66%) and 20–24 years old (67%) is heterosexual transmission. Injection drug use is less common among adolescent girls 13–19 years old (19%) compared to young women 20–24 years old (29%). Many young women are unaware of both their own risk of HIV infection and their sexual partners' risk factors for HIV infection. Adolescent girls are disproportionately affected by HIV compared to older women. For example, among 13–19-year-olds with AIDS, 48% are female. However, women represent only 41% of AIDS cases in the 20–24 year age range and 25% of AIDS cases among those over 25 years of age [1].

HIV seroprevalence rates for adolescents vary greatly depending on the population being tested. For example, seroprevalence among young MSM in homeless shelters has been reported to be as high as 16% to 17% [5]. Sexually transmitted infection (STI) clinics have reported rates of 0% to 3.5% among adolescents. Minorities are disproportionately affected by HIV in the USA. For example, 61% of AIDS cases in 13–19-year-olds were among blacks in 2001, although only 15% of the adolescent population in the USA is black [1]. This trend appears to be continuing, based on data from those states that report HIV infection.

Adolescent development

Effective care of the HIV-infected adolescent requires an understanding of the unique psychosocial and physical stages of adolescence. Adolescence can be divided roughly into three stages of intellectual, social, and emotional development: early, middle, and late adolescence [6] (Table 8.1). An understanding of adolescent physical development provides essential background for the care of adolescents. The Tanner sexual maturation scale is used to stage sexual maturation [6] (Table 8.2). Girls begin pubertal development between 8–13 years (compared to 9.5–13.5 years for boys). Sexual maturation in girls usually begins with thelarche, or breast development; testicular enlargement is the first sign of puberty in boys. Girls begin menstruation around Tanner Stage 4; boys begin ejaculation at Tanner Stage 3, although sperm are produced around Tanner Stage 4. Understanding the stages of sexual development helps the clinician to understand

Table 8.1. Stages of adolescent social and psychosocial development

| Adolescent stage | Early adolescence | Mid adolescence | Late adolescence |
Age (years)	12–14	15–17	18–19
Social orientation	Family oriented	Increasing independence	Adult relationships
Peer relations	Striving for autonomy	Alliance to peer group	Intimacy in friendships
Thought processes	Concrete	Abstract thinking begins; concrete thinking under stress	Abstract thinking; future orientation
Psychosexual development	Concerned about physical development	Sexual experimentation	Romantic relationships

Table 8.2. Stages of adolescent genital development

Stage	Characteristics
Males	
1	Prepubertal
2	Testes become larger, scrotum coarsens, downy hair at base of penis
3	Lengthening of penis, increase in coarseness and amount of pubic hair
4	Penis continues to enlarge, pigmentation of scrotum, adult type hair – not on thighs
5	Adult type hair extending to medial part of thighs
Females	
1	Prepubertal
2	Sparse downy hair on sides of labia
3	Increased amount of hair and increased coarsness
4	Adult type hair not yet on medial part of thighs
5	Adult type hair extending onto medial thighs

After Tanner, for review see [6].

when there are abnormalities in development that require investigation, and understanding sexual development in the context of psychosocial development helps the clinician guide counseling.

Sexual experimentation often accompanies normal adolescent sexual development, but it can carry a significant risk of HIV infection. A large proportion of youth are potentially at risk for HIV infection: 45.6% of US high school students report ever having had sexual intercourse [7]. Observational data regarding HIV-infected and -uninfected high-risk youth in the USA indicate 43% of HIV-infected girls and 68% of HIV-infected boys reported eight or more lifetime sexual partners [8]. In the high-risk but uninfected group, condom use was sporadic; only 48% of uninfected girls and 56% of uninfected boys reported condom use at last intercourse.

Homosexual identity formation is a staged process [9]. In the first stage (sensitization), the adolescent feels different from his or her peers and may first sense attraction to the same sex. The next stage (sexual identity confusion) is a stage where the adolescent is confused, not about his or her attractions, but about how to reconcile his or her feelings with negative societal stereotypes. In the sexual identity assumption phase, the adolescent explores his or her own gay identity, and the adolescent considers the options of a homosexual lifestyle. This phase usually lasts several years and may extend beyond late adolescence. In the final stage, integration and commitment, the individual incorporates his or her homosexual identity into a positive self-acceptance. It is during this final stage that an individual is ready not only to accept his or her homosexuality but also to share it with others. Some may never reach this final stage and some only reach it in adulthood. Understanding the adolescent's stages of sexual identity formation helps the clinician to provide optimal care and to support the youth through the subsequent stages.

Counseling and testing

Part of good, comprehensive adolescent care for sexually active and needle-using youth must include HIV counseling and testing. Epidemiologic data indicate that only a fraction of HIV-infected youth have been identified and engaged in care, partly due to the lack of counseling and testing [2,4]. Often, providers have relied on reported "high-risk" behavior to identify patients at risk for HIV infection, but studies have shown that many HIV-infected adolescents do not fall into a particular high-risk group. Early in the epidemic, D'Angelo and colleagues found that, if only those youth who were perceived to fall into a high-risk group were offered HIV counseling and testing, only 38% of infected youth would be diagnosed [10]. Among pregnant adolescents in Atlanta, 59% of those infected reported no risk factor [11]. HIV counseling and testing provides two important benefits: (i) it is the only way to identify HIV-infected adolescents and link them into care; and (ii) it reduces sexual risk taking when testing and client-centered prevention counseling are linked [12]. Unfortunately, in a US study of 1500 adolescents, only 27% of those who were sexually active reported that they had been tested for HIV [13].

In most of the USA, adolescents can provide consent to HIV counseling and testing such as they can for other STIs. Key elements that should be included in such counseling include:

- what HIV/AIDS is
- how HIV is transmitted
- how HIV infection is diagnosed
- what a positive, negative, and indeterminant HIV test means
- what will happen if the HIV test is positive
- identification of a support person with whom the youth could share his/her HIV results
- the adolescent's plans should an HIV test result be positive or negative.

This last point is especially important in HIV counseling of adolescents and young adults. Many adolescents seek care and treatment for conditions during periods of crisis. Assessment for depression and suicide is part of good adolescent primary health-care. In cases where an adolescent is overwhelmed and an HIV diagnosis could enhance depression and risk for suicide, HIV counseling and testing is not indicated until the adolescent is more emotionally stable. The CDC recommends voluntary HIV counseling and testing for all at-risk patients and in all healthcare settings where the HIV prevalence is over 1% or the AIDS diagnosis rate is over 0.1%. Thus, many sites that care for at-risk adolescents should make HIV counseling and testing available and developmentally appropriate [14].

Clinicians providing HIV counseling and testing must have a treatment referral plan for patients who are determined to be HIV-infected. In addition, clinicians should be aware of treatment centers with programs for HIV-infected youth or clinical sites with clinicians experienced in caring for youth. Adolescents often require tremendous support to link them into care and often require active efforts to engage them at the time of post-test counseling. Youth should ideally be treated in HIV centers with adolescent-specific programs where there are providers versed in adolescent development who can provide the needed psychosocial support.

Prevention

HIV prevention is an important part of good adolescent healthcare and is essential for adolescents who are sexually active, or who use needles for injecting drugs (including steroids) or for tattooing. Although primary healthcare providers are likely to screen adolescents for such things as risk for homicide or suicide and risky behaviors such as smoking and alcohol, risks for HIV infection such as illicit drug use and lack of condom use are less likely to be addressed [15]. For those adolescents already infected with HIV, prevention is equally important. Infection with new strains of HIV could lead to accelerated disease progression or greater drug resistance problems, and prevention of other STIs is important for potentially immunosuppressed adolescents. Unplanned pregnancies can have a potentially negative impact on the HIV-infected adolescent, both physically and emotionally, and risk infection of the infant. The provision of effective prevention counseling to HIV-infected adolescents can halt further spread of

HIV infection. Practitioners must offer intensive psychosocial support to HIV-infected adolescents to help them to negotiate safer sex. Peer support, both one-on-one and in support groups, can serve as an important vehicle for providing adolescents with the ability to negotiate condom use.

All prevention counseling for the HIV-infected adolescent should be done in a caring, supportive atmosphere, rather than in an authoritarian manner. Before beginning prevention counseling for an HIV-infected adolescent, it is often helpful to have a good assessment of the adolescent's living situation. The SHADSSS assessment provides a framework for discussions of all areas of the life of the adolescent [16], enabling the clinician to provide appropriate counseling and prevention services. SHADSSS is an acronym representing:

S = school;

H = home;

A = activities;

D = depression/self-esteem;

S = substance abuse;

S = sexuality;

S = safety.

The SHADSSS assessment provides the opportunity to identify particularly troubling areas of the adolescent's life and helps the clinician identify services the adolescent may require. For example, if a history of substance abuse is obtained during the interview, it must be dealt with along with other issues, such as depression, to optimally benefit the adolescent. Such an assessment provides at least an initial means for the provider to identify important issues in the adolescent's life which must be addressed. Many youth face problems that generally require more extensive interventions, such as alcohol and drug dependence, abusive home relationships, poor self-esteem, and failure at school. It is important that the adolescent understand that all information is confidential, except for information that may indicate that the adolescent is a threat to himself or herself, or to another person. Setting the stage for good, confidential counseling is essential at every encounter with the adolescent.

Some adolescents are at particular risk for HIV infection. Youth who have run away from home or who live on the street often trade sex for food, housing, and protection. Such survival sex becomes a basic part of that adolescent's existence. Adolescents who survive through the exchange of sex may be unwilling or unable to negotiate safer sex because they fear losing access to their basic needs. These youth must be presented with options, which enable them to provide for themselves without the exchange of sex before issues around safer sex can even begin to be addressed. Similarly, young gay male youth have unique issues related to their sexual orientation. Homosexual identity formation is a process; the youth must gain a degree of acceptance of his sexual orientation before he can begin to plan for safer sex. It is not uncommon to find young homosexual men involved in relationships with older men, which may add additional barriers to negotiating safer sex [17]. Clinicians must respect the confidentiality of, and should strive to understand the special concerns of, homosexual, bisexual, and transgendered youth in order to provide the best care possible to these groups [18].

Clinicians must ensure that adolescents receive counseling concerning safer sex. Abstinence counseling should be provided to all adolescents, even those who are already sexually active. Some adolescents who are sexually active subsequently may decide to refrain from intercourse until they are more comfortable with negotiating safer sex. For these youth, it is helpful to discuss sexual acts such as kissing and touching, which hold no risk for disease transmission. Counseling both persons involved in a relationship may help to open up communication between the partners and lead to a more mature and thoughtful attitude. Peer counselors can be particularly helpful in assisting adolescents negotiate safer sex. For the provider, it is important to focus not only on knowledge but also on practice. All adolescents should come away from prevention counseling with knowledge of the following: correct use of a condom for oral, vaginal, and anal sex; proper use of an internal or "female" condom; correct and incorrect lubrication for use with a condom; the common STIs and their symptoms; strategies for negotiating safer sex and abstaining from sex; and the potential consequences of unsafe sex. It is also important for the provider to understand the dynamics of the couple and how that may influence risk taking. In one study of adolescent girls, current partners were, on average, older by 4 to 6 years [19]. This age difference was somewhat greater for the HIV-infected girls compared to the uninfected girls. Abusive relationships also can pose a particular challenge to the adolescent who is being counseled about how to negotiate safer sex. For the adolescent who continues in high-risk behavior despite counseling, such issues may be pertinent and should be investigated.

All counseling should be done in a supportive, non-judgmental manner. It is also very important for the provider counseling an adolescent to have a clear understanding of the differences between sexuality and sexual behaviors. When counseling about sexuality, it is important to consider emotional as well as physical dimensions. Discussions of sexuality should include issues related to peer and societal norms, as well as the adolescent's response to feelings as a sexual being. Such discussions can uncover problems such as internalized homophobia, feelings of disempowerment, and issues of abstinence and self-esteem. Addressing these issues requires an ongoing dialogue between the adolescent and the clinician, and may necessitate the involvement of a psychologist or sex counselor. Sexual curiosity can lead to risk-taking behavior; discussing sex with an adult may provide an answer to very key questions a young person may feel they can obtain only from an actual sexual encounter. It also has been shown that discussing sex does not encourage non-sexually active youth to initiate sex. Most providers are more accustomed to discussing sexual behaviors with their adolescent patients. For some youth, the first attempt by the provider to discuss such issues may be poorly received. The provider should explain to the youth why he or she is discussing such issues with them and also should stress the confidentiality of the conversation. The provider must speak in terms understood by the youth and should be as specific as possible to ensure the adolescent is learning as much as possible from the session. Repeated reinforcement of the key points of negotiating safer sex is essential.

Care of the HIV-infected adolescent

General

Good, comprehensive HIV care includes not only the prescribing of antiretroviral drugs, but also must include other key elements: general healthcare; ongoing psychosocial support and counseling; care for other STIs; and gynecologic care and family planning. Before initiating treatment of HIV infection, it is essential to confirm the HIV infection. Uninfected adolescents have presented for HIV care [20]. Retesting provides an opportunity for a thorough discussion of HIV infection and AIDS, and the need for good medical care. After confirmation of infection, a comprehensive medical history and physical examination should be performed. The medical history should include a good psychosocial history, using the SHADSSS assessment. Determination of the timing of infection, although often difficult, can be useful. For example, if a youth presents with an acute retroviral infection syndrome, early initiation of antiretroviral therapy can decrease total viral burden and theoretically can improve the long-term outcome through good viral suppression before significant immunologic deterioration develops. The history and results of previous HIV tests should be obtained. In addition, any history of receipt of blood or blood products should be obtained because of the possibility that early infection through these routes might present during adolescence. The family history should pay special attention to the health of the parents, since individuals infected through mother-to-child transmission (MTCT) can present, albeit rarely, during adolescence. Finally, some adolescents are infected with HIV through early childhood sexual abuse; any history of sexual abuse should be included in the assessment.

During an acute infection, the ELISA and Western Blot may not detect infection, since it can take up to 6 months from the time of infection until there are sufficient HIV antibodies to yield positive results. In this situation, other diagnostic assays (e.g., HIV culture, HIV DNA PCR, or HIV RNA PCR) should be performed. Staging of HIV infection (according to CD4+ lymphocyte measurements, HIV RNA PCR assays, and clinical examination) should be performed. The decision to initiate antiretroviral therapy in an HIV-infected adolescent must take into account a number of factors (see Chapter 15), including adherence (see Chapter 7 and the metabolic complications associated with antiretroviral therapy (see Chapter 13).

Clinicians should be careful to prescribe drugs, including antiretroviral drugs, correctly. For those adolescents who are either Tanner Stage 1 or 2, pediatric dosing should be followed. For adolescents who are either Tanner Stage 3 or 4, pediatric or adult dosing guidelines should be followed depending on the weight of the young person and comparing the standard adult dose to that based on weight for pediatric dosing. For adolescents who are Tanner stage 5, the adult dosing guidelines should be followed (see Chapter 15).

Care and treatment of other STIs, and gynecologic care for adolescent girls and young women, are essential, and are addressed in further detail below. Since a youth's sexual activities provide an important guide for STI screening, clinicians should take a careful sexual history, which should include questions about oral, vaginal, and anal sex for all patients, and about the possibility of both receptive and insertive anal sex for MSM. Diagnosing STIs of the anus/rectum or pharynx is important, since such infections can cause significant morbidity. For example, in young MSM, anal infections with human papillomavirus (HPV) can cause anal warts and cancer. In one study of HIV-infected and -uninfected adolescents in the USA, anal HPV infection was noted in 48% of males [21]. Anal cytology tests, performed using a thin preparation technique, revealed anal dysplasia in 50% of the young men. In multivariate analyses, males with anal HPV infection were more likely to be MSM and to have anal warts, anal dysplasia, and HIV infection. Some experts advocate routine screening for anal HPV or anal dysplasia. If screening for anal dysplasia is conducted, clinicians should refer patients with anal HPV infection or concerning cytology for anoscopy and biopsy.

The care of HIV-infected adolescents is complex and often requires a team of clinicians with diverse expertise. Multidisciplinary teams of clinicians caring for HIV-infected adolescents often include case managers and psychologists to provide ongoing counseling and support and to help address the complex psychosocial issues facing these young people.

Each HIV-infected adolescent may have a unique set of problems, but many share similar concerns. Disclosure of HIV infection to a sexual partner or partners is often the most challenging and disturbing issue facing the adolescent. All too frequently the sexual partner is the only supportive or loving person in that adolescent's life. The fear of rejection after disclosure can be great. Some youth may be concerned about physical and emotional abuse following disclosure. In a study of adolescents with HIV infection in the USA, HIV-infected youth enrolled in the study disclosed their HIV infection status to 242 sexual partners (47.5%) [22]. Males and females were equally likely to disclose their HIV status to their sexual partner. Subjects were most likely to disclose to partners whom they considered their "main" partner and to partners who were also HIV-infected, as compared to those who were HIV-uninfected or whose HIV serostatus was uncertain. It is important that the adolescent see the care team as supportive rather than authoritarian, particularly surrounding the problems of disclosure. When the adolescent has accepted disclosure, the team can offer the youth assistance. Some adolescents will want to bring their sexual partners in to see the care team following disclosure to assist with answering questions regarding HIV infection and its transmission. Others may choose to disclose their HIV infection status in the clinic setting with a member of the care team present. This latter option serves different purposes: (i) it gives some protection to the adolescent should they fear that the partner might react violently; (ii) it provides a good opportunity for counseling the couple together. It is also important that sexual partners be made aware of availability of HIV counseling and testing.

HIV infection presents the adolescent with an as yet incurable disease. It is essential for the adolescent to understand that HIV can be manageable, given good medical and psychosocial care. HIV-infected youth need a sense of hope and control over their disease, and clinicians need to provide this message.

Adolescent gynecology/reproductive health

The most practical approach when considering the most common reproductive and gynecological disorders of HIV-infected adolescents is to identify if the adolescent is sexually active or not. Among non-sexually active girls with HIV infection acquired through MTCT, the most common conditions include delayed pubertal development and menstrual disorders related to an immature hypothalamic–pituitary axis. Sexually active adolescents, both HIV-infected and -uninfected, experience other conditions such as STIs, pregnancy, and abnormal uterine bleeding.

Most reproductive health disorders among HIV-infected adolescent girls are best managed by an adolescent medicine physician. Certain patients, such as those with delayed puberty, amenorrhea, and hyperandrogenism should be managed in collaboration with an endocrinologist. Finally, referral to an obstetrician/gynecologist is required for complications of pregnancy and for pelvic infections.

Non-infectious

Delayed puberty

Pubertal maturation in girls begins with the acceleration of growth followed by onset of breast development (thelarche) between the ages of 8 and 13 years. Later signs of pubertal maturation include development of pubic or axillary hair (adrenarche), which generally occurs after age 8 years (mean age: 12.5 years, range: 10–15 years) and onset of menses (menarche) between 9.1 and 17.7 years (median 12.8) [23, 24]. The failure to have breast budding by age 13 years or menarche by age 15 years is considered indicative of delayed sexual maturation.

The differential diagnosis of delayed puberty in girls, including those with HIV infection, can be divided between those processes associated with short stature and those associated with normal stature (Table 8.3) [25]. Delayed onset of puberty is often reported in young women suffering from many chronic conditions, including HIV infection. In general, the earlier the onset and the longer and more severe the illness, the greater are the repercussions on pubertal development [24, 25].

Medical assessment is required for any girl with delayed sexual maturation or with extremely slow pubertal progression (e.g., breast development but persistent amenorrhea for 5 years). Such an assessment should include a complete history and physical examination, and initial laboratory studies are driven by the history and physical examination findings. Consultation with an endocrinologist is highly recommended [27–29]. The goals of therapy are to induce a pubertal growth spurt, to prevent potential

Table 8.3. Differential diagnosis of delayed puberty in HIV-infected girls

Pubertal delay with short stature

1. **Chronic diseases:** HIV-infected teens with other HIV-associated chronic conditions (such as wasting syndrome, chronic infections, respiratory illnesses, chronic anemia gastrointestinal disease, and renal disturbances) may be at highest risk for pubertal delay and short stature
2. **Constitutional delay of puberty and normal variant short stature**
3. **Panhypopituitarism:** congenital or acquired infections; viral infection, tuberculosis, sarcoidosis, histiocytosis, posttraumatic, central tumors
4. **Congenital syndromes:** an array of genetic disorders, and syndromes of primary gonadal dysfunction with hypergonadotropic hypogonadism, including Turner syndrome, and a group of acquired and genetic abnormalities
5. **Glucocorticoid excess**

Pubertal delay without short stature

1. **Constitutional delay of puberty**
2. **Chronic diseases** (HIV, hyperthyroidism, asthma, inflammatory bowel disease, celiac disease, juvenile rheumatoid arthritis, systemic lupus erythematosus)
3. **Acquired gonadotropin deficiency**
   - CNS infections: viral encephalitis, tuberculosis
   - Central hypothalamic–pituitary tumors: craniopharyngioma, hypothalamic glioma, astrocytoma, pituitary adenomas
   - Head trauma
   - Histiocytosis X
   - Sarcoidosis
4. **Congenital gonadal disorders** (enzyme defects on androgen and estrogen production)
5. **Androgen receptor defects** ("testicular feminization")

short- and long-term psychological and social handicaps, and to achieve full functional sexual maturation. If hormonal substitution therapy is considered, consultation with an endocrinologist should occur (see Chapter 28) [30–32].

Menstrual disorders

Abnormal uterine bleeding

Abnormal uterine bleeding is defined as a significant variation from normal menstrual bleeding patterns. Although abnormal uterine bleeding occurs among women of all ages, it is a particularly common problem within 1 to 2 years after menarche. Abnormal uterine bleeding is responsible for approximately 50% of gynecologic visits among adolescents [33]. Neither HIV infection nor the associated immunosuppression appears to have clinically relevant effects on menstruation [34].

Amenorrhea

There are two types of amenorrhea: primary amenorrhea, or lack of onset of menses by age 15 years, and secondary amenorrhea, defined as the absence of menses for a period longer than 3 months at any time after the onset of regular menses. Primary amenorrhea is associated with pubertal delay, discussed earlier, and is likely to be more common among girls with HIV infection acquired through MTCT [35].

Most amenorrhea among HIV-infected adolescent girls is secondary amenorrhea, which falls into two categories: amenorrhea associated with low body weight and wasting syndrome, and amenorrhea common to adolescents in general, associated with pregnancy, with long-acting hormonal contraceptives, and with endocrine and hypothalamic pituitary dysfunction. Most HIV-infected adolescent girls have acquired HIV during adolescence, are at early stages in their HIV disease progression, and have not experienced significant body fat loss. They may experience secondary amenorrhea, as do their uninfected peers [36, 37].

Pregnancy is the most common cause of amenorrhea in sexually active adolescents and the clinician must be suspicious of pregnancy in any adolescent presenting with amenorrhea. The second most common cause of amenorrhea is long-acting hormonal contraceptive use. Endocrine conditions associated with amenorrhea include thyroid dysfunction, hyperprolactinemia, and pituitary tumors. In addition, polycystic ovary syndrome (PCOS), an endocrine disorder frequently associated with obesity, is also associated with amenorrhea. This disorder is characterized by high levels of androgens, which can be converted to estrogens in peripheral and hepatic tissue [33]. Marijuana can produce amenorrhea, which is reversible after marijuana use is discontinued [38].

The initial workup for amenorrhea should include a history, a physical examination, including a pelvic examination, and a pregnancy test. A maturation index of a vaginal smear also can be obtained by introducing, if patient permits, a cotton-tipped applicator to the vagina, which is then fixed with a Papanicolaou fixative. Superficial cells predominate with increasing estrogen effect and parabasal cells predominate in the absence of estrogen [39]. In adolescent girls who are not sexually active, a speculum examination with a Huffman speculum should be attempted to visualize the vagina and cervix. If the hymenal opening is too small to permit a vaginal bimanual examination, a recto-abdominal examination in the lithotomy position may permit palpation of uterine and adnexal masses. In sexually active girls, a full pelvic examination should be performed, to identify signs of pregnancy such as softening and discoloration (purple or hyperemic) of the cervix and uterine enlargement, in addition to a pregnancy test [35].

Laboratory evaluation of the adolescent with amenorrhea should be based on diagnoses suggested by the history and physical examination. If the results of the pregnancy test are negative and there is absence of menses for over 6 months, a more extensive workup is conducted, in consultation with an endocrinologist, to identify androgen excess or hypothalamic–pituitary dysfunction. In general, more extensive evaluation of amenorrhea is recommended if neoplasia is suspected or if signs and symptoms related to other organ systems accompany the amenorrhea.

Management of amenorrhea depends on whether it is primary or secondary. Primary amenorrhea should be managed in consultation with an endocrinologist and will not be the focus of this discussion. In young women with secondary amenorrhea associated with weight loss, bone mineral density loss can occur soon after amenorrhea develops. Therefore, these patients may be at highest risk of developing osteoporosis and stress fractures. The efficacy of estrogen replacement therapy in this setting is an area of debate. However, estrogen has beneficial effects on bone and other tissues [37]. The use of combination estrogen and progesterone is indicated after pregnancy and neoplasias have been excluded. In addition to the bone effect, cyclic estrogen and progesterone therapy also can be beneficial through restoration of the menstrual pattern desired by the adolescent. Patients with secondary amenorrhea due to hypothalamic–pituitary failure and ovarian failure should be managed in collaboration with an endocrinologist [35].

Oligomenorrhea and hyperandrogenism

Oligomenorrhea is defined as abnormal menses that are infrequent or irregular, of variable duration, and characterized by painless scanty bleeding. Usually the result of anovulatory cycles, oligomenorrhea is one of the signs and symptoms of androgen excess (hyperandrogenism) along with hirsutism, acne, weight gain, and, if severe, virilization or masculinization. Adolescents with hyperandrogenism are often worried about their appearance and the potential relationship to infertility. Androgen excess can be associated with metabolic disturbances such as insulin resistance [40]. The differential diagnosis of hyperandrogenism is summarized in Table 8.4.

Polycystic ovary syndrome (PCOS) is the most common cause of hyperandrogenism, accounting for 80%–90% of all cases of androgen excess in adolescent girls and women. A diagnosis of PCOS is important, particularly in HIV-infected adolescents, because the metabolic defects of PCOS (glucose intolerance leading to type 2 diabetes and dyslipidemia leading to cardiovascular disease) have major implications for antiretroviral therapy management [41,42]. Patients with PCOS often present with hirsutism, obesity, acne, and acanthosis nigricans [41, 43,44]. PCOS includes its variant, the hyperandrogenic-insulin resistant acanthosis nigricans (HAIRAN) syndrome. The HAIRAN syndrome is characterized by acanthosis nigricans, fasting glucose levels that are relatively normal despite extremely high circulating levels of insulin, and androgen excess [44]. PCOS is often a diagnosis of exclusion. Criteria for diagnosis include chronic anovulation with a premenarcheal onset of menstrual irregularities [45], and biochemical or clinical evidence of androgen excess (primarily ovarian in origin). Approximately 50% of women with PCOS are insulin resistant with or without obesity (40, 44).

Initial laboratory evaluation includes measurements of LH, FSH, LH:FSH ratio, free testosterone, DHEAS, prolactin, thyroid function tests, glucose and insulin levels, and a lipid profile. As a rule, all anovulatory women who are hyperandrogenic should be

Table 8.4. Differential diagnosis of hyperandrogenism

Endocrine disorders	Characteristics
Ovarian	
PCOS	Chronic anovulation with menstrual irregularities, with or without skin manifestations and absence of other androgen disorders. Supportive labs include LH:FSH ratio >2:1 provided that LH level is not below 8 mIU/mL; mild elevation of testosterone and DHEAS and hyperprolactinemia (25%).
HAIRAN	Insulin resistance, and acanthosis nigricans. Similar metabolic features of PCOS, myocardial hypertrophy, insulin receptor mutations, circulating antibodies to the insulin receptor, postreceptor signaling defects. Fasting basal insulin levels of >80 μU/mL compared with reference range of about 7–8 μU/mL, peaks of >1000 μU/mL (60 μU/mL in healthy individuals).
Ovarian tumors	Palpation of ovarian mass; testosterone level >200 ng/mL; DHEAS (level >700 μU/mL suggests an ovarian or adrenal tumor); non-suppression of androgens with dexamethasone.
Adrenal	
Late onset 21-hydroxylase (21-OH)	Presentation similar to PCOS, onset in adolescence. Elevated serum 17-OHP (17-hydroxyprogesterone), large increase after 0.25 mg single-dose injection of adrenocorticotropin hormone (ACTH) is diagnostic. Elevated 11-deoxycortisol or DHEAS and 17-hydroxypregnenolone levels are found in 11-hydroxylase and 3 β-hydroxysteroid dehydrogenase deficiencies.
Cushing's syndrome	Lack of cortisol suppression after dexamethasone (0.5mg q.i.d. for 5–7 days).
Adrenal tumors	Rare and associated with rapid virilization. Palpable mass; elevated 17-KS, DHEAS, and DHEA levels. No suppression with dexamethasone administration. Mass on ultrasound or CT scan.
Other	
Idiopathic hirsutism	Ovulation regularly, normal levels of androgens. Mechanism remains to be determined.
Exogenous: androgenic drugs	Anabolic steroids, testosterone, DHEAS, androgenic protestins, danazol, corticotropin, high-dose corticosteroids, metyrapone, derivates of phenothiazine, acetazolamide.
Exogenous: non-androgenic drugs	Phenytoin, valproate, cyclosporine, diazoxide, minoxidil, hexachlorobenzene, psoralens.
Central nervous system lesions	Encephalitis.

assessed for insulin resistance and glucose tolerance with measurements of the fasting glucose:insulin ratio. Alternatively, the glucose level in the bloodstream 2 hours after ingestion of a 75-gram glucose load can be assessed. Follow-up evaluation of hyperandrogenic patients requires frequent monitoring of glucose intolerance, insulin resistance, and dyslipidemia. Further evaluation to rule out an ovarian or adrenal tumor is required for any girl with severe acne, hirsutism, virilization, or markedly elevated levels of serum testosterone and DHEAS. This evaluation requires imaging studies and consultation with an endocrinologist [40,41, 44, 46].

Specific management strategies for PCOS [41, 42, 44, 47, 48] include the following.

(a) Weight loss to reduce circulating androgen levels and decrease unbound testosterone [49];

(b) Hormonal management with combination oral contraceptives with low androgenic progestins (desogestrel and gestodine) for abnormal uterine bleeding and endometrial hyperplasia [40];

(c) Management of hirsutism: cosmetic approaches such as chemical depilatories, electrolysis, and laser photodermodestruction can be utilized. In addition to combination oral contraceptives, antiandrogenic agents such as spironolactone can be used [40,44];

(d) Management of diabetes: insulin-sensitizing agents such as metformin, can be used for overt diabetes and are the focus of current research. Initial trials with metformin have shown promising results in terms of lowering insulin secretion, improving insulin sensitivity, restoring normal menstrual cycles, and correcting lipid abnormalities. Primary prevention of diabetes and cardiovascular lifestyle modifications, regular exercise, and a balanced diet are also important, especially for those HIV-infected young women taking HAART [40,48];

(e) Treatment with clomiphene to induce ovulation: such treatment is reserved for patients with infertility. These patients should be referred to a reproductive endocrinologist.

Dysfunctional uterine bleeding (DUB)

DUB is defined as irregular, painless bleeding of endometrial origin that can be excessive, prolonged, or unpatterned. The bleeding is related to endometrial sloughing in the absence of structural pathology and is usually due to anovulation. Ovulatory DUB occurs secondary to defects in local endometrial hemostasis. Anovulatory DUB, a systemic disorder occurring secondary to endocrinologic, neurochemical, or pharmacologic mechanisms, is the most common form and may result from prolonged amenorrhea leading to endometrial hypertrophy [50, 51]. DUB is a diagnosis of exclusion. The differential diagnosis of DUB is shown in Table 8.5 [50].

As part of the evaluation, a menstrual and sexual history, a history of hormonal contraceptive use, and a family history, including a history of PCOS or bleeding disorders,

Table 8.5. Differential diagnosis of dysfunctional uterine bleeding (DUB)

Category	Comments
Pregnancy and complications of pregnancy	• Spontaneous and incomplete abortion • Ectopic pregnancy
Use of exogenous hormones leading to anovulatory breakthrough or withdrawal bleeding	• Estrogen breakthrough bleeding that occurs when excess estrogen stimulates the endometrium to proliferate • Estrogen withdrawal bleeding occurs after stopping exogenous estrogen therapy or just before ovulation in the normal menstrual cycle and is usually self-limited • Progesterone breakthrough bleeding: occurs when the ratio of progesterone to estrogen is high, the endometrium becomes atrophic and more prone to frequent, irregular bleeding. This occurs with the use of progesterone-only contraceptive methods
Infections	• Sexually transmitted infections
Local pathology	• Trauma • Foreign body • Lesions of the cervix or vagina
Hormonal imbalance	• Hypothyroidism • Hyperthyroidism • Androgen excess • Insulin resistance • Obesity
Coagulopathies and hematologic conditions	• Thrombocytopenic disorders related or unrelated to HIV infection • Idiopathic thrombocytopenic purpura • Abnormal platelet function due to drugs (aspirin) • Systemic illness or anticoagulant therapy • Von Willebrand's disease (diagnosed when patient presents with excessive vaginal bleeding upon menarche)
Neoplasia	• Rare, but screening for cervical dysplasia highly recommended

should be obtained. The review of systems should include specific questions about tachycardia, palpitations, fatigue, lightheadedness, easy bruises, and epistaxis or gum bleeding [51–53].

The physical examination should include an assessment of hemodynamic stability. In addition, height, weight, and sexual maturity rating should be evaluated. A skin examination is performed to identify signs of hyperandrogenicity or bleeding disorders, the thyroid should be palpated to detect enlargement and nodularities, and the breasts should be examined for galactorrhea. A pelvic examination is essential to identify structural abnormalities and to assess the amount of bleeding [50,54].

The initial laboratory evaluation of DUB includes assessment of hematologic status with a complete blood count to detect anemia and thrombocytopenia and a pregnancy test to rule out pregnancy. STI screening is indicated for sexually active adolescents. No further laboratory testing is necessary in adolescents with mild anovulatory DUB associated with physiological immaturity. A bleeding time and other tests to diagnose von Willebrand's disease should be performed before initiation of any hormonal therapy, since hormonal therapy may slightly prolong bleeding time. A transabdominal pelvic ultrasonography is recommended to evaluate uterine and ovarian anatomy in patients who do not tolerate a pelvic examination. Transvaginal ultrasonography is indicated if the pregnancy test is positive or if a mass is palpated on pelvic examination, and tubo-ovarian abscess (TOA) or ectopic pregnancy should be ruled out. Endometrial sampling is rarely recommended in adolescents [55, 56].

The treatment of DUB depends on the severity of the bleeding. Once DUB is diagnosed, hormonal management with oral contraceptives is frequently successful. Low-dose oral contraceptives are as effective as contraceptives with higher estrogen doses. They establish regular menses with decreased menstrual flow, preventing long intervals of amenorrhea and subsequent endometrial hyperplasia with resultant profuse bleeding. The dosage of combined oral contraceptives (OCs) is guided by the severity of the bleeding. For immediate treatment of moderate bleeding, oral contraceptives may be administered up to one tablet four times a day, with antiemetics prescribed with these high doses. The dose is reduced slowly based on daily assessment of bleeding. Depot medroxyprogesterone acetate (DMPA) 150 mg intramuscularly every 12 weeks also has been used to produce amenorrhea in these cases but has not been traditionally the first choice for the initial management of moderate to severe dysfunctional uterine bleeding. Severe bleeding (heavy flow and hemoglobin <10 g/DL) usually requires intravenous estrogen and hospitalization. Surgical management is rarely required and is reserved for situations in which medical therapy has been unsuccessful or is contraindicated [52, 55–57].

Hormonal contraceptives also are used in the management of ovulatory DUB. The management is directed at decreasing menstrual frequency or inducing endometrial atrophy. Combined OCs (21-day packet), one pill daily continuously, is recommended. Discontinuation of the pill for 1 week every 3 months prevents excessive endometrial proliferation. Endometrial atrophy also can be induced by administration of DMPA 150 mg IM every 3 months once the endometrial stability has been achieved and the bleeding is controlled. GnRH (gonadotropin releasing hormone) analogs are reserved for severe cases and should not be used for more than 6 months [51, 53, 56, 58].

Dysmenorrhea

Dysmenorrhea, characterized by lower abdominal pain that is usually cramping in nature, is categorized as primary or secondary. Primary dysmenorrhea refers to cyclic pain associated with the menstrual flow without evidence of pelvic pathology. It is associated with ovulatory cycles and is due to myometrial contractions induced by prostaglandins originating in the secretory endometrium. Secondary dysmenorrhea refers to pain associated with menses due to organic disease such as endometriosis, outflow tract obstruction or pelvic infections. Dysmenorrhea is a common gynecological disorder affecting 60% of menstruating adolescents, 14% of whom report it as the cause of school absenteeism [59].

The most common type of dysmenorrhea in adolescents is primary dysmenorrhea. It appears within 1 to 2 years of menarche, when ovulatory cycles have been established, and may persist through adulthood as long as the patient is ovulating. The pain of primary dysmenorrhea usually begins a few hours prior to the onset of menstrual bleeding and may last as long as 2 to 3 days. The pain of dysmenorrhea is described as suprapubic cramping and can be accompanied by nausea, vomiting, diarrhea, dizziness or syncope, and lumbosacral back pain. Signs include suprapubic tenderness without rebound on palpation. Bimanual examination reveals uterine tenderness but absence of cervical motion tenderness.

Secondary dysmenorrhea, usually developing years after menarche, is rare in adolescents [60]. The most common causes of secondary dysmenorrhea in adolescents include salpingo-oophoritis, endometriosis, adhesions, imperforate hymen, transverse vaginal septum, cervical stenosis, and uterine anomalies. Less frequent causes of secondary dysmenorrhea are gastrointestinal disorders (e.g., irritable bowel syndrome, ulcerative colitis, and Crohn's disease), genitourinary disorders (e.g., ureteral obstruction and pelvic kidney); and neurologic disorders. Musculoskeletal causes, including scoliosis, kyphosis, spondylolysis, and spondylolisthesis, are rare [60]. The pain of secondary dysmenorrhea can be diffused in the pelvic or localized in areas outside the pelvis such as the rectum or the back. The examination may show cervical motion tenderness such as with PID. Tenderness or nodularity of the uterosacral ligaments and cul-de-sac or ovary can be found in patients with endometriosis [61].

The diagnosis depends on the history of the cyclic nature of the pain and presence or absence of underlying pelvic pathology as determined by pelvic examination. Cigarette smoking has been associated with increased duration of dysmenorrhea [62]. The review of systems should include a complete review of gastrointestinal, genitourinary, neurological, and musculo-skeletal systems. Screening for pregnancy and for STIs, and obtaining a complete blood cell count and an erythrocyte sedimentation rate, are essential to rule out pregnancy, PID, and inflammatory bowel disease, respectively. Ultrasound is indicated when complications of pelvic infections or a müllerian abnormality are suspected, and when masses are palpated [60].

The most effective treatments for primary dysmenorrhea are prostaglandin synthetase inhibitors such as non-steroidal anti-inflammatory drugs (NSAIDs) and OCs. NSAIDs are the most common pharmacologic treatment for dysmenorrhea and are effective in approximately 80% of primary dysmenorrhea cases. They should be taken before, or at the onset of, pain and then every 6 to 8 hours for the first 3 days of the menstrual period. The benefit depends on dose and duration of treatment. A loading dose of NSAIDs (typically twice the regular dose) should be used as initial treatment for dysmenorrhea in adolescents followed by a regular dose until symptoms abate. For those adolescents who also desire contraception or those who do not respond after 3 months of treatment with NSAIDs, combined OCs represent the agent of choice for treating dysmenorrhea. Compared to placebo, treatment with desogestrel-containing low-dose oral contraceptives also reduces the severity of menstrual pain and cramping among women with dysmenorrhea. However, no significant change in bloating, anxiety, weight gain, or acne was reported in the treatment group [63]. If dysmenorrhea is not relieved by the above measures, a trial of up to 6 months is indicated, with necessary changes in doses and medications before the therapy is considered a failure. If symptoms persist after 6 months, the clinician should suspect secondary causes of dysmenorrhea such as endometriosis and the patient should be referred to a gynecologist [58, 60].

PMS

PMS is characterized by behavioral, somatic, affective, and cognitive disorders appearing in the luteal phase of the menstrual cycle and usually disappearing a few days after the onset of menses. It is estimated that up to 85% of women have some degree of symptoms before menses, and 5%–10% have severe symptoms and restrictions of daily activities [64]. Studies in adolescents have reported prevalences ranging from 14% to 96% [65, 66]. Common complaints of adolescents experiencing PMS include physical symptoms (e.g., abdominal bloating, breast tenderness, weight gain, edema of lower extremities, headaches and joint or muscle pain, fatigue, increased appetite) and food cravings) and psychological symptoms (e.g., emotional instability, irritability, anxiety, depression, decreased concentration, clumsiness, insomnia or hypersomnia, tearfulness, a sense of being out of control, social withdrawal, and changes in libido) [66]. The most severe form of PMS is the premenstrual dysphoric disorder (PMDD), in which the symptoms markedly interfere with work, school, usual activities, or relationships with others, and are not the exacerbation of another disorder [67].

The differential diagnosis for PMS includes exacerbation of existing psychiatric conditions such as major depression, dysthymia, panic or personality disorders, and medical disorders such as seizures, migraine headaches, irritable bowel syndrome, asthma, and allergies. Menstrual exacerbation of existing psychiatric or medical disorders does not constitute PMS [68]. Confirmation of the diagnosis of PMS requires obtaining a history of the patient's symptoms over at least two menstrual cycles, as well as a physical examination. The patient history should include an assessment of the patient's lifestyle, diet, stress level, and a history of previous psychiatric disorders [69]. The diagnosis of PMS is made by prospectively charting the cyclic nature of the symptoms, which occur in the luteal phase and resolve within a few days after onset of menses. The symptoms must be recurrent and severe enough to disrupt normal activities.

Stress management, dietary changes, and increased exercise have relieved symptoms of PMS in some adolescents. Treatment to suppress ovulation with combined OCs, depot medroxyprogesterone, and GnRH analogues also have been shown to alleviate PMS symptoms. However, the use of GnRH analogs in adolescents is limited due to the hypoestrogenic effects and the risks of bone density. Selective serotonin reuptake inhibitors (SSRIs) such as fluoxetine and sertraline are the drugs of choice for severe PMS and for PMDD. In some cases, the use of these drugs only during the luteal phase has resulted in improvement of symptoms [69–71].

Contraception

There are numerous types of contraception. Barrier methods include male and female condoms, diaphragms, cervical caps, and vaginal sponges. The latter three barrier methods are not widely used in the adolescent population, and will not be addressed in detail in this chapter. Hormonal contraceptives, either combined estrogen/progestin or progestin-only contraceptives, are taken orally, or in certain cases injected. Intrauterine devices (IUDs), natural methods (such as coitus interruptus), and voluntary sterilization also exist as contraceptive methods, but are not used often in the adolescent population [33] and will not be addressed in detail in this chapter. Other methods in development include biodegradable implants, pellets, microspheres, and microcapsules [33]. Microbicides are being extensively researched as a means of developing a safe, acceptable chemical barrier to prevent HIV transmission during sexual intercourse [72]. Patient-focused interactive counseling is likely to encourage adherence to a desired contraceptive method [73]. Regardless of the contraceptive method chosen, ideally the clinician should discuss emergency contraception options with the adolescent, and together develop a plan for responding to situations in which she may have unprotected sex [74, 75]. Adolescents infected with HIV also require intense counseling concerning their reproductive health including their desire for pregnancy, contraceptive practice, and decisions and choices if an unintended pregnancy occurs.

Besides abstinence, only condoms, if used consistently and correctly, offer protection against HIV transmission and may substantially reduce the risk for many STIs. Condoms do not offer as much protection against HPV and genital herpes, which can be transmitted by contact with infected skin areas not covered by the condom [33]. Sexually active adolescents should be informed of, and strongly encouraged to use, male or female condoms to protect themselves from STIs, including HIV, no matter what other method they may use to prevent pregnancy.

Barrier methods
Condoms
Condoms are designed for one-time use. The recommended male condom is made of latex and its integrity should be protected by avoiding use of oil-based lubricants and by educating the patient in proper application techniques, including appropriate

lubricants, and storage strategies to prevent punctures and heat damage. The female condom consists of a lubricated polyurethane sheath with loose soft rings at each end; it is available in one size, and should be used in conjunction with a lubricant. The inner ring is placed as high as possible in the vagina. The outer ring covers the perineum and thus provides protection against perineal contact with infectious organisms. The conscious decision at each episode of sexual activity required for effective use of either male or female condoms for contraception or infection prevention is a major disadvantage. Although growing numbers of young women are choosing to rely on condoms for contraception, pregnancy and STI rates among those choosing condoms suggest that many do not use them with each sexual encounter, or have difficulties in using them correctly [76].

Vaginal spermicides

Vaginal spermicides containing nonoxynol-9 (N-9) enhance the contraceptive effectiveness of barrier methods. They are not effective in preventing infections with *Neisseria gonorrheae, Chlamydia trachomatis*, and HIV. In addition, frequent use of N-9-containing products has been associated with genital lesions and sloughing of epithelial cells, which may be associated with an increased risk of HIV transmission. N-9-containing products have more damaging effects upon the rectal mucosa than upon the vaginal mucosa. Adolescent women who engage in anal intercourse, a strategy sometimes used by young women to avoid the risk of conception or to maintain "technical virginity," should be cautioned against the use of N-9-containing products as sexual lubricants. Spermicide use has been associated with an increased risk of bacterial urinary tract infection in girls [77].

Hormonal contraception

Hormonal contraceptives include combined or single drug oral contraceptive, long-acting hormonal contraceptive methods, and emergency contraception. Table 8.6 summarizes the currently available hormonal contraceptive methods [75, 78, 79]. With the numerous medications required by HIV-infected individuals, drug interactions between OCs (estrogen–progestin combinations or progestin-only products) and other drugs, including antiretroviral drugs and drugs for prevention or treatment of opportunistic infections (OIs), are likely. Such interactions can result in either an increase or decrease in plasma concentrations of OCs and other drugs. (See Chapter 12). Counseling about acquisition and transmission of STIs, including HIV, prior to prescribing and during use of hormonal contraceptive methods is essential to minimize the incidence of STIs. Clinicians should emphasize that hormonal contraceptives do not protect against STIs, including HIV [80].

Oral contraceptives (OCs)

OCs are divided in two groups: (i) combination OCs that include an estrogen and a progestin; and (ii) progestin-only pills. Combination OCs come in monophasic packs

Table 8.6. Hormonal contraceptive methods

	Oral contraceptive pill (OCP)	Depo-provera (DMPA)	Monthly injectable Lunelle©	Patch OrthoEvra©	Ring NuvaRing©	Intrauterine system (IUS) Mirena©	Subdermal implants Levonorgestrel Rod Implants©	Emergency contraception (EC)
Description	The two types of OCP are: (i) combination pills containing both estrogen (ethinyl estradiol and menstranol) and progestins (norethindrone, norethindrone acetate, ethynodiol diacetate, norgestrel, levonorgestrel, noretgynodrel, desogestrel, norgestimate, and gestodene) (ii) Progestin-only pills.	150-mg depot medroxyprogesterone acetate injections every 3 months.	A single 0.5-ml monthly intra-muscular injection with a combination of progestin and estrogen (medroxyprogesterone acetate and estradiol cypionate injectable suspension).	A one-and-three-quarter inch square skin patch consisting of three layers containing progesterone and estrogen. It delivers continuous levels of norelgestromin and ethinyl estradiol for a 7-day period. Each cycle contains three hormone-releasing patches.	A flexible, transparent, colorless vaginal ring about 2.1 inches in diameter containing the hormones etonogestrel and ethinyl estradiol. Women insert it into the vagina and leave in place for three weeks. It releases daily doses of progestin and estrogen.	A small device that is inserted and left inside the uterus and releases progestin (levonorgestrel).	A two-rod system containing levonorgestrel-filled capsules that are inserted subdermally in the upper arm. A single rod system that contains progestin.	A one-time oral contraceptive that can be used after intercourse to prevent pregnancy. Treatment initiated within 72 hours of unprotected intercourse. EC reduces the risk of pregnancy by at least 75%.
Efficacy	High	High	High	High	High	High	High	High <72 hrs
Dosing frequency	Daily	Every 3 months	Monthly	Weekly	Monthly	Every 5 years	Every 3 years	Once

Office visits	Prescription	Every three months	Monthly	Prescription	Prescription	For insertion and removal (requires trained clinicians)	For insertion and removal (requires trained clinicians)	Once
Easy reversibility	Yes	No	Yes	Yes	Yes	Yes	No	Yes
User controlled	Yes	No	No	Yes	Yes	Yes	No	Yes
Discreet	Yes	Yes	Yes	Sometimes	Yes	Yes	Sometimes	Yes
Side effects	In some cases: unwanted menstrual cycle changes, nausea and vomiting, headaches, effects on depression, decreased libido, increased cervical ectopy, risk of cardiovascular disease, effects on glucose intolerance, gallbladder disease acceleration, hepatocellular adenoma.	Weight gain, depression, breast tenderness, menstrual irregularities (may take up to 8 months after last injection to discontinue side effects), lipid changes, bone density decreases.	Bleeding between periods, weight gain or loss, breast tenderness; nausea — rarely, vomiting; changes in mood or sex drive.	Same as oral contraceptives, include nausea, vomiting, mastalgia, headaches, menstrual cramps and abdominal pain; irregular bleeding, and skin irritation.	Risks and side effects are the same as oral contraceptives. Also may include vaginal discharge, vaginitis, and irritation.	Most commonly reported side effects include menstrual changes, lower abdominal pain, mastalgia; headache, vaginal discharge, mood changes, and nausea.	Irregular bleeding or spotting, headache, weight gain, breast tenderness.	Nausea (30–50%); Vomiting (15–25%); Menstrual change (10–15%). Also breast tenderness, headache, abdominal pain, fatigue, dizziness.
Protection against HIV and other STDs	No	No	No	No	No	No	No	No

Sources: [74, 78–80, 82–84]

that contain the same dosage of estrogen and progestin in every pill and multiphasic packs that contain different dosages of estrogen, progestin, or both during the cycle. The latter offers no significant benefit over the former. The pills are packaged in 21- and 28-day packs. The 28-day pack contains seven placebo pills and is preferred because adolescents are less likely to lose track of the pill-free interval. Newer products include a shortened placebo interval followed by a low-dose estrogen to reduce breakthrough bleeding. OCs with 20 to 30 μg of ethinyl estradiol are referred to as "low dose" OCs. The progestins in OCs can be classified in two families: (i) the estrane family, including norethindrone, norethindrone acetate, ethynodiol diacetate, and norethynodrel; and (ii) the gonane family, including norgestrel, levonorgestrel, norgestimate, desogestrel, and gestodene. Norgestimate and desogestrel have the lowest androgenicity effect and have less of an adverse impact on lipoprotein metabolism than levonorgestrel and norgestrel. These lower androgenic progestins may be more appropriate for youth with hyperandrogenism, excessive acne, and hirsutism [75].

In general, low dose OCs containing gonane progestins decrease the incidence of estrogen-related side effects, and are associated with lower rates of breakthrough bleeding. Low dose OCs have a low margin for error; pregnancy may result if doses are taken at different times of day or if a dose is missed. Despite the obvious disadvantage of the daily requirement for taking a pill, OCs are popular among teenagers [81]. Additional non-contraceptive benefits of OCs, such as improvement of acne and dysmenorrhea, increase the adherence of adolescents to the method [80].

Progestin-only OCs are usually reserved for those adolescents for whom combination OCs are contraindicated and who do not desire injectable, implantable, or dermal methods. The advantages include lack of interference with breastfeeding quality, or quantity of milk production, and decreased menstrual cramps, menstrual flow, PMS, and breast tenderness. The major disadvantage is that progestin-only OCs have a shorter half-life than do combination OCs, causing unpredictable pattern of menstrual bleeding and breakthrough bleeding, the most common side effect and reason for discontinuation. This method requires daily dosing without hormone free intervals. Other side effects include weight gain, increased appetite with subsequent weight gain, headaches, moodiness, fatigue, and breast enlargement [80, 81].

Long-acting hormonal contraceptive methods
Depot medroxyprogesterone acetate (DMPA, or Depo-Provera) injections administered every three months (150 mg) has become a more popular hormonal contraceptive method for adolescents [82]. As with OCs, discontinuation rates are high. Adolescents will often discontinue the use of DMPA unless close medical supervision is possible and side effects (primarily menstrual irregularities and weight gain) are carefully monitored and aggressively managed [72, 82].

The contraceptive patch is a one-and-three quarter inch square skin patch consisting of three layers, and it delivers continuous levels of norelgestromin and ethinyl estradiol for a 7-day period. Three hormone-releasing patches, used in successive weeks, comprise one cycle. The patch can be worn in several areas of the body, and it is recommended that different areas of skin be used for consecutive patches, to avoid skin irritation. The patches adhere well to the skin, allowing young women to continue any athletic activities includings wimming. It has demonstrated efficacy and safety, and a side effect profile similar to that of combination OCs. Additionally, the once-weekly dosing results in statistically better adherence than with OCs. A common complaint among adolescents about the patch is its visibility [83, 84].

Hormonal implants involve a two-rod system containing levonorgestrel-filled capsules that are inserted subdermally in the upper arm. A single rod system also contains progestin. Left in place, implants can protect against pregnancy for 3 years. However, implants are not very popular among adolescents because they require insertion, and discontinuation requires removal by a trained clinician [82].

Emergency contraception (EC)

EC is extremely safe and highly effective [74,85,86]. Two hormone regimens (ethinyl estradiol with levonorgestrel; high-dose levonorgestrel) given within 72 hours of intercourse and repeated 12 hours later are available for this purpose. These regimens are packaged as labeled US Food and Drug Administration dedicated products or they can be adapted for use from standard OCs. Levonorgestrel and mifepristone (not yet licensed for use as EC in the USA) seem to offer the highest effectiveness with an acceptable side-effect profile. For young women with a past history of deep vein thrombosis, pulmonary embolism, stroke, or heart attack, progestin-only regimens may be the preferred EC method. A history of ectopic pregnancy is not a contraindication for EC use. However, these patients require more careful follow-up because they are at risk for repeat ectopic pregnancies. All EC patients require follow-up for several reasons, including determination of the success of the EC and provision of additional education about other contraceptive methods [74].

Pregnancy

The main clinical issues confronting HIV-infected adolescent girls regarding pregnancy are the possibility of transmitting the virus to their child or to their uninfected sexual partner, and the potential impact of a pregnancy on disease progression. Rates of MTCT have decreased substantially with the use of antiretroviral drugs, cesarean section before labor and before ruptured membranes, and avoidance of breastfeeding (see Chapter 4). Current evidence suggests that pregnancy does not exacerbate the progression of the HIV infection [87]. Many pregnant young women appear to be more conscientious in adhering to HIV treatment regimens than they had been before becoming pregnant, suggesting that pregnancy may indirectly improve their clinical status [87].

The subject of future pregnancy and childbearing should be discussed proactively with any HIV-infected adolescent. HIV-infected adolescent girls may be anxious to have a baby after learning their diagnosis, believing themselves to be under a death warrant and therefore having limited time for motherhood, or believing that it would be much better for them to have a baby sooner rather than later when their disease may be more serious. Family and friends and healthcare professionals may project the opposite attitudes, that HIV infection should preclude pregnancy and childbearing. A major goal of any comprehensive program for HIV-infected adolescents and young adults is to encourage and facilitate their living normal lives. More than other teens, adolescents with HIV infection need to be encouraged to envision and plan for a future, since many assume they have no future. Adolescents with HIV infection should be encouraged to work together with their clinician if they do intend to become pregnant, or if they experience an unplanned pregnancy, so as to optimize the likelihood of the best possible outcomes for themselves and for their children [76].

Pregnant HIV-infected adolescents should be counseled about all of their options regarding pregnancy and child bearing. Providers can help the adolescent to identify individuals who can be truly supportive in helping her to make a decision and understand the implications of her decision for her and her family [88]. It is important to avoid assumptions about the supportiveness of family members, friends, and partners, especially if the girl is contemplating an abortion, and in some cases when she is planning to continue the pregnancy and raise her child. The adolescent should be referred to appropriate counseling and social service facilities.

Sexually transmitted infections (STIs)

Adolescents with HIV, particularly those who acquired HIV sexually, are at increased risk of acquiring other STIs. HIV-infected adolescent girls have high rates of STIs [89]. HIV-infected girls also have high HPV infection rates (77.4%) [90]. STIs characterized by inflammation, such as gonorrhea and chlamydia, can increase vulnerability to HIV infection from sexual activity with an HIV-infected partner [91–93]. The increased vulnerability to HIV infection caused by inflammatory STIs is also an important issue for adolescents who are already HIV-infected, as they can become super-infected with additional HIV strains, some of which may be resistant to various antiretroviral drugs, seriously complicating effective management of the HIV infection [94].

Among HIV-infected youth, STIs can be particularly problematic. Adolescent girls have the highest age-specific rates of complications of STIs; immunosuppression due to HIV dramatically increases the severity of these complications [91,92, 95,96). PID is likely to be more difficult to diagnose and treat in HIV-infected young women [97]. HPV infections among HIV-infected young women (even those not severely immunosuppressed) are more likely to involve strains associated with dysplasia and cervical cancer than those occurring among young women without HIV infection [90,98]. Not only does the HIV infection affect the body's response to STIs, but STIs and other infections are associated with increases in viral loads and with decreases in CD4+ lymphocyte counts as the already challenged immune system confronts additional pathogens.

The health education about their condition, which should be an integral component of primary and HIV care for any HIV-infected adolescent, should include a candid discussion about the serious implications of STIs to their health and to effective management of their HIV infection. Screening for STIs should be included in routine quarterly examinations of HIV-infected youth, and the youths should also be encouraged to call for appointments at the first sign of an STI, rather than waiting in the hopes that it will improve on its own [99, 100].

Vulvovaginitis

Vulvovaginitis, inflammation of the vulva and vagina characterized by symptoms such as vaginal discharge, odor, irritation, vulvar or vaginal itching, burning, and dyspareunia, is frequently caused by infection. The primary infectious causes of vulvovaginitis in adolescent girls are bacterial vaginosis (BV), vulvovaginal candidiasis (VVC), and trichomoniasis. Given the significant differences in pH, leukocyte count on wet mount (a microscopic examination of a vaginal smear after the addition of one to two drops of normal saline to the specimen), and Gram stain appearance, these three common infections are easy to distinguish and differentiate [99,101]. Other, non-infectious causes of vulvovaginitis include: physiologic causes such as menses, ovulation, hypoestrogenism, physiologic leukorrhea; foreign bodies; cervicitis [99, 102,103]; hypersensitivity, irritant, or allergic vulvovaginitis, including cases resulting from intravaginal medications or personal hygiene products or cases representing latex condom allergy; idiopathic focal vulvovestibulitis; and cytolytic vaginosis [101].

Bacterial vaginosis (BV)

Vulvovaginitis due to BV is common, resulting from overgrowth of bacteria (a mixed flora consisting of *Mycoplasma hominis*, *Bacteroides* sp., *Gardnerella* sp.) replacing the normal vaginal flora (*Lactobacillus*). The prevalence of BV varies by population, ranging from 10%–31% in sexually inexperienced adolescents in the USA [101]. BV has been associated with a variety of gynecologic and obstetric complications, including PID, prolonged rupture of membranes, preterm birth, low birthweight, and postpartum endometritis. In longitudinal studies using clinical criteria, women with HIV infection were more likely than uninfected women to have persistent BV, and those with greater immunosuppression (CD4+ cell counts less than 200 cells/mm^3) were more likely to have persistent and severe BV infections [104,105]. Because HIV infection may predispose these patients to more severe BV infections, perhaps leading to PID, and because the risk of HIV transmission may be greater among women with BV, clinicians should consider treating asymptomatic BV in HIV-infected adolescent girls [101].

The clinical and laboratory characteristics associated with BV are shown in Table 8.7. When symptomatic, the primary symptom is malodorous vaginal discharge (non-viscous homogeneous, white, uniformly adherent) with an amine odor that is more noticeable after menses or intercourse. Pruritus and irritation also are present in 67% of the cases [101]. BV can be diagnosed clinically based on three of the four Amsel's criteria [106,107] (Table 8.7). Cultures for *Gardnerella* or *Mycoplasma* sp. have little use in the diagnosis of BV and more expensive tests are not necessary [99]. As some patients

Table 8.7. Vulvovaginitis: clinical and laboratory characteristics, treatment

	Normal	Bacterial vaginosis (BV)	Vulvovaginal candidiasis (VVC)	*Trichomonas vaginalis* infection (trichomoniasis)
Etiology		Bacterial overgrowth with organisms such as *Mycoplasma hominis*, *Bacteroides* sp., *Gardnerella* sp.	80% *C. albicans*, 20% other *Candida* sp.	Flagellated anaerobic protozoa
Symptoms		Odor, discharge, pruritus (50% asymptomatic)	Pruritus, discomfort, dysuria, thick discharge, soreness	Pruritus, discharge (50% asymptomatic)
Discharge	Clear to white	Homogeneous, adherent, thin, milky white; malodorous ('fishy' odor)	Thick, clumpy, white, "cottage cheese"	Frothy, gray or yellow–green; malodorous
Physical examination findings		more vaginal mucosal inflammation	Inflammation and erythema. more vaginal mucosal inflammation	Cervical petechiae ("strawberry cervix") in 5–10% of cases; can cause cervical inflammation
Vaginal pH	3.8–4.2	>4.5 very sensitive but not specific	≤4.5	>4.5
KOH "whiff" test	Negative	Positive	Negative	Often positive
	Lactobacilli	Clue cells; no/few WBCs	Few WBCs, pseudohyphae or budding cells	Motile flagellated protozoa; many WBCs; Sensitivity 60%
Diagnostic criteria		**Amsel criteria (three of four)** 1. White adherent discharge 2. pH > 4.5 3. Fishy odor; positive KOH whiff 4. >20% clue cells on microscopy	See text	See text

| **Treatment strategies** | Metronidazole 500 mg PO BID × 7 d, or 2 g PO in single dose, or 0.75%, 5 g InV BID × 5 d, or Clindamycin 2% Cream 5 g InV QHS × 7 d, or 300 mg PO BID × 7 d. *If pregnant: No creams or gels Can use oral medications.* | Treatment of *Candida* vaginitis requires individualization. A new classification of VVC into uncomplicated and complicated vaginitis has simplified choice and duration of antifungal therapy. Uncomplicated VVC due to *C. albicans*: Oral agent: Fluconazole 150mg PO in single dose (For severe *Candida* vaginitis: two sequential 150-mg doses of fluconazole given 3 days apart). Topical agents: Miconazole 2% cream 5 g InV for 7 days 200 mg InV (suppository) for 3 days 100 mg InV (suppository) for 7 days. Other available agents include butoconazole, clotrimazole, tioconazole, and terconazole | Metronidazole 2 g PO in single dose, or 500 mg PO BID × 7 d, or 250 mg PO TID × 7 d, or clindamycin 300 mg PO BID × 7 d. *If pregnant, use 2 grams PO in single dose —* |

InV = Intravaginal; PO = oral. Adapted from [99, 103].

with BV are asymptomatic, screening using pH strips, wet mount and KOH should be performed routinely in HIV-infected adolescent girls.

Suggested treatment regimens for BV are shown in Table 8.7. Acceptable treatment options include metronidazole or clindamycin [99,101]. Because of the interaction between metronidazole and alcohol, adolescents needing treatment for BV should be screened for alcohol abuse, and those who are unlikely to be able to abstain from alcohol as needed should be treated with an alternative treatment, e.g., clindamycin. High rates of recurrence after treatment have been reported [108,109]. Preventive interventions include abstinence and avoidance of douching and/or the use of intravaginal soaps. Routine treatment of sex partners is not recommended [99].

Vulvovaginal candidiasis (VVC)

VVC, one of the most common infections of the female genital tract, is most commonly caused by *Candida albicans*. Although uncommon before age 17 years, the incidence of VVC increases rapidly with age thereafter; by age 25 years, 55% of women have been diagnosed with VVC [110]. Factors that increase the risk of VVC include pregnancy, contraceptive use, diabetes, antibiotics (such as tetracycline, ampicillin, and oral cephalosporins), and sexual activity including receptive oral sex [110]. *Candida* vaginitis infection rates in HIV-infected women are unknown, and reports of refractory fungal vaginitis have not been substantiated [111]. HIV-infected women appear more likely to have non-*C. albicans* isolates than women without HIV infection. In one study, oral and vaginal isolates were recovered prospectively over a period of 2 years. Among those with *C. albicans* isolates, resistance of the isolate to antifungal agents (such as fluconazole) was rare. In contrast, non-*C. albicans* isolates frequently had reduced susceptibility to fluconazole, and subjects with non-*C. albicans* isolates had more infections. The non-*C. albicans* species most closely associated with the development of fluconazole resistance were *C. glabrata* and *C. tropicalis* [112].

The clinical and laboratory characteristics associated with VVC are shown in Table 8.7. VVC symptoms include vulvar/vaginal pruritus, soreness or discomfort, dysuria, and thick discharge. The thick vaginal discharge is clumpy, white, and resembles "cottage cheese." Examination frequently reveals vulvar and/or vaginal inflammation and erythema. The diagnosis of VVC requires the combination of clinical and laboratory (microscopy, culture) findings. Patients with vaginitis symptoms can be diagnosed with VVC by examining the vaginal secretions under the microscope. A wet mount or saline preparation should show yeast cells and mycelia and few WBCs. If large numbers of WBCs are present along with yeast cells and mycelia, there is likely a mixed infection. Patients with signs and symptoms of VVC and negative microscopy should have a vaginal culture. Although vaginal cultures are the most sensitive for detecting *Candida* organisms, a positive test does not indicate that yeast is responsible for the vaginal symptoms since *Candida* organisms are isolated from the lower genital tract of an estimated 20% of asymptomatic healthy women. Among women with symptoms of VVC, 29.8% had yeast isolated, confirming the diagnosis of VVC [110]. Patients are treated when there is clinical evidence of yeast infection, or when the wet mount test with saline shows budding yeast with pseudohyphae. Culture is expensive and time consuming. The culture may be useful in the individual with recurrent symptoms consistent with *Candida* vulvovaginitis but negative results from KOH preparation.

Treatment options for VVC are listed in Table 8.7. An estimated 5% of women experience complicated VVC, defined as recurrent VVC (more than four episodes per year), VVC with severe symptomatology, or VVC caused by non-*C. albicans* isolates. This diagnosis should be confirmed by cultures before therapy is instituted. Vaginitis due to *C. albicans* responds well to available therapy. In contrast, vaginitis due to *C. glabrata* is associated with a high treatment failure rate [112] and requires a longer duration of therapy (i.e., 10–14 days) with either topical or oral azoles [99,113]. The management of recurrent VVC requires an induction course of either oral or vaginal antimycotic therapy, which must be continued daily until the patient is completely asymptomatic or the culture becomes negative. Failure to initiate a maintenance regimen will result in a clinical relapse of VVC in 50% of cases. Maintenance suppressive therapy with ketoconazole, fluconazole, or clotrimazole are effective. The treatment of sexual partners adds no benefit. The role of yogurt in preventing VVC remains unproven.

Trichomoniasis

T. vaginalis infection has been reported in 12.6% of HIV-infected adolescents and in 3.4% of HIV-uninfected adolescents [110]. Sexual activity is the most common predisposing factor for trichomoniasis. An increased risk of this infection is described in women with multiple sexual partners, poor personal hygiene, and low socioeconomic status.

The clinical and laboratory characteristics associated with trichomoniasis are delineated in Table 8.7. The symptoms of *T. vaginalis* infection include vaginal pruritus and a frothy, malodorous, and gray or yellow–green colored discharge. In HIV-infected women, *T. vaginalis* also can infect Skene's ducts, Bartholin's glands and the urethra, where organisms may not be susceptible to topical therapy [114]. The clinical manifestations of vaginal trichomoniasis vary from asymptomatic carriage to severe vaginitis. This range of clinic symptoms is influenced by host factors, which vary during the course of the menstrual cycle and may influence the expression of T. *vaginalis* virulence. The proportion of women who are symptomatic ranges from 20%–50% [115]. Physical examination may demonstrate cervical petechiae ("strawberry cervix") in 5%–10% of cases, and the cervix, urethra, and bladder can be inflamed. Definitive diagnosis of *T. vaginalis* infection requires microscopic and/or laboratory examination, since other pathogens cause similar symptoms. In addition, women with trichomoniasis are more likely to be colonized by *Gardnerella vaginalis* and with other organisms such as *Bacteriodes* sp. (90%), *Ureaplasma urealyticum* and/or *Mycoplasma hominis* (over 90%), *N. gonorrhoeae* (30%), yeast (20%), and *C. trachomatis* (15%). Culture has greater diagnostic sensitivity than wet mount and DNA probe. A special "Trich pouch" has been developed to facilitate culturing and isolating *T. vaginalis* in the clinic setting.

However, clinicians must still be proficient at microscopic examination. Although *T. vaginalis* may be identified on Pap smear, Pap smears have low levels of sensitivity and specificity for *T. vaginalis* and should not be relied on for diagnosis [115]. *T. vaginalis* infection of the lower genital tract is associated with a significantly higher risk of PID. If *T. vaginalis* infection is present, the risk of PID is significantly higher among HIV-infected compared with uninfected patients [116].

Treatment regimens for trichomoniasis are shown in Table 8.7 [99]. Treatment generally involves one of two agents: metronidazole or clindamycin. These agents should not be used together because of possible toxicities. Metronidazole is the treatment of choice for both men and women. If the patient is pregnant, the recommended treatment is a single 2-gram oral dose of metronidazole. This treatment is highly effective, with cure rates ranging from 82%–88%. Simultaneous therapy for sexual partners increases the cure rate to 95% or more with single dose treatment. Infected women should avoid sexual intercourse until they are cured. Because *T. vaginalis* often infects the urethra and periurethral glands, systemic therapy is superior to topical regimen.

Metronidazole can produce malaise, nausea, and occasionally vomiting; the nausea and vomiting may be particularly problematic with the 2-g dose. However, for those who can tolerate the one-time larger dose, malaise tends to disappear quickly, whereas those taking smaller doses for a week may feel varying degrees of malaise during the entire time, a factor likely to interfere with compliance. Since metronidazole can produce nausea, flushing, headaches, and seizures in individuals who consume alcohol while taking the medication, women given the single dose therapy should be alcohol free for 72 hours afterwards. Those taking the 7-day regimens must be prepared to abstain from alcohol for the entire period and through 72 hours after the last dose [99].

If treatment failure occurs, the patient should be retreated with the same agent and an extra effort should be made to ensure treatment of sex partner(s). If the sexual partner(s) are treated and intercourse has been halted, then oral metronidazole 2 g QD for 3 to 5 days should be considered for patients experiencing previous treatment failure. Metronidazole resistance is rare. HIV-infected individuals with trichomoniasis are treated in the same manner as HIV-uninfected patients [115].

Cervicitis

There are two main types of cervicitis: endocervicitis, also called mucopurulent cervicitis (owing to characteristic yellowish mucopurulent exudates from the endocervix), and ectocervicitis, characterized by inflammation of the outside of the cervix. Ectocervicitis is usually caused by infections with *T. vaginalis* or *Candida* species. Among adolescent girls, ectocervicitis may be easily confused during a gynecologic speculum examination with cervical ectopy [99]; the brighter red color of the columnar epithelium can easily be mistaken for inflammation. Mucopurulent cervicitis, common in sexually active women and adolescent girls, is usually caused by sexually transmitted pathogens, including *C. trachomatis* and *N. gonorrhoeae*. Sexual activity is the main risk factor for cervicitis. Symptomatic infection is common. Other pathogens causing cervicitis include *T. vaginalis, Candida* species, and HSV.

The clinical and laboratory characteristics of mucopurulent cervicitis are delineated in Table 8.8. A presumptive diagnosis of chlamydial or gonorrheal endocervicitis may be made based on the presence of mucopurulent endocervical discharge, cervical friability, and more than 15 WBCs per high-power field seen on either wet mount or Gram stain of endocervical specimens. The diagnosis is definitive if a culture, direct fluorescent antibodies (DFA), DNA probe, or nucleic acid amplification test (NAAT) shows positive results for *C. trachomatis* and/or *N. gonorrhoeae*. The latter two are the most sensitive diagnostic tests currently available to detect both pathogens. Ectocervicitis is usually associated with vaginitis and the diagnosis is often made with the identification of *T. vaginalis* and *Candida* species on wet mount. HSV infection is highly correlated with cervical ulcers or necrotic lesions, whereas *T. vaginalis* is correlated with colpitis macularis or "strawberry cervix". A positive cervical culture for HSV confirms the diagnosis of HSV cervicitis and viral isolation permits the differentiation between HSV-1 and HSV-2, which has prognostic importance, since HSV-1 is less likely than HSV-2 to produce recurrent episodes [101].

Treatment options for mucopurulent cervicitis due to *C. trachomatis* or *N. gonorrhoeae* are shown in Table 8.8 [99]. If a symptomatic adolescent is an unreliable historian or resides in an area of high prevalence for both *C. trachomatis* and *N. gonorrhoeae*, she should be treated presumptively for both organisms. HIV-infected girls should receive the same treatment as HIV-uninfected girls. It is important that any male sex partner during the 60 days preceding the cervicitis diagnosis be referred for evaluation and treatment. Patients and their partners should refrain from sexual intercourse until their infections have been cured. Treatment of gynecologic infections with HSV, *Candida* sp., and *T. vaginalis* are addressed elsewhere in this chapter.

When considering prevention of cervicitis, it is important to note that nonoxynol-9 (N-9) has no antimicrobial effects against pathogens such as *N. gonorrhoeae* or *C. trachomatis* causing common STIs. Importantly, the repeated use of this spermicide increases the likelihood of HIV infection [117].

Pelvic inflammatory disease (PID)

PID represents an acute clinical syndrome resulting from ascending spread of microorganisms from the vagina or cervix to the endometrium, fallopian tubes, ovaries, and contiguous structures. PID is the most common serious complication of STIs, with its long-term sequelae including ectopic pregnancy, chronic pelvic pain, and tubal infertility [118]. Sexually active adolescents are more vulnerable to PID than older women, with sexually active 15-year-old girls estimated to have ten times the risk of developing PID in a given year than 24-year-old women in the USA [119, 120]. Women with STIs (especially infections due to *N. gonorrheae, C. trachomatis*, and BV) are at greater risk of developing PID; having had a previous PID infection increases the risk of another episode. The more sexual partners an adolescent has, the greater her risk of developing

Table 8.8. Mucopurulent cervicitis: clinical and laboratory characteristics, treatment

	Mucopurulent cervicitis	*Chlamydia trachomatis*	*Neisseria gonorrhoeae*
Etiology	C. trachomatis, N. gonorrhoeae		
Signs symptoms	Women may be symptomatic or asymptomatic	Women may be symptomatic or asymptomatic	Abnormal vaginal discharge, spotting, abnormal menses, dysuria
	Yellow mucopurulent endocervical exudates	Dysuria, yellow mucopurulent vaginal discharge	Women may be asymptomatic
			Anorectal and pharyngeal infections are common and may or may not be symptomatic
Discharge	1. Yellow, mucopurulent endocervical exudate on white cotton-tipped swab 2. Presence of increased number of polymorphonuclear leukocytes on Gram stain specimen has low predictive value	Presence of yellow, mucopurulent endocervical exudate on white cotton-tipped swab	Gram stain is not sensitive and should be confirmed by culture, DNA probe, or NAAT; Mucopurulent discharge
Diagnosis	Positive *Chlamydia* (culture, DFA, DNA probe, or NAAT) or *Gonorrhea* (culture, DNA probe, or NAAT) test results	Positive *Chlamydia* (culture, DFA, DNA probe, or NAAT)	Growth on selective medium demonstrating typical colonial morphology, positive oxidase reaction, and typical Gram stain morphology
Treatment	Based on testing results. If patient is unreliable or in a high prevalence area, treat presumptively covering for both organisms.	Azithromycin 1 gram PO in a single dose, or Doxycycline 100 mg PO BID for 7 days, or	Cefixime 400 mg PO in a single dose, or Ceftriaxone 125 mg IM in a single dose, or

Table 8.8. (*cont.*)

	If pregnant: avoid tetracycline and quinolones	Erythromycin base 500 mg PO QID for 7 days *If pregnant*: Azithromycin 1 gm PO × Amoxicillin 500ng PO TID for 7 days, or Erythromycin base 500 mg PO QID for 7 days	Ciprofloxacin 500 mg PO in a single dose, or Ofloxacin 400 mg PO in a single dose *If pregnant*: avoid quinolones
Complications	Untreated infections may ascend causing endometritis, salpingitis, and subsequent infertility		10–20% of women develop PID if untreated
Follow-up	As appropriate	No need for retesting after therapy completion unless symptoms persist or reinfection is suspected. Rescreening is recommended in 3–4 months since reinfection is common, especially in adolescents.	No need for retesting after therapy for patients with uncomplicated gonorrhea. Treatment failure most likely due to reinfection.
Partner treatment	Sex partners should be referred for evaluation and treatment. Referral of partners within the last 60 days is recommended. Sexual intercourse should be avoided until patient and partners are cured.	Same	Same

DFA = direct immunofolurescence assay; NAAT = nucleic acid amplification test. Adapted from [99, 101].

PID. Smoking, alcohol use, and use of other drugs also have been identified as risk factors. More frequent douching is associated with PID. Douching also may relieve discharge caused by an infection, leading the woman to delay seeking health care [119].

PID may have a more complicated course in HIV-infected women [121]. HIV-infected women with PID appear to be more likely than women without HIV infection to present with sonographically diagnosed adnexal masses (tubo-ovarian abscesses) [121], to require hospitalization, and to require surgery for PID [97,99,122]. In general, HIV-infected women with acute salpingitis respond well to appropriate antibiotic therapy [123,124], although duration of hospitalization tends to be longer among women with CD4 percentages of <14% [124]. General immune suppression may contribute to the altered pathogenesis of PID in HIV-infected women, but there also appear to be some specific, local, genital tract defects in host defenses in HIV-infected women that predispose them to more serious PID.

The etiology of PID is usually polymicrobial (both aerobic and anaerobic). The most common organisms detected in cultures of cervical secretions include *C. trachomatis*, *N. gonorrhoeae*, and genital *Mycoplasma* species. Although the prevalence of *C. trachomatis* and *N. gonorrhoeae* is similar between HIV-infected and uninfected women with PID, *Mycoplasma* organisms and streptococci have been isolated more commonly from HIV-infected women with PID than from HIV-uninfected women [121]. In the most serious cases, *N. gonorrhoeae* and *C. trachomatis* have been isolated from the upper genital tract in less than one-third of women with PID undergoing laparotomy. Other microorganisms causing PID include anaerobic bacteria (e.g., *Peptococcus, Peptostreptococcus, Bacterioides*, and *Provetella* species)and facultative aerobes (e.g., *Escherichia coli*, group B streptococcus, *Gardnerella vaginalis*, and *Haemophilus influenzae*). As discussed earlier, trichomoniasis has also been associated with PID. Women with PID due to gonorrhea usually present with acute (less than three days) and severe symptoms, leading to rapid diagnosis. In contrast, women with PID due to *C. trachomatis* may be asymptomatic or have only mild symptoms, resulting in a longer period of time until diagnosis, usually more than one week [119].

Diagnostic criteria for PID include: (i) uterine or adnexal tenderness or cervical motion tenderness (CMT); (ii) an oral temperature greater than 38.3 °C (101 °F); (iii) mucopurulent cervical or vaginal discharge; (iv) WBCs on wet mount preparations of vaginal secretions; (v) elevated erythrocyte sedimentation rate (ESR) or C-reactive protein (CRP) levels; and (vi) positive test results for chlamydial and gonorrheal infection [119]. If the cervical discharge appears normal and there are no WBCs noted on wet mount, the diagnosis of PID is unlikely and alternative causes of pain should be considered and investigated. Elevated levels of CRP are a more sensitive and specific predictor than an elevated ESR [118,119].

Additional procedures are required for a definitive diagnosis: ultrasound to view the pelvic area to determine whether the fallopian tubes are enlarged or whether there is an abscess, laparoscopy to allow for visual inspection and to collect specimens for cultures and pathology, laparotomy when scarring or abnormal conditions make laparoscopy technically difficult, and endometrial biopsy to document endometritis. Definitive criteria include: (i) histopathologic evidence of endometritis on endometrial biopsy; (ii) thickened fluid-filled fallopian tubes with or without free pelvic fluid or a TOA on ultrasound or other radiologic tests; and (iii) laparoscopic abnormalities consistent with PID. Sonography is indicated in patients in whom a TOA is suspected. Patients with a palpable adnexal mass or persistent fever should be evaluated for TOA. Many adolescents with PID have unrecognized TOAs [99,102–103,125–127]. Indications for hospitalization include: (i) the inability to exclude surgical emergencies (e.g., appendicitis, ectopic pregnancy); (ii) TOA; (iii) pregnancy; (iv) immunosuppression; (v) inability to follow or tolerate outpatient oral antibiotic therapy; (vi) failure to respond clinically to oral antibiotic therapy; and (vii) severe illness including severe nausea and vomiting or high fever.

Treatment regimens for PID are shown in Table 8.9. Inadequate treatment of PID in adolescents may lead to serious complications, long-term sequelae, or recurrent infections. HIV-infected adolescents who are not significantly immunocompromised and who are clinically stable may be treated as outpatients, but the clinician should have a low threshold for hospitalization if the patient's condition fails to improve or if the patient does not adhere to the prescribed outpatient therapy [97,99,118].

HPV infection

HPV infection is the most prevalent STI in the USA. HPV causes external genital warts, cervical intraepithelial and invasive neoplasia, low- and high-grade squamous intraepithelial lesions (SILs), and genital squamous cell cancers. Numerous HPV subtypes have been described and are categorized into low-risk (types 6, 11, 42, 43, and 44) or high-risk (types 16, 18, 31, 33 and 35) types depending on their oncogenic potential.

The prevalence of HPV infection among sexually active adolescent girl ranges from 20–83% [128]. HIV-infected women have a higher prevalence of HPV infections [129–132] than uninfected women. HPV infections among HIV-infected women and adolescent girls differ from those of uninfected women in several ways: they persist for a longer period of time [131,133]; they are more likely to involve multiple HPV subtypes [134]; and they are more likely to include oncogenic subtypes, particularly subtypes 16 and 18 [129,135].

HIV, HPV and cervical dysplasia

Several varieties of abnormal cervical cytologies are associated with HPV infection, especially in the presence of HIV infection. The risk for the development of SILs among women with HPV is most closely associated with infection by high- and intermediate-risk HPV types. In contrast to dysplasias among women, associated with CD4 levels and viral loads indicative of advanced HIV disease [136–138], the degree of immune suppression is not highly predictive of SIL. HIV-infected and high-risk HIV-uninfected adolescent girls have comparable rates of HPV infection and SILs. However, among HIV-infected adolescent girls, increasing severity of HPV infection, evidenced by dysplasia,

Table 8.9. Treatment regimens for pelvic inflammatory disease (PID)

Inpatient therapy

Parenteral regimen A	• **Cefotetan** 2 g IV every 12 hours, or • **Cefoxitin** 2 g IV every 6 hours, PLUS **doxycycline** 100 mg PO or IV every 12 hours
Parenteral regimen B	• **Clindamycin** 900 mg IV every 8 hours, PLUS **gentamicin** loading dose IV or IM (2 mg/kg), followed by maintenance dose (1.5 mg/kg) every 8 hours
Alternative regimens	• **Oflaxacin** 400 mg IV every 12 hours, or • **Levofloxacin** 500 mg IV QD with or without **metronidazole** 500 mg IV every 8 hours, or • **Ampicillin/sulfbactam** 3 g IV every 6 hours, PLUS **doxycycline** 100mg PO or IV every 12 hours
Comments	Both parenteral regimens (A and B) offer excellent coverage for polymicrobial infections, with Regimen B more appropriate when anaerobic coverage is desired. Parenteral therapy may be discontinued 24 hours after patient's condition improves clinically. Oral therapy with doxycycline should continue until completion of 14-day course. When TOA is present, anaerobic coverage is better achieved by combining clindamycin or metronidazole with doxycycline

Outpatient therapy

Oral regimen A	• **Oflaxacin** 400 mg PO BID for 14 days, or • **Levofloxacin** 500 mg PO QD, with or without **metronidazole** 500 mg PO BID for 14 days
Oral regimen B	• **Ceftriaxone** 250 mg IM once, or • **Cefoxitin** 2 g IM, plus **probenicid** 1g PO in a single concurrent dose, or • Other parenteral third-generation cephalosporin (ceftizoxime or cefotaxime) PLUS **doxycycline** 100 mg PO BID for 14 days, with or without **metronidazole** 500 mg PO BID for 14 days
Comments	Regimen A covers gonorrhea and chlamydia effectively, but also provides excellent anaerobic coverage. Patients need to return to clinic in 72 hrs to assure improvement has occurred and to assess compliance with therapy.

Sources: [99, 127].

appears to be independent of HIV disease progression. Therefore, in adolescents, it appears that HIV infection may have a synergistic effect on the HPV infection through additional mechanisms not directly linked to low CD4 cell counts, particularly early in the course of HIV infection [90].

HIV-infected women who are highly immunocompromised are more likely to experience progression of their dysplasias than HIV-uninfected women. All HIV-infected women, except those with exceptionally well-controlled disease, are less likely to show regression of dysplasia than uninfected women [137].

Uncomplicated HPV infections
External genital warts (EGW) or condylomata are the most common manifestation of HPV in the vulvar area and are often caused by HPV types 6, 11, and 42–44. These lesions usually manifest as hyperkeratotic or warty type lesions in the vulva and peri-anal areas, and can easily be detected after the application of 5% acetic acid to the area. After this application, the cells undergo dehydration and this produces the characteristic "acetowhite" changes. Although rare, both vulvar SIL and cancers can occur and can present as hyperpigmented raised lesions in the vulva. This is of particular importance in patients with HIV infection. The treatment of EGW includes application of trichloroacetic acid (TCA) directly into the lesion as first line therapy. Podophylin is a potent antimitotic agent but TCA seems to work better on keratotic lesions. Self-applied therapy also should be offered to patients. They include imidazoquinolone compounds such as imiquimod (5% cream, single dose packets). It is applied directly to the lesion at bedtime for up to 16 weeks on a schedule of three alternate days/week. The cream is washed off in six to 10 hours. Unfortunately, these therapies are costly and improvement may not be noted for several weeks [139].

Invasive cervical cancer in HIV disease
In 1993, the case definition of AIDS was expanded by the CDC to include invasive cervical cancer. Although high-grade changes in cervical cytology and progression to invasive disease are still relatively uncommon among HIV-infected women [137], there is some evidence that the invasive cervical cancer rate in HIV-infected women is higher than in uninfected women [140–142]. Invasive cervical cancer is more severe in HIV-infected women; HIV-infected women are more likely than uninfected women to have cervical cancer which presents at a younger age [143], presents at more advanced stages, metastasizes to unusual sites (e.g., psoas muscle, clitoris, meninges), responds poorly to standard therapy, has higher recurrence and death rates, and has shorter intervals to recurrence or death [144, 145].

Papanicolaou (Pap) smear screening and colposcopy
Screening tests include the traditional Pap smear, which has a false negative rate of 10%–25%. Newer Pap smear screening techniques, such as those modified to employ liquid-based media and other modifications to increase sensitivity and decrease inadequate

smears, help to reduce, but not eliminate, false negative results. These modified techniques also offer the opportunity to perform direct testing for both oncogenic and non-oncogenic types of HPV. The reliability of Pap testing to detect cervical abnormalities is significantly increased with regular, periodic screening. Results should be reported according to the Bethesda System [146].

HIV-infected women and sexually active adolescents should have a complete gynecologic evaluation including a Pap smear and pelvic exam as part of an initial evaluation when the diagnosis of HIV infection is first made [99]. A Pap smear should then be obtained twice in the first year after the diagnosis of HIV infection. If Pap results are normal, annual examinations are recommended. Indications for more frequent Pap smears are: (i) a previously abnormal Pap smear; (ii) an HPV infection; (iii) previous treatment of cervical dysplasia; or (iv) more advanced HIV disease including CD4+ cell counts < 200 cells/mm^3. The American College of Obstetricians and Gynecologists (ACOG) recommends Pap smears every three to four months for the first year after treatment of preinvasive cervical lesions, followed by Pap smears every 6 months [147]. The role of anal cytology is currently under study.

Atypical squamous cells of undetermined significance (ASCUS) represent the mildest cytologic abnormality in the Bethesda system. HIV-uninfected patients with an initial report of ASCUS should have a prompt repeat Pap smear. If the repeat Pap smear also shows ASCUS, the patient should be referred for colposcopy. Studies in HIV-infected women with ASCUS have found a higher frequency of underlying dysplasia than in uninfected women [148, 149]. Therefore, in HIV-infected women, colposcopy should be performed with any ASCUS result. Women with a diagnosis of atypical glandular cells of undetermined significance (AGCUS) have a significantly higher risk of underlying pathology than patients with ASCUS. Approximately 17%–34% of patients with AGCUS have associated significant intraepithelial or invasive lesions [150–152]. Colposcopy and endocervical and endometrial sampling is indicated with any AGCUS result.

Recent studies suggest that HIV-infected women are at increased risk for the development of invasive vulvar carcinoma. Women with any degree of vulvar abnormality, except for typical exophytic condylomata acuminata, should be referred for colposcopy and biopsy so that pre-invasive or invasive disease can be ruled out. The studies have not targeted specific adolescent female populations, therefore no conclusive adolescent-specific data can be given [149]. For HIV-infected women, a thorough examination of the entire lower genital tract (vagina, vulva, and perianal region) should be performed whenever colposcopy is done.

Management of cervical lesions

High-grade cervical lesions require treatment with standard excisional or ablative therapy. HIV-infected women are more likely to have recurrent disease after treatment (over 50%) than HIV-uninfected women, and HIV-infected women with immunosuppression are even more likely to have recurrent disease [153, 154]. Cryotherapy leads to the highest rate of recurrences and should be avoided if other treatment methods are available. Topical vaginal 5-fluorouracil 5-FU) cream (2 grams biweekly for 6 months) has been shown to reduce recurrence rates after standard treatment for high-grade cervical dysplasia in HIV-infected women. Disease also has been shown to recur more slowly in HIV-infected women who receive effective antiretroviral therapy [155]. HIV-infected adolescent girls and young women with a history of abnormal Pap smears or a history of cervical dysplasia should continue to be followed closely for evidence of lower genital tract neoplasia, regardless of antiretroviral therapy or stage of HIV disease.

HSV infection

There are two herpes virus subtypes that cause genital infections, HSV-1 and HSV-2. HSV infections are discussed in more detail in Chapter 34. HSV infections are the most prevalent cause of genital ulcers in the United States. Approximately 22% of individuals aged 12 years or older in the USA are infected [156]. The majority of genital herpes lesions (60%–95%) are caused by HSV-2. Transmission of herpes simplex infections likely occurs through close contact with a person who is shedding the virus, e.g., in genital or oral secretions.

For HIV-infected patients, HSV infections can be more frequent, prolonged, and severe, especially with progressive immunosuppression. Lesions also can be atypical in appearance or location. Viral shedding increases in individuals with lower CD4 cell counts [157], in those using oral contraceptives or depot-medroxyprogesterone, and in individuals with severe vitamin A deficiency [158].

The lesions are typically single or multiple vesicles that are painful, that ulcerate and heal without scarring, and that can appear anywhere on the genitalia. As with most other herpes viruses, HSV causes lifelong infection. Following a primary infection, the virus can remain latent within cells. The latent virus can reactivate when the patient experiences certain stimuli or triggering events including stress, worsening immunosuppression, or even hormonal changes. Some women experience periodic recurrences in association with menses. The primary, or initial, infection can produce systemic symptoms such as fever, photophobia, malaise, and headache. However, primary infections can be sub-clinical such that an individual could experience a first, clinically apparent infection when antibodies to HSV are present. The lesions accompanying primary infection can last longer (mean duration, 12 days) than those accompanying reactivated disease, and viral shedding following a primary infection can continue for days to weeks or more. Recurrent episodes, representing reactivated disease, are generally milder and shorter, with a mean duration of four to five days. They can occur at variable frequency and consist of more localized lesions. Viral shedding and sexual transmission can occur during asymptomatic, latent periods. Reactivated disease can sometimes be quite serious, even life-threatening, in patients with severe immunosuppression. The lesions can sometimes have an atypical appearance, particularly in immunosuppressed patients, so the practitioner should be alert to the possibility of HSV disease [157, 158].

Table 8.10. Recommended treatment of herpes simplex virus infections

Drug and dose	
First clinical episode	• **Acyclovir** 400 mg PO tid for 7–10 days, or
	• **Acyclovir** 200 mg PO 5x/day for 7–10 days, or
	• **Famciclovir** 250 mg PO tid for 7–10 days, or
	• **Valacyclovir** 1 g PO bid for 7–10 days
Recurrent episodes	• **Acyclovir** 400 mg PO tid for 5 days, or
	• **Acyclovir** 200 mg PO 5x/day for 5 days, or
	• **Acyclovir** 800 mg PO bid for 5 days, or
	• **Famciclovir** 125 mg PO bid for 5 days, or
	• **Valacyclovir** 500 mg PO bid for 3–5 days, or
	• **Valacyclovir** 1 g PO qd for 5 days
Daily suppressive therapy	• **Acyclovir** 400 mg PO bid, or
	• **Famciclovir** 250 mg PO bid, or
	• **Valacyclovir** 500 mg PO qd, or
	• **Valacyclovir** 1 g PO qd
Severe disease	• **Acyclovir** 5–10 mg/kg body weight IV q 8 hours for 5–7 days or until clinical resolution is achieved
Acyclovir-resistant HSV	• **Foscarnet** 40 mg/kg body weight IV q 8 hours or 60 mg/kg IV every 12 hours for 3 weeks
	• **Cidofovir** 1% gel topical application to lesions q day for 5 consecutive days

Source: [99].

A presumptive diagnosis of HSV infection can be made on the basis of clinical presentation with or without one of the following: direct identification of multinucleated giant cells with intranuclear inclusions on a scraping from a lesion (Tzanck preparation), direct immunofluorescent assay performed on material scraped from lesions, or detection of HSV antigens by monoclonal antibody detection systems. Definitive diagnosis can be made using an HSV tissue culture. Observation of typical HSV morphology with electron microscopy of material scraped from lesions or other clinical specimens can also be used for diagnosis [99].

Treatment of HSV infections is outlined in Table 8.10. Systemic administration of antiviral drugs (acyclovir, valacyclovir, and famciclovir) can be used to treat primary and recurrent infections. For troublesome, recurrent disease, the drugs can be used as daily suppressive therapy. However, these drugs neither eradicate latent virus nor affect the risk, frequency, or severity of recurrences after the drug is discontinued [99]. For severe, clinically apparent infections with HSV (severe infections generally requiring hospitalization, such as disseminated infection, pneumonitis, or hepatitis). If lesions persist or recur in a patient receiving antiviral treatment, HSV resistance should be suspected and a viral isolate obtained for sensitivity testing. Such patients should be managed in consultation with a specialist, and alternate therapy should be administered. The CDC has reported a 6.4% resistance rate to acyclovir among HIV-infected patients, as well as cross-resistance to famciclovir and valacyclovir [159]. Factors associated with acyclovir resistance include low CD4 counts and long-term acyclovir exposure. Most of these isolates are susceptible to other antiviral drugs such as foscarnet or cidofovir. Foscarnet has several potentially serious side effects and should only be used in severe cases in consultation with specialists, and patients should be monitored carefully for signs of toxicity. Topical cidofovir gel 1% is not commercially available and must be compounded at a pharmacy [99].

Because HSV infection can recur more frequently and with greater severity in HIV patients, suppressive therapy may be needed. Daily suppressive therapy reduces recurrence frequency by more than 75% among patients who suffer from frequent HSV episodes (i.e., six or more recurrences per year). Suppressive therapy can reduce but may not eliminate viral shedding. Suppressive therapy is delineated in Table 8.10, as are recommended regimens for episodic (recurrent) HSV infection [99].

Secondary prevention of STIs

HIV-infected adolescents have high STI rates, suggesting that they continue to engage in risky sexual behaviors. HIV-infected adolescent patients should receive careful counseling on a continuing basis aimed at promoting healthy behaviors and at decreasing their risks for further infections. In counseling HIV-infected adolescents, providers should assess their sexual practices, the presence of substance abuse, and their understanding of their HIV disease and other STIs. Patients should be carefully informed of the risks of STIs and of super-infection with HIV [89, 122, 160].

Many adolescents erroneously believe that, if they have unprotected sexual encounters with a steady sexual partner, they are not at risk for acquiring STIs and, consequently, they do not take precautions against acquiring STIs [160–162]. When counseling adolescents, providers should carefully assess their mental health. Substance abuse has been associated with an increased risk of acquiring STIs. Depression and anxiety were associated with frequent alcohol use and with a previous history of unprotected sex [161]. Prevention-oriented interventions aimed at reducing risky behaviors and preventing the development of more significant health, mental health, or substance abuse disorders are needed [160–162].

Appropriate HIV prevention interventions are based on a solid understanding of developmental, societal, cultural, and gender issues affecting each individual. Gender inequality is an important consideration when, in many cases, adolescent girls feel inferior to adolescent boys. Intimate relationships may then result in increased vulnerability to HIV among the adolescent female. Violence and sexual abuse may also prevent girls from expressing their desires to practice preventative behaviors. Many behavioral interventions involve the development of self-efficacy and equipping the young woman with negotiating skills to encourage condom use or to abstain from sexual intercourse. These approaches may not be appropriate in certain cultures where negotiating is unlikely and unacceptable for girls. Therefore, other means of HIV prevention and behavior interventions must be used. The female condom is becoming more popular because it does not necessarily require negotiation by the female [163].

HIV-infected adolescents have limited knowledge of the impact of HIV on their STIs and vice versa [90]. Clear explanation of these interactions as well as prevention messages, early detection, and management of STIs are crucial elements to improve the health of these adolescents. HIV-seropositive adolescents have little understanding of the concept of secondary infection with new HIV strains and the risk of being secondarily infected with drug-resistant strains of HIV [94]. Reducing the risk of transmission of drug-resistant HIV requires careful assessment of the HIV-infected adolescent's sexual practices and health education messages that include discussion about the possibility of acquiring a new, potentially drug-resistant virus.

Care programs for the HIV-infected adolescent

The care of the HIV-infected adolescent requires a skilled team of providers with broad expertise, including clinicians skilled in medical care and psychological care, and social workers, educators, and case managers who can help the patient navigate through many bureaucratic and logistical challenges. Ideally, these providers can offer basic gynecologic care or have links to gynecologic providers who are also versed in the care of adolescents. Practitioners must emphasize health education and the essential messages concerning safer sex. Health educators can help youth overcome the many barriers to practicing safer sex, help improve self-esteem, and emphasize the critical importance of medication adherence. Peer educators can serve to reinforce information provided by the physicians and professional educators, casting the information in terms better understood by the youth. Many other services are often necessary. Mental health care for those youth grappling with depression, substance abuse, or other major mental health disorders is integral to the general care of the adolescent. All too often HIV-infected adolescents are not in school or do not have jobs. Job readiness training can help the youth to achieve their maximum potential in the work place. Finally, outreach to at-risk youth is essential. Youth need to become aware of their personal risk for HIV and must begin to see how early intervention can help to sustain life. Outreach into the community, partnerships with community service agencies, and work with agencies providing adolescent-specific HIV services can help facilitate entry of youth into HIV counseling, testing and care.

Conclusions

Care of the HIV-infected adolescent requires not only experience with HIV infection, but also an understanding of the psychosocial, physical development, and social issues that confront every adolescent. With the help of a dedicated care staff, the adolescent can confront HIV and learn to live with the infection. Through education, support, and understanding, those providing care to the HIV-infected adolescent can help that youth to better care for themself and live a longer and healthier life.

REFERENCES

1. Centers for Disease Control and Prevention. HIV/AIDS Surveillance Report 2001; **13**(2): 1–44.
2. Rotheram-Boris, M. J., Futterman, D. Promoting early detection of HIV infection among adolescents. *Arch. Pediatr. Adolesc. Med.* 2000; **154**:435–439.
3. Rosenberg, P. R., Biggar, R. J., Goedert, J. J. Declining age at HIV infection in the United States. *N. Engl. J. Med.* 1994;**330**:789.
4. Valleroy, L. A., Mackellar, D. A., Karon, J. M. *et al.* HIV prevalence and associated risks in young men who have sex with men. *J. Am. Med. Assoc.* 2000;**284**: 198–204.
5. Sweeney, P., Lindegren, M. L., Buehler, J. W., Onorato, I. M., Janssen, R. S. Teenagers at risk of human immunodeficiency virus type I infection. *Arch. Pediatr. Adolesc. Med.* 1995;**149**:521–528.
6. Slap, G. B. Normal physiological and psychosocial growth in the adolescent. *J. Adolesc. Hlth Care* 1986;**7**:13S–23S.
7. Centers for Disease Control and Prevention. *CDC Surveillance Summaries* 2002;**51**(SS04):1–64.
8. Wilson, C. M., House, J., Partlow, C. *et al.* The REACH (Reaching for Excellence in Adolescent Care and Health) Project: study design, methods, and population profile. *J. Adolesc. Hlth* 2001;**29**(3S):8–18.
9. Troiden, R. R. Homosexual identity development. *J. Adolesc. Hlth Care* 1988;**9**:105–113.
10. D'Angelo, L. J., Getson, P. R., Luban, N. L. C., Gayle, H. D. Human immunodeficiency virus infection in urban adolescents: can we predict who is at risk? *Pediatrics* 1991;**88**:982–986.
11. Lindsay, M. K., Johnson, N., Peterson, H. B., Willis, S., Williams, H., Klein, L. Human immunodeficiency virus infection among inner-city adolescent parturients undergoing routine voluntary screening, July 1987 to March 1991. *Am. J. Obstet. Gynecol.* 1992;**167**(4):1096–1099.
12. Futterman, D. C., Peralta, L., Rudy, B. J. *et al.* The ACCESS (Adolescents Connected to Care, Evaluation, and Special Services) Project: social marketing to promote HIV testing to adolescents, methods and first year results from a six city campaign. *J. Adolesc. Hlth* 2001; **29**(3S):19–29.
13. Kaiser Family Foundation. National Survey of Teens on HIV/AIDS. 2000:1–8.
14. Centers for Disease Control and Prevention. Recommendations for HIV testing services for in-patients and outpatients in acute care hospital settings. *Morb. Mortal. Wkly Rep.* 1993;**42**:1–17.
15. Centers for Disease Control and Prevention. HIV testing among populations at risk for HIV in nine cities: results from the HIV Testing Survey (HITS) 1995–96. *Morbid. Mortal. Wkly Rep.* 1998;**47**: 1086–1091.
16. Clark, L. R., Ginsburg, K. R. How to talk to your teenage patients. *Contemp. Adolesc. Gynecol.* 1995–96;**1**:23–27.

17. Remafedi, G. Adolescent homosexuality: psychosocial and medical implications. *Pediatrics* 1987;**79**:331–337.

18. Ginsburg, K. R., Winn, R. J., Rudy, B. J., Crawford, J., Zhao, H., Schwarz, D. F. How to reach sexual minority youth in the health care setting: The teens offer guidance. *J. Adolesc. Hlth* 2002;**31**:407–416.

19. Strurdevant, M. S., Belzer, M., Weissman, G. *et al.* The relationship of unsafe sexual behavior and the characteristics of sexual partners of HIV infected and HIV uninfected adolescent females. *J. Adolesc. Hlth* 2001;**29**(3S):64–71.

20. Joseph-Di Caprio, J., Remafedi, G. J. Adolescents with factitious HIV disease. *J. Adolesc. Hlth Care* 1997;**21**:102–106.

21. Moscicki, A. B., Houser, J., Ma, Y., Murphy, D., Wilson, C. M. Adolescent males and females with HIV at high risk for anal squamous intraepithelial lesions. *XIII Int. AIDS Conf.* Durban, South Africa, July 9–14, 2000 (abstract number TuOrB305).

22. D'Angelo, L. J., Abdalian, S. E., Sarr, M., Hoffman, N., Belzer, M., and The Adolescent Medicine HIV/AIDS Research Network. Disclosure of serostatus by HIV infected youth: The experience of the REACH Study. *J. Adolesc. Hlth*, 2001;**29**(3S)72–79.

23. Harlan, W. R., Harlan, E. A., Grillo, G. P. Secondary sex characteristics of girls 12 to 17 years of age: The US health examination survey. *J. Pediatr.* 1980;**96**(6):1074–1078.

24. Zacharias, L., Rand, W. M., Wurtman, R. J. A prospective study of sexual development and growth in American girls: the statistics of menarche. *Obstet. Gynecol. Survey* 1976;**31**:325.

25. Sedlmeyer, I. L., Palmert, M. R. Delayed puberty: Analysis of a large case series from an academic center. *J. Clin. Endocrinol. Metab.* 2002;**87**(4):1613–1620.

26. Frisch, R. E., Revelle, R. Menstrual cycles: fatness as a determinant of minimum weight-for-height for their maintenance or onset. *Science* 1974;**185**:949.

27. Albanese, A., Stanhope, R. Investigation of delayed puberty. *Clin. Endocrinol.* 1995;**43**:105–110.

28. Mahoney, C. P. Evaluating the child with short stature. *Pediatr. Clin. North Am.* 1987;**34**:825–849.

29. Oerter, K. E., Uriarte, M. M., Rose, S. R., Barnes, K. M., Cutler, G. B., Jr. Gonadotropin secretory dynamics during puberty in normal girls and boys. *J. Clin Endocrinol. Metab.* 1990;**71**(5):1251–1258.

30. Finkelstein, J. W., Susman, E. J., Chinchilli, V. M. *et al.* Effects of estrogen or testosterone on self-reported sexual responses and behaviors in hypogonadal adolescents. *J. Clin. Endocrinol. Metab.* 1998;**83**(7):2281–2285.

31. Susman, E. J., Finkelstein, J. W., Chinchilli, V. M. *et al.* The effect of sex hormone replacement on behavior problems and moods in adolescents with delayed puberty. *J. Pediatr.* 1998;**133**(4):521–525.

32. Palmert, M. R., Malin, H. V., Boepple, P. A. Unsustained or slowly progressive puberty in young girls: initial presentation and long-term follow-up of 20 untreated patients. *J. Clin. Endocrinol. Metab.* 1999;**84**:415–423.

33. Carpenter, S. *Pediatric and Adolescent Gynecology.* Philadelphia: Lippincott Williams and Wilkins; 2000.

34. Chirgwin, K. D., Feldman, J., Muneyyirci-Delale, O., Landesman, S., Minkoff, H. Menstrual function in human immunodeficiency virus-infected women without acquired immunedeficiency syndome. *Obstet. J. Acquir. Immune Defic. Syndr. Hum. Retrovirol.* 1996;**12**(5):489–494.

35. Pletcher, J. R., Slap, G. B. Menstrual disorders. Amenorrhea. *Pediatr. Clin. North Am.* 1999;**46**(3):505–518.

36. Grinspoon, S., Corcoran, C., Miller, K. *et al.* Body composition and endocrine function in women with acquired immunodeficiency syndrome wasting. *J. Clin. Endocrinol. Metab.* 1997;**82**(5):1332–1337J.

37. Golden, N. H. A review of the female athlete triad (amenorrhea, osteoporosis and disordered eating). *Int. J. Adolesc. Med. Hlth* 2002;**14**(1):9–17.

38. Block, R. L., Farinpour, R., Schlechte, J. A., Effects of chronic marijuana use on testosterone, luteinizing hormone, follicle stimulating hormone, prolactin and cortisol in men and women. *Drug Alcohol Depend.* 1991;**28**(2):121–128.

39. Efstratiades, M., Panitsa-Faflia, C., Batrinos, M. Vaginal cytology in endocrinopathies. *Acta Cytol.* 1983;**27**(4):421–425.

40. Speroff, L., Glass, R. H., Kase, N. G. Anovulation and the polycystic ovary. In *Clinical Gynecology Endocrinology and Infertility*. Philadephia: Lippincott Williams and Wilkins; 1999:487–513.

41. Lobo, R. A., Carmina, E. The importance of diagnosing the polycystic ovary syndrome. *Ann. Intern. Med.* 2000;**132**(12):989–993.

42. Stafford, D. E., Gordon, C. M. Adolescent androgen abnormalities. *Curr. Opin. Obstet. Gynecol.* 2002 Oct:**14**(5):445–451.

43. Balen, A. Pathogenesis of polycystic ovary syndrom – the enigma unravels? *Lancet* 1999;**354**(9183):966–967.

44. McKenna, T. J. Pathogenesis and treatment of polycystic ovary syndrome. *N. Engl. J. Med.* 1988; **318**:558.

45. Avyad, C. K., Holeuwerger, R., Silva, V. C., Bordallo, M. A., Breitenbach, M. M. Menstrual irregularity in the first postmenarchal years: an early clinical sign of polycystic ovary syndrome in adolescence. *Gynecol. Endocrinol.* 2001;**15**(3):170–177.

46. Carmina, E., Wong, L., Chang, L., Paulson, R. J., Sauer, M. V., Stanczyk, F. Z., Lobo, R. A. Endocrine abnormalities in ovulatory women with polycystic ovaries on ultrasound. *Hum. Reprod.* 1997;**12**(5):905–909.

47. Gordon, C. M. Menstrual disorders in adolescents: excess androgens and the polycystic ovary syndrome. *Pediatr. Clin. North Am.* 1999; **46**:519–543.

48. Arslanian, S. A., Lewy, V., Danadian, K., Saad, R. Metformin therapy in obese adolescents with polycystic ovary syndrome and impaired glucose tolerance: amelioration of exaggerated adrenal response to adrenocorticotropin with reduction of insulinemia/insulin resistance. *J. Clin. Endocrinol. Metab.* 2002;**87**(4):1555–1559.

49. Legro, R. S., Detection of insulin resistance and its treatment in adolescents with polycystic ovary syndrome. *J. Pediatr. Endocrinol. Metab.* 2002 Dec;**15** Suppl 5:1367–1378.

50. Bravender, T., Emans, S. J. Menstrual disorders. Dysfunctional uterine bleeding. *Pediatr. Clin. North Am.* 1999;**46**(3):545–553, viii.

51. Munro, M. G. Dysfunctional uterine bleeding: advances in diagnosis and treatment. *Curr. Opin. Obstet. Gynecol.* 2001;**13**(5):475–489.

52. Munro, M. G. Abnormal uterine bleeding in the reproductive years. Part I – pathogenesis and clinical investigation. *J. Am. Assoc. Gynecol. Laparosc.* 1999;**6**(4):393–416.

53. Munro M. G. Abnormal uterine bleeding in the reproductive years. Part II – medical management. *J. Am. Assoc. Gynecol. Laparosc.* 2000;**7**(1):17–35.

54. Kilbourn, C. L., Richards, C. S. Abnormal uterine bleeding. Diagnostic considerations, management options. *Postgrad. Med.* 2001;**109**(1):137–138, 141–4, 147–150.

55. Shah, P. N., Smith, J. R., Well, C., Barton, S. E., Kitchen, V. S., Steer, P. J. Menstrual symptoms in women infected by the human immunodeficiency virous. *Obstet. Gynecol.* 1994;**83**(3):397–400.

56. Dealy, M. F. Dysfunctional uterine bleeding in adolescents. *Nurse Pract.* 1998;**23**(5): 2–3,16,18–20.

57. Minjarez, D. A., Bradshaw, K. D. Abnormal uterine bleeding in adolescents. *Obstet. Gynecol. Clin. North Am.* 2000;**27**(1):63–78.

58. Speroff, L., Glass, R. H., Kase, N. G. Dysfunctional uterine bleeding. In *Clinical Gynecologic Endocrinology and Infertility*. Philadephia: Lippincott Wiliams and Wilkins; 1999: 575–593.

59. Klein J. R., Litt, I. F. Epidemiology of adolescent dysmenorrhea. *Pediatrics* 1981. **68**(5):661–664.

60. Harel, Z. A contemporary approach to dysmenorrhea in adolescents. *Pediatr. Drugs* 2002;**4**(12):797–805.

61. Fedele, L., Bianchi, S., Bocciolone, L., Di Nola, G., Parazzini, F. Pain symptoms associated with endometriosis. *Obstet. Gynecol.* 1992;**79**(5 (Pt 1)):767–769.

62. Hornsby, P. P., Wilcox, A. J., Weinberg, C. R. Cigarette smoking and disturbance of menstrual function. *Epidemiology* 1998;**9**(2):193–198.

63. Hendrix, S. L., Alexander, N. J. Primary dysmenorrhea treatment with a desogestrel-containing low-dose oral contraceptive. *Contraception* 2002;**66**(6):393–399.

64. Chakmakjian Z. H. A critical assessment of therapy for the premenstrual tension syndrome. *J. Reprod. Med.* 1983;**28**(8):532–538.

65. Raja, S. N., Feehan, M., Stanton, W. R., McGee, R. Prevalence and correlates of the premenstrual syndrome in adolescence. *J. Am. Acad. Child Adolesc. Psychiatry* 1992;**31**(5):783–789.

66. Fisher, M., Trieller, K., Napolitano, B. Premenstrual symptoms in adolescents. *J. Adolesc. Hlth Care* 1989;**10**(5):369–375.

67. American Psychiatric Association. *Diagnostic and Statistical Manual of Mental Disorders*, 4th edn. DSM-IV Text Revision. R. R. Washington, DC: American Psychiatric Association, 2000.

68. Steiner, M., Pearlstein, T. Premenstrual dysphoria and the serotonin system: pathophysiology and treatment. *J. Clin. Psychiatry* 2000;**61** Suppl 12:17–21.

69. Freeman, E. W. Premenstrual syndrome: current perspectives on treatment and etiology. *Curr. Opin. Obstet. Gynecol.* 1997;**9**(3):147–153.

70. Wenning J. Premenstrual syndrome. In McAnarney, E., Kreipe, R., Orr, D., Comerci, G. *Textbook of Adolescent Medicine*. Philadelphia, PA: W.B. Saunders Company; 1992: 670–671.

71. Johnson, S. R. Premenstrual syndrome therapy. *Clin. Obstet. Gynecol.* 1998;**41**(2):405–421.

72. Stone, A. Microbicides: a new approach to preventing HIV and other sexually transmitted infections. *Nat. Rev. Drug Discov.* 2002;**1**(12):977–985.

73. Guest, F. Education and Counseling: Factors influencing education and counseling. In Kowal, D., ed. *Contraceptive Technology* 17th edn. New York: Ardent Media Inc; 1998: 249–261.

74. Derman, S., Peralta, L. Postcoital contraception: present and future options. RU486 (Mifepristone) *J. Adolesc. Hlth* 1995;**16**:6–11.

75. Hatcher, R., Trussel, J., Stewart, F. *et al.* In Kowal, D., ed. Contraceptive *Technology* 17th edn. New York: Ardent Media Inc; 1998.

76. Belzer, M., Rogers, A. S., Camarca, M. *et al.* Contraceptive choices in HIV-infected and HIV at-risk adolescent females. *J. Adolesc. Hlth* 2000;**29**S: 93–100.

77. Hatcher, R., Trussel, J., Stewart, F. *et al.* HIV/AIDS and Reproductive Health. In Kowal, D., ed. *Contraceptive Technology* 17th edn. New York: Ardent Media Inc; 1998: 141–178.

78. Sivin, I., Moo-Yong, A. Recent developments in contraceptive implants at the Population Council. *Contraception* 2002;**65**(1):113–119.

79. Smallwood, G. H., Meador, M. L., Lenihan, J. P., Shangold, G. A., Fisher, A. C., Creasy, G. W. Efficacy and safety of a transdermal contraceptive system. *Obstet. Gynecol.* 2001;**98** (5 Pt 1):799–805.

80. Hatcher, R. A., Guillebaud, J. The pill: combined oral contraceptive. In Kowal, D. ed. *Contraceptive Technology*, 17th edn. New York: Ardent Media Inc; 1998: 405–466.

81. Everett, S. A. Warrem, C. W., Santelli, J. S., Kann, L., Collins, J. L., Kolbe, L. J. Use of birth control pills, condoms, and withdrawal among US high school students. *J. Adolesc. Hlth* 2000;**27**(2):12–18.

82. Hatcher, R. A. Depo-Provera, Norplant, and progestin-only pills (minipills). In Kowal, D. ed. *Contraceptive Technology* 17th edn. New York: Ardent Media Inc; 1998, 467–509.

83. Audet, M. C., Moreau, M., Koltun, W. D. *et al.* Evaluation of contraceptive efficacy and cycle control of a transdermal contraceptive patch vs an oral contraceptive: a randomized controlled trial. *J. Am. Med. Assoc.* 2001;**285**(18):2347–2354.

84. Abrams, L. S., Skee, D., Matarajan, J., Wong, F. A. Pharmacokinetic overview of Ortho Evra/Evra. *Fertil. Steril.* 2002;**77**(2 Suppl 2): S3–S12.

85. Johansson, E., Brache, V., Alvarez, F. *et al.* Pharmacokinetic study of different dosing regimes of levonorgestrel for emergency contraception in healthy women. *Hum. Reprod.* 2002;**17**(6):1472–1476.

86. Sivin, I., Mishell, D. R. Jr, Victor, A. *et al.* A multicenter study of levonorgestrel-estradiol contraceptive vaginal rings. II-Subjective and objective measures of effects. An international comparative trial. *Contraception* 1981;**24**(4):359–376.

87. Ahdieh, L. Pregnancy and infection with human immunodeficiency virus. *Clin. Obstet. Gynecol.* 2001;**44**(2):154–166.

88. Levin, L., Henry-Reid, L., Murphy, D. A. *et al.* Adolescent Medicine HIV/AIDS Research Network. Incident pregnancy rates in HIV-infected and HIV uninfected at-risk-adolescents. *J. Adolesc. Hlth* 2001;**29**S:101–108.

89. Vermund, S. H., Wilson, C. M., Rogers, A. S., Partlow, C., Moscicki, A. B. Sexually transmitted infections among HIV-infected and HIV uninfected high-risk youth in the REACH study. *J. Adol. Hlth* 2001;**9**S:49–56.

90. Moscicki, A. B., Ellenberg, J. H., Vermund, S. H. *et al.* Prevalence of and risks for cervical human papillomavirus infection and squamous intraepithelial lesions in adolescent girls: impact of infection with human immunodeficiency virus. *Arch. Pediatr. Adolesc. Med.* 2000;**54**(2):127–134.

91. Wasserheit, J. N. Epidemiological synergy. Inter-relationships between human immunodeficiency virus infection and other sexually transmitted diseases. *Sex. Transm. Dis.* 1992;**19**(2):61–77.

92. Laga, M., Manoka, A., Kivuvu, M. *et al.* Non-ulcerative sexually transmitted diseases as risk factors for HIV transmission in women: results from a cohort study *AIDS* 1993;**7**(1): 95–102.

93. Fleming, D. T., Wasserheit, J. N. From epidemiological synergy to public health policy and practice: The contribution of other sexually transmitted diseases to sexual transmission of HIV infection. *Sex. Transm. Infect.* 1999;**75**(1):3–17.

94. Pilon, R., Sandstrom, P., Burchell, A. *et al.* Transmitted HIV reverse transcriptase inhibitor resistance mutation stability in ART-naive recent seroconverters: results of the polaris HIV seroconversion study. *XIV Int. AIDS Conf.*; 2002 July 9; Barcelona. Abstract TuPeB4611.

95. Robertson, D., McMillan, A., Young, H. *Clinical Practice in Sexually Transmissible Diseases.* 2nd edn. Edinburgh: Churchill Livingstone; 1989.

96. Goldenberg, R. L., Andrews, W. W., Yuan, A. C., MacKay, H. T., St Louis, M. E. Sexually transmitted diseases and adverse outcomes of pregnancy. *Clin. Perinatal.* 1997;**24**(1): 23–41.

97. Korn, A. P. Pelvic inflammatory disease in women infected with HIV. *AIDS Patient Care STDs* 1998;**12**(6):431–434.

98. Moscicki AB, Ma Y, Holland C, Vermund SH. Cervical ectopy in adolescent girls with and without human immunodeficiency virus infection. *J. Infect. Dis.* 2001;**183**(6):865–870.

99. Centers for Disease Control and Prevention. Sexually transmitted diseases treatment guidelines 2002. *Morbid. Mortal. Wkly Rep.* 2002;**51**(R6):1–78.

100. Ahmed, S., Lutalo, T., Wawer, M. *et al.* HIV incidence and sexually transmitted disease prevalence associated with condom use: a population study in Rakai, Uganda. *AIDS* 2001;**15**(16):2171–2179.

101. Holmes, K., Stamm, W. Lower genital tract infection syndromes in women. In Holmes, K., Sparling, F., Lemon, S. *et al.* eds. *Sexually Transmitted Diseases.* 3rd edn. New York: McGraw-Hill; 1999: 766.

102. Neinstein, L. S. ed. *Adolescent Health Care. A Practical Guide.* 4th edn. Lippincott Williams and Wilkins, Philadelphia, PA. 2002.

103. California STD/HIV Prevention Training Center. Core STD Curriculum: Comprehensive Outlines for Clinical STD Management. 1999.

104. Ledru, S., Meda, N., Ledru, E., Bazie, A. J., Chiron, J. P. HIV-1 infection associated with abnormal vaginal flora morphology and bacterial vaginosis. *Lancet* 1997;**350**(9086): 1251–1252.

105. Jamieson, D. J., Duerr, A., Klein, R. S. *et al.* Longitudinal analysis of bacterial vaginosis: findings from the HIV epidemiology research study. *Obstet. Gynecol.* 2001;**98**(4): 656–663.

106. Hillier, S., Holmes, K. K. Bacterial vaginosis. In Holmes, K., Sparling, F., Lemon, S. *et al. Sexually Transmitted Diseases.* 3rd edn. New York: McGraw-Hill; 1999: 563–586.

107. Amsel, R., Totten, P. A., Spiegel, C. A., Chen, K. C., Eschenbach, D., Holmes, K. K. Nonspecific vaginitis: diagnostic criteria and microbial and epidemiologic associations. In Holmes, K., Sparling, F., Lemon, S. *et al.* eds. *Sexually Transmitted Diseases.* 3rd edn. New York: NcGraw-Hill; 1999: 569.

108. Schwebke, J. R. Asymptomatic bacterial vaginosis: response to therapy. *Am. J. Obstet. Gynecol.* 2000;**183**(6):1434–1439.

109. Hay, P. Sr. National guideline for the management of bacterial vaginosis. Clinical Effectiveness Group (Association of Genitourinary Medicine and the Medical Society for the Study of Venereal Diseases). *Sex. Transm. Infect.* 1999;**75** (Suppl 1):S16–S18.

110. Sobel, J. D. Vulvovaginal candidiasis. In Holmes, K., Sparling, F., Lemon, S. *et al.* eds. *Sexually Transmitted Diseases*. 3rd edn., New York: McGraw-Hill;1999:629–639.

111. Sobel, J. D., Ohmit, S. E., Schuman, P. *et al.* The evolution of *Candida* species and fluconazole susceptibility among oral and vaginal isolates recovered from human immunodeficiency virus (HIV)-seropositive and at-risk HIV-seronegative women. *J. Infect. Dis.* 2000;**183**(2):286–293.

112. Sobel, J. D. Treatment of vaginal *Candida* infections. *Expert Opin. Pharmacother.* 2002;**3**(8):1059–1065.

113. Sobel, J. D., Kapernick, P. S., Zervos, M. *et al.* Treatment of complicated Candida vaginitis: comparison of single and sequential doses of fluconazole. *Am. J. Obstet. Gynecol.* 2001;**185**(2):363–369.

114. Jackson, D. J., Rakwar, J. P., Bwayo, J. J., Kreiss, J. K., Moses, S. Urethal *Trichomonas vaginalis* infection and HIV transmission. *Lancet* 1997;**350**(9084):1076.

115. Krieger, J., Alderete, J. *Trichomonas vaginalis* and trichomoniasis. In Holmes, K., Sparling, F., Lemon, S. *et al. Sexually Transmitted Diseases*. 3rd edn, New York: McGraw-Hill; 1999:587–604.

116. Moodley, P., Wilkinson, D., Connolly, C., Moodley, J., Sturm, A. W. *Trichomonas vaginalis* is associated with pelvic inflammatory disease in women infected with human immunodeficiency virus. *Clin. Infect. Dis.* 2002;**34**(4):519–22.

117. Van Damme, L., Ramjee, G., Alary, M. *et al.* COL-1492 study group. Effectiveness of COL-1492, a nonoxynol-9 vaginal gel, on HIV transmission in female sex workers: a randomized controlled trial. *Lancet* 2002; **360**(9338):971–977.

118. Igra, V. Pelvic inflammatory disease in adolescents. *AIDS Patient Care STDs* 1998;**12**(2):109–124.

119. Westrom, L., Eschenbach, D. Pelvic inflammatory disease. In Holmes, K., Sparling, F., Lemon, S. *Sexually Transmitted Diseases*. 3rd edn, New York: McGraw-Hill; 1999: 783–809.

120. HRP Annual Technical Report 1995: Executive Summary. Available at: www.who.int/reproductive-health/publications/HRP–ATRs/1995/execsum.html. Acessed November 11, 2005.

121. Irwin, K. L., Moorman, A. C., O'Sullivan, M. J. *et al.* Influence of human immunodeficiency virus infection on pelvic inflammatory disease. *Obstet. Gynecol.* 2000;**95**(4):525–534.

122. Bersoff-Matcha, S. J., Horgan, M. M., Fraser, V. J., Mundy, L. M., Stoner, B. P. Sexually transmitted disease acquisition among women infected with human immunodeficiency virus type 1. *J. Infect. Dis.* 1998; **78**(4): 1174–1177.

123. Irwin, K. L., Moorman, A. C., O'Sullivan, M. J. *et al.* Influence of human immunodeficiency virus infection on pelvic inflammatory disease. *Obstet. Gynecol.* 2000;**95**(4):525–534.

124. Cohen, C. R., Sinej, S., Reilly, M. *et al.* Effect of human immunodeficiency virus type 1 infection upon acute salpingitis: a laparoscopic study. *J. Infect. Dis.* 1998;**178**(5): 1352–1358.

125. Rice, P. A., Schachter, J. Pathogenesis of pelvic inflammaotory disease: what are the questions? *J. Am. Med. Assoc.* 1991;**266**(18): 2587–2593.

126. Slap, G. B., Forke, C. M., Cnaan, A. *et al.* Recognition of tubo-ovarian abscess in adolescents with pelvic inflammatory disease. *J. Adolesc. Hlth.* 1996;**18**(6):397–403.

127. Walker, C. K., Workowski, K. A., Washington, A. E., Soper, D., Sweet, R. L. Anaerobes in pelvic inflammatory disease: implications for the Centers for Disease Control and Prevention's guidelines for treatment of sexually transmitted diseases. *Clin. Infect. Dis.* 1999;**28**(Suppl 1):S29–S36.

128. Jacobson, D., Mizell, S., Peralta, L. *et al.* Concordance of human papilloma virus in the cervix and urine of adolescents with a high prevalence of HPV. *Pediatr. Infect. Dis. J.* 2000;**19**(8):722–728.

129. Minkoff, H., Feldman, J., DeHovitz, J., Landesman, S., Burk, R. A longitudinal study of human papillomavirus carriage in human immunodeficiency virus-infected and human immunodeficiency virus-uninfected women. *Am. J. Obstet. Gynecol.* 1998;**178**(5):982–986.

130. Palefsky, J. M., Minkoff, H., Kalish, L. A. *et al.* Cervicovaginal human papillomavirus infection in human immunodeficiency virus-1 (HIV)-positive and high-risk HIV-negative women. *J. Natl Cancer Inst.* 1999;**337**(3):22–236.

131. Sun, X. W., Kuhn, L., Ellerbrock, T. V., Chiasson, M. A., Bush, T. J., Wright, T. C. Human papillomavirus infection in women infected with the human immunodeficiency virus. *N. Engl. J. Med.* 1997;**337**(19):1343–1349.

132. Jamieson, D. J., Duerr, A., Burk, R. *et al.* Characterization of genital human papillomavirus infection in women who have or who are at risk of having the HIV infection. *Am. J. Obstet. Gynecol.* 2002;**186**(1):21–27.

133. Ahdieh, L., Munoz, A., Vlahov, D., Trimble, C., Timpson, L., Shah, K. Cervical neoplasia and repeated positivity of human papillomavirus infection in human immunodeficiency virus-seropositive and -seronegative women. *Am. J. Epidemiol.* 2000;**151**(12): 1148–1157.

134. Brown, D. R., Bryan, J. T., Cramer, H., Katz, B. P., Handy, V., Fife, K. H. Detection of multiple human papillomavirus types in condylomata acuminata from immunosuppressed patients. *J. Infect. Dis.* 1994;**70**:759–765.

135. Uberti-Foppa, C., Origoni, M., Maillard, M. *et al.* Evaluation of the detection of human papillomavirus genotypes in cervical specimens by hybrid capture as screening for precancerous lesions in HIV-infected women. *J. Med. Virol.* 1998;**56**:133–137.

136. Garzetti, G. G., Ciavattini, A., Butini, L., Vecchi, A., Montroni, M. Cervical dysplasia in HIV-seropositive women: role of human papillomavirus infection and immune status. *Gynecol. Obstet. Invest.* 1995;**40**(1):52–56.

137. Massad, L. S., Riester, K. A., Anastos, K. M. *et al.* Prevalence and predictors of squamous cell abnormalities in Papanicolaou smears from women infected with HIV. Women's Interagency HIV Study Group. *J. Acquir. Immune Defic. Syndr.* 1999;**21**(1):33–41.

138. Delmas, M. C., Larsen, C., van Benthem, B. *et al.* Cervical squamous intraepithelial lesions in HIV-infected women: prevalence, incidence, and regression. *AIDS* 2000;**14**(12):1775–1784.

139. Kiviat, N., Kovtsky, L. A., Paavonen, J. Cervical neoplasia and other STD related genital tract neoplasias. In Holmes, K., Sparling, F., Lemon, S. *et al.* eds. *Sexually Transmitted Diseases.* 3rd edn. New York: McGraw-Hill; 1999: 811–831.

140. Chiasson, M. A., Declining AIDS mortality in New York City. New York City Department of Health. *Bull. N Y Acad. Med.* 1997;**74**(1):151–152.

141. Weber, T., Chin, K., Sidhu, J. S., Janssen, R. S. Prevalence of invasive cervical cancer among HIV-infected and uninfected hospital patients, 1994–1995. *Program Abstracts of 5th Conf. Retroviruses Opportunistic Infect.* (Chicago, IL; 1998). Abstract 717.

142. Phelps, R., Smith, D. K., Gardner, L. *et al.* Incidence of lung and invasive cervical cancer in HIV-infected women. *Program Abstracts 13th Int. Conf. AIDS* (Durban, South Africa; July 9–14, 2000). Abstract number TuPeB3168.

143. Lomalisa, P., Smith, T., Guidozzi, F. Human immunodeficiency virus infection and invasive cervical cancer in South Africa. *Gynecol. Oncol.* 2000;**77**(3):460–463.

144. Maiman, M., Fruchter, R. C., Serur, E., Remy, J. C., Feurer, G., Boyce, J. Human immunodeficiency virus infection and cervical neoplasia. *Gynecol. Oncol.* 1990;**38**(3): 377–382.

145. Klevens, R. M., Fleming, P. L., Mays, M. A., Frey, R. Characteristics of women with AIDS and invasive cancer. *Obstet Gynecol.* 1996;**88**(2):269–273.

146. Solomon, D., Darvey, D., Kurman, R. *et al.* The 2001 Bethesda System: terminology for reporting results of cervical cytology. *J. Am. Med. Assoc.* 2002;**287**(16):2114–2119.

147. American College of Obstetricians and Gynecologists. Cervical cytology: evaluation and management of abnormalities (Technical Bulletin No. 183). Practice Guidelines August 1993.

148. Wright, T. C., Moscarelli, R. D., Dole, P., Ellerbrock, T. V., Chiasson, M. A., Vandevanter, N. Significance of mild cytologic atypia in women infected with human immunodeficiency virus. *Obstet. Gynecol.* 1996;**87**(4):515–519.

149. Holcomb, K., Abulafia, O., Matthews, R. P. *et al.* significance of ASCUS sytology in HIV-infected women. *Gynecol. Oncol.* 1999;**75**(1):118–121.

150. Duska, L. R., Flynn, C. F., Chen, A., Whall-Strojwas, D., Goodman, A. Clinical evaluation of atypical glandular cells of undetermined significance on cervical cytology. *Obstet. Gynecol.* 1998;**91**(2):278–282.

151. Kennedy, A. W., Salmieri, S. S., Wirth, S. L., Biscotti, C. V., Tuason, L. J., Travarca, M. J. Results of the clinical evaluation of atypical glandular cells of undetermined significance (AGCUS) detected on cervical cytology screening. *Gynecol. Oncol.* 1998;**63**(1):14–18.

152. Korn, A. P., Judson, P. L., Zaloudek, C. J. Importance of atypical glandular cells of uncertain significance in cervical cytologic smears. *J. Reprod. Med.* 1998;**43**(9):774–778.

153. Fruchter, R., Maiman, M., Sedlis, A., Bartley, L., Camilien, L., Arrastia, C. D. Multiple recurrences of cervical intraepithelial neoplasia in women with the human immunodeficiency virus. *Obstet. Gynecol.* 1996;**87**(3):338–344.

154. Holcomb, K., Matthews, R. P., Chapman, J. E. *et al.* The efficacy of cervical colonization in treatment of cervical intraepithelial neoplasia in HIV-infected women. *Gynecol. Oncol.* 1999;**74**(3):428–431.

155. Maiman, M., Watts, D. H., Andersen, J., Clax, P., Merino, M., Kendall, M. A. Vaginal 5-fluorouracil for high-grade cervical dysplasia in human immunodeficiency virus infection: a randomized trial. *Obstet. Gynecol.* 1999;**94**(6):954–961.

156. Fleming, D. T., McQuillan, G. M., Johnson, R. E. *et al.* Herpes simplex virus type 2 in the United States, 1976 to 1994. *N. Engl. J. Med.*1997;**337**(16):1105–1111.

157. Augenbraun, M., Feldman, J., Chirgwin, K. *et al.* Increased genital shedding of herpes simplex virus type 2 in HIV-seropositive women. *Ann. Int. Med.* 1995;**123**(11):845–847.

158. Mostad, S. B., Kreiss, J. K., Ryncarz, A. J. *et al.* Cervical shedding of herpes simplex virus in human immunodeficiency virus-infected women: effects of hormonal contraception, pregnancy and vitamin A deficiency. *J. Infect. Dis.* 2000;**181**(1):58–63.

159. Retesm, M., Graber, J., Reeves, W. Acyclovir-resistant HSV: preliminary results from a national surveillance system. *Program and Abstracts of the Int. Conf. Emerging Infect. Dis.* 1998 Mar 10; Atlanta, GA (Abstract 55).

160. Tapert, S. F., Aarons, G. A., Sedlar, G. R., Brown, S. A. Adolescent substance use and sexual risk-taking behavior. *J. Adolesc. Hlth.* 2001;**28**(3):181–189.

161. Nyrphy, D. A., Durako, S. D., Moscicki, A. B. *et al.* and the Adolescent Medicine HIV/AIDS Research Network. No change in health risk behaviors over time among HIV-infected adolescents in care: role of psychological distress. *J. Adolesc. Hlth* 2001;**29S**:57–63.

162. Boyer, C. B., Shafer, M., Wibbelsman, C. J., Seeberg, D., Teitle, E., Lovell, N. Associations of sociodemographic psychosocial and behavioral factors with sexual risk and sexually transmitted diseases in teen clinic patients. *J. Adolesc. Hlth* 2000;**27**(2):102–111.

163. Sanders-Phillips K. Factors influencing HIV/AIDS in women of color. *Public. Hlth Rep.* 2002;**117** Suppl 1:S151–S156.

9 Growth, nutrition, and metabolism

Caroline J. Chantry, M.D.

Department of Clinical Pediatrics, University of California Davis Medical Center, Sacramento, CA

Jack Moye, Jr., M.D.

Pediatric, Adolescent, and Maternal AIDS Branch, National Institute of Child Health and Human Development, NIH, Bethesda, MD

In recent years, growth, nutrition and metabolism of HIV-infected children have received increased attention for several reasons. It has been recognized for the past decade that HIV-infected children generally do not grow as well as their uninfected counterparts, but more recent evidence suggests that this is often true even in the face of adequate virologic control. Given also that growth is a predictor of survival, there has been closer scrutiny of nutritional and metabolic factors that can contribute to poor growth. Additionally, potentially serious metabolic complications of HIV infection and/or antiretroviral therapies overlap with nutritional aspects of the infection and have prompted attention to the pathophysiology of malnutrition in these children.

The current state of knowledge regarding the complex interrelationships of nutrition, HIV disease, antiretroviral therapy, and growth is reviewed in this chapter. Recommendations for nutritional monitoring and support are discussed, as are therapies for certain recognized causes of malnutrition in HIV-infected children. Briefly described are the complications and recommended treatments for fat redistribution, hyperlipidemia, insulin resistance, osteonecrosis, and mitochondrial toxicity. Finally, nutritional issues most germane to resource-poor settings are highlighted.

Definitions: malnutrition, growth failure

Pediatric HIV disease may lead to multiple nutritional deficiencies. Deficiencies of adequate macronutrients (protein or calories) and/or micronutrients (vitamins, minerals) to maintain optimal health status is referred to as undernutrition or, more commonly, malnutrition. Many definitions for growth failure or failure to thrive (FTT) exist. In this chapter, the terms are used interchangeably and refer to a child who is failing to grow (gain weight and/or height) as expected for age, or who is losing weight. Children with growth failure or FTT can be further classified into those who have decreased weight for height or length (wasting) and those who have reduced linear growth or decreasing

Handbook of Pediatric HIV Care, ed. Steven L. Zeichner and Jennifer S. Read.
Published by Cambridge University Press. © Cambridge University Press 2006.

height or length for age (stunting). Mechanistically, growth failure can be defined as any of the following:

(a) serial weight or height measurements which downwardly cross two major centile lines (e.g., 95th, 75th, 50th, etc.) on reference growth charts (freely available for downloading via the Internet from the National Center for Health Statistics (NCHS) at http://www.cdc.gov/growthcharts), or the equivalent z-score (distance in standard deviation units above or below the reference median z-score of 0.0 (50th percentile) for a given age and sex) decrease of 1.4 or more;

(b) failure of the slope of serial growth measurements to parallel or better the standard growth curve in a child previously below the 5th percentile of weight for age;

(c) loss of 5% or more of body weight;

(d) growth velocity below the 3rd percentile for weight or height measurements taken 6 months apart; or

(e) weight for height below the 5th percentile.

The use of growth velocities or z-scores is particularly useful to assess change in children whose growth percentile values are near the tails of the distribution (e.g., below the 5th percentile). Reference curves are available to quantify 6-month growth velocities [1]. A minimum interval of three months between measurements is recommended to determine growth velocity, as shorter intervals may not be accurate due to the saltatory nature of growth. Z-scores provide a standardized measure of the relative magnitude of weight or height change, regardless of location on or off the curve. Growth failure is considered clinically significant if the above criteria are met within 3 months in an infant or 6 months in a child 1 to 3 years of age, but even more gradual changes should prompt concern in children at high-risk for malnutrition, such as those with HIV infection.

It should be noted that the NCHS reference growth charts represent children in the United States, and may not ideally represent children of all genetic backgrounds. Nevertheless, the World Health Organization (WHO) has adopted them as the international standard, based on evidence that growth patterns of well-nourished preschool children from different ethnic backgrounds are similar, i.e., genetic variations are relatively minor compared to the effects of malnutrition. The World Health Organization has a global database of child growth and malnutrition which details growth data and references from many individual countries. It can be found at http://www.who.int/nutgrowthdb/en/./

Effects of malnutrition

General

The term malnutrition covers a broad array of situations and can present variably, largely dependent upon which nutrients are deficient. Deficiencies can impact a wide variety of metabolic functions. Nutrition plays important roles in immune function, central nervous system (CNS) maturation, and physical growth. Malnutrition can cause a broad array of immunodeficiencies, globally referred to as nutritionally-acquired immune deficiency syndromes. Chronic protein-calorie malnutrition (PCM) adversely affects T-lymphocyte number and function, delayed type hypersensitivity, complement levels, and new primary antibody responses. PCM causes atrophy of lymphoid tissue, especially in children. Single-nutrient deficiencies, particularly of vitamins A and C, and of trace metals iron and zinc, often coexist with PCM. Alone or in conjunction with PCM, they affect cell-mediated immunity and immunoglobulin G responses [2, 3].

Malnutrition in the first two years of life can cause deficient myelinization and abnormal growth of neurons potentially resulting in irreversibly impaired intelligence or behavior. Both the CNS and peripheral nervous system (PNS) remain susceptible beyond 2 years of age to PCM as well as to micronutrient deficiencies (most notably of B vitamins).

Caloric deficiency impairs growth. Initially, ponderal (weight) growth alone is affected, but with chronic malnutrition, linear (height) growth also is affected, as is head growth in young children. Micronutrient deficiencies also can result in poor growth, and zinc supplements have been noted to improve both ponderal and linear growth, with greater response seen when initial weight-for-age and height-for-age are more severely affected [4]. Additionally, iron, copper, vitamin D, and iodine deficiencies can result in impaired growth.

HIV infection

HIV-infected children can present with FTT. Both mean weight and height are affected within the first 6 months of life [5–8]. Weight for length is also decreased, but less so than weight and length for age. Brain growth as reflected by head circumference may also be affected in the first months of life. On average, body mass index (BMI) decreases in the first six months and then recovers to normal by 12 months. Children with AIDS are more stunted than children with less severe illness [2]. Chronic malnourishment can be associated with pubertal delay during adolescence. Wasting syndrome is an AIDS-defining illness and contributes significantly to morbidity and mortality in HIV-infected children [9].

The immunodeficiency of HIV can be exacerbated by malnutrition. Survival in HIV infection, as in other chronic diseases, is directly related to nutritional status. Survival in HIV-infected adults is correlated with body cell mass [10], visceral protein status [11], and micronutrient status, including zinc inadequacy and copper:zinc ratio [12]. Higher vitamin E levels have been shown to protect against disease progression [13], and reduced vitamin A and B_{12} levels are associated with lower CD4+ cell counts [13, 14]. Magnesium has been shown to have a direct impact on immune response during HIV infection [15].

In HIV-infected children, height growth velocity predicts survival, regardless of plasma viral load, age, or $CD4^+$ cell count [16]. Low weight-for-age also is associated with increased disease progression and mortality [17, 18], but an association between weight and disease progression has not been described independent of factors previously considered to confound this effect, such as plasma viral load. Weight growth velocity has been described as an independent predictor for disease progression or death [19], but this finding was confounded by inclusion of weight growth failure as a clinical endpoint.

Selenium deficiency has been shown to be a significant independent predictor of mortality in HIV-infected children [20]. HIV-infected children have been found to exhibit lower mean serum levels of lycopene, retinol, beta-carotene, and vitamin E and lower plasma glutathione levels, and are more likely to have low serum levels of vitamin B_6, vitamin B_{12}, and zinc compared with uninfected children [21]. Several of these vitamins and minerals in adults can affect CD4+ cell counts. While effects of such deficiencies in children are not entirely clear, lower plasma glutathione levels were associated with higher plasma viral load and lower CD4+ cell counts [22], and beta-carotene levels in children with AIDS are half those of HIV-infected children without AIDS [23]. Glutathione removes hydrogen peroxide from cells, and beta-carotene scavenges free radicals directly, as do vitamins A and E. Increased oxidative stress from these deficiencies can play an indirect role in the immunodeficiency of HIV through multiple mechanisms. Few micronutrient supplementation trials in HIV-infected children have been undertaken. Vitamin A supplements given to children in Tanzania reduced mortality in those with HIV more than in those without [24].

The association between HIV morbidity and malnutrition can be bidirectional. Malnourishment appears to affect progression of HIV disease, but HIV infection can itself affect nutritional status via decreased nutrient intake, malabsorption, increased utilization of nutrients, and/or dysregulation of metabolism, particularly when HIV disease is complicated by opportunistic and other infections.

HIV infection can alter body composition, a more accurate measure of nutritional status than weight growth velocity. Conflicting data about preservation of lean body mass (LBM) in HIV-infected children exist [6, 7, 25]. There appears to be a significant inverse correlation between fat free mass (FFM) and viral load [26] (suggesting that dynamics of viral replication and/or the associated host immune response impair anabolism). Infected children may have decreased arm muscle mass and resistance index (an indirect measure of total lean body mass measured by bioelectrical impedance analysis (BIA)) [27].

The relation between HIV viral load, antiretroviral therapy, and growth remains ambiguous. There is some suggestion that patients on antiretroviral therapy with lower viral loads have better growth velocities than those with higher viral loads [26, 28, 29], although CD4+ T-cell count may be a better predictor for normal growth [30]. Improved growth is sometimes seen when patients are treated with highly active antiretroviral therapy (HAART, generally combination antiretroviral treatment regiments including a protease inhibitor) [31, 32], but the mechanisms responsible for the improved growth remain unclear.

Importance of prevention and early intervention

Nutritional support should be an integral component of all medical management for children with HIV disease. The goals include maintenance of normal growth and development; provision for catch-up growth as necessary; correction of nutritional deficiencies; prevention of further immunologic compromise; enhancement of a sense of well-being and ability to maintain age-appropriate activities; lessened morbidity from secondary infections; and treatment of underlying gastrointestinal and infectious disease.

Prevention of malnutrition is facilitated by regular nutritional assessment of all HIV-infected children. Prevention of specific causes of malnutrition is important. For example, enteric infections increase metabolic needs and can impair absorption of nutrients and therapeutic agents. Enteric infections can be prevented by avoiding ingestion of contaminated water or ice, swimming in contaminated water, and eating undercooked meat, and by carefully following food safety precautions. Fever increases metabolic needs and should be treated aggressively in these children. Other components of prevention include routine provision of up to 200% of the appropriate dietary reference intake (e.g., recommended dietary allowance, not to exceed tolerable upper intake level) for vitamins and minerals and 150% for calories and protein. The cultural and ethnic background of the family is important to consider when assisting with food choices. As developmental delays and multiple caretakers have been reported with greater frequency in children with HIV infection and FTT [33], availability of a primary caretaker and screening for developmental delays can be important components of prevention. If the parent(s) is HIV-infected, anticipation of their health care needs, including nutritional support, should be considered as part of the child's management.

Routine nutritional assessment

Nutritional assessment should be begun in infancy and performed regularly in all HIV-infected children, in an effort to prevent malnutrition and growth failure. The baseline nutritional evaluation should be performed by a registered dietitian at the first or second visit. Thorough follow-up evaluation every 4–6 months is sufficient if no signs of faltering growth develop. For children with growth abnormalities, poor intake, vomiting, diarrhea, or disease progression, nutritional follow-up should be more frequent, such as every 1 to 3 months, depending on clinical severity [34]. Guidelines for nutritional assessment are summarized in Table 9.1.

Anthropometric measurements

Height, weight, head circumference, triceps skinfold thickness (TSF) and mid-arm circumference (MAC) should be measured on a regular basis. Older children should also

Table 9.1. Recommended Nutritional Assessment for HIV-infected Children[a,b]

Anthropometric measurements
- a. Height, weight, head circumference, TSF, MAC, waist circumference, hip circumference, truncal skin fold (e.g., sub-scapular, abdominal)
- b. Weight and height growth velocities, weight and height for age, weight for height

Comprehensive dietary history
- a. Calorie and protein intake
- b. Symptoms of gastrointestinal disturbances
- c. Access to food and food preparation facilities
- d. Available diet (including food frequencies)
- e. Food safety

Laboratory studies
- a. Protein status [c] (Short term: pre-albumin or retinol-binding protein; long term: albumin or transferrin)
- b. Complete blood count with differential
- c. Other studies based on clinical features and dietary history[c]

Assessment of body composition and fat distribution
- a. TSF, MAC, and sub-scapular or abdominal skin fold
- b. Waist circumference or waist/hip ratio, body mass index calculation
- c. BIA and/or DEXA scan

Estimation of energy and protein requirements

[a] Abnormal results:
  Estimate and counsel regarding requirements
  Multidisciplinary evaluation: intake, loss, requirements
  Early intervention[c]
  Nutritional follow-up every 1–3 months.

[b] Normal results:
  Anthropometrics and nutritional follow-up every 4–6 months.

[c] = Individualize (see text)
  TSF = triceps skinfold thickness
  MAC = midarm circumference
  BIA = bioelectrical impedance analysis
  DEXA = dual energy X-ray absorptiometry

have waist and hip circumferences and truncal (subscapular and/or abdominal) skinfolds measured. Serial measurements of height, weight and head circumference (for children less than three years old) are essential and should be performed at every routine visit. More frequent weight checks are needed in the presence of weight loss or lack of weight gain. Skinfold and arm circumference evaluate adipose and muscle (somatic protein) mass and should be measured every 4–6 months and any time significant weight loss (>5%) or growth faltering occurs. Reference values for arm circumference and triceps skinfold measurements are available in Table 9.2. For sites unable to measure skinfold thickness, the BMI, calculated as weight (in kilograms) divided by height (in meters) divided by height (in meters), or (weight in kilograms)/[height in meters × height in meters]) gives indirect information about body composition. Normal BMI values for children are presented in Table 9.3. The child's weight and height growth velocities, weight and height for age, BMI, and fat and muscle mass should be assessed, abnormalities evaluated, and comparisons made with previous measures. Children who are crossing percentile lines downwardly on reference growth charts, or who are below the fifth percentile and not paralleling the curve, need to be identified promptly. Establishing trends in a child's growth, lean body mass, and fat stores is more valuable than any individual measurement. Standardized procedures for anthropometric measurement accuracy and reproducibility are described in Table 9.4.

Comprehensive dietary history

A comprehensive diet history includes an evaluation of: (a) calorie and protein intake; (b) symptoms of gastrointestinal disturbances (e.g., anorexia, dysphagia, nausea, vomiting, diarrhea, early satiety, heartburn, fever); (c) access to food and food preparation facilities (e.g., electricity, refrigeration, cooking appliances and utensils, resources for food transport); (d) available diet (including type and frequency of food and beverage consumption); and (e) food safety (i.e., knowledge and facilities to provide safe food preparation and storage).

Current nutrient intake can be calculated using a 24-hour dietary recall along with food and beverage frequency questionnaires. Reasons for decreased intake or feeding problems should be explored and an assessment of the parent-child interaction should be made. The dietary history is used as a basis for comparing current intake with estimated energy and protein needs (see Estimation of Energy and Protein Requirements).

Laboratory studies

Visceral protein status can be assessed by use of short-term markers, such as prealbumin (half-life of 2 days) and retinol-binding protein (half-life of 11 hours) levels, or more long-term markers, such as albumin and transferrin (half-lives of 21 and 20 days) levels. Serum iron, total iron-binding capacity or transferrin, folate and B_{12} levels should be evaluated in patients with anemia. A more extensive laboratory evaluation, guided by history (symptoms, disease progression, and diet including vitamin, mineral and other dietary supplements) and physical examination findings, can be helpful when suboptimal nutrition is suspected. For example, children with diarrhea should be monitored for electrolyte imbalance and deficiencies of magnesium and zinc. If there is significant fat malabsorption, vitamins A and E levels should be checked. Additional clinical signs on physical examination that may signal deficiency include dermatitis (vitamin A, zinc, biotin, essential fatty acids), cheilosis (riboflavin, biotin, zinc) or peripheral neuropathy (vitamins B_6 or B_{12}).

Table 9.2. Reference arm measurements

Percentiles of upper arm circumference (mm) and estimated upper arm muscle circumference (mm) for whites of the United States Health Examination Survey 1 of 1971 to 1974

Age (yr)	Arm circumference (mm)						Arm muscle circumference (mm)					
	5th	50th Males	95th	5th	50th Females	95th	5th	50th Males	95th	5th	50th Females	95th
1–1.9	142	159	183	138	156	177	110	127	147	105	124	143
2–2.9	141	162	185	142	160	184	111	130	150	111	126	147
3–3.9	150	167	190	143	167	189	117	137	153	113	132	152
4–4.9	149	171	192	149	169	191	123	141	159	115	136	157
5–5.9	153	175	204	153	175	211	128	147	169	125	142	165
6–6.9	155	179	228	156	176	211	131	151	177	130	145	171
7–7.9	162	187	230	164	183	231	137	160	190	129	151	176
8–8.9	162	190	245	168	195	261	140	162	187	138	160	194
9–9.9	175	200	257	178	211	260	151	170	202	147	167	198
10–10.9	181	210	274	174	210	265	156	180	221	148	170	197
11–11.9	186	223	280	185	224	303	159	183	230	150	181	223
12–12.9	193	232	303	194	237	294	167	195	241	162	191	220
13–13.9	194	247	301	202	243	338	172	211	245	169	198	240
14–14.9	220	253	322	214	252	322	189	223	264	174	201	247
15–15.9	222	264	320	208	254	322	199	237	272	175	202	244
16–16.9	244	278	343	218	258	334	213	249	296	170	202	249
17–17.9	246	285	347	220	264	350	224	258	312	175	205	257
18–18.9	245	297	379	222	258	325	226	264	324	174	202	245
19–24.9	262	308	372	221	265	345	238	273	321	179	207	249

Table 9.2. (cont.)

Percentiles for triceps skinfold for whites of the United States Health and Nutrition Examination Survey 1 of 1971 to 1974

Age (yr)	Triceps skinfold percentiles (mm)															
	Males								Females							
	N	5	10	25	50	75	90	95	N	5	10	25	50	75	90	95
1–1.9	228	6	7	8	10	12	14	16	204	6	7	8	10	12	14	16
2–2.9	223	6	7	8	10	12	14	15	208	6	8	9	10	12	15	16
3–3.9	220	6	7	8	10	11	14	15	208	7	8	9	11	12	14	15
4–4.9	230	6	6	8	9	11	12	14	208	7	8	8	10	12	14	16
5–5.9	214	6	6	8	9	11	14	15	219	6	7	8	10	12	15	18
6–6.9	117	5	6	7	8	10	13	16	118	6	6	8	10	12	14	16
7–7.9	122	5	6	7	9	12	15	17	126	6	7	9	11	13	16	18
8–8.9	117	5	6	7	8	10	13	16	118	6	8	9	12	15	18	24
9–9.9	121	6	6	7	10	13	17	18	125	8	8	10	13	16	20	22
10–10.9	146	6	6	8	10	14	18	21	152	7	8	10	12	17	23	27
11–11.9	122	6	6	8	11	16	20	24	117	7	8	10	13	18	24	28
12–12.9	153	6	6	8	11	14	22	28	129	8	9	11	14	18	23	27
13–13.9	134	5	5	7	10	14	22	26	151	8	8	12	15	21	26	30
14–14.9	131	4	5	7	9	14	21	24	141	9	10	13	16	21	26	28
15–15.9	128	4	5	6	8	11	18	24	117	8	10	12	17	21	25	32
16–16.9	131	4	5	6	8	12	16	22	142	10	12	15	18	22	26	31
17–17.9	133	5	5	6	8	12	16	19	114	10	12	13	19	24	30	37
18–18.9	91	4	5	6	9	13	20	24	109	10	12	15	18	22	26	30
19–24.9	531	4	5	7	10	15	20	22	1060	10	11	14	18	24	30	34

Adapted from Frisancho AR. New norms of upper limb fat and muscle areas for assessment of nutritional status. *Am J Clin Nutr 1981*; **34**: 2540.

Table 9.3. Body mass index reference values (Percentile Values of Body Mass Index*)

Age (yr)	Percentile						
	5	10	25	50	75	90	95
Males							
1	14.6	15.4	16.1	17.2	18.5	19.4	19.9
2	14.4	15.0	15.7	16.5	17.6	18.4	19.0
3	14.0	14.6	15.3	16.0	17.0	17.8	18.4
4	13.8	14.4	15.0	15.8	16.6	17.5	18.1
5	13.7	14.2	14.9	15.5	16.3	17.3	18.0
6	13.6	14.0	14.7	15.4	16.3	17.4	18.1
7	13.6	14.0	14.7	15.5	16.5	17.7	18.9
8	13.7	14.1	14.9	15.7	17.0	18.4	19.7
9	14.0	14.3	15.1	16.0	17.6	19.3	20.9
10	14.2	14.6	15.5	16.6	18.4	20.3	22.2
11	14.6	15.0	16.0	17.2	19.2	21.3	23.5
12	15.1	15.5	16.5	17.8	20.0	22.3	24.8
13	15.6	16.0	17.1	18.4	20.8	23.3	25.8
14	16.1	16.6	17.7	19.1	21.5	24.4	26.8
15	16.6	17.1	18.4	19.7	22.2	25.4	27.7
16	17.2	17.8	19.1	20.5	22.9	26.1	28.4
17	17.7	18.4	19.7	21.2	23.4	27.0	29.0
18	18.3	19.1	20.3	21.9	24.0	27.7	29.7
19	19.0	19.7	21.1	22.5	24.4	28.3	30.1
Females							
1	14.7	15.0	15.8	16.6	17.6	18.6	19.3
2	14.3	14.7	15.3	16.0	17.1	18.0	18.7
3	13.9	14.4	14.9	15.6	16.7	17.6	18.3
4	13.6	14.1	14.7	15.4	16.5	17.5	18.2
5	13.5	14.0	14.6	15.3	16.3	17.5	18.3
6	13.3	13.9	14.6	15.3	16.4	17.7	18.8
7	13.4	14.0	14.7	15.5	16.7	18.5	19.7
8	13.6	14.2	15.0	16.0	17.2	19.4	21.0
9	14.0	14.5	15.5	16.6	18.0	20.8	22.7
10	14.3	15.0	15.9	17.1	19.0	21.8	24.2
11	14.6	15.3	16.2	17.8	19.8	23.0	25.7
12	15.0	15.6	16.7	18.3	20.4	23.7	26.8
13	15.4	16.0	17.1	18.9	21.2	24.7	27.9
14	15.7	16.4	17.5	19.4	21.8	25.3	28.6
15	16.1	16.8	18.0	19.9	22.4	26.0	29.4
16	16.4	17.1	18.4	20.2	22.8	26.5	30.0
17	16.9	17.6	18.9	20.7	23.3	27.1	30.5
18	17.2	18.0	19.4	21.1	23.7	27.4	31.0
19	17.5	18.4	19.8	21.4	24.0	27.7	31.3

From National Health and Nutritional Examination Survey, 1971 to 1974 (NHANES 1); and Hammer LD, Kraemer HC, Wilson DM, *et al.* Standardized percentile curves of body-mass index for children and adolescents. *Am J Dis Child* 1991;**145:**972.

Table 9.4. Anthropometric measurement guidelines

General rules of measurement technique

1. Always document measurement conditions. For example, indicate the scale used, whether a length or height measure was taken, or if a child was unstable or moving during the measurement.
2. Calibrate equipment according to individual facility policy.
3. Remember that accuracy of measurements is directly dependent on subject cooperation.
4. Measurements of weight, height/length, and head circumference should be plotted on NCHS growth charts and followed closely, monitoring trends.

Weight

1. Use an electronic scale or beam scale with non-detachable weights.
2. Zero scale prior to each measure. Calibrate scales when needed.
3. Weigh infants and young children lying down with infants wearing only a dry diaper during measurement and small children in a gown or very light clothing.
4. Weigh children who can stand on a beam scale, preferably ones with "handle bars" for support. Calm children and reduce movement as much as possible for accurate measurements. Take a child's weight while in a gown or very light clothing.
5. For children too large for the infant scale who have disabilities that prevent them from standing on a beam scale, using a bed scale is most accurate. However, if equipment is not available, a staff member or caretaker can hold the child on a beam scale, take his/her own weight on the same scale, and subtract to calculate the child's estimated body weight. When using this method, take the average of two measures.

Length

1. Measure children's recumbent length up to 24 months of age and, for those unable to stand, up to 36 months of age on a calibrated length board with a stable headboard and a sliding footboard.
2. Two people are required to perform an accurate length measurement. One person holds the head in place with two hands while the other slides the footboard and takes the reading. The child's foot should be flat against the footboard with toes pointing straight upward and legs should be straight at the time of measurement.
3. If a child has hypertonicity and cannot be held in the above position, other forms of measurement should be performed (e.g., tibial length, below).

Tibial length[a]

1. With child sitting or lying down, use a non-stretchable, flexible measuring tape to measure the distance from the tip (superomedial edge) of the tibia to the lower edge of the medial malleolus. In lay terms, measure the inner lower leg from the middle of the knee where the tibia inserts to the bottom edge of the ankle bone.
2. Measure the left leg whenever possible.
3. Measure to the nearest 0.1 centimeter.
4. Take the average of two measures on the same leg.
5. Calculate estimated height using the following equation:

$$S = (3.26 \times TL) + 30.8$$

S: Stature in centimeters

TL: Tibial length in centimeters

Table 9.4. (*cont.*)

6. Consistently measure individual patients and plot on NCHS growth charts.
7. In children less than 3 years of age, a crown–rump measure can be used:
   Using a length board, hold head in place at head board. Have a second measurer slide the foot board up to the infant's buttocks, holding the torso as straight as posible. Average crown rump measures and normal increments are available in the literature [51] or an individual's trends can be used.

Height
1. Once a child is greater than 24 months of age and can stand upright, stature is measured using a calibrated stadiometer.
2. For best results, measure child while he/she wears a gown or clothing in which one can visualize body position. Children need to stand with bare feet close together, body and legs straight, arms at sides, relaxed shoulders, and head, back, buttocks, and heels up against the wall or shaft of the stadiometer.
3. Instruct child to look straight ahead and stand tall, keeping heels on the ground.
4. Bring headboard down to top of the child's head while at eye to eye level with child and record measure to nearest 0.1 centimeter.
5. Take the average of three measures.

Head circumference
1. Measure head circumference in children regularly at routine physical examination appointments up until 36 months of age or according to study parameters.
2. Have the infant or child sit on caretaker's lap or stand if capable.
3. Remove any hair pieces that could interfere with measurement.
4. Place non-stretchable measuring tape just above the eyebrow and ears and straight around the occipital bulge in the back of the child's head.
5. Compress hair with tape and record measure to the nearest 0.1 centimeter.

Mid-arm circumference
1. Use a non-stretchable centimeter tape, with millimeters delineated. On the non-dominant arm bent at a 90 degree angle with palm facing up, mark the midpoint between the acromion and olecranon processes. Make sure clothing is pushed up above the shoulder or removed if interfering with arm tissue.
2. Measure the distance around the arm at the mark and record to the nearest 0.1 centimeter.

Triceps skinfold thickness
1. Grasp vertical fold of fat about 1–2 centimeter above the midpoint using forefinger and thumb.
2. Measure skinfold with calipers at the midpoint after needle stabilizes while continuing to hold fold with hand.
3. Average three measures.
4. Edematous tissue and very squirmy children are two main factors that prevent accuracy of this measurement.
5. Measure to the nearest 0.5 millimeter.

Mid-arm muscle circumference
1. Use the following equation to calculate mid-arm muscle circumference:
   $MAMC = MAC - (TSF \times 3.14)/10$
   MAC = mid-arm circumference in centimeters, $MAMC$ = mid-arm muscle circumference in centimeters, TSF = triceps skinfold thickness in millimeters

---

[a] Validated only in children over 3 years of age [117]

Monitoring of micronutrients such as selenium, zinc, copper:zinc ratios, beta-carotene, and vitamins A, B_{12}, and E can be beneficial in patients with evidence of malnutrition or disease progression, as deficiencies have been associated with disease progression in children and/or adults. Finally, deficiencies of other micronutrients have been reported among HIV-infected patients and consideration therefore should be given to monitoring carnitine, as well as vitamins C and D, in addition to those micronutrients mentioned above [35–37]. There is little information and less consensus regarding contribution of most of these deficiencies to clinical manifestations of disease in pediatric patients. One report suggests deficiencies of selenium, zinc and vitamin A are uncommon in USA children infected with HIV [38]. In HIV-infected adults, however, deficiencies of vitamins A, E, B_6, B_{12} and zinc are reported to be common [39].

Baseline evaluation should be performed when the patient is clinically stable because acute illness can affect levels of these micronutrients. Furthermore, plasma levels are not always indicative of mild deficiency, particularly in the case of zinc. In the case of vitamin A, levels should be obtained in conjunction with retinol-binding protein to assess the cause of abnormal values.

Assessment of body composition

As discussed above (see 'Effects of malnutrition – HIV infection'), the bulk of evidence suggests that children with HIV infection lose lean body mass early in the course of the disease. LBM is known to correlate with survival in many diseases, including adult HIV infection. Therefore, assessment of body composition should be performed routinely, at least in children with any evidence of malnutrition or other significant symptoms of HIV infection, to see if changes in LBM are beginning to occur. Anthropometric measurements of MAC and TSF provide rough measures of body composition. Bioelectrical impedance analysis (BIA) is another simple, non-invasive method to determine body composition and equations have been developed for use with HIV-infected children [40]. Dual energy x-ray absorptiometry (DEXA) scans are one of the most reliable measures of body composition. While the latter methods are currently used most commonly in research settings, consideration should be given to clinical use of these measures – particularly when deviations from the norm are clinically suspected. For sites unable to measure body composition, calculation of BMI gives indirect information about body fat. Trends observed in body composition are more important than any single isolated measure.

Body fat distribution also should be monitored. Accumulation of central fat and loss of limb fat can occur in HIV-infected children (discussed more fully under Metabolic Abnormalities and Associated Therapies). In children as in adults, a relative central or abdominal distribution of body fat has been associated with adverse lipid and insulin concentrations independently of weight, height and age [41]. Truncal fat can be measured by various anthropometric or imaging methodologies. Accumulating data suggest that waist circumference itself can be a good measure of central adiposity. Waist circumference (adjusted for weight, height, and age) has shown the most consistent and generally strongest association with adverse risk factors, but the association is similar in magnitude when quantified by waist:hip ratio or comparison of the waist circumference to the sum of hip circumference and triceps skinfold thickness [41]. Differentiation of abdominal and visceral adiposity is aided by measures of abdominal and subscapular skinfold thicknesses, in addition to waist circumference, height, and ethnicity [42].

While DEXA accurately measures body composition, it is unable to differentiate between intraabdominal and subcutaneous fat. Nevertheless, truncal fat mass as measured by DEXA has been shown to strongly correlate with intraabdominal fat in young children and correlation between lipid profiles and fat distribution is similar whether measured by central fat on DEXA or visceral fat on MRI images.

Estimated energy and protein requirements

Recommended daily allowances for children infected with HIV are not well established because energy requirements engendered by HIV infection itself are not defined. Asymptomatic HIV-infected adults have increased resting and total energy expenditure, but clinical experience and research in children suggest that energy requirements are relatively normal when children are well [26, 43]. At minimum, there are increased energy requirements during periods of stress such as infection, and these children may not compensate well for these increased needs. Accordingly, some recommend estimating both energy and protein requirements at 150% of the recommended dietary allowance for healthy children. Alternatively, a range can be calculated using weight for actual height as the minimum and median (50th percentile) reference weight for actual age as the maximum.

The following formula can be used to grossly estimate caloric requirements for normal children: 100 kcal/kg for the first 10 kg of body weight; 50 kcal/kg for the second 10 kg of body weight; 20 kcal/kg for each kg over 20 kg of body weight. This simple method produces estimates towards the lower end of the range of normal needs. Age-specific energy and protein requirements for normal children are found in Table 9.5.

Children often have increased energy and protein requirements during illness, particularly during periods of fever or infection. Caloric needs are increased as follows: 12% for each degree centigrade rise, 25% for acute diarrhea, and 60% for sepsis. It has been estimated that increasing the Recommended Dietary Allowance for protein by 50 to 100% will provide for increased protein requirements during illness. These estimates of energy and protein requirements are generic recommendations for children under stressful conditions, and applicability to HIV infection has not been confirmed. Early treatment for fever and infection can limit the metabolic impact. As a child recovers from illness, they often enter a period of catch-up growth. The following formula can be used to estimate caloric and protein requirements during this phase:

Table 9.5. Recommended daily energy and protein intake by age

Age/years	kcal/kg	Protein/kg(grams)
0–0.5	108	2.2
0.5–1	98	1.6
1–3	102	1.2
4–6	90	1.2
7–10	70	1.2
11–14 (males)	55	1.0
11–14 (females)	47	1.0
15–18 (males)	45	0.8
15–18 (females)	40	0.8

From: Food and Nutrition Board, National Academy of Sciences National Research Council. Recommended Dietary Allowances. Washington, DC: National Academy Press, 1989.

Daily energy requirement, in kcal per kg of body weight

$$= \frac{(\text{RDA kcal for weight age}^a) \times (\text{ideal weight for height})^b}{(\text{actual weight})}$$

Daily protein requirement, in grams protein per kg of body weight

$$= \frac{(\text{RDA protein for weight age}^a) \times (\text{ideal weight for height})^b}{(\text{actual weight})}$$

[a] Weight age is the age at which the patient's present weight would be at the 50th percentile

[b] For those children recovering from acute illness who tend to have a weight for height greater than the 50th percentile, the "ideal weight for height" in the catch-up equation can be goal weight based on 90th percentile weight growth velocity averages for age added to current weight. Tables are available for both younger and older children [44, 45].

Causes of malnutrition and associated therapies

There are many potential causes of malnutrition in HIV-infected children, such as decreased intake, increased nutrient losses, increased nutrient requirements, and metabolic dysregulation. The relative contribution of each of these to the problem of malnutrition among HIV-infected children is not well understood. Malabsorption, increased energy expenditure, and endocrinopathies have been postulated but not documented as etiologic in most HIV-infected children with growth failure [26, 43, 46, 47]. Specific causes of malnutrition and suggested therapies are summarized in Table 9.6. Appropriate interventions can be divided into those that treat the underlying problem (e.g., identifying and removing a drug that is causing anorexia),

Table 9.6. Causes of malnutrition and associated therapies

Part 1: Decreased oral intake	
Cause	**Intervention**
All causes	*Referral to registered dietitian*
1. Anorexia	Supportive: Increase nutrient density of foods, high kcal infant formula, small frequent meals, calorie boosting instructions, nutritional supplements (per tube if needed). Symptomatic: appetite stimulants[a]
Nutritional deficiency	Treat deficiency (zinc, carnitine, vitamin A, B_6)
Depression/despair	Treat depression
Pain	Acute and chronic pain management
Drug-induced[a]	Remove offending agent if possible
Cytokine production	Control primary and secondary infections; cytokine modulators untested
Neurologic dysfunction	See below
2. Food aversion/refusal symptom avoidance: (nausea, vomiting diarrhea, abdominal pain)	Referral to feeding/speech therapy
Drug-induced[a]	Remove offending agent if possible; medications after or between meals
Infections	Treat infection
Behavioral	Reinforce parenting skills;[a] self-feeding
Upper GI tract lesions	
Oral lesions: gingivitis, aphthous ulcers, stomatitis, dental abscesses	Treat infections (CMV, HSV, *Candida*); symptomatic relief (see text); meticulous oral hygiene
Esophagitis: reflux, infectious	Antacids, H_2 blockers; soft diet; treat infection (CMV, HSV, *Candida*)
Gastritis, duodenitis: infectious, peptic	Treat infection; antacids, H_2 blockers if peptic
3. Barriers to food access or preparation	Coordinate with social work; Refer: WIC, soup kitchens, food pantries, food stamps, meal delivery programs
Caretaker limitation	As above; home health assistance
Limited food availability (money, transportation, etc.)	Evaluate food availability[a]
4. Altered taste (dysgeusia)	
Zinc deficiency	Zinc supplements
Neurologic dysfunction	See below
Drug-induced*	Remove offending agent if possible

Table 9.6. (*cont.*)

5.	Early satiety	Small frequent meals
	Cytokine-related and /or dysmotility	Consider trial of agent to improve GI motility
6.	Neurologic dysfunction:	
	Developmental delay	Modify consistency of food and bottle or spoon feed as necessary; reduce inconsistencies in care; daily routine; 1 or 2 caretakers.
	Dysphagia	As above for developmental delay
	Dysguesia	As above for developmental delay; Consider zinc deficiency
	Gastroesophageal reflux	Standard reflux therapies.

Part 2: Increased nutrient losses

Cause		**Intervention**
All causes		*Referral to registered dietitian; parenteral nutrition indicated if enteral nutrition not tolerated*
1.	Vomiting	
	Gastritis	See above
	Pancreatitis	Standard supportive care
	Drug-induced (ddI, ddC, d4T, pentamidine)	Remove offending agent
	Infectious (CMV, MAC)	Treat infection
	Drug-related[a]	Remove offending agent as necessary
2.	Diarrhea	
	Enteric infection[a]	Treat infection
	Drug-related[a]	Symptomatic: loperamide, Kaopectate; remove agent as necessary
	Idiopathic	Symptomatic (as above)
3.	Malabsorption[a]	Dietary management;[a] antibiotics for bacterial overgrowth

Part 3: Increased nutrient requirements

Cause		**Intervention**
All Causes		*Referral to registered dietitian; supportive care: increase intake to meet requirements as for anorexia*
1.	Fever	Fever control, identify source
2.	Secondary infection	Treat infection
3.	End-organ complications (cardiac, neurologic, dermatologic, hematologic, renal)	Supportive care

Table 9.6. (*cont.*)

Part 4: Metabolic and endocrine dysregulation	
Cause	**Intervention**
Cytokine production	Cytokine modulators untested; consider oxandrolone for wasting
TNF, interleukins 1 and 6	Control primary disease (antiretroviral therapy)
Endocrine dysregulation (thyroid, adrenal, growth hormone, IGF-1)	Treat deficiencies; Growth hormone may improve growth in the absence of deficiency

a See text for further details.

symptomatic interventions (e.g., use of appetite stimulants for anorexia), and supportive interventions (e.g., use of nutritional supplements to achieve adequate intake despite anorexia). Understanding the difference between starvation and cachexia can be helpful in determining the appropriate intervention. Starvation is weight loss from inadequate intake or malabsorption of nutrients. It normally results in loss of fat mass initially. Cachexia is loss of weight or growth retardation with preferential catabolism of LBM over fat mass. Why this occurs is not clear, but it could be secondary to increased cytokine production by macrophages. For example, tumor necrosis factor (TNF) and interleukin-1 (IL-1) have both been shown to result in inefficient use of energy substrates. TNF specifically causes peripheral lipolysis and resultant increased circulation of free fatty acids which are then cycled from liver back to adipose tissue, i.e. futile cycling. IL-1 has catabolic effects on several tissues including liver and connective tissues, resulting in loss of both visceral and somatic protein stores.

Because malnutrition in this population is often multifactorial in etiology, a multidisciplinary team approach to evaluation and management is important. Family-centered care is ideal. The assistance of community agencies is of particular importance. For example, home health nurses and aides, or community organizations that provide services such as meal delivery can be of tremendous benefit.

Decreased oral intake

As noted above, many factors can contribute to malnutrition in HIV-infected children, and often more than one etiology is present in an individual child. Many of these causes result in decreased oral intake, frequent in HIV-infected children [26, 48]. Decreased oral intake, in turn, can result from diverse causes including anorexia, food aversion or refusal (often to avoid symptoms such as vomiting, diarrhea, oral pain, etc.), barriers to food access or preparation, dysgeusia, early satiety, or neurologic dysfunction.

Anorexia is associated with many of the medications used in this population, including reverse transcriptase inhibitors (e.g., zidovudine (ZDV), stavudine (d4T), lamivudine (3TC)), PIs (e.g., ritonavir, indinavir, nelfinavir), dapsone, antifungal drugs (e.g., fluconazole, ketoconazole), and antiviral medications (e.g., ganciclovir, acyclovir). Additionally, clarithromycin has been associated with dysgeusia. If anorexia or other side effects are debilitating and alternative therapeutic options exist, consideration should be given to changing therapies. Additional causes of anorexia in this population include micronutrient deficiency, pain, and depression.

Several appetite stimulants can be considered for anorectic children. Megestrol acetate (Megace) results in weight gain primarily by increasing body fat mass. Almost no data are available on the use of this progestational hormone in children. Doses of megestrol acetate that have been used to increase weight gain include 7.9 mg/kg per day (median dose) [49], 4 to 15 mg/kg per day, and 200 to 400 mg/m^2 per day. Megestrol acetate has known glucocorticoid activity [50], and adrenal suppression [51, 52] as well as glucose intolerance [53] has been observed among HIV-infected children receiving this medication. Cyproheptadine (Periactin) (0.25 to 0.5 mg/kg per day or 8 mg/m^2 per day divided in two to three daily doses) has been used with anecdotal reports of limited success. Dronabinol (Marinol; 2.5 mg twice daily before meals) also has been used for appetite stimulation although psychological side effects may limit its use in children.

Micronutrient deficiencies can exacerbate malnutrition by causing anorexia, dysgeusia, etc. and must be addressed. Recognizing that therapy should be individualized, recommended doses for some of the more commonly supplemented micronutrients are provided in Table 9.7. Excesses as well as deficiencies of micronutrients, particularly zinc, iron, and selenium, are harmful to the immune system, and extremely large doses are not recommended. Children with low iron-binding capacity should not be given supplemental iron. Caution should be exercised with vitamin A supplements in the presence of low retinol-binding protein.

The child may eat less to avoid exacerbation of symptoms such as nausea, vomiting, diarrhea, or oral or abdominal pain. One or more of these symptoms can be caused by medications that the child is taking. For example, abdominal pain may be associated with dideoxyinosine (ddI), 3TC, dideoxycytidine (ddC), ritonavir, saquinavir, nelfinavir, indinavir, pentamidine, or antibiotics such as sulfonamides and macrolides. ZDV alone can cause nausea, vomiting, and esophageal ulcers. Stomatitis, esophagitis, and gastritis all can be caused by opportunistic infections, in addition to the etiologies in healthy children. Food aversion or refusal can be behavioral in origin, and particular attention should be paid to the parent-child interaction.

Symptomatic relief for painful oral lesions often can be achieved by avoiding irritating foods such as orange juice and hot spices, using a straw to bypass the lesions, giving cold foods such as popsicles before meals, and using topical medications before meals. In older children, viscous lidocaine 2% (20 mg/ml) can be applied directly to the lesions at a maximum dose of 3 mg/kg, not to be repeated before 2 hours. Diphenhydramine

Table 9.7. Recommended therapeutic doses for selected micronutrient deficiencies

Nutrient	Dose	Comments
Zinc	0.5–1.0 mg elemental Zn/kg per day po with food.	
Selenium	50 micrograms/day	
Carnitine	25–350 mg/kg/day PO ÷ bid-tid (maximum 3g daily dose)	Begin with 50 mg/kg per day if cardiomyopathy present, 25 mg/kg/day if absent; titrate to clinical response and levels; consider if suspect mitochondrial toxicity; may give IV for adjunctive therapy for lactic acidosis
Copper	Infants: 2–3 mg Copper sulfate/day (400–600 mcg copper)	
Folate	Infants: 15 mcg/kg/day: max 50 mcg/day; children 1mg/day	(PO, IM, IV, SC)
Magnesium	Mg oxide salt: 65–130 mg/kg/day ÷ qid po, $MgSO_4$ salt: 100–200 mg/kg/dose qid PO	
Vitamin A	100 000 IU/ dose 6–12 mos. 200 000 IU/dose >1 yr. Give 2 doses PO qd × 2 + repeat 1 dose 1–4 weeks later;	Malabsorption syndrome prophylaxis: >8 yrs: 10 000–50 000 IU/d water miscible product
Vitamin B1 (thiamine)	Children: 5mg po qd for mild disease; 10 mg po bid for severe disease	Consider if suspect mitochondrial toxicity; high adult dose is 100 mg/day
Vitamin B2 (riboflavin)	Infants: 0.5 mg PO twice weekly Children: 1 mg PO tid for several weeks Adults: 2 mg po tid for several weeks	Consider if suspect mitochondrial toxicity; may give IV for adjunctive therapy for lactic acidosis; high adult dose is 50 mg/day
Vitamin B6 (pyridoxine)	5–250mg/day for 3 weeks	Up to 50 mg/day for drug-induced neuritis; (PO preferred, may give IM or IV).
Vitamin B12	Hematologic signs: 30–50 mcg /24 h IM or SC for ≥14 days to total of 1000–5000 mcg. Follow with maintenance. Neurologic signs: 100mcg/24 h IM or SC qd × 10–15 days then once or twice weekly for several months. Taper to 250–1000mcg monthly by one year. Maintenance treatment after deficiency: 100–250 mcg/dose IM or SC q 2–4 weeks	
Vitamin C	100–300 mg/day ÷ qd-bid for at least 2 weeks	PO preferred, can give IM, IV, SC
Vitamin E	Preterm and newborn infants: 25–50 IU/day × 6–10 weeks. Older children: 1 IU/kg/day PO	1mg DL-tocopherol acetate = 1 IU, use water miscible form with malabsorption; follow levels
Ubidecarenone (Ubiquinone, Coenzyme Q)	1 –10 mg/kg/day PO ÷qd-qid	Consider if suspect mitochondrial toxicity; may give IV for adjunctive therapy for lactic acidosis

syrup can be used as a swish and swallow in the usual dose of 5 mg/kg per day in divided doses before meals.

Additionally, "non-organic" causes of malnutrition such as food availability should be evaluated (e.g., with the food sufficiency questionnaire [54]), ideally by a visiting nurse in the home, and social service agencies involved as necessary. Barriers to food preparation can increase with parental illness common to these families. The absence of a primary caretaker or adequate parenting skills should be noted. Family difficulties and behavioral problems of the child can adversely affect the child's nutritional intake.

Neurologic dysfunction is common in HIV-infected children, and even subtle neurologic involvement can result in feeding difficulties. This can take the form of oral-motor dysfunction or prolonged feeding duration. Frank developmental delay may require significant modification of food consistency and routines.

Regardless of the cause of decreased oral intake, enteral formulas can constitute an important form of supplemental nutritional support and should be considered to supply unmet nutritional requirements. There are many commercially available formulas. The daily quantity of a given enteral feeding formula necessary to provide for the child's caloric or protein needs can be calculated and prescribed. The following factors should be considered when choosing a formula:

- Integrity of the gastrointestinal tract;
- Type of protein, fat, and carbohydrate required;
- Density of protein and energy provided and the relative ratio;
- Sodium, potassium, and phosphorous content (especially for patients with cardiac, renal, or hepatic dysfunction);
- Palatability;
- Taste preference;
- Cost.

Enteral feeding formulas for adults can be used for older children but may have too much sodium or protein for younger children, especially those younger than four years. Instant breakfast powders added to whole milk and supplements such as Ensure, Sustacal, or Nutren have similar nutritional values. These supplements are appropriate for older children with intact gastrointestinal tracts. Supplements with higher protein content, such as Sustacal or Ensure High Protein or Ensure Plus (also more calories) may be necessary. Alternatively, children with high-protein needs can use powdered skim milk or protein supplements (e.g., ProMod, Casee) directly mixed with food or beverages, including supplemental formulas. Toddler formulas are available for use in younger children, such as Kindercal (high in fiber), Pediasure (with or without fiber), and Nutren Jr, and are appropriate for those without specialized nutrient needs.

For children with evidence of malabsorption, supplements which maximize absorption should be chosen. Specialized supplements are available with hydrolyzed protein and medium-chain triglycerides with or without lactose or sucrose. These are discussed in more detail below under "Increased nutrient losses."

In addition to commercial supplements, other calorie-boosting tips include use of whole milk or cream rather than water (e.g., when cooking hot cereals or soups) if lactose intolerance is not an issue and use of fats such as peanut butter, cheese, or butter when serving vegetables, fruits, and breads. Calorie content can be boosted further by direct addition of powdered glucose polymers (e.g., Polycose, Moducal) to food or beverages.

Children who are unable to ingest sufficient calories by mouth may require tube feedings. Tube feedings increase fat mass but may not increase LBM significantly [55]. Such weight gain is associated nonetheless with decreased hospitalization and mortality rates [56]. Nasogastric tube feedings are painful, increase the likelihood of sinusitis, and limit oral intake. However, they can supplement nutritional intake acutely and help to evaluate the potential efficacy of long-term gastrostomy feedings. Gastrostomy tubes generally are better tolerated than nasogastric tube feedings, do not restrict normal activities, and can result in improved quality of life in children with nutritional difficulties.

There are a variety of different feeding progression schedules available, with little information to support one regimen over another. Generally tube feeding is begun with a hypo-osmolar concentration, which is gradually increased to full concentration formula over one to several days. Increases in volume follow, assessing tolerance of bolus volumes by measuring remaining volume in the stomach prior to the next feed. If the residual volume is less than 50% of the prior feed, volume can be increased by 25% to 30% until the desired volume is attained. Continuous feedings are used if bolus feeds are not tolerated, or for overnight feeding when necessary. Residuals also are checked when advancing continuous feeds, at least every 2 to 4 hours. If residual volume is greater than that infused during the previous two hours, the infusion should be stopped for 1 to 2 hours. When residuals are not a problem, the volume can be increased 1–5 ml/h. An alternative method to begin tube feedings uses very small volumes of full concentration formula from the start, with slow increases in volume thereafter as tolerated [57].

Increased nutrient losses

Despite adequate intake, malnutrition can result from increased nutrient loss as occurs with chronic vomiting, diarrhea, or malabsorption. Nausea, vomiting, and diarrhea are extremely common side effects of medications used in HIV-infected children. Examples of such drugs are antiretroviral medications (ZDV, ddI, 3TC, and most of the PIs), antibiotics, antifungal medications, and antiviral drugs. Vomiting also can be an indirect result of drugs *via* pancreatitis caused by antiretroviral medications or pentamidine. Vomiting and/or diarrhea may be the result of gastrointestinal infections such as gastritis, gastroenteritis, or pancreatitis. Besides organisms that cause vomiting and diarrhea in the normal host, opportunistic pathogens can cause chronic gastrointestinal disease in children with HIV infection. In addition, chronic diarrhea may be either the cause or the result of malabsorption.

Malabsorption occurs more commonly in HIV-infected children than healthy controls. It can result from enteric infections, malnutrition, small bowel bacterial overgrowth, or HIV enteropathy, which is villous atrophy associated with HIV infection in the absence of other detectable pathogens. Drug-induced diarrhea can result in malabsorption if transit time is substantially reduced. Carbohydrate (particularly lactose), fat and protein malabsorption have been described in 32–40%, 30–39% and 17% of HIV-infected children, respectively [46, 58, 59]. Although exocrine pancreatic insufficiency is often cited as a possible cause of fat malabsorption in this population, adequate pancreatic function was documented in the 39% of HIV-infected children demonstrating qualitative steatorrhea in one study [46]. The authors recommend that evaluation of fat malabsorption in HIV-infected children focus on other potential causes such as bacterial overgrowth. Cross-sectional analyses have not demonstrated an association between malabsorption and growth failure.

Appropriate dietary therapy or supplementation or both should be instituted for children with evidence of malabsorption. Enteral feeding formulas containing fewer simple carbohydrates present less osmotic load and have better gastrointestinal tolerance. Carbohydrate intolerance requires reduction or removal of the specific sugar from the diet. For lactase deficiency, there are many lactose-free supplements for all ages, such as Kindercal, Nutren Jr, and Pediasure for toddlers and young children, and similarly, Ensure, Sustacal, and Nutren for older children. Alternatively, microbial-derived lactase (e.g., Lactaid) can be added directly to milk and milk products or ingested with meals. Milk containing lactase is commercially available. Formulas with no sucrose are available for those with other (non-lactase) disaccharidase deficiency. Examples are Lactofree and Vivonex Pediatric for younger children and Isocal, Peptamen, and Vivonex for older children.

Children with fat malabsorption should be placed on low-fat diets with medium-chain triglyceride oil used directly as a dietary additive for supplementation or as the primary lipid in supplements modified specifically for them (e.g. Lipisorb). Calories also can be increased in patients with fat malabsorption by addition of glucose polymers (Polycose or Moducal) to the diet. While exocrine pancreatic sufficiency was not the cause in patients with steatorrhea in one report noted previously, it was found in 9% of the patients not presenting with steatorrhea [46]. Pancreatic enzymes (e.g., Cotazym, Pancrease, and others) can be offered in doses of lipase of 1000 U/kg/meal, generally not to exceed 20 000 U, with frequent evaluation for improvement. Doses can be titrated to eliminate diarrhea and steatorrhea and to avoid signs of excessive dosage, such as perianal irritation, occult gastrointestinal bleeding, hyperuricemia, and others. Enzymes should be discontinued if there has not been symptomatic improvement within two weeks of consistent administration with meals and snacks. Fat-soluble vitamins (A, D, E and K) may be deficient in the presence of fat malabsorption, and annual monitoring of their levels should be considered (particularly vitamins A and E, those that have associations with HIV disease progression).

Protein malabsorption generally necessitates supplements with hydrolyzed protein (e.g., Peptamen or Peptamen Jr) or amino acids (e.g., Vivonex, Vivonex Pediatric, or Neonate One Plus), depending on the severity. Specialized infant formulas for carbohydrate, fat, or protein malabsorption are available also. Absorption may be further enhanced by continuous gravity tube feedings, if necessary.

Parenteral nutrition can provide essential nutrition for children unable to maintain growth with enteral support alone. However, because of the expense and risks, including infectious complications, total parenteral nutrition should be used only in children unable to tolerate enteral feedings.

Increased nutrient requirements

The third major category of conditions which may result in malnutrition is increased nutritional requirements. A child may not grow despite apparently adequate intake and absorption of normal requirements if their individual requirements are in excess of the norm.

It has been postulated that total energy expenditure is increased in children with HIV secondary to basal metabolic increases, as demonstrated in HIV-infected adults [60]. Lack of a demonstrable hypermetabolic state in clinically stable HIV-infected children notwithstanding, increased requirements may occur periodically during acute febrile illnesses to which these children are prone. Marginal intake when patients are well may not allow for the extra nutrition required for catch-up growth after acute illnesses. End-organ complications, such as HIV encephalopathy or cardiomyopathy, may result in extra caloric requirements.

In addition to increasing enteral or parenteral intake to account for increased energy requirements, therapy for malnutrition due to increased requirements should be directed at treatment of the underlying cause (e.g., congestive heart failure). Fevers and infections should be aggressively treated to minimize nutritional impact.

Metabolic and endocrine dysregulation

Poor growth may be a manifestation of endocrine disease, which can complicate HIV infection. In particular, thyroid abnormalities, adrenal insufficiency, and classic growth hormone (GH) deficiency have been described [61–64]. Other abnormalities of the GH axis also occur. Reduced insulin-like growth factor-1 (IGF-1) levels have been described in malnourished adults with AIDS and in HIV-infected children, particularly those with FTT [65]. IGF-1 stimulates protein accretion in normal individuals, as does GH, and is probably the best-integrated indicator of GH action [66]. IGF actions at the target tissue level are modulated by high-affinity IGF binding proteins (BPs), abnormalities of which have been detected in children with HIV. Specifically, catabolic patients with AIDS have increased proteolysis of and therefore diminished serum levels of IGFBP-3, which tracks with growth [65, 67]. In HIV-infected adolescents, linear growth failure may be due in part to delayed sexual maturation [68]. Therefore, appropriate endocrinologic evaluation should be performed if FTT does not readily respond to nutritional interventions (see Chapter 28).

It is hypothesized that, in some cases, the malnutrition associated with HIV infection in children is secondary to metabolic dysregulation produced by inflammatory cytokines, analogous to HIV wasting syndrome in adults, which has been related to overproduction of tumor necrosis factor [69]. Cytokine-mediated malnutrition may overlap with endocrine dysregulation of the growth hormone axis. There is some suggestion that growth failure may be related to increased interleukin 6 activity which results in increased IGFBP-1 [43, 70]. In turn, diminished IGF-1 availability at the tissue level may impair protein accretion and affect anabolism and growth.

Effective therapeutic strategies have yet to be developed for growth failure not amenable to traditional nutritional interventions. Cytokine modulators (e.g., thalidomide) and treatment with IGF-1 may have a role but are untested in children.

In addition to growth failure, wasting syndrome remains a significant contributor to morbidity and mortality in HIV-infected children. For children with clearly diminished LBM, consideration therefore can be given to oxandrolone, but anabolic response requires adequate energy intake [71]. The maximum recommended pediatric dose is 0.1 mg/kg daily. Therapy can be repeated intermittently, as indicated.

Trials of GH in HIV-infected children are ongoing, but no definitive information is available and its use is investigational. GH, in supraphysiologic doses, does result in increases in both body weight and LBM in HIV-infected adults [72], and has an anabolic effect in HIV-infected adolescent wasting [73]. The anabolic response to GH in adults with HIV decreases with advancing disease.

Metabolic abnormalities and associated therapies

Lipodystrophy syndrome

Fat redistribution has been noted to occur in HIV-infected adults and children. It may be associated with metabolic abnormalities, most notably hyperlipidemia (with increases in low density lipoprotein (LDL) cholesterol and triglyceride levels) and insulin resistance. This triad of findings has been referred to in adults as the "fat redistribution" or "lipodystrophy" syndrome. There can be lipoatrophy (loss of subcutaneous fat) in the face, buttocks and extremities, with concomitant increase in abdominal visceral fat, increased breast size in women, and sometimes development of a dorsocervical fat pad ("buffalo hump"). Cross-sectional clinical studies find that these signs can occur in isolation, e.g., fat redistribution without metabolic changes and vice versa. Specifically, hyperlipidemias are known to occur with increased frequency in HIV-infected persons, and can occur prior to antiretroviral treatment and without noticeable body shape changes.

Those affected with any or all of the three components (insulin resistance, hyperlipidemia, and visceral adiposity) may be at increased risk of cardiovascular disease, particularly children. The etiology of this syndrome likely is multifactorial, and research into potential causes, associations and treatments continues. A complete discussion of the current state of knowledge of these metabolic alterations is beyond the scope of this chapter. More information on these abnormalities, including pathophysiology, is found in Chapter 9.

Studies in children

Research in children thus far has focused primarily on defining the prevalence of these abnormalities and associated clinical findings. Care is needed in interpreting and comparing research findings as different authors use various definitions. Fat redistribution has been reported with highly variable prevalence (18%–100%) in HIV-infected children, depending on population and methodology. Clinically evident changes have been noted in 4% to 33% in the same populations [74–78]. The prevalence of hyperlipidemia in HIV-infected children is also highly variable and depends on the definition used. Twenty-six to 73% of subjects have abnormal lipid values; hypercholesterolemia is much more common than hypertriglyceridemia, and appears to be exaggerated in those patients receiving PI therapy [75–78]. Insulin resistance, measured by fasting glucose, insulin, C-peptide levels and/or insulin:glucose ratios, has been reported in 8% to 35% of HIV-infected children, depending on the population studied [75, 77, 78].

Potential treatments

No trials in children for treatment of fat redistribution or associated metabolic abnormalities have been reported, nor is there consensus regarding whether and when fat redistribution, insulin resistance without glucose intolerance, or hyperlipidemia should be treated. A variety of treatments have been studied in HIV-infected adults with lipodystrophy syndrome, with varying success. GH administration improves morphologic abnormalities in adults with fat redistribution syndrome. It has been shown to increase LBM, reduce excess visceral adipose tissue and buffalo hump size, and increase mid-thigh circumferences [73, 79]. Metformin, an insulin-sensitizing agent, was successful in reducing abdominal adiposity and insulin resistance [80]. Trials of substituting and interrupting PI therapies have been undertaken. One randomized trial of PI substitution led to improvement in lipid levels and decreased intraabdominal fat, but peripheral lipoatrophy was exacerbated and insulin resistance unchanged [81]. Interruption of therapy for 5 to 10 weeks was noted to improve lipid levels, but had no effect on insulin resistance or anthropometric measures [82].

Preliminary guidelines for the evaluation and management of dyslipidemias in the HIV-infected adult population have been made by the Adult AIDS Clinical Trials Group Cardiovascular Disease Focus Group [83]. Their recommendations are to evaluate and treat on the basis of existing guidelines for hyperlipidemia in the general population, with the additional caveat that drug interactions with antiretrovirals should be avoided. Dietary interventions have been successful in some patients, and drug therapy with pravastatin had a similar magnitude of effect as with endogenous hyperlipidemia [84]. Atorvastatin also probably is safe in combination with PIs. Experience with these drugs in children is very limited. Fibrates are the drug of choice if hypercholesterolemia and hypertriglyceridemia both are present. Combined aerobic and resistance training in adults over 10 weeks achieved an 18% reduction in cholesterol and 25% reduction in triglyceride levels [85].

Osteopenia and osteonecrosis

Adults and children with HIV infection have been reported to be at increased risk of osteopenia. Specifically, there are three reports of decreased total bone mineral content (BMC) or bone mineral density (BMD) in HIV-infected children [86–88]. Decreased BMD was significant at all ages studied (4–17 years) and the decrement increased in magnitude with age. Association with PI therapy has not been clearly demonstrated for children, although studies in adults report increased osteopenia on HAART. No correlation between osteoporosis and fat redistribution has been demonstrated in adults, but one study documents decreased BMD in children on HAART with lipodystrophy compared to those without lipodystrophy [88].

Decreased BMD may be secondary in part to increased bone resorption as evidenced by increased serum and urine markers of bone turnover. Increased bone turnover has been reported in HIV-infected adults, both those who are untreated and in association with PI use [89]. Other evidence suggests that a decrease in bone formation may be primary [90, 91]. Calcium insufficiency may contribute to increased bone resorption in HIV-infected girls [86].

Osteonecrosis has been described with increased frequency in HIV-infected children and adults compared with the general population. The most common form of osteonecrosis in children is Legg–Calvé–Perthes disease, or osteonecrosis of the capital femoral epiphysis. Perinatally infected children have been shown to have a 4.8-fold increase in age-adjusted incidence of Legg–Calvé–Perthes disease [92]. As with studies in adults, there was no clear association with antiretroviral therapy in these children. Abnormal growth has been reported as a risk factor in the general population, and this may explain the increased risk in HIV-infected children. Thrombophilia also can be a risk factor for osteonecrosis [93], and decreased free protein S has been reported to be common in HIV-infected children [94].

Mitochondrial toxicity

An additional metabolic complication noted in HIV-infected patients who receive antiretroviral treatment is mitochondrial toxicity and a subsequent decrease in oxidative phosphorylation. A more complete discussion of this phenomenon is found in Chapter 9. Briefly, NRTI agents have been established to cause some of their toxicity *via* inhibition of the human DNA polymerase γ, the enzyme that replicates mitochondrial DNA, leading to depletion of the same [95]. As more mitochondria are affected, there may be cellular and organ dysfunction, affecting brain, peripheral nerves, kidney, heart, liver, endocrine glands, the gastrointestinal system, and bone marrow. There may be intracellular accumulation of lipids and increased lactic acid due to anaerobic metabolism. Muscle or liver biopsy is considered definitive to diagnose mitochondrial toxicity. Screening with random venous lactate levels is currently performed by some experts, but it is unclear how useful this is (due to lack of specificity, and technical and biologic variability).

Mitochondrial dysfunction is felt to contribute to NRTI side effects in adults as diverse as lactic acidosis, pancreatitis, proximal renal tubular dysfunction, hepatic steatosis, myopathy, cardiomyopathy, peripheral neuropathy, and perhaps lipodystrophy, lipoatrophy, bone marrow toxicity, and osteopenia [96]. Additionally, possible signs and symptoms in children of mitochondrial dysfunction include encephalopathy, developmental delay, hyper- or hypotonia, seizures, ataxia, blindness, retinopathy, ophthalmoplegia, deafness, and growth failure [97]. Hyperlactatemia without frank lactic acidosis can be asymptomatic (lactate levels 2.1–5 mmol/l) or symptomatic (lactate levels of 5–10 mmol/l), which in adults includes fatigue, weight loss, abdominal pain, nausea, shortness of breath, hepatic steatosis, and lipid abnormalities [95]. Asymptomatic hyperlactatemia does not appear to be a risk for more severe forms, but it is unknown if the milder symptomatic forms are at risk of progressing to fatal lactic acidosis.

Potential treatments

Management of potential mitochondrial toxicity during NRTI therapy remains a challenge. A range of treatments which protect mitochondria have been suggested by *in vitro* studies. Substitution of better tolerated alternative NRTIs or drugs of other antiretroviral classes for the probable causative agent represents the current mainstay of management for mitochondrial toxicity [98]. However, significantly lower mortality rate among patients with nucleoside-associated lactic acidosis who received therapy with an essential cofactor has been described [99]. Cofactor therapies included thiamine, riboflavin, L-carnitine, prostaglandin E or coenzyme Q, all of which have been used for congenital mitochondrial diseases.

Resource-poor settings

Discussed earlier in this chapter (see "Effects of malnutrition") was the bi-directional association between HIV morbidity and malnutrition, with most data from and recommendations primarily fashioned for resource-rich settings. Discussed below is what is known about the interaction of malnutrition and HIV infection in children in resource-poor settings, both the effect of malnutrition on HIV disease as well as the effect of HIV on malnutrition.

Malnutrition is more common by far in resource-poor compared with resource-rich settings, with associated greater risk of morbidity and mortality. Many of the excess deaths in children under 5 years of age in resource-poor settings, regardless of HIV, are attributed to nutritional immunodeficiencies, and the synergistic effect of malnutrition and infectious diseases [24]. This synergy undoubtedly contributes to more rapid disease progression and heightened mortality among HIV-infected children in resource-poor settings. The probability of death for HIV-infected children in sub-Saharan Africa aged 12 months and five years, respectively, is 0.23–0.35 and 0.57–0.68, with malnutrition one of the three most common causes of death. This compares with data from Europe prior to HAART of 0.1 and 0.2, for the same ages.

Relationships between micronutrient status and morbidity and mortality among HIV-infected and uninfected children may be different in resource-poor settings, where deficiencies are more common and/or severe. For example, perinatally HIV-exposed infants in Malawi were more likely to have growth failure or die when their mothers had low plasma vitamin A concentrations, but a study in the United States revealed no association in the general population between vitamin A status and childhood growth or mortality. HIV-infected children in the USA have been shown to have more rapid disease progression when maternal vitamin A stores were lower. As would be expected, results of vitamin A and zinc supplementation trials vary by population and risk of deficiency. Some, but not all, studies of vitamin A supplementation show dramatically reduced mortality. Incidence and severity of infections also vary by site. For example, supplemented children were hospitalized less frequently than control children in Ghana but not in Brazil. There are several trials of vitamin A supplementation in HIV-infected children. Periodic supplementation provided to HIV-infected children in Tanzania has demonstrated a large reduction in mortality in HIV-infected children [100], and a 50% reduction in diarrheal morbidity in South Africa. Vitamin A, when given prenatally to women in South Africa, had the effect of preventing subsequent deterioration of gut integrity in their HIV-infected infants [101]. Pooled analysis of randomized zinc supplementation trials in resource-poor settings has shown decreased incidence of both diarrhea and pneumonia, but the effect specifically on HIV-infected children has not been reported. Although multivitamin administration in HIV-infected pregnant women in Tanzania was shown to substantially improve CD4+ cell counts, this study has yet to be done in children [102].

HIV infection may alter the presentation of malnutrition in resource-poor settings. Zambian children who were HIV-seropositive had lower weight-for-age scores than their seronegative counterparts, but were also more likely to have marasmus compared with seronegative children, who were more likely to have kwashiorkor. Marasmus was associated with higher mortality [103].

No discussion of nutrition and pediatric HIV infection in resource-poor settings would be complete without mention of the controversy surrounding recommendations for feeding infants of HIV-infected mothers. This topic is beyond the scope of this chapter and is discussed in Chapter 4.

Future research

Despite the dramatic gains in the past decade in knowledge in many areas of pediatric HIV disease, such as prevention of mother-to-child transmission of HIV and treatment of HIV-infected children with antiretroviral drugs our understanding of the causes, effects, and appropriate interventions for malnutrition and growth failure in this population remains incomplete [104].

Little is known about prevalence of micronutrient deficiencies in HIV-infected children, or the effects of such deficiencies on disease progression. Vitamin A supplementation in resource-poor settings has been demonstrated clearly to affect mortality in these children, but it is likely that additional micronutrient and early protein/calorie supplementation could affect disease progression as well. This may be true in both resource-rich and resource-poor settings. Interventions should be studied with the aim to maintain the best possible quality of life for as long as possible.

The pathophysiology of growth failure is elusive. Our understanding even of the major determinants of poor growth remains largely speculative. Conceivably, adjunctive interventions that may improve growth, e.g., anticytokine therapies or treatment with IGF-1, may affect anabolism generally and hence disease progression and survival. More research to understand the mechanisms and consequences of poor growth in HIV-infected children and to identify safe and effective therapies clearly is needed.

The incidence, nature, and etiology of metabolic disturbances related to HIV infection and/or antiretroviral therapy are even less well understood in children than in adults. Hyperlipidemia, glucose intolerance, fat redistribution and osteopenia all have potential to affect morbidity and mortality significantly in HIV-infected children.

REFERENCES

1. Baumgartner, R. N., Roche, A. F., Himes, J. H. Incremental growth tables: supplementary to previously published charts. *Am. J. Clin. Nutr.* 1986;**43**:711–722.
2. Miller, T. L. Nutrition in paediatric human immunodeficiency virus infection. *Proc. Nutr. Soc.* 2000;**59**:155–162.
3. Beisel, W. R., Nutrition and immune function: overview. *J. Nutr.* 1996;**126**:2611–2615S.
4. Brown, K. H., Peerson, J. M., Rivera, J., Allen, L. H. Effect of supplemental zinc on the growth and serum zinc concentrations of prepubertal children: a meta-analysis of randomized controlled trials. *Am. J. Clin. Nutr.* 2002;**75**:1062–1071.
5. McKinney, R. E., Robertson, W. R. Effect of human immunodeficiency virus infection on the growth of young children. *J. Pediatr.* 1993;**123**:579–582.
6. Miller T. L., Evans, S., Morris, V., Orav, E. J., McIntosh, K., Winter, H. S. Growth and body composition in children with human immunodeficiency virus-1 infection. *Am. J. Clin. Nutr.* 1993;**57**:588–592.
7. Moye, J., Jr, Rich, K. C., Kalish, L. A. *et al.* Natural history of somatic growth in infants born to women infected by human immunodeficiency virus. *J. Pediatr.* 1996;**128**:58–67.
8. Saavedra, J. M., Henderson, R. A., Perman, J. A., Hutton, N., Livingston, R. A., Yolken, R. H. Longitudinal assessment of growth in children born to mothers with human immunodeficiency virus infection. *Arch. Pediatr. Adolesc. Med.* 1995;**149**:497–502.
9. Lindegren, M. L., Steinberg, S., Byers, R. H. Epidemiology of HIV/AIDS in children. *Pediatr. Clin. North Am.* 2000;**47**:1–20.

10. Kotler, D. P., Tierney, A. R., Wang, J., Pierson, R. N. Magnitude of body cell mass depletion and the timing of death from wasting in AIDS. *Am. J. Clin. Nutr.* 1989;**50**:444–447.

11. Chlebowski, R. T., Grosvenor, M. B., Berhard, N. H., Morales, L. S., Bulcavage, L. M. Nutritional status, gastrointestinal dysfunction, and survival in patients with AIDS. *Am. J. Gastroenterol.* 1989;**84**:1288–1293.

12. Lai, H., Lai, S., Shor-Posner, G., Ma, F., Trapido, E., Baum, M. K. Plasma zinc, copper, copper:zinc ratio, and survival in a cohort of HIV-1-infected homosexual men. *J. Acquir. Immune Defic. Syndr.* 2001;**27**:56–62.

13. Tang, A. M., Graham, N. M. H., Semba, R. D., Saah, A. J. Association between serum vitamin A and E levels and HIV-1 disease progression. *AIDS* 1997;**11**:613–620.

14. Baum, M. K., Shor-Posner, G., Lu, Y. *et al.* Micronutrients and HIV-1 disease progression. *AIDS* 1995;**9**:1051–1056.

15. Cunningham-Rundles, S., Ahrn, S., Abuav-Nussbaum, R., Dnistrian, A. Development of immunocompetence: role of micronutrients and microorganisms. *Nutr. Rev.* 2002;**60**:S68–S72.

16. Chantry, C., Byrd, R., Englund, J., Baker, C., McKinney, R., PACTG 152 Team. Growth, survival. and viral load in childhood HIV infection. *Pediatr. Infect. Dis. J.* 2003;**22**(12):1033–1039.

17. McKinney, R. E., Jr, Wilfert, C. Growth as a prognostic indicator in children with human immunodeficiency virus infection treated with zidovudine. AIDS Clinical Trials Group Protocol 043 Study Group. *J. Pediatr.* 1994; **125**: 728–733.

18. Berhane, R., Bagenda, D., Marum, L. *et al.* Growth failure as a prognostic indicator of mortality in pediatric HIV infection. *Pediatrics* 1997;**100**:e7.

19. Yong, F. H., Stanley, K., McKinney, R. E. *et al.* Prognostic value of plasma RNA, CDR, and growth markers for clinical disease progression in children with HIV disease. *Intersci. Conf. Antimicrob. Agents Chemother.* (ICAAC) 1998;**38**:364 [Abstract I-7].

20. Campa, A., Shor-Posner, G., Indacochea, F. *et al.* Mortality risk in selenium-deficient HIV-positive children. *J. Acquir. Immune Defic. Syndr. Hum. Retrovirol.* 1999;**20**:508–513.

21. Duggan, C., Fawzi, W. Micronutrients and child health: studies in international nutrition and HIV infection. *Nutr. Rev.* 2001;**59**:358–369.

22. Rodríguez, J. F., Cordero, J., Chantry, C. J. *et al.* Glutathione levels in HIV-infected children. *Pediatr. Infect. Dis. J.* 1998;**17**:236–241.

23. Omene, J. A., Easington, C. R., Glew, R. H., Prosper, M., Ledlie, S. Serum beta-carotene deficiency in HIV-infected children. *J. Natl Med. Assoc.* 1996;**88**:789–793.

24. Fawzi, W. W., Mbise, R. L., Hertzmark, E. *et al.* A randomized trial of vitamin A supplements in relation to mortality among human immunodeficiency virus-infected and uninfected children in Tanzania. *Pediatr. Infect. Dis. J.* 1999;**18**:127–133.

25. Fontana, M., Zuin, G., Plebani, A. *et al.* Body composition in HIV-infected children: relations with disease progression and survival. *Am. J. Clin. Nutr.* 1999;**69**:1282–1286.

26. Arpadi, S. M., Cuff, P. A., Kotler, D. P. *et al.* Growth velocity, fat-free mass and energy intake are inversely related to viral load in HIV-infected children. *J. Nutr.* 2000;**130**:2498–2502.

27. Moye, J., Frederick, M., Chantry, C. *et al.* for the Women and Infants Transmission Study. 10-year follow-up of somatic growth in children born to women infected by human

immunodeficiency virus. *8th Conference on Retroviruses Opportunistic Infections* 2001 Feb 4–8; [Abstract 514].

28. Pollack, H., Glasberg, H., Lee, E. *et al.* Impaired early growth of infants perinatally infected with human immunodeficiency virus: correlation with viral load. *J. Pediatr.* 1997;**130**:915–922.

29. Miller, T. L., Easley, K. A., Zhang, W. *et al.* for the Pediatric Pulmonary and Cardiovascular Complications of Vertically Transmitted HIV Infection (P2C2 HIV) Study Group, Maternal and infant factors associated with failure to thrive in children with vertically transmitted human immunodeficiency virus-1 infection: The prospective, P2C2 human immunodeficiency virus multicenter study. *Pediatrics* 2001;**108**:1287–1296.

30. Hilgartner, M. W., Donfield, S. M., Lynn, H. S. *et al.* The effect of plasma human immunodeficiency virus RNA and CD4+ T lymphocytes on growth measurements of hemophilic boys and adolescents. *Pediatrics* 2001;**107**:e56.

31. Buchacz, K., Cervia, J. S., Lindsey, J. C. *et al.* for the Pediatric AIDS Clinical Trials Group 219 Study Team. Impact of protease inhibitor-containing combination antiretroviral therapies on height and weight growth in HIV-infected children. *Pediatrics* 2001;**108**:e72.

32. Verweel, G., van Rossum, A. M. C., Hartwig, N. G., Wolfs, T. F., Scherpbier, H. J., de Groot, R. Treatment with highly active antiretroviral therapy in human immunodeficiency virus type-1-infected children is associated with a sustained effect on growth. *Pediatrics* 2002;**109**:e25.

33. Dunn, A. M., Cervia, J., Burgess, A. *et al.* Failure to thrive in the HIV-infected child. *11th Int Conf AIDS* 1996; **1**:319. [Abstract 2312]

34. Heller, L. S. Nutritional support for children with HIV / AIDS. *AIDS Reader* 2000;**10**:109–114.

35. Allard, J. P., Aghdassi, E., Chau, J., Salit, I., Walmsley, S. Oxidative stress and plasma antioxidant micronutrients in humans with HIV infection. *Am. J. Clin. Nutr.* 1998;**67**:1443–1447.

36. Mintz, M.. Carnitine in human immunodeficiency virus type 1 infection/acquired immune deficiency syndrome. *J. Child. Neurol.* 1995;**10**:2S40–2S44.

37. Haug, C. J., Aukrust, P., Haug, E., Morkrid, L., Muller, F., Froland, S. S. Severe deficiency of 1,25-dihydroxyvitamin D3 in human immunodeficiency virus infection: association with immunological hyperactivity and only minor changes in calcium homeostasis. *J. Clin. Endocrinol. Metab.* 1998;**83**:3832–3838.

38. Henderson, R. A., Talusan, K., Hutton, N., Yolken, R. H., Caballero, B. Serum and plasma markers of nutritional status in children infected with the human immunodeficiency virus. *J. Am. Diet. Assoc.* 1997;**97**:1377–1381.

39. Skurnick, J. H., Bogden, J. D., Baker, H. *et al.* Micronutrient profiles in HIV-1-infected heterosexual adults. *J. Acquir. Immune Defic. Syndr.* 1996;**12**:75–83.

40. Horlick, M., Arpadi, S. M., Bethel, J. *et al.* Bioelectrical impedance analysis models for prediction of total body water and fat-free mass in healthy and HIV-infected children and adolescents. *Am. J. Clin. Nutr.* 2002;**76**:991–999.

41. Freedman, D. S., Serdula, M. K., Srnivasan, S. R., Berenson, G. S. Relation of circumferences and skinfold thicknesses to lipid and insulin concentrations in children and adolescents: the Bogalusa Heart Study. *Am. J. Clin. Nutr.* 1999;**69**:308–317.

42. Goran, M. I., Gower, B. A., Treuth, M., Nagy, T. R. Prediction of intra-abdominal and subcutaneous abdominal adipose tissue in healthy pre-pubertal children. *Int. J. Obes. Relat. Metab. Disord.* 1998;**22**:549–568.

43. Johann-Liang, R., O'Neill, L., Cervia, J. *et al.* Energy balance, viral burden, insulin-like growth factor-1, interleukin-6 and growth impairment in children infected with human immunodeficiency virus. *AIDS* 2000;**14**:683–690.

44. Guo, S., Roche, A. F., Foman, S. J. *et al.* Reference data on gains in weight and length during the first two years of life. *J. Pediatr.* 1991;**119**:355–362.

45. Karlberg, P., Taranger, J., Engstrom, I. *et al.* I. Physical growth from birth to 16 years and longitudinal outcome of the study during the same age period. *Acta Pediatr. Scand. Suppl.* 1976;**258**:7–76.

46. Sentongo, T. A., Rutstein, R. M., Stettler, N. *et al.* Association between steatorrhea, growth, and immunologic status in children with perinatally acquired HIV infection. *Arch. Pediatr. Adolesc. Med.* 2001;**155**:149–153.

47. Alfaro, M. P., Siegel, R. M., Baker, R. C., Heubi, J. E. Resting energy expenditure and body composition in pediatric HIV infection. *Pediatr. AIDS HIV Infect* 1995;**6**: 276–280.

48. Henderson, R. A., Talusan, K., Hutton, N., Yolken, R. H., Caballero, B. Resting energy expenditure and body composition in children with HIV infection. *J. Acquir. Immune Defic. Syndr. Hum. Retrovirol.* 1998;**19**:150–157.

49. Clarick, R. H., Hanekom, W. A., Yogev, R., Chadwick, E. G. Megestrol acetate treatment of growth failure in children infected with human immunodeficiency virus. *Pediatrics* 1997;**99**:354–357.

50. Mann, M., Koller, E., Murgo, A., Malozowski, S., Bacsanyi, J., Leinung, M. Glucocorticoid like activity of megestrol: a summary of Food and Drug Administration experience and a review of the literature. *Arch. Intern. Med.* 1997;**15**:1651–1656.

51. Stockheim, J. A., Daaboul, J. J., Yogev, R., Scully, S. P., Binns, H. J. Chadwick, E. G. Adrenal suppression in children with the human immunodeficiency virus treated with megestrol acetate. *J. Pediatr.* 2000;**137**(1):141–142.

52. Chantry, C., González de Pijem, L., Febo, I., Lugo, L. Adrenal suppression secondary to megestrol acetate in HIV-infected children. *12th International Conference on AIDS* 1998;**610**. [Abstract 32445].

53. Brady, M. T., Korany, K. I., Hunkler, J. A. Megestrol acetate for the treatment of anorexia associated with human immunodeficiency virus infection in children. *Pediatr. Inf. Dis. J.* 1994;**13**:754–756.

54. Briefel, R. R., Woteki, C. E. Development of food sufficiency questions for the Third National Health and Nutrition Examination Survey. *J. Nutr. Education* 1992;**24**:24S–28S.

55. Henderson, R. A., Saavedra, J. M., Perman, J. A., Hutton, N., Livingston, R. A., Yolken, R.H. Effect of enteral tube feeding on growth of children with symptomatic immunodeficiency virus infection. *J. Pediatr. Gastroenterol. Nutr.* 1994;**18**:429–434.

56. Miller, T. L., Awnetwant, E. L., Evans, S., Morris, V. M., Vazquez, I. M., McIntosh, K. Gastrostomy tube supplementation for HIV infected children. *Pediatrics* 1995;**96**:696–702.

57. Sinden, A. A., Dillard, V. L., Sutphen, J. L. Enteral nutrition. Chapter 41, Part 5. Walker, W. A., Durie, P. R., Hamilton, J. R., Walker-Smith, J. A., Watkins, J. B., eds. *Pediatric Gastrointestinal Disease.* Philadelphia, PA, USA: BC Decker, Inc., 1991;1636.

58. Miller, T. L., Orav, E. J., Martin, S. R. *et al.* Malnutrition and carbohydrate malabsorption in children with vertically-transmitted human immunodeficiency virus-1 infection. *Gastroenterology* 1991;**100**:1296–1302.

59. The Italian Pediatric Intestinal/HIV Study Group. Intestinal malabsorption of HIV-infected children: relationship to diarrhea, failure to thrive, enteric micro-organisms and immune impairment. *AIDS* 1993;**7**:1435–1440.

60. Mulligan, K., Tai, V. W., Schambelan, M. Energy expenditure in human immunodeficiency virus infection [letter]. *N. Engl. J. Med.* 1997;**70**:70–71.

61. Chiarelli, F., Galli, L., Verrotti, A., diRocco, L., Vierucci, A., de Martino, M. Thyroid function in children with perinatal human immunodeficiency virus type 1 infection. *Thyroid* 2000;**10**:499–505.

62. Laue, L., Pizzo, P. A., Butler, K., Cutler, G. B., Jr. Growth and neuroendocrine dysfunction in children with acquired immunodeficiency syndrome. *J. Pediatr.* 1990;**117**:541–545.

63. Jospe, N., Powell, K. R. Growth hormone deficiency in an 8-year old girl with human immunodeficiency virus infection. *Pediatrics* 1990;**86**:309–312.

64. Cieslak, T. J., Ascher, D. P., Zimmerman, P. A. *et al.* Adrenal insufficiency presenting as HIV wasting syndrome in a child: initial successful response to megestrol. *Pediatr. AIDS HIV Infect.* 1991;**2**:279–283.

65. Frost, R. A., Nachman, S. A., Lang, C. H., Gelato, M. C. Proteolysis of insulin-like growth factor-binding protein-3 in human immunodeficiency virus-positive children with failure to thrive. *J. Clin. Endocrinol. Metab.*, 1996;**81**:2957–2962.

66. Guyda, H. J. How do we best measure growth hormone action? *Horm. Res.* 1997; **48** Suppl 5:1–10.

67. Gelato, M. C., Frost, R. A. IGFBP-3. Functional and structural implications in aging and wasting syndromes. *Endocrine* 1997;**7**(1): 81–85.

68. Mahoney, E. M., Donfield, S. M., Howard, C., Kaufman, F., Gerner, J. M. HIV-associated immune dysfunction and delayed pubertal development in a cohort of young hemophiliacs. Hemophilia Growth and Development Study. *J. Acquir. Immune Defic. Syndr.* 1999;**21**:333–337.

69. Arnalich, F., Martinez, P., Hernanz, A. *et al.* Altered concentrations of appetite regulators may contribute to the development and maintenance of HIV-associated wasting. *AIDS* 1997;**11**:1129–1134.

70. de Martino, M., Galli, L., Chiarelli, F. *et al.* Interleukin-6 release by cultured peripheral blood mononuclear cells inversely correlates with height velocity, bone age, insulin-like growth factor-I, and insulin-like growth factor binding protein-3 serum levels in children with perinatal HIV-1 infection. *Clin. Immunol.* 2000; **94**:212–218.

71. Fox-Wheeler, S., Heller, L., Salata, C. M. *et al.* Evaluation of the effects of oxandrolone on malnourished HIV-positive pediatric patients. *Pediatrics* 1999;**104**:e73.

72. Lo, J. C., Mulligan, K., Noor, M. A. *et al.* The effects of recombinant human growth hormone on body composition and glucose metabolism in HIV-infected patients with fat accumulation. *J. Clin. Endocrinol. Metab.* 2001;**8**:3480–3487.

73. Dreimane, D., Gallagher, K., Nielsen, K. *et al.* Growth hormone exerts potent anabolic effects in an adolescent with human immunodeficiency virus wasting. *Pediatr. Infect. Dis. J.* 1999;**18**:167–169.

74. Brambilla, P., Bricalli, D., Sala, N. *et al*. Highly active antiretroviral-treated HIV-infected children show fat distribution changes even in absence of lipodystrophy. *AIDS* 2001;**15**:2415–2422.

75. Arpadi, S. M., Cuff, P. A., Horlick, M., Wang, J., Kotler, D. R. Lipodystrophy in HIV-infected children is associated with high viral load and low CD4+-lymphocyte count and CD4+-lymphocyte percentage at baseline and use of protease inhibitors and stavudine. *J. Acquir. Immune Defic. Syndr.* 2001;**27**:30–34.

76. Melvin, A. J., Lennon, S., Mohan, K. M., Purnell, J. Q. Metabolic abnormalities in HIV type 1-infected children treated and not treated with protease inhibitors. *AIDS Res. Hum. Retroviruses* 2001;**17**:1117–1123.

77. Amaya, R. A., Kozinetz, C. A., McMeans, A., Schwarzwald, H., Kline, M. W. Lipodystrophy syndrome in human immunodeficiency virus-infected children. *Pediatr. Infect. Dis. J.* 2002;**21**:405–410.

78. Jaquet, D., Levine, M., Ortega-Rodriguez, E. *et al*. Clinical and metabolic presentation of the lipodystrophic syndrome in HIV-infected children. *AIDS* 2000;**14**:2123–2128.

79. Wanke, C., Gerrior, J., Kantaros, J., Coakley, E., Albrecht, M. Recombinant human growth hormone improves the fat redistribution syndrome (lipodystrophy) in patients with HIV. *AIDS* 1999;**13**:2099–2103.

80. Hadigan, C., Corcoran, C., Basgoz, N., Davis, B., Sax, P., Grinspoon, S. Metformin in the treatment of HIV lipodystrophy syndrome: a randomized controlled trial. *J. Am. Med. Assoc.* 2000;**284**:472–477.

81. Carr, A., Hudson, J., Chuah, J. *et al*. HIV protease inhibitor substitution in patients with lipodystrophy: a randomized, controlled, open-label, multicentre study. *AIDS* 2001;**15**:1811–1822.

82. Hatano, H., Miller, K. D., Yoder, C. P. *et al*. Metabolic and anthropometric consequences of interruption of highly active antiretroviral therapy. *AIDS* 2000;**14**:1935–1942.

83. Dube, M. P., Sprecher, D., Henry, W. K. *et al*. Preliminary guidelines for the evaluation and management of dyslipidemia in adults infected with human immunodeficiency virus and receiving antiretroviral therapy: recommendations of the Adult AIDS Clinical Trial Group Cardiovascular Disease Focus Group. *Clin. Infect. Dis.* 2000;**31**:1216–1224.

84. Moyle, G. J., Lloyd, M., Reynolds, B., Baldwin, C., Mandalia, S., Gazzord, B. G. Dietary advice with or without pravastatin for the management of hypercholesterolaemia associated with protease inhibitor therapy. *AIDS* 2001;**15**:1503–1508.

85. Jones, S. P., Doran, D. A., Leatt, P. B., Maher, B., Pirmohamed, M. Short-term exercise training improves body composition and hyperlipidaemia in HIV-positive individuals with lipodystrophy. [letter] *AIDS* 2001;**15**:2049–2051.

86. O'Brien, K. O., Razavi, M., Henderson, R. A., Caballero, B., Ellis, K. J. Bone mineral content in girls perinatally infected with HIV. *Am. J. Clin. Nutr.* 2001;**73**:821–826.

87. Arpadi, S. M., Horlick, M., Thornton, J. *et al*. Bone mineral content is lower in prepubertal HIV-infected children. *J. Acquir. Immune Defic. Syndr.* 2002;**29**:450–454.

88. Mora, S., Sala, N., Bricalli, D. *et al*. Bone mineral loss through increased bone turnover in HIV-infected children treated with highly active antiretroviral therapy. *AIDS* 2001;**15**:1823–1829.

89. Tebas, P., Powderly, W. G., Claxton, S. *et al*. Accelerated bone mineral loss in HIV-infected patients receiving potent antiretroviral therapy. *AIDS* 2000;**14**:F63–F67.

90. Aukrust, P., Haug, C. J., Ueland, T. *et al*. Decreased bone formative and enhanced resorptive markers in human immunodeficiency virus infection: indication of normalization of the bone-remodeling process during highly active antiretroviral therapy. *J. Clin. Endocrinol. Metab.* 1999;**84**:145–150.

91. Tan, B. M., Nelson, R. P., James-Yarish, M., Emmanuel, P. J., Schurman, S. J. Bone metabolism in children with human immunodeficiency virus infection receiving highly active anti-retroviral therapy including a protease inhibitor. *J. Pediatr.* 2001;**139**:447–451.

92. Gaughan, D. M., Mofenson, L. M., Hughes, M. D., Seage, G. R. 3rd, Ciupak, G. L., Oleske, J. M. Osteonecrosis of the hip (Legg–Calve–Perthes disease) in human immunodeficiency virus-infected children. *Pediatrics* 2002;**109**:e74.

93. Sugerman, R. W., Church, J. A., Goldsmith, J. C., Ens, G. E. Acquired protein S deficiency in children infected with human immunodeficiency virus. *Pediatr. Infect. Dis. J.* 1996; **15**: 106–111.

94. Eldridge, J., Dilley, A., Austin, H. *et al*. The role of protein C, protein S, and resistance to activated protein C in Legg–Perthes disease. *Pediatrics* 2001; **107**: 1329–1334.

95. Cote, H. C., Brumme, Z. L., Craib, K. J. *et al*. Changes in mitochondrial DNA as a marker of nucleoside toxicity in HIV-infected patients. *N. Engl. J. Med.* 2002;**346**:811–820.

96. Glesby, M. J. Overview of mitochondrial toxicity of nucleoside reverse transcriptase inhibitors. *Top. HIV Med.* 2002;**10**:42–46.

97. The Perinatal Safety Review Working Group. Nucleoside exposure in the children of HIV-infected women receiving antiretroviral drugs: absence of clear evidence for mitochondrial disease in children who died before 5 years of age in five United States cohorts. *J. Acquir. Immune Defic. Syndr.* 2000;**25**:261–268.

98. Moyle, G. Clinical manifestations and management of antiretroviral nucleoside analog-related mitochondrial toxicity. *Clin. Ther.* 2000;**22**:911–936.

99. Falco, V., Rodriguez, D., Ribera, E. *et al*. Severe nucleoside-associated lactic acidosis in human immunodeficiency virus-infected patients: report of 12 cases and review of the literature. *Clin. Infect. Dis.* 2002;**34**:838–846.

100. Fawzi, W. W., Mbise, R. L., Hertzmark, E. *et al*. A randomized trial of vitamin A supplements in relation to mortality among human immunodeficiency virus-infected and uninfected children in Tanzania. *Pediatr. Infect. Dis. J.* 1999;**18**:127–133.

101. Filteau, S. M., Rollins, N. C., Coutsoudis, A., Sullivan, K. R., Willumsen, J. F., Tomkins, A. N. The effect of antenatal vitamin A and beta-carotene supplementation on gut integrity of infants of HIV-infected South African women. *J. Pediatr. Gastroenterol. Nutr.* 2001;**32**:464–470.

102. Fawzi, W. W., Msamanga, G. I., Spiegelman, D. *et al*. Randomised trial of effects of vitamin supplements on pregnancy outcomes and T cell counts in HIV-1 infected women in Tanzania. *Lancet* 1998;**351**:1477–1482.

103. Amadi, B., Kelly, P., Mwiya, M. *et al*. Intestinal and systemic infection, HIV, and mortality in Zambian children with persistent diarrhea and malnutrition. *J. Pediatr. Gastroenterol. Nutr.* 2001;**32**:550–554.

104. Stevenson, R. Use of segmental measures to estimate stature in children with cerebral palsy. *Arch. Pediatr. Adolesc. Med.* 1995;**149**:658–662.

10 Neurobehavioral function and assessment of children and adolescents with HIV-1 infection

Pamela L. Wolters, Ph.D. and Pim Brouwers, Ph.D.

HIV and AIDS Malignancy Branch, National Cancer Institute and Medical Illness Counseling Center, Bethesda, MD

Texas Children's Cancer & Sickle Cell Centers and Baylor College of Medicine, Houston, TX

Children infected with human immunodeficiency virus-type 1 (HIV-1) are at increased risk for central nervous system (CNS) disease characterized by cognitive, language, motor, and behavioral impairments. The severity of HIV-related CNS manifestations in children ranges from subtle impairments in selective domains to severe deterioration of global developmental skills.

HIV-related CNS dysfunction in children is primarily the result of HIV-1 infection in the brain [1, 2]. Various host or viral neurotoxic factors are postulated as the main cause of neurologic damage as neurons seem to remain largely uninfected [1, 3]. Secondary CNS complications due to immune deficiency, such as brain tumors, other infections, or cerebrovascular diseases, also may cause CNS manifestations but are less common and usually occur in older children [4].

Early in the epidemic, approximately 50% to 90% of children with HIV-1 infection exhibited severe CNS manifestations [5, 6] termed HIV encephalopathy. More recent studies, however, report that the prevalence of encephalopathy in HIV-infected children is approximately 13% to 23% percent [7–10]. This decline in the prevalence of severe HIV-related CNS manifestations may be related in part to the earlier and more generalized use of combination antiretroviral treatment (ART), including highly active antiretroviral therapy (HAART) [11–14]. HAART is effective in suppressing systemic viral replication [15], which in turn may reduce the number of HIV-infected cells entering the CNS. However, the CNS is a separate compartment from the rest of the body and it may serve as a reservoir for persistent HIV-1 infection [16]. Many antiretroviral agents, including protease inhibitors (PIs), do not penetrate well into the CNS [17, 18]. Thus, combination ART may provide systemic benefits but not be as effective in treating the CNS [19] so that HIV-infected patients with well-controlled systemic disease may still be at risk for developing CNS manifestations.

Handbook of Pediatric HIV Care, ed. Steven L. Zeichner and Jennifer S. Read.
Published by Cambridge University Press. © Cambridge University Press 2006.

In addition to the effects of HIV-1 on the developing brain, other medical and environmental risk factors can contribute to neurobehavioral abnormalities in infected children. Thus, the assessment of neurobehavioral functioning throughout childhood and adolescence is warranted to monitor these effects, evaluate response to antiretroviral therapy, and plan interventions.

Clinical presentation of HIV-related CNS disease in children

Pediatric HIV-related encephalopathy has characteristic features and distinct patterns although it varies in onset, severity, and prevalence in different subgroups. Factors associated with variations in the presentation of HIV-related CNS manifestations include age at infection, route and timing of transmission, maternal and child disease status, genetic factors, treatment history, and other medical and environmental conditions.

Infants and young children tend to exhibit the highest rates of HIV-related CNS disease and the most severe neurodevelopmental impairments [20–22], while older children and adolescents tend to have the lowest rates and less severe manifestations [7, 22, 23]. The greatest risk for encephalopathy occurs during the first year of life, when it is often the initial AIDS-defining symptom [8–10, 24]. Children with early onset of HIV encephalopathy, before the age of 1 year, have smaller head circumference and lower body weight at birth, suggesting a different pathophysiology compared to later occurring encephalopathy [10]. Older children and adolescents may develop CNS complications several years after infection during more advanced stages of the disease [24, 25].

Vertically infected children with in utero transmission (positive HIV-1 cultures or DNA PCR at birth) display more severe HIV disease [26] and poorer neurodevelopmental function [27] compared to children with presumed intrapartum infection. Children with vertically acquired infection tend to have more severe CNS manifestations than children who were infected via blood or blood products, even in the neonatal period [24]. Adolescents infected with HIV, often through sexual transmission, also appear to have fewer CNS symptoms with a clinical presentation resembling that seen in adults [25].

The risk of encephalopathy is higher in HIV-infected children born to mothers with more advanced disease as measured by CD4 cell count and viral load at the time of delivery [28]. In addition, high plasma viral loads [9, 10, 29, 30], more severe immunodeficiency early in life [8–10, 26], and genetic factors in the child [31, 32] are associated with more rapid HIV disease progression, including encephalopathy. HIV-1-infected children who are naive to ART [22] or who might be on monotherapy [23] appear to be at greater risk of developing CNS manifestations than children on combination ART, such as HAART [14]. However, children with HIV-1 infection exposed to zidovudine in utero and for 6 weeks after birth did not differ in the incidence of encephalopathy or level of cognitive function compared to children who had not been treated [10, 33].

Finally, other medical and environmental conditions, such as substance abuse during pregnancy, low birthweight, preterm birth, exposure to toxic substances (i.e., lead), other CNS infections, impoverished socioeconomic and environmental background, and psychosocial difficulties, also may negatively influence the development of children with HIV-1 infection. As vertically-infected children live longer, such conditions will have a greater impact on neurobehavioral function and need to be considered when assessing the effects of HIV-1 on the developing CNS.

Patterns of HIV-related CNS disease in children

Despite variations in the presentation of CNS disease among different subgroups of children with HIV-1 infection, three main patterns have been described: encephalopathy, CNS compromise, and apparently not compromised [34, 35].

HIV-related encephalopathy is characterized by pervasive and severe CNS dysfunction. Children with HIV-related encephalopathy exhibit global impairments in cognitive, language, motor, and social skills as well as significant neurologic impairments that affect their day-to-day functioning. Differential deficits may be observed in selective functions such as expressive language or gross motor skills. HIV-related encephalopathy can be progressive (subacute or plateau subtypes) or static [36–38]. Subacute progressive encephalopathy, the most severe subtype, is characterized by progressive, global deterioration and loss of previously acquired abilities and skills. In the plateau course of progressive encephalopathy, the acquisition of new skills significantly slows or stops, but previously acquired milestones are not lost. Both subacute and plateau subtypes result in a significant decline in standardized scores on repeated neurodevelopmental testing. Children with static encephalopathy continue to consistently gain new skills and abilities but at a slower rate than normal, thus, their standardized tests scores are below average but remain stable over time. Pediatric HIV encephalopathy appears to be less prevalent in the HAART era, with new cases of encephalopathy seen mostly in very young children [7–10], particularly those naive to ART [22], and older children in advanced stages of HIV disease [25]. In the revised CDC classification system for HIV infection in children less than 13 years of age, encephalopathy is a condition listed in Category C [39].

HIV-related CNS compromise is characterized by overall cognitive functioning that is within normal limits but with a significant decline in psychometric test scores or deficit in one or more selective neurobehavioral functions [35, 40]. Patients who were functioning within normal limits but exhibited significant improvements after initiation or change in antiretroviral therapy also are included in this category. Children with HIV-related CNS compromise continue to have adequate functioning in school and activities of daily living. With the widespread availability of HAART, children displaying CNS disease are more likely to exhibit this more subtle form of CNS compromise rather than the more severe and pervasive encephalopathy that was frequently seen during the first decade of the AIDS epidemic. CNS compromise is not yet a condition listed in the revised CDC classification system for HIV infection in children [39].

The CNS of children is considered to be *apparently not compromised* by HIV when their cognitive functioning is at least within the normal range and without evidence of HIV-associated significant deficits, decline in functioning, neurological abnormalities that affect day-to-day functioning, or therapy-related improvements.

When review of medical, developmental, and family history suggests that factors other than HIV most likely explain the neurobehavioral deficits, children also may have non-HIV-related CNS impairments. It is possible for children to exhibit both HIV and *non-HIV-related impairments*. Determining whether developmental deficits are related to HIV-1 disease or other etiologies is complex but important for making treatment decisions.

The specific criteria used by the neurobehavioral team at the HIV and AIDS Malignancy Branch of the National Cancer Institute to classify the above patterns of CNS disease in children with HIV-1 infection is presented in Table 10.1. These criteria were developed to determine a child's CNS classification in a consistent and objective manner to help standardize neurobehavioral research efforts in pediatric AIDS.

Domains of neuropsychological impairment
General cognitive function
In children with frank HIV encephalopathy, the effects of the disease on the CNS tend to be generalized with cognitive function and brain structures severely and globally affected [35, 37, 41] although some domains (i.e., receptive/expressive language, gross/fine motor) may be differentially impaired. Furthermore, overall measures of general cognitive functioning are sensitive to HIV-related changes in the CNS and correlate well with biological data, such as brain imaging [41, 42], cerebrospinal fluid (CSF) analysis [2, 43] and virological and immunological parameters [44]. However, in children with less severe CNS manifestations, mild atrophy tends to be more anterior than posterior [45]. Thus, selective functions may be differentially affected by HIV while general cognitive ability is preserved, particularly in less advanced stages of disease. Neuropsychological features characteristic of pediatric HIV disease are described below by various domains of functioning.

Language
Children with symptomatic HIV-1 disease frequently exhibit speech and language deficits [6, 46–48], which may appear prior to declines in general cognitive function [46, 49] and even when receiving ART [49]. Expressive language is significantly more impaired than receptive language. Although children with encephalopathy exhibit more deficient overall language skills than non-encephalopathic children, the discrepancy between receptive and expressive language is similar for both these groups [48]. Uninfected siblings score higher than their HIV-positive siblings on both expressive

Table 10.1. Specific criteria for classification of HIV-related CNS disease in children used at the HIV and AIDS Malignancy Branch of the National Cancer Institute

HIV-related encephalopathy
(One or more of the following criteria must be met):
- loss of previously acquired skills;
- significant drop in cognitive test scores, generally to the borderline/delayed range with functional deficits (deficits in day-to-day functioning);
- cognitive test scores are in the borderline delayed range with functional deficits (and no history of significant drop or previous testing available);
- significantly abnormal neurologic examination with functional deficits (i.e., significant tone, reflex, cerebellar, gait, or movement abnormalities);
- significant improvement in cognitive test scores over approximately a 6-month period associated with a new treatment when baseline scores are in the borderline to delayed range (no history of previous testing) with or without significant brain imaging or neurologic abnormalities (retrospective classification).

Subtypes of HIV encephalopathy:

- *Progressive*:
  - *Subacute*–children exhibit a loss of previously acquired skills, resulting in a significant decline in raw and standard score on psychometric tests, and new neurologic abnormalities.
  - *Plateau*–children either do not gain further skills or exhibit a slowed rate of development compared to their previous rate of development, resulting in a significant drop in standard scores on psychometric tests.
- *Static*: children exhibit consistent but slower than normal development in the delayed range or their neuropsychological functioning remains stable for at least 1 year after a significant decline (IQ scores remain below average and without significant decline for at least 1 year).

HIV-related CNS compromise
(One or more of the following criteria must be met):
- significant drop in cognitive test scores, but generally still above the delayed range, with or without mild brain imaging abnormalities, with no loss of previously acquired skills and no apparent functional deficits (adaptive behavior and school performance stable); or
- cognitivetest scores in the borderline range, with no significant functional deficits (and no history of significant drop or previous testing);
- cognitive test scores within normal limits (low average range or above) with no significant functional deficits and moderate to severe brain imaging abnormalities consistent with HIV-related changes;
- abnormal neurologic findings but not significantly affecting function;
- significant improvement in cognitive test scores over approximately a 6-month period associated with a new treatment when **baseline** scores are in the low average to average

(*cont.*)

Table 10.1. (*cont.*)

range (no history of previous testing) and no neurologic or brain imaging abnormalities (retrospective classification).

<u>Non-HIV-related CNS condition</u>

– overall cognitive scores or selective areas of deficits below the low average range, but careful review of medical and family history suggests factors other than HIV disease most likely explain the low scores.

<u>Considerations for classification of HIV encephalopathy or CNS compromise</u>

– no other factors can reasonably explain the drop in cognitive test scores, compromised/delayed cognitive functioning, and/or abnormal neurologic exam (such as myopathy, neuropathy, cord lesions, CNS opportunistic infections, neoplasms, or vascular diseases, non-HIV-related developmental or learning disabilities, behavioral problems, or psychosocial/environmental circumstances), and the impairments are considered most likely due to HIV, classify as either HIV-related encephalopathy or CNS compromise (depending on the criteria met).

– if other factors (i.e., behavioral, acute illness, other infection, etc.) may *possibly* explain the drop in scores or low cognitive functioning, do *not* classify as HIV-related CNS compromise or encephalopathy and re-evaluate at a later time.

<u>Definitions used in the criteria:</u>
<u>Significant decline in cognitive function:</u>
For infants from birth to 42 months (on the Bayley Scales)[a]

• a decline of 2 standard deviations (30 points) in the Mental Developmental Index (MDI) on the Bayley Scales, or
• a decline of 1 standard deviation (15 points) in the MDI to the mildly delayed range or below on the Bayley Scales (< 85), maintained over 2 assessments (separated by at least 1 month), or
• a loss of raw score over any period greater/equal to 2 months.

For children > 30 months (on IQ tests)[a]

• a loss of $\geq$ 1 standard deviation in McCarthy GCI (16 points) or Wechsler (WISC-III & WAIS-R) Full Scale IQ (15 points) *and* at least 15%, or
• a loss of $\geq$ 20 IQ points in *either* the Verbal or Performance IQ,
[a] the significant drop in scores occurs within approximately 1 year.
[a] cannot attribute the decline in cognitive functioning to other factors (such as change in test, behavioral/emotional factors, lack of appropriate schooling, acute illness, medication effects, other diseases of the CNS, etc.)

<u>Significant improvement in cognitive function:</u>
For infants from birth to 42 months (on the Bayley Scales)[b]

• an increase of 1 to 2 standard deviations in the MDI (15 to 30 points) maintained over at least 2 assessments, dependent in part on the age of the child.

For children > 30 months (on IQ tests)[b]

• the same degree of change as with a significant decline, except test scores increase rather than decrease.
[b] occurs within approximately 6 months of starting a new antiretroviral treatment.
[b] cannot be attributed to other factors, such as a change in environment of caregivers, effect of other medications, improvement in test behavior, etc.

Table 10.1. (*cont.*)

Ranges used in the Criteria:

Cognitive Functioning:		Brain Imaging:
Average range	90–110	–Degree of cortical atrophy (mild = 1, moderate = 2, severe = 3)
Low average range	80–89	–Absence = 0/presence = 1 of basal ganglia calcifications
Borderline range	70–79	
Delayed range	< 70	*Rating of severity*:
		Mild = 1
		Moderate = 2
		Severe = 3 +

This pediatric HIV CNS classification system was developed by Wolters, Brouwers, and Civitello.

and receptive language tests and do not exhibit a discrepancy between these two language components [48] suggesting that the deficit is related to HIV disease and not environmental factors.

Attention

Attention deficits have been frequently noted in children with HIV-1 infection, however, it is unclear whether these deficits are directly related to the effects of HIV on the CNS [50, 51]. Elevated attention problems have been found in HIV-positive children but also in various uninfected control groups [50–52], suggesting an etiology other than HIV. On the other hand, studies assessing attention using computerized laboratory measures found deficits in sustained attention in children and adults with HIV-1 infection [53, 54] that were not found in uninfected control groups, suggesting that the attention problems are related to HIV disease. Attention deficits in children with HIV-1 may contribute to school and learning problems and may respond to stimulant medication.

Memory

Memory impairments have been found in children with vertically acquired HIV-1 infection [55–57] but not in children with transfusion acquired HIV infection, either for hemophilia or neonatal problems [51, 52, 58, 59]. However, HIV-infected hemophiliacs with low CD4 counts had declines in memory functioning over time [60]. Children with HIV CNS compromise exhibited significantly poorer verbal learning and recall compared to children without CNS compromise, who performed in the average range, but the two groups had similar scores on a recognition task [61, 62]. This pattern suggests a retrieval deficit, similarly found in HIV-infected adults, and may indicate subcortical pathology [63–65].

Behavioral functioning

In addition to cognitive deficits, children with HIV-1 infection also may display behavioral abnormalities. The etiology of these abnormalities may be related to the effects of HIV disease on the CNS and/or the psychological stresses of living with a chronic illness. Parents reported that children with encephalopathy exhibit more severe impairments in everyday behaviors, such as daily living skills and socialization skills, compared to children without encephalopathy [66]. Futhermore, deficits in adaptive behavior were associated with CT brain scan abnormalities [44] and immune status [67], and improved with ART [66], suggesting that they are related to the effects of HIV-1 on the CNS. In contrast, levels of emotional and behavioral problems, including hyperactivity, were similar for HIV-infected and HIV-exposed but uninfected children as rated by the primary caregiver on behavior checklists [50, 68]. These findings suggest that some behavior problems are not related to the effects of HIV on the CNS but rather to other etiologies, such as environmental conditions, biological factors, or psychosocial difficulties.

Motor functioning

Motor impairments often coexist with cognitive deficits in children with HIV-1 CNS disease [22, 69, 70], particularly in infants and in children naive to antiretroviral therapy [22]. Children with encephalopathy exhibit the most severe motor involvement and may lose previously attained motor milestones [36]. Gross motor function, particularly running speed and agility, tends to be more impaired than fine motor skills [71]. Oral–motor functioning also may be affected, resulting in articulation problems, expressive language deficits, and feeding and swallowing difficulties [47]. Furthermore, motor dysfunction is highly predictive of later disease progression [72]. Thus the evaluation of motor skills is an important part of the neurobehavioral assessment. Refer to Chapter 19 for more information on motor dysfunction in pediatric AIDS.

Neurobehavioral assessment of children and adolescents with HIV-1 infection purposes of neurobehavioral assessment

Psychological assessment is a critical component of the comprehensive multidisciplinary evaluation of children and adolescents with HIV-1 disease and serves three main purposes: (a) to determine whether neurobehavioral deficits may be attributed to HIV-associated factors, which is important when considering therapeutic options; (b) to monitor neurobehavioral growth over time to assess the longitudinal effects of HIV on the CNS and evaluate the effectiveness and possible toxicities of antiretroviral therapies; and (c) to identify strengths and weaknesses in neurobehavioral functioning to assist the multidisciplinary team with planning for rehabilitative, educational, adherence and psychosocial interventions [73]. Furthermore, deficient scores on neuropsychological tests and motor dysfunction are predictive of later disease progression, beyond information obtained from medical surrogate markers [72, 74], and thus, may be useful to predict long-term outcomes in children with HIV infection.

Methodological issues in longitudinal neurobehavioral assessment

Several methodological issues that need to be considered when conducting longitudinal neurobehavioral assessments of children and adolescents with HIV-1 disease are discussed below.

Specific domains to assess

Many abilities may be affected by HIV and should be evaluated in the neurobehavioral assessment or by professionals from other disciplines, including neurology, neuroradiology, and rehabilitation medicine.

Neurobehavioral assessment

The neurobehavioral assessment battery should include an age appropriate measure of general cognitive abilities as well as tests that evaluate specific abilities such as language (receptive, expressive), attention (sustain, shift), visuospatial function, motor (fine, gross), memory (visual, verbal), and executive function, which may identify the more subtle effects of HIV on the CNS [49]. In addition to evaluating neurocognitive functioning, assessment of adaptive behavior, socioemotional functioning, and academic achievement also is recommended. Table 10.2 lists the neurobehavioral functions to be assessed and representative tests to be used as part of a comprehensive psychological assessment for different ages of children and adolescents with HIV-1 infection.

Referral for assessment by other disciplines

Deterioration in gait or speech, a slowed rate of development, or decline in neurobehavioral test scores, may suggest HIV-related CNS disease and a child with any of these symptoms should be referred to a neurologist for further evaluation. Focal neurobehavioral deficits or abrupt changes in mental status, even in those with pre-existing HIV-related CNS disease, may indicate secondary CNS complications, including opportunistic infections, stroke, and neoplastic processes [40]. Such changes in functioning should prompt immediate and thorough medical, neuroimaging, and neurologic evaluations. Children who exhibit oral–motor or speech deficits should be referred to a speech pathologist [47] while children with motor dysfunction should be referred to a physical and occupational therapist for further evaluation and rehabilitation services [75].

Assessing developmental change over time

When longitudinally assessing children, it is imperative to use standardized tests with reliable age norms to compare the rate of growth of neurobehavioral functions with

Table 10.2. List of the neurobehavioral functions to be assessed and psychometric tests that can be used as part of a comprehensive psychological assessment of children with HIV infection

Function	Psychometric test	Age range[a]
General Intelligence	Bayley Scales of Infant Development (Mental)–2nd edn.[101]	1–3.5
	Mullen Scales of Early Learning [102]	0–5.8
	Differential Abilities Scale – Preschool and School Age Levels [103]	2.6–17.11
	McCarthy Scales of Children's Abilities [104]	2.4–8.6
	Wechsler Preschool and Primary Scale of Intelligence–III [105]	2.6–7.3
	Wechsler Intelligence Scale for Children IV. [106]	6–16.11
	Wechsler Adult Intelligence Scale–III [107]	16–74
Language	Peabody Picture Vocabulary Test–III [108]	2.5–90
	Expressive Vocabulary Test [109]	2.6–90
	Verbal Fluency [110]	> 2.5
	Preschool Language Scale–3 [111]	0–6
	Clinical Evaluation of Language Fundamentals– IV [112]	5–21
Visuospatial	Developmental Test of Visual-Motor Integration – 4R [113]	4–17.11
Memory and learning	Children's Memory Scale [114]	5–16.11
	California Verbal Learning Test–Children's Version [115]	5–16.11
	McCarthy Memory Scale [104]	2.4–8.6
	Stanford–Binet Memory Scale–5th edn. [116]	2–90
Attention	Digit Span Subtest [106, 107]	≥ 6
	Trail Making Test [117]	≥ 6
	Connors' Continous Performance Task II [118]	≥ 6
Concept formation	Ravens Progressive Matrices [119]	≥ 5.5
Motor function	Bayley Scales of Infant Development (Motor)-2nd edn. [101]	0–2 1/2
	Peabody Developmental Motor Scales – 2 [120]	0.5–6
	Bruininks–Oseretsky Test of Motor Proficiency [121]	> 5.5
	Grooved Pegboard [122]	> 5
Behavior	Vineland Adaptive Behavior Scales – II [123]	0–90.11
	Achenbach Child Behavior Checklist [124]	2–16
	Connors' Rating Scales – R [125]	3–17
	Behavior Assessment System for Children – II[126]	2.0–21.11
	Behavior Rating Inventory of Executive Function [127]	5–18

[a] age range in years, for which the test is standardized.

Based on a table previously published in Wolters & Brouwers, 1998.

the normative group over time. Differences in these growth rates will be reflected by changes in the standardized test scores of the HIV-infected child. As the child grows older, test instruments need to be changed to utilize age-appropriate measures and norms since most standardized psychometric tests for children have restricted age ranges [76]. It is helpful to continue administering the same test to the child for as long as possible so congruent comparisons can be made over time. When a new test needs to be administered, it is often difficult to interpret an interval change in scores, so if possible, the change to a new instrument should be done when the child is relatively healthy with no new developmental concerns. Minimal effects have been found when transitioning from the child to the adult version of the Wechsler intelligence test [77], so a significant decline in test scores may be due to HIV-related CNS disease. In this situation, the new test or the one that was previously given should be re-administered as soon as repeat testing is considered valid for a chronically ill population (i.e., in six months) to continue monitoring the child's CNS status.

Frequency of repeated testing and practice effects

When planning for a follow-up neurobehavioral evaluation, several factors need to be considered, including the child's potential risk of developing CNS disease, the rate of disease progression, possible treatment effects, and potential practice effects. Shorter intervals between testing are recommended for infants and young children with HIV-1 infection since they have the highest risk of developing severe CNS disease, the effects of an antiretroviral drug regimen often occur shortly after the initiation of treatment, and practice effects are less of a concern for a young age group. On the other hand, school-age children and adolescents with HIV-1 infection have a lower probability of developing CNS disease, tend to exhibit more subtle neurocognitive changes, and are more likely to demonstrate practice effects. Thus, test-retest intervals need to be longer in older children and adolescents, particularly in those without evidence of HIV-related CNS disease or those with higher IQs who may show more benefit from repeated assessments [77]. However, IQ scores from the Wechsler Intelligence Scales were found to be highly reliable and free of significant practice effects over several years, supporting their use in longitudinal pediatric evaluations [77]. In consideration of these assessment issues, the recommended neurobehavioral testing schedule for children with HIV-1 is presented in Table 10.3.

Special test administration procedures

Some children with HIV-1 infection may exhibit motor dysfunction, sensory defects, limited speech, short attention spans, high activity levels, or extreme fatigue that require modification of the psychological test battery or procedures to obtain a valid assessment of their cognitive function. Also, some children may not be fluent in English. When a child cannot be assessed with the standard assessment battery, alternative tests, specifically designed for children with visual, hearing, or physical impairments, or who speak another language, or non-standard assessment procedures (i.e., use of

Table 10.3. Recommended neurodevelopmental serial assessment schedule for children with HIV-1 infection at various ages

Age of child	Serial assessment schedule
< 2 year	Evaluate every 6 months due to a higher risk of developing CNS disease
2–8 years	Evaluate every year unless they exhibit neurodevelopmental deficits, in which case they should be assessed every 6 months[a]; and
> 8 years	Evaluate every 2 years if child exhibits stable functioning in the average range; otherwise, evaluate every year[a]

[a] Shorter batteries of individual subtests and specific function tests can be administered between the major evaluations to further decrease the testing burden on children while still monitoring the effects of the disease.

interpreters or eye gaze instead of a pointing response) should be used. For a child who exhibits attention or behavioral difficulties, the examiner may need to use behavior management techniques or multiple test sessions. Testing should be conducted when the child is in an optimal state and not when the child is febrile, hungry or fatigued, or after certain medical procedures, such as sedation, eye dilation, or those that are upsetting to the child.

Differential diagnosis

The determination of whether a child's neurobehavioral deficits or change in functioning is related to HIV disease or other factors is critical for the formulation of an effective treatment plan. If a change in neurobehavioral functioning is abrupt or the manifestations are focal or lateralized, the etiology may be due to non-HIV-related medical causes, such as opportunistic infections, stroke, or neoplastic processes [40]. In such cases, immediate referral for a neurologic evaluation, neuroimaging studies, and examination of CSF is criticial for determining the appropriate diagnosis and treatment. If a change in neurobehavioral functioning is attributed to HIV-1 infection, then the selection of a treatment regimen that may be relatively more effective at inhibiting viral replication within the CNS is important. If the changes or deficits are more consistent with other non-HIV associated factors, such as birth trauma, or are considered a static expression of earlier HIV-associated CNS insult, then specific treatments targeting CNS viral replication are less of a concern. Determining the etiology of CNS manifestations in children with HIV infection is challenging due to the wide range of functions that may be affected, the progressive nature of the disease, and the pre-existing medical conditions or environmental factors that may confound the effects of HIV on the CNS. Following is a brief description of information to be considered when interpreting neurobehavioral test results and changes in CNS function.

Birth and medical history

Birth trauma, hypoxia, severe prematurity, low birth weight, maternal substance abuse, exposure to toxic substances (i.e., lead), CNS infections other than HIV, and chronic illnesses may alter neurobehavioral development, resulting in delays and deficits.

Developmental and educational history

A loss or no substantial gain over previously acquired developmental milestones in young children or declining school performance in older children may indicate HIV-related CNS effects. Lack of appropriate environmental stimulation or schooling, however, also may result in a gradual decline in psychometric test scores over time [78].

Psychometric test results

Comparing current test scores with previous results is important for evaluating whether changing neurobehavioral functioning may be related to HIV-1 infection and its treatment. A significant decline in test scores may indicate a progression in HIV-related CNS disease [21], suggesting the need for a possible adjustment of antiretroviral treatment, while a significant improvement may suggest a reversal of deficits related to treatment effects. Inspection of the neuropsychological profile also is useful to identify patterns of deficits that have been related to HIV disease.

Environment and family factors

Various environmental factors, such as culture, education, and socioeconomic status can influence the development of a child's cognitive abilities [78, 79] as well as their response to brain injury [80, 81]. The general cognitive abilities of children and their parents and siblings are strongly correlated [82] and some behavioral and learning problems are hereditary [83]. Thus, environmental and family factors should be considered, but used cautiously, when interpreting psychometric test results since many other factors may influence cognitive development.

Neuroimaging findings

Children with HIV-related CNS disease often exhibit neuroimaging abnormalities that may be correlated with their level of neurocognitive functioning [41, 45]. Furthermore, the presence and severity of cortical atrophy may be a good indicator of the degree of HIV-related CNS compromise in children [84, 85]. On computed tomography (CT) brain scans, intracerebral calcifications in young vertically-infected children have been associated with poor prognosis and encephalopathy, particularly when moderate to severe cortical atrophy is also noted. Minor white matter abnormalities detected on MRI have not been associated with altered cognitive function [86], but more extensive white matter changes evident on CT scans have been associated with cognitive impairments [42].

Neurological findings

Motor and cognitive deficits are each frequent indicators of HIV-related CNS disease but may be found independent of one another [36]. Tone abnormalities, such as spastic diplegia and central hypotonia, and movement disorders, such as rigidity, bradykinesia, and dystonia that affect day-to-day functioning suggest HIV-related encephalopathy. Neuropathies as potential side effects of treatment or manifestations of HIV disease also need to be evaluated. As stated earlier, if changes in neurobehavioral function are acute, focal, or lateralized, the patient should be referred immediately for further medical and neurological evaluations to investigate non-HIV-related etiologies. See Chapter 19 for more details.

Behavioral observations

Direct observation by the examiner of the child's behavior during the interview and testing, including affect, attention, activity level, response style, dealing with difficulties on various subtests, and parent–child interaction is critical for interpreting neuropsychological test results. Ratings of the child's functioning in the home and school environment obtained from parent, teacher, and self-report questionnaires, can provide additional information about the effects of HIV and treatment on behavior.

Immunological and virological testing

Low CD4+ T-lymphocyte counts and high plasma HIV-1 RNA concentrations strongly predict HIV disease progression [87, 88] and have been associated with more severe cognitive impairments and brain imaging abnormalities [30, 44]. Furthermore, a decrease in the fraction of lymphocytes that are CD4+ T-cells has been associated with increases in cognitive dysfunction and brain imaging abnormalities [84]. The concentrations of HIV-1 RNA in the CSF were higher and detected more often in encephalopathic children than those without encephalopathy [2, 89] and were associated with the degree of cortical atrophy [85]. However, the level of HIV-1 RNA in the plasma is not consistently correlated with such levels in the CSF and may not be a good indicator of the effects of HIV on the CNS in children [2, 85]. These data seem to suggest that the CNS may be a distinct compartment with regard to viral replication. Immune and plasma virologic measures can thus be utilized to evaluate the significance of neurobehavioral test data but should be used with caution due to inter- and intrapatient variability, compartmentalization of the CNS, and the modifying factor of treatment, which may act differently on the markers of the immunologic, virologic [90], and neurologic domains.

Other evaluations

Since opportunistic infections may impair the vision and hearing of children with HIV disease, which in turn can negatively affect cognitive test performance, audiological and ophthalmological evaluations are important for monitoring such impairments and interpreting psychometric test results. Physical, occupational, and speech therapy evaluations provide additional information regarding the child's functioning. Social workers can supply useful information regarding the child's family history and current home environment and nurses can inquire about medication adherence. All members of the multidisciplinary team contribute data that can be useful for determining if the child's neurobehavioral functioning has been affected by HIV or other factors.

Effects of antiretroviral treatment on neurobehavioral function

Antiretroviral treatment may be preventative and/or therapeutic for HIV-associated CNS disease. With the availability of effective HAART, the prevention of CNS disease appears to be related to the suppression of systemic viral replication, which reduces or eliminates the invasion of HIV-carrying cells into the CNS. However, the CNS is a separate compartment from the rest of the body and it may serve as a reservoir for persistent HIV-1 infection [16]. Some antiretroviral agents have been found to penetrate the blood–brain barrier [3, 18, 91, 92], inhibit viral replication in the CNS [93, 94], and reduce the neurotoxic effects of the virus on the brain [3, 95]. In children with evidence of HIV-associated CNS manifestations, treatment studies have shown that some antiretroviral drugs, particularly used in combination [19], may improve neurobehavioral functioning [96–98] as well as cortical atrophy [99]. These improvements in CNS functioning are likely due to treatment-related decreases in viral replication in the brain [94, 100]. Thus, children with HIV-related neurobehavioral deficits should be given antiretroviral therapy that includes at least one agent that has adequate CNS penetration, such as zidovudine (ZDV) or stavudine. Treatment for HIV disease is discussed in more detail in Chapters 11 and 15.

Summary

Neurobehavioral deficits can be a significant morbidity of pediatric HIV-1 infection. Since no current measure can predict which children may develop HIV-related CNS disease, regular psychometric testing can identify early neurobehavioral changes in functioning. The development of HIV-related neurobehavioral deficits indicates the need for antiretroviral therapy that is active within the CNS. Longitudinal neurobehavioral assessments also are important for evaluating response to treatment and planning appropriate individual educational, rehabilitative, adherence and psychosocial interventions. Thus, periodic monitoring of neurobehavioral functioning is critical for the appropriate management of HIV-1 infection in children and adolescents and should be used in conjunction with other data to plan an effective treatment strategy for the child or adolescent and their family.

Acknowledgments

Support for this chapter was provided to Pam Wolters by HIV and AIDS Malignancy Branch, National Cancer Institute Research Contract #NO1-SC-07006 awarded to the

Medical Illness Counseling Center, Chevy Chase, MD and to Pim Brouwers by National Institute of Allergy and Infectious Disease grant U01-A127551-15 awarded to Baylor College of Medicine, Houston, TX.

REFERENCES

1. Zheng, J., Gendelman, H. E. The HIV-1 associated dementia complex: a metabolic encephalopathy fueled by viral replication in mononuclear phagocytes. *Curr. Opin. Neurol.* 1997;**10**(4):319–325.

2. Sei, S., Stewart, S. K., Farley, M. *et al.* Evaluation of human immunodeficiency virus (HIV) type 1 RNA levels in cerebrospinal fluid and viral resistance to zidovudine in children with HIV encephalopathy. *J. Infect. Dis.* 1996;**174**(6):1200–1206.

3. Gendelman, H. E., Zheng, J., Coulter, C. L. *et al.* Suppression of inflammatory neurotoxins by highly active antiretroviral therapy in human immunodeficiency virus-associated dementia. *J. Infect. Dis.* 1998;**178**:1000–1007.

4. Sharer, L. R., Mintz, M. Neuropathology of AIDS in children. In Scaravilli, F., ed. *AIDS: The Pathology of the Nervous System.* Berlin: Springer Verlag, 1993: 201–214.

5. Belman, A. L., Diamond, G., Dickson, D. *et al.* Pediatric acquired immunodeficiency syndrome: neurologic syndromes. *Am. J. Dis. Child.* 1988;**142**(1):29–35.

6. Epstein, L. G., Neurologic manifestations of HIV infection in children. *Pediatrics* 1986;**78**(4):678–687.

7. Blanche, S., Newell, M., Mayaux, M. *et al.* Morbidity and mortality in European children vertically infected by HIV-1. *J. Acquir. Immune Defic. Syndr. Hum. Retrovirol.* 1997;**14**:442–450.

8. Lobato, M. N., Caldwell, M. B., Ng, P., Oxtoby, M. J. Encephalopathy in children with perinatally acquired human immunodeficiency virus infection. *J. Pediatr.* 1995;**126**(5 – Part I):710–715.

9. Cooper, E. R., Hanson, C., Diaz, C. *et al.* Encephalopathy and progression of human immunodeficiency virus disease in a cohort of children with perinatally acquired human immunodeficiency virus infection. Women and Infants Transmission Study Group. *J. Pediatr.* 1998;**132**(5):808–812.

10. Tardieu, M., Chenadec, J. L., Persoz, A., Meyer, L., Blanche, S., Mayaux, M. J. HIV-1-related encephalopathy in infants compared with children and adults. *Neurology* 2000;**54**:1089–1095.

11. Brodt, H. R., Kamps, B. S., Gute, P., Knupp, B., Staszewski, S., Helm, E. B. Changing incidence of AIDS-defining illnesses in the era of antiretroviral combination therapy. *AIDS* 1997;**11**:1731–1738.

12. d'Arminio, Monforte, A., Duca, P. G., Vago, L., Grassi, M. P., Moroni, M. Decreasing incidence of CNS AIDS-defining events associated with antiretroviral therapy. *Neurology* 2000;**54**:1856–1859.

13. Palella, F. J., Delaney, K. M., Moorman, A. C. *et al.* Declining morbidity and mortality among patients with advanced human immunodeficiency virus infection. *N. Engl. J. Med.* 1998;**338**(13):853–860.

14. Tardieu, M., Boutet, A., HIV-1 and the central nervous system. In *Current Topics Microbiology Immunology.* Berlin: Springer Verlag, 2002: 183–195.

15. Deeks, S. G., Smith, M., Holodniy, M., Kahn, J. O. HIV-1 Protease Inhibitors. *J. Am. Med. Assoc.* 1997;**277**(2):145–153.

16. Sonza, S., Crowe, S. Reservoirs for HIV infection and their persistence in the face of undetectable viral load. *AIDS Patient Care STDs* 2001;**15**(10):511–518.

17. Aweeka, F., Jayewaardene, A., Staprana, S. *et al.* Failure to detect nelfinavir in the cerebrospinal fluid of HIV-1-infected patients with and without AIDS dementia complex. *J. Acquir. Immune Defic. Syndr. Hum. Retrovirol.* 1999;**20**:39–43.

18. Swindells, S., Therapy of HIV-1. *In Infection: A Practical Guide for Providers.* New York: Chapman & Hall; 1998.

19. Raskino, C., Pearson, D. A., Baker, C. J. *et al.* Neurologic, neurocognitive, and brain growth outcomes in human immunodeficiency virus-infected children receiving different nucleoside antiretroviral regimens. *Pediatrics* 1999;**104**(3):e32.

20. Chase, C., Vibbert, M., Pelton, S., Coulter, D., Cabral, H. Early neurodevelopmental growth in children with vertically transmitted human immunodeficiency virus infection. *Arch. Pediatr. Adolesc. Med.* 1995;**149**:850–855.

21. Chase, C., Ware, J., Hittelman, J. *et al.* Early cognitive and motor development among infants born to women infected with human immunodeficiency virus. *Pediatrics* 2000;**106**(2):1–10.

22. Englund, J. A., Baker, C. J., Raskino, C., McKinney, R. *et al.* Clinical and laboratory characteristics of a large cohort of symptomatic, human immunodeficiency virus-infected infants and children. *Pediatr. Infect. Dis. J.* 1996;**15**:1025–1036.

23. McKinney, R. E., Johnson, G. M., Stanley, K. *et al.* A randomized study of combined zidovudine-lamivudine versus didanosine monotherapy in children with symptomatic therapy-naive HIV-1 infection. The Pediatric AIDS Clinical Trials Group Protocol 300 Study Team. *J. Pediatr.* 1998;**133**(4):500–508.

24. Mintz, M., Clinical comparison of adult and pediatric neuroAIDS. *Adv. Neuroimmunol.* 1994;**4**:207–221.

25. Mitchell, W., Neurological and developmental effects of HIV and AIDS in children and adolescents. *Ment. Retard. Developm. Disabil. Res. Rev.* 2001;**7**:211–216.

26. Mayaux, M. J., Burgard, M., Teglas, J.-P. *et al.* Neonatal characteristics in rapidly progressive perinatally acquired HIV-1 disease. *J. Am. Med. Assoc.* 1996;**275**(8):606–610.

27. Smith, R., Malee, K., Charurat, M. *et al.* Timing of perinatal human immunodeficiency virus type 1 infection and rate of neurodevelopment. *Pediatr. Infect. Dis. J.* 2000;**19**:862–871.

28. Blanche, S., Mayaux, M. J., Rouzioux, C. *et al.* Relation of the course of HIV infection in children to the severity of the disease in their mothers at delivery. *N. Engl. J. Med.* 1994;**330**(5):308–312.

29. Lindsey, J. C., Hughes, M. D., McKinney, R. E. *et al.* Treatment-mediated changes in human immunodeficiency virus (HIV) Type I RNA and CD4 cell counts as predictors of weight growth failure, cognitive decline, and survival in HIV-infected children. *J. Infect. Dis.* 2000;**182**:1385–1393.

30. Pollack, H., Kuchuk, A., Cowan, L. *et al.* Neurodevelopment, growth, and viral load in HIV-infected infants. *Brain, Behav. Immun.* 1996;**10**:298–312.

31. Just, J., Abrams, E., Louie, L. *et al.* Influence of host genotype on progression to acquired immunodeficiency syndrome among children infected with human immunodeficiency virus type 1. *J. Pediatr.* 1995;**127**:544–549.

32. Sei, S., Boler, A. M., Nguyen, G. T. *et al*. Protective effect of CCR5 delta32 heterozygosity is restricted by SDF-1 genotype in children with HIV-1 infection. *AIDS* 2001;**15**:1343–1352.

33. Culnane, M., Fowler, M., Lee, S. *et al*. Lack of long-term effects of in utero exposure to zidovudine among uninfected children born to HIV-infected women. *J. Am. Med. Assoc.* 1999;**281**(2):151–157.

34. Working Group of the American Academy of Neurology AIDS Task Force. Nomenclature and research case definitions for neurologic manifestations of human immunodeficiency virus-type 1 infection. *Neurology* 1991;**41**:778–785.

35. Wolters, P. L., Brouwers, P. Evaluation of neurodevelopmental deficits in children with HIV infection. In Gendelman, H. E., Lipton, S. A., Epstein, L., Swindells, S., eds. *The Neurology of AIDS*. New York: Chapman & Hall, 1998: 425–442.

36. Belman, A. L. HIV-1 associated CNS disease in infants and children. In Price, R. W., Perry, S. W., eds. *HIV, AIDS and the Brain*. New York: Raven Press, 1994: 289–310.

37. Brouwers, P., Belman, A. L., Epstein, L. Central nervous system involvement: manifestations, evaluation, and pathogenesis. In Pizzo, P. A., Wilfert, C. M., eds. *Pediatr. AIDS: The Challenge of HIV Infection in Infants, Children and Adolescents*. 2nd edn. Baltimore: Williams & Wilkins, 1994: 433–455.

38. Epstein, L., Sharer, L. R., Joshi, V. V., Fojas, M. M., Koenigsberger, M. R., Oleske, J. Progressive encephalopathy in children with acquired immune deficiency syndrome. *Ann. Neurol.* 1985;**17**:488–496.

39. Centers for Disease Control. 1994 Revised classification system for human immunodeficiency virus infection in children less than 13 years of age; official authorized addenda: human immunodeficiency virus infection codes and official guidelines for coding and reporting ICD-9-CM. *Morbid. Mortal. Wkly Rep.*: Centers for Disease Control; 1994.

40. Brouwers, P., Wolters, P., Civitello, L., *Central Nervous System Manifestations and Assessment*. 3rd edn. Philadelphia: Williams & Wilkins, 1998.

41. Brouwers, P., DeCarli, C., Civitello, L., Moss, H. A., Wolters, P. L., Pizzo, P. A. Correlation between computed tomographic brain scan abnormalities and neuropsychological function in children with symptomatic human immunodeficiency virus disease. *Arch. Neurol.* 1995;**52**:39–44.

42. Brouwers, P., van der Vlugt, H., Moss, H. A., Wolters, P. L., Pizzo, P. A. White matter changes on CT brain scan are associated with neurobehavioral dysfunction in children with symptomatic HIV disease. *Child Neuropsychol.* 1995;**1**(2):93–105.

43. Brouwers, P., Heyes, M. P., Moss, H. A. *et al*. Quinolinic acid in the cerebrospinal fluid of children with symptomatic human immunodeficiency virus type 1 disease: Relationship to clinical status and therapeutic response. *J. Infect. Dis.* 1993;**168**:1380–1386.

44. Brouwers, P., Tudor-Williams, G., DeCarli, C. *et al*. Relation between stage of disease and neurobehavioral measures in children with symptomatic HIV disease. *AIDS* 1995;**9**:713–720.

45. DeCarli, C., Civitello, L. A., Brouwers, P., Pizzo, P. A. The prevalence of computed axial tomographic abnormalities of the cerebrum in 100 consecutive children symptomatic with the human immune deficiency virus. *Ann. Neurol.* 1993;**34**(2):198–205.

46. Coplan, J., Contello, K. A., Cunningham, C. K. *et al*. Early language development in children exposed to or infected with human immunodeficiency virus. *Pediatrics*, 1998: 102–105.

47. Pressman, H., Communication disorders and dysphagia in pediatric AIDS. *ASHA* 1992;**34**:45–47.

48. Wolters, P. L., Brouwers, P., Moss, H. A., Pizzo, P. A. Differential receptive and expressive language functioning of children with symptomatic HIV disease and relation to CT scan brain abnormalities. *Pediatrics* 1995;**95**:112–119.

49. Wolters, P. L., Brouwers, P., Civitello, L., Moss, H. A. Receptive and expressive language function of children with symptomatic HIV infection and relationship with disease parameters: a longitudinal 24 month follow-up study. *AIDS* 1997;**11**(9):1135–1144.

50. Havens, J., Whitaker, A., Feldman, J., Ehrhardt, A. Psychiatric morbidity in school-age children with congenital human immunodeficiency virus infection: a pilot study. *Developm. Behav. Pediatr.* 1994;**15**(3):S18–S25.

51. Whitt, J. K., Hooper, S. R., Tennison, M. B. *et al.* Neuropsychologic functioning of human immunodeficiency virus-infected children with hemophilia. *J. Pediatr.* 1993;**122**:52–59.

52. Loveland, K. A., Stehbens, J., Contant, C. *et al.* Hemophilia growth and development study: baseline neurodevelopmental findings. *J. Pediatr. Psychol.* 1994;**19**(2):223–239.

53. Law, W. A., Mapou, R. L., Roller, T. L., Martin, A., Nannis, E. D., Temoshok, L. R. Reaction time slowing in HIV-1 infected individuals: role of the preparatory interval. *J. Clin. Exp. Neuropsychol.* 1995;**17**(1):122–133.

54. Watkins, J. M., Cool, V. A., Usner, D. *et al.* Attention in HIV-infected children: results from the Hemophilia Growth and Development Study. *J. Int. Neuropsychol. Soc.* 2000;**6**(4):443–454.

55. Boivin, M., Green, S., Davies, A., Giordani, B., Mokili, J., Cutting, W. A preliminary evaluation of the cognitive and motor effects of pediatric HIV infection in Zairian children. *Hlth Psychol.* 1995;**14**(1):13–21.

56. Fundaro, C., Miccinesi, N., Baldieri, N., Genovese, O., Rendeli, C., Segni, G. Cognitive impairment in school-age children with asymptomatic HIV infection. *AIDS Patient Care STDs* 1998;**12**(2):135–140.

57. Levenson, R., Mellins, C., Zawadzki, R., Kairam, R., Stein, Z. Cognitive assessment of human immunodeficiency virus-exposed children. *AJDC* 1992;**146**:1479–1483.

58. Cohen, S. E., Mundy, T., Kaarassik, B., Lieb, L., Ludwig, D. D., Ward, J. Neuropsychological functioning in children with HIV-1 infection through neonatal blood transfusion. *Pediatrics* 1991;**88**(1):58–68.

59. Smith, M. L., Minden, D., Netley, C., Read, S., King, S., Blanchette, V. Longitudinal investigation of neuropsychological functioning in children and adolescents with hemophilia and HIV infection. *Dev. Neuropsychol.* 1997;**13**(1):69–85.

60. Loveland, K., Stehbens, J., Mahoney, E. *et al.* Declining immune function in children and adolescents with hemophilia and HIV infection: effects on neuropsychological performance. *J. Pediatr. Psychol.* 2000;**25**(5):309–322.

61. Klaas, P., Wolters, P. L., Martin, S., Civitello, L., Zeichner, S. Verbal learning and memory in children with HIV [Abstract]. *J. Int. Neuropsychol. Soc.* 2002;**8**:187.

62. Perez, L. A., Wolters, P. L., Moss, H. A., Civitello, L. A., Brouwers, P. Verbal learning and memory in children with HIV infection [Abstract]. *J. Neurovirol.* 1998;**4**:362.

63. Brouwers, P., Mohr, E., Hildebrand, K. *et al.* A novel approach to the determination and characterization of HIV dementia. *Can. J. Neurol. Sci.* 1996;**23**(2):104–109.

64. Stout, J. C., Salmon, D. P., Butters, N. *et al.* Decline in working memory associated with HIV infection. *Psychol. Med.* 1995;**25**:1221–1232.

65. White, D., Taylor, M., Butters, N. *et al*. Memory for verbal information in individuals with HIV-associated dementia complex. *J. Clin. Exp. Neuropsychol*. 1997;**19**(3):357–366.

66. Wolters, P., Brouwers, P., Moss, H., Pizzo, P. Adaptive behavior of children with symptomatic HIV infection before and after zidovudine therapy. *J. Pediatr. Psychol*. 1994;**19**(1):47–61.

67. Nichols, S., Mahoney, E., Sirois, P. *et al*. HIV-associated changes in adaptive, emotional, and behavioral functioning in children and adolescents with hemophilia: results from the hemophilia growth and development study. *J. Pediatr. Psychol*. 2000;**25**(8):545–556.

68. Mellins, C. A., Smith, R., O'Driscoll, P. *et al*. High rates of behavioral problems in perinatally HIV-infected children are not linked to HIV disease. *2003; Pediatrics* iii: 384–393.

69. Aylward, E. H., Butz, A. M., Hutton, N., Joyner, M. L., Vogelhut, J. W. Cognitive and motor development in infants at risk for human immunodeficiency virus. *Am. J. Disabled Child*. 1992;**146**:218–222.

70. Gay, C. L., Armstrong, F. D., Cohen, D. *et al*. The effects of HIV on cognitive and motor development in children born to HIV-seropositive women with no reported drug use: birth to 24 months. *Pediatrics* 1995;**96**:1078–1082.

71. Parks, R. A., Danoff, J. V. Motor performance changes in children testing positive for HIV over 2 years. *Am. J. Occupat. Ther*. 1999;**53**(5):524–528.

72. Pearson, D. A., McGrath, N. M., Nozyce, M. *et al*. Predicting HIV disease progression in children using measures of neuropsychological and neurological functioning. *Pediatrics*, 2000; **106** (6): 1–10.

73. Wolters, P. L., Brouwers, P., Moss, H. A. Pediatric HIV disease: effect on cognition, learning, and behavior. *School Psychol. Quart*. 1995;**10**(4):305–328.

74. Llorente, A. M., Brouwers, P., Charurat, M. *et al*. Early neurodevelopmental markers predictive of morbidity and mortality in HIV-1 infected infants: findings from the Women and Infant Transmission Study (WITS). *Dev. Med. Child Neurol*. 2003;**45** (2):76–84.

75. Lord, D., Danoff, J., Smith, M. Motor assessment of infants with human immunodeficiency virus infection: a retrospective review of multiple cases. *Pediatr. Physi. Ther*. 1995;**7**:9–13.

76. Lindsey, J. C., O'Donnell, K., Brouwers, P. Methodological issues in analyzing psychological test scores in pediatric clinical trials. *J. Dev. Behav. Pediatr*. 2000;**21**:141–151.

77. Sirois, P. A., Posner, M., Stehbens, J. A. *et al*. Quantifying practice effects in longitudinal research with the WISC-R and WAIS-R: a study of children and adolescents with hemophilia and male siblings without hemophilia. *J. Pediatr. Psychol*. 2002;**27**(2):121–131.

78. Burchinal, M. R., Campbell, F. A., Bryant, D. M., Wasik, B. H., Ramey, C. T. Early intervention and mediating processes in cognitive performance of children of low-income African-American families. *Child Dev*. 1997;**68**:935–954.

79. Neisser, U., Boodoo, G., Bouchard, T. J. *et al*. Intelligence: knowns and unknowns. *Am. Psychol*. 1996;**51**:77–101.

80. Wade, S. L., Drotar, D., Taylor, H. G., Stancin, T. Assessing the effects of traumatic brain injury on family functioning: conceptual and methodological issues. *J. Pediatr. Psychol*. 1995;**20**(6):737–752.

81. Yeates, K. O., Taylor, H. G., Drotar, D. *et al*. Preinjury family environment as a determinant of recovery from traumatic brain injuries in school-age children. *J. Inte. Neuropsychol Soc*. 1997;**3**(6):617–630.

82. Erlenmeyer-Kimling, L., Jarvik, L. F. Genetics and intelligence: a review. *Science* 1963;**142**:1477–1479.

83. Pennington, B. F., Smith, S. D. Genetic influences on learning disabilities and speech and language disorders. *Child Dev.* 1983;**54**:369–387.

84. Brouwers, P., DeCarli, C., Tudor-Williams, G., Civitello, L., Moss, H. A., Pizzo, P. A. Inter-relations among patterns of change in neurocognitive, CT brain imaging, and CD4 measures associated with antiretroviral therapy in children with symptomatic HIV infection. *Adv. Neuroimmunol.* 1994;**4**:223–231.

85. Brouwers, P., Civitello, L., DeCarli, C., Wolters, P., Sei, S. Cerebrospinal fluid viral load is related to cortical atrophy and not to intracerebral calcifications in children with symptomatic HIV disease. *J. NeuroVirol.* 2000;**6**(5):390–396.

86. Tardieu, M., Blanche, S., Brunelle, F., Cerebral magnetic resonance imaging studies in HIV-1 infected children born to seropositive mothers [Abstract] Neuroscience of HIV-1 Infection. In *Satellite Conf. Seventh Int. Conf. AIDS*; 1991; Padova, Italy, 1991: 60.

87. Mellors, J. W., Munoz, A., Giorgi, J. V. *et al.* Plasma viral load and CD4+lymphocytes as prognostic markers of HIV-1 infection. *Ann. Int. Med.* 1997;**126**:946–954.

88. Mofenson, L., Korelitz, J., Meyer, W. A. *et al.* The relationship between serum human immunodeficiency virus type 1 (HIV-1) RNA level, CD4 lymphocyte percent, and long-term mortality risk in HIV-1-infected children. *J. Infect. Dis.* 1997;**175**:1029–1038.

89. Pratt, R. D., Nichols, S., McKinney, N., Kwok, S., Dankner, W., Spector, S. Virologic markers of human immunodeficiency virus type 1 in cerebrospinal fluid of infected children. *J. Infect. Dis.* 1996;**174**:288–293.

90. Jacobson, L. P., Li, R., Phair, J. *et al.* Evaluation of the effectiveness of highly active antiretroviral therapy in persons with human immunodeficiency virus using bio-marker-based equivalence of disease progression. *Am. J. Epidemiol.* 2002;**155**(8):760–770.

91. Haas, D. W., Clough, L. A., Johnson, B. W. *et al.* Evidence of a source of HIV type 1 within the central nervous system by ultraintensive sampling of cerebrospinal fluid and plasma. *AIDS Res. Hum. Retroviruses* 2000;**16**:1491–1502.

92. Haworth, S. J., Christofalo, B., Anderson, R. D., Dunkle, L. M. A single dose study to assess the penetration of stavudine into human cerebrospinal fluid in adults. *J. Acquir. Immune Defic. Syndr. Hum. Retrovirol.* 1998;**17**:235–238.

93. Foudraine, N. A., Hoetelmans, R. M. W., Lange, J. M. A. *et al.* Cerebrospinal-fluid HIV-1 RNA and drug concentrations after treatment with lamivudine plus zidovudine or stavudine. *Lancet* 1998;**351**:1547–1551.

94. McCoig, C., Castrejon, M. M., Castano, E. *et al.* Effect of combination antiretroviral therapy on cerebrospinal fluid HIV RNA, HIV resistance, and clinical manifestations of encephalopathy. *J. Pediatr.* 2002;**141**:36–44.

95. Mueller, B. U., Pizzo, P. A. Therapy for HIV infection of the central nervous system in children. In Gendelman, H., Lipton, S., Epstein, L., Swindells, S., eds. *Neurological and Neuropsychiatric Manifestations of HIV-1 Infection*. New York: Chapman & Hall, 1998.

96. Brouwers, P., Moss, H., Wolters, P. *et al.* Effect of continuous-infusion zidovudine therapy on neuropsychologic functioning in children with symptomatic human immunodeficiency virus infection. *J. Pediatr.* 1990;**117**(6):980–985.

97. McKinney, R. E., Maha, M. A., Connor, E. M. *et al*. A multicenter trial of oral zidovudine in children with advanced human immunodeficiency virus disease. *N. Engl. J. Med.* 1991;**324**(15):1018–1025.

98. Pizzo, P., Eddy, J., Falloon, J. *et al*. Effect of continuous intravenous infusion of zidovudine (AZT) in children with symptomatic HIV infection. *N. Engl. J. Med.* 1988;**319**(14):889–896.

99. DeCarli, C., Fugate, L., Falloon, J. *et al*. Brain growth and cognitive improvement in children with human immune deficiency virus-induced encephalopathy after six months of continuous infusion zidovudine therapy. *J. Acquir. Immune Defic. Syndr.* 1991;**4**:585–592.

100. Yarchoan, R., Berg, G., Brouwers, P. *et al*. Preliminary observations in the response of HTLV-III/LAV (human immunodeficiency virus) – associated neurological disease to the administration of 3-azido-3-deoxythymidine. *Lancet* 1987;**i**:131–135.

101. Bayley, N. *Bayley Scales of Infant Development*. 2nd edn. San Antonio, TX: Psychological Corporation, 1993.

102. Mullen, E. *Mullen Scales of Early Learning*. Circle Pines, MN: American Guidance Service, 1995.

103. Elliott, C. *Differential Ability Scales*. San Antonio, TX: Psychological Corporation, 1990.

104. McCarthy, D. *McCarthy Scales of Children's Abilities*. San Antonio, TX: Psychological Corporation, 1972.

105. Wechsler, D. *Wechsler Preschool and Primary Scale of Intelligence*. 3rd edn. San Antonio, TX: Psychological Corporation, 2002.

106. Wechsler, D. *Wechsler Intelligence Scale for Children*. 3rd edn. San Antonio, TX: Psychological Corporation, 1991.

107. Wechsler, D. *Wechsler Adult Intelligence Scale*. 4th edn. San Antonio, TX: Psychological Corporation, 2003.

108. Dunn, L. M., Dunn, L. M., *Peabody Picture Vocabulary Test*. 3rd edn. Circle Pines, MN: American Guidance Service, 1997.

109. Williams, K. *Expressive Vocabulary Test*. Circle Pines, MN: American Guidance Service, Inc., 1997.

110. Spreen, O., Strauss, E. A. *A Compendium of Neuropsychological Tests: Administration, Norms, and Commentary*. New York: Oxford University Press, 1991.

111. Zimmerman, I., Steiner, V., Pond, R. *Preschool Language Scale*. 3rd edn. San Antonio, TX: Psychological Corporation, 1992.

112. Semel, E., Wiig E. H., Secord, W. *Clinical Evaluation of Language Fundamentals*. 4th edn. San Antonio, TX: Psychological Corporation, 2003.

113. Beery, K. *The Developmental Test of Visual–Motor Integration*. 4th edn. Cleveland, OH: Modern Curriculum Press, 1997.

114. Cohen, M. *Children's Memory Scale*. San Antonio, TX: Psychological Corporation, 1997.

115. Delis, D., Kramer, J., Kaplan, E. *California Verbal Learning Test, Children's Version*. San Antonio, TX: Psychological Corporation, 1994.

116. Roid, G. H., *Stanford–Binet Intelligence Scale*. 5th edn. Itasca IL: Riverside Publishing Company, 2003.

117. Reitan, R., Davidson, L. *Clinical Neuropsychology: Current Status and Applications*. New York: Winston/Wiley, 1974.

118. Conners, C. K. *MHS Staff. Conners' Continuous Performance Test II for Windows*. North Tonawanda, NY: MHS, Inc., 2000.

119. Raven, J., Summers, B., Birchfield, M. *et al. Manual for the Raven's Progressive Matrices and Vocabulary Scales. Res. Suppl. No.3: A Compendium of North American Normative and Validity Studies*. London: HK Lewis, 1984.

120. Folio, M., Fewell, R. *Peabody Developmental Motor Scales* 2nd edn. Chicago, IL: Riverside, 2001.

121. Bruininks, R., *Bruininks–Oseretsky Test of Motor Proficiency*. Circle Pines, MN: American Guidance Service, 1978.

122. Klove, H. Clinical neuropsychology. *Med. Clin. North Am.* 1963;**26**:592–600.

123. Sparrow, S., Cicchetti, D. Balla, D., *Vineland Adaptive Behavior Scales*. 2nd edn. Circle Pines, MN: American Guidance Service, 2005.

124. Achenbach, T., Edelbrock, C. *Manual for the Child Behavior Checklist and Revised Child Behavior Profile*. Burlington, VT: University of Vermont, 1983.

125. Conners, C. K., *Conners' Rating Scales-Revised*. North Tonawanda, NY: Multi-Health Systems, 1997.

126. Reynolds, C., Kamphaus, R. *Behavior Assessment System for Children-2*. Circle Pines, MN: American Guidance Service, Inc., 2004.

127. Gioia, G., Isquith, P., Guy, S., Kenworthy, L. *Behavior Rating Inventory of Executive Function*: Psychological Assessment Resources, Inc., 1996.

Part III
Antiretroviral therapy

11 Antiretroviral therapy

Ross McKinney, Jr., M.D.

Department of Pediatrics, Duke University School of Medicine, Durham, NC

The biology of HIV and antiretroviral therapy

Chapter 1 describes the HIV life cycle and outlines the steps in the life cycle targeted by antiretroviral drugs. The viral targets of antiretroviral agents are outlined in Chapter 1 Fig. 1.3, and Table 1.6. The antiretroviral drugs in current clinical use inhibit either the viral reverse transcriptase, the viral protease, or block the fusion of the virus with the membrane of its would-be future host cell. Additional viral targets (e.g., the viral integrase or chemokine receptors) are the subject of drug development efforts, but there are no currently approved antiviral drugs directed at these other targets

There are two classes of reverse transcriptase inhibitors (RTIs), the nucleoside analogue RTIs (NRTIs) and the non-nucleoside RTIs (NNRTIs). Nucleoside-analogue reverse transcriptase inhibitors (NRTIs) are modified nucleosides that are designed to lack a 3′OH group (see Chapter 1, Fig. 1.4). (Tenofovir is a nucleotide analagon, see below.) They are phosphorylated by host cell kinases and then incorporated into the elongating polynucleotide chain. Their incorporation produces a prematurely terminated cDNA molecule because another nucleotide cannot add to the chain due to the absent 3′OH. The viral reverse transcriptase has a greater relative affinity for the modified nucleosides than does the human DNA polymerase, which is why nucleoside analogues have a tolerable therapeutic index. The non-nucleoside RT inhibitors, NNRTIs, act through a different mechanism than the NRTIs. The NNRTIs interfere with binding at the active site of the reverse transcriptase. The NNRTIs have no effect on cellular DNA polymerases and have no effect on the reverse transcriptase of HIV-2. NNRTIs and NRTIs have very different side effect profiles. NNRTIs can be used in combination with NRTIs, often with synergistic activity (see also Chapter 14).

HIV's Gag virion structural proteins and the Pol proteins are synthesized as a long preprotein. The preprotein must be cleaved into many smaller proteins by the viral protease to produce a fully mature and infectious virion. The HIV protease, an aspartyl protease with similarities to cellular aspartyl proteases, has been a prominent target

Handbook of Pediatric HIV Care, ed. Steven L. Zeichner and Jennifer S. Read.
Published by Cambridge University Press. © Cambridge University Press 2006.

for drug development. Several of the resulting protease inhibitors (PIs) have excellent antiviral activity.

The fusion inhibitors (like enfuvirtide, also known as T-20, Fuzeon) bind to the gp41 envelope glycoprotein and inhibit the formation of the gp41 structure required for insertion of the gp41 fusion peptide into the host cell plasma membrane, inhibiting the fusion of the lipid bilayer of the virus and that of the host cell membrane. These drugs are peptides, and require parenteral, rather than oral, administration.

Suboptimal antiretroviral dosing or lack of adherence permits continued viral replication in the presence of low concentrations of drug, promoting the development of resistance to the agents, with important implications for the long'-term efficacy of antiretroviral therapeutic regimens (see chapter 14).

Doses of antiretroviral agents are provided in the formulary (Appendix 1). The formulary includes doses both for drugs approved by the FDA for use in pediatrics, and so that readers may have some appreciation of drugs currently under development, the doses for antiretroviral drugs that are in advanced stages of clinical development. Some of the drugs are not specifically approved for use in pediatrics and dosing recommendations for those drugs represent estimates that are based on the available literature and clinical experience, and may not be correct. Dosing and indications may change. New side effects and drug interactions may become known. Clinicians should take care to consult a current version of the package insert when prescribing antiretroviral agents, particularly newer agents. Many antiretroviral drugs have serious side effects and potentially harmful interactions with other drugs. Patients must be carefully monitored for these potential problems. Antiretroviral therapy should be managed by or in close consultation with an expert in the care of pediatric HIV disease.

Antiretroviral agents

Nucleoside analogue reverse transcriptase inhibitors (NRTIs)

The NRTIs were the first class of antiretroviral drugs developed. They can be divided into two categories: the thymidine derivatives and non-thymidine NRTIs. The two thymidine derivatives are zidovudine (ZDV) and stavudine (D4T). These two agents are antagonistic. In general, most combination regimens include at least two NRTIs, beginning with either ZDV or D4T. The second agent is generally selected from among lamivudine (3TC), didanosine (ddI), and zalcitabine (ddC). There has been an increasing trend toward the use of abacavir (ABC) (GlaxoSmithKline) in first line regimens, often in combination with 3TC or ZDV and 3TC (marketed as a fixed ratio combination tablet, Trizavir), although results from recent clinical trials suggest that the use of the fixed ABC/ZDV/3TC combination alone may be less effective than combination therapies that also include an NNRTI or a PI. The role of nucleotide analogs like tenofovir (Gilead Sciences), which has assumed an increasingly important role in HIV therapy for adults, has yet to be established in pediatrics. More details concerning the choice of antiretroviral agents, and the recommended criteria for starting and changing antiviral therapy can be found in Chapter 15.

The effective pharmacokinetic properties of the NRTIs are determined by the pharmacokinetic properties of the intracellular tri-phosphate form of the drug. The serum half-life of the unphosphorylated native drugs is relatively short, and most are rapidly excreted, some after hepatic glucuronidation. However, within the cell, the phosphorylated forms of the drugs may have a prolonged half-life, which allows for less frequent dosing intervals than the serum half-life would suggest.

Zidovudine (ZDV)

Overview

Zidovudine, (AZT or ZDV, Retrovir – GlaxoSmithKline; Combivir, as a fixed dose combination with lamivudine – GlaxoSmithKline; Trizivir, as a fixed dose combination with lamivudine and abacavir – GlaxoSmithKline), was the first FDA-approved antiretroviral drug [1]. It is a chain-terminating, thymidine-derived NRTI. The drug has substantial, although tolerable, side effects, and demonstrated clinical efficacy in children [2]. However, while ZDV monotherapy has clinical benefits, resistance develops over time, so the drug is now used only in combination regimens, except in the setting of regimens designed to interrupt vertical transmission (see Chapters 4 and 15). ZDV is available as both liquid and capsules.

Antiviral activity

As monotherapy, ZDV typically produces a 0.7 to 0.8 $\log_{10}$ decline in RNA copy number. The effect lasts for several months to years. In children, ZDV monotherapy produces only mild improvements in CD4+ lymphocyte counts [2]. It improves weight growth, at least in the short term, and can improve cognitive function in children with HIV encephalopathy.

The primary resistance mutations to ZDV are at codons 41, 67, 70, 210, 215, and 219. The first to appear is at codon 70, while the most important site is 215. Both contribute to multidrug resistance against nRTIs. A complex of mutations including codon 151 may also produce multinucleoside resistance.

Pharmacokinetics

ZDV has a short serum half-life (roughly 1 hour) in children beyond the first few months of life. The drug is first glucuronidated in the liver, then renally excreted. In young infants, the half-life is prolonged, both because of limited glucuronidation capability, and because of immature renal function. The active form of ZDV is zidovudine triphosphate. The drug is phosphorylated by cellular kinases. The intracellular half-life is approximately 3 hours, explaining why ZDV can be given as infrequently as twice per day.

Adverse effects

Alone or in combination, ZDV has a significant adverse event profile [2]. The most common problems are hematologic: anemia and neutropenia. These may respond to dose adjustment, although care should be taken to remain in a therapeutic range. Some physicians use erythropoietin or g-CSF to combat these side effects. Thrombocytopenia is rarely produced by ZDV. ZDV reliably produces increase in red cell volume (MCV), and can lead to an erythrocytic macrocytosis, with MCVs >100 fl. Indeed, the absence of an increase in MCV in patients for whom ZDV has been prescribed can be a clinically useful indication of poor compliance. ZDV has been associated with myopathy and cardiomyopathy. The drug can also produce restlessness, mild headaches, nausea, and fatigue, particularly in older children. There are some theoretical concerns regarding potential long-term and transplacental carcinogenicity of ZDV and presumably other NRTIs and, while ZDV has mutagenic and carcinogenic potential in certain animal models, there are no human data to support these concerns. Long-term follow-up studies of children exposed to ZDV in utero and as newborns as a component of strategies to prevent mother to infant transmission have not exhibited any significant long-term toxicities (see Chapter 4).

Didanosine (DDI)

Overview

Didanosine (DDI, Videx – Bristol Myers Squibb) is an NRTI that is metabolized from dideoxyinosine (DDI) to its active form, dideoxyadenosine (DDA). It has a good side effect profile in children; its use in young children is limited primarily by inconvenient dosage regimens, principally caused by its chemical instability in acid conditions such as those found in the stomach, and its consequent requirement for oral co-administration of substantial buffering, and by taste problems [3, 4]. DDI is available as a liquid mixed in antacid (usually Maalox), as a chewable/dispersible tablet, and as an extended release, enteric-coated capsule (Videx EC).

Antiviral effects

DDI monotherapy has antiviral effects similar to ZDV, as measured by surrogate markers. It has somewhat better durability as a monotherapy than ZDV, but it is now almost always given in combinations [5, 6].

The resistance mutations most often associated with DDI are at codons 65 and 74, although it is difficult to demonstrate antiviral resistance to DDI in vitro.

Pharmacokinetics

DDI is acid labile, and is administered simultaneously with an antacid. The intracellular half-life of DDA-triphosphate is quite long (more than 24 hours), so that it may be possible to administer DDI once daily, a considerable advantage given the complexity of many antiretroviral regimens. The concept of once-daily dosing has yet to be demonstrated to be effective in children, although early adult trials appear promising.

Didanosine should be given, when possible, on an empty stomach, ideally one hour before or two hours after a meal. However, with small children who eat often this may not be possible, and the importance of the daily schedule for compliance should be weighed against a relatively small loss in absorption due to food.

Didanosine liquid is not stable at ambient temperatures. It needs to be stored under refrigerated conditions, and some clinics give patients ice chests to use in transporting DDI suspension home from the pharmacy. The shelf-life, even refrigerated, is only 30 days. The chewable tablets are somewhat more convenient, but the taste can be challenging for children. If tablets are used, the minimum dose is two tablets at a time, since the tablets contain an antacid and two tablets are needed to supply enough antacid to provide adequate buffering capacity. The enteric-coated preparation is by far the most convenient, but young children may not be large enough for the minimum size capsule (and may not be able to swallow capsules in any case).

Adverse effects

Didanosine is generally well tolerated, although some patients have difficulty taking the drug because of its taste. The most common adverse events are peripheral neuropathy and pancreatitis. The neuropathy usually presents as paresthesias, most often of the feet, and may appear as a gait disturbance in younger children. Pancreatitis typically presents as abdominal pain, nausea, and vomiting. As opposed to other causes of abdominal pain, pancreatitis is usually associated with a rise in amylase and lipase levels, and may be confirmed in some instances through the use of ultrasonography. There is, however, no utility in routinely monitoring serum amylase levels for patients on DDI, since most episodes of pancreatitis are relatively acute and signaled first by pain. In addition, high amylase concentrations are often released by the salivary glands in children with HIV. In order to determine whether an elevated serum amylase is attributable to pancreatitis or parotitis, a fractionated amylase can be performed to distinguish between pancreatic and salivary isoenzymes. However, the isoenzyme assays have some overlap, so that a very high salivary amylase will give a falsely elevated pancreatic fraction. To improve the predictive value of amylase measurements, a serum lipase can be obtained. In most instances where both enzyme concentrations are high, pancreatitis should be suspected.

Some children experience abdominal symptoms such as diarrhea, pain, or nausea during treatment with DDI. Some of the effects may be from the antacid.

Stavudine (d4T)

Clinical overview

Stavudine (D4T, Zerit – Bristol Myers Squibb) is a thymidine-derived nucleotide with clinical potency roughly equivalent to ZDV [6, 7]. The advantages of D4T are that it can be given on a twice-daily dosing schedule, side effects are relatively uncommon in children, and timing around food is not an issue. D4T is available in an FDA approved liquid preparation, as well as capsules.

Antiviral effects

Stavudine is similar to ZDV in effect, producing a 0.7–0.8 $\log_{10}$ decrease in viral RNA concentration when used as monotherapy. Resistance to D4T involves mutations at essentially the same reverse transcriptase amino acid residues as ZDV, although mutations at amino acid 75 can also contribute to resistance. As with DDI, in vitro resistance is hard to document, although clinical exhaustion of potency is clearly demonstrable using surrogate markers.

Pharmacokinetics

Stavudine has a relatively long intracellular half life (3–4 hours) and can be given on a twice daily schedule. No special arrangements for mealtime are required since it is well absorbed on a full or empty stomach. Because D4T is renally excreted, dosage adjustment may be required in patients with renal problems. As with all of the nucleoside analogue drugs, D4T is phosphorylated intracellularly to the active triphosphate form. ZDV competes with D4T for the kinase that accomplishes the phosphorylations, so ZDV inhibits D4T phosphorylation. Therefore, ZDV and D4T should not be used simultaneously. In December 2002, an extended release form of D4T was FDA approved, which gives larger children the option of once-daily dosing.

Adverse effects

Stavudine is generally well tolerated by children. In adults, D4T is associated with peripheral neuropathy in a high proportion of patients. However, neuropathy appears to be less common in children. D4T is also associated rarely with anemia, pancreatitis, headache, and gastrointestinal disturbances. A major concern with D4T has been an interaction with DDI. There appears to be an increased rate of lactic acidosis, at times with fatal outcome, in all patients, although the incidence is still uncommon. In pregnant women, however, the incidence of lactic acidosis appears to be markedly elevated, which has meant the combination of D4T with DDI in pregnant women is now contraindicated. Some anecdotal evidence also suggests that the risks of pancreatitis may be worse when D4T and DDI are used together.

Lamivudine (3TC)

Overview

Lamivudine (3TC, Epivir – GlaxoSmithKline; Combivir, as a fixed dose combination with zidovudine – GlaxoSmithKline; Trizivir, as a fixed dose combination with zidovudine and abacavir – GlaxoSmithKline) is a well-tolerated cytosine analogue and is a relatively potent NRTI in the absence of resistance, but a single nucleotide substitution in RT dramatically increases resistance to the drug. The drug is well tolerated, and frequently is used together with ZDV and D4T as the "nucleoside backbone" component of combination regimens. Liquid and tablet preparations are available.

Antiviral effect

As monotherapy, 3TC can produce up to 1 $\log_{10}$ decreases in plasma concentrations of HIV RNA. However, resistance to 3TC monotherapy occurs quickly and requires only a single point mutation at amino acid 184 in the RT gene. 3TC is virtually always used in combination with another NRTI, particularly D4T or ZDV (the two thymidine-analogue NRTIs). The benefits of 3TC were confirmed in Pediatric ACTG protocol 300, where ZDV/3TC was clinically superior to monotherapy DDI [8]. 3TC also appears to make tenofovir more effective, particularly when the M184V mutation is present. In order to maintain the M184V mutation and its tenofovir hypersensitizing effect, 3TC should be continued even when resistance appears to be present. Resensitization and hypersusceptibility are discussed in more detail in Chapter 14.

Pharmacokinetics

3TC has a relatively long half-life and is renally excreted. It may be given every 12 hours, and has recently been approved in adults for once daily dosing. There are no food-related interactions. The dosage should be reduced in patients with renal impairment.

Adverse effects

3TC is a well-tolerated compound. The only major side effect has been pancreatitis, which was primarily seen in a very ill, multiply antiretroviral treated group of children at the National Cancer Institute. Subsequent studies have demonstrated that pancreatitis is quite rare. For example, there were no instances of 3TC-associated pancreatitis in PACTG 300 (patients followed a median of 11 months), while there were eight cases of pancreatitis in patients treated with DDI-containing regimens. 3TC can occasionally cause headaches, gastrointestinal upset, fatigue, and elevated hepatic transaminases. None of these is a common reason for dosage adjustment.

Zalcitabine (DDC)

Overview

Zalcitabine (DDC, Hivid – Roche) has been used relatively sparingly in children, because there is no liquid formulation, because of its side effects profile and because there is extensive cross resistance between DDC and other NRTIs, notably DDI and 3TC (see below). The available capsule formulation is geared toward adult dosing.

Antiviral effects

DDC is roughly comparable to DDI in activity [9, 10]. HIV exhibits a considerable degree of cross-resistance between DDI and DDC, and between 3TC and DDC. In general, once a patient has had DDI experience, there will be little benefit from a shift to DDC. The most important resistance mutations occur at RT amino acid residues 65, 69, 74, and 184.

Pharmacokinetics

Zalcitabine is given every 8 hours. There are some medications that affect DDC's renal clearance (cimetidine, amphotericin, foscarnet, and aminoglycosides). Antacids may decrease absorption.

Adverse effects

Zalcitabine has been associated with a peripheral neuropathy affecting the distal extremities, especially the feet. The symptoms usually begin with numbness or paresthesias, can be quite painful, and may persist for several weeks after discontinuation of the ddC. Zalcitabine is rarely associated with pancreatitis or painful oral ulcerations. Headache and fatigue can sometimes occur.

Abacavir (ABC)

Overview

Abacavir (ABC, Ziagen – GlaxoSmithKline; Trizivir, as a fixed dose combination with zidovudine and lamivudine – GlaxoSmithKline) is a relatively potent novel carbocyclic guanosine analogue nucleoside that has excellent activity when used as initial antiviral therapy [11, 12]. Both capsule and liquid preparations are available. Its major drawback has been a hypersensitivity syndrome, generally seen in the first few weeks of dosing. Those patients who have rash, fever, and abdominal pain during their first few weeks on ABC should, in most cases, have it stopped immediately. They should not be rechallenged, since profound hypotension has been seen in some patients on reinstitution of ABC after interruption.

Antiviral effects

ABC is probably the most potent of current NRTI compounds as initial therapy, but resistance to it has been observed even when patients have not been exposed to ABC, presumably due to cross-resistance with other NRTIs (see below). Most studies have evaluated abacavir in combination with other antiretroviral agents. When used with PIs in therapy-naïve adults, ABC produced 2 $\log_{10}$ decreases in RNA copy number.

There is substantial cross-resistance between ABC and other nucleosides, particularly the thymidine analogs. Resistance sites also include the DDI resistance codons like 65, 74, and 115, and the 3TC resistance codon 184, although the relative importance of each remains to be determined. There has been considerable interest in the Trizivir fixed dose combination as an all NRTI regimen, particularly in adolescents, but recent results suggest that this combination may be inferior to combination regimens that include a PI or NNRTI.

Pharmacokinetics

ABC is administered on an every 12-hour schedule. The drug is cleared by glucuronidation and by the alcohol dehydrogenase system, which produces a carboxylic acid metabolite. The serum half-life is approximately 1 hour. There is no food effect on absorption. ABC crosses the blood-brain barrier in a manner similar to ZDV, with a CSF/plasma ratio of approximately 0.2.

Adverse effects
The main concern with ABC is an idiosyncratic allergic reaction manifested by rash, fever, abdominal pain, nausea, and vomiting. This reaction seems to occur most often in the first 3 weeks of therapy, and if it occurs there should be no ABC rechallenge. Patients have progressed to shock and even death as a result of rechallenge after an episode of hypersensitivity. This reaction can be difficult to distinguish from the rash syndrome of nevirapine and even from some infectious conditions (adenovirus, scarlet fever). There appears to be a definable genetic risk for predisposition to the reaction in that patients with certain HLA subtypes may have an increased risk of developing the hypersensitivity reaction.

Tenofovir (TDF)
Overview
Tenofovir disoproxil fumarate (TDF, Viread – Gilead Sciences) is a nucleo*tide* analogue reverse transcriptase inhibitor, unlike the other members of the class, which are nucleoside analogues. A nucleotide is a phosphorylated nucleoside, which means that TDF, as administered, is already monophosphorylated. Both the nucleoside analogue reverse transcriptase inhibitors and TDF must be phosphorylated by cellular kinases to the triphosate form before they can function as substrates for reverse transcriptase, but TDF bypasses the first phosphorylation step. (Thus, as a nucleotide analogue the active form of the drug is tenofovir diphosphate.) Since the kinases that catalyze phosphorylation to the monophosphate may be less active in resting cells, TDF may offer some advantages in that it may have greater activity in resting cells.

Antiviral effects
TDF is similar to ZDV in potency. As monotherapy, it produces a 0.6 to 1.5 log_{10} decrease in plasma HIV RNA concentration [13]. Resistance is conferred by mutations at RT codons K65R, although there are probably contributions from M41L and L210W. Virus with several nucleoside analogue-associated mutations (NAMS, see also Chapter 14) appears to be relatively resistant. Codon T69D, may also play a role in resistance, although data are still preliminary. The 69 insertion mutation complex that confers high level resistance to the nucleoside analogue reverse transcriptase inhibitors also confers high level resistance to tenofovir.

TDF is also active against hepatitis B, although studies in pediatric patients are limited.

Pharmacokinetics
Tenofovir disoproxil fumarate is a pro-drug which is converted to tenofovir in the gastrointestinal tract. Oral bioavailability in adults is roughly 25% (fasted), and the

drug is better absorbed when taken with food. Tenofovir is cleared renally, with no involvement of the cytochrome P450 system. Its long intracellular half-life means the drug can be administered once a day.

TDF interacts with DDI, causing increased ddI exposure. When the drugs are used in combination, a reduced ddI dose is probably indicated. TDF causes decreases in atazanavir levels (see below) and the combination of atazanavir and TDF should either be avoided or atazanavir should be boosted with ritonavir.

Adverse effects

Gastrointestinal problems (diarrhea, nausea, vomiting) can occur, but are not frequent. Liver transaminase elevations have been reported. Nephrotoxicity may rarely occur. As with the nucleoside RT inhibitors, lactic acidosis has been reported with TDF. In studies of young animals, higher doses of TDF have caused decreases in bone mineral density, a finding that suggests that if the drug is used in children there should be careful consideration given to this potential toxicity.

Emtricitabine (FTC)

Overview

Emtricitabine (FTC, Emtriva – Gilead Sciences) is a nucleoside analogue reverse transcriptase inhibitor very similar in its resistance profile to 3TC. Studies are in progress in children (for example, Pediatric AIDS Clinical Trials Group Protocol 1021), and while it appears to have predictable pharmacokinetics and activity, now approved.

Antiviral effects

FTC is similar to 3TC in potency. Resistance is conferred by mutations at RT codon M184V/I, as is 3TC. Cross resistance with 3TC and zalcitabine is present in most FTC resistant isolates.

Pharmacokinetics

While studies in children are still preliminary, FTC pharmacokinetics appear to be relatively predictable in children. Food does not affect absorption, and the oral bioavailability of capsule FTC is 93% in adult studies (according to the Emtriva package insert). The half-life is approximately 10 hours, and clearance is renal (a mix of filtration and active tubular secretion). Dosage should be downwardly adjusted in renal failure. Drug interactions have been minimal to date. A dose of 6 mg/kg per day gave an AUC comparable to the standard adult dose of 200 mg/day [14].

Adverse effects

Adverse effects of FTC have been relatively uncommon. The most notable adverse effect has been hyperpigmentation of the palms and/or soles. The mechanism is unknown. Lactic acidosis and severe hepatomegaly with steatosis is a rare but severe problem for all NRTIs.

Non-nucleoside reverse transcriptase inhibitors (NNRTIs)

There are three licensed NNRTIs, nevirapine (NVP), delavirdine (DLV), and efavirenz (EFU), which are similar in their activity. Efavirenz is the most widely used NNRTI, but there is little data on its use in children under the age of 3 years. Nevirapine is the most widely used NNRTI in young children, since there is a liquid formulation of nevirapine. Efavirenz has an investigational liquid formulation, but that formulation is not approved in the USA and pediatric dosing in the USA is based on giving multiples of small capsules. Because it lacks a liquid preparation and is probably less potent, DLV is the least used and studied of the three. Single amino acid change mutations, for example mutations at codon 103, confer high level resistance to all the available NNRTIs. Cross-resistance among these three agents is almost complete, so if a patient becomes unresponsive to one NNRTI another NNRTI should not be substituted.

Nevirapine (NVP)

Overview

Nevirapine (NVP, Viramune – Roxane/Boehringer Ingelheim) was developed simultaneously in children and adults, although the adult preparation was FDA-approved substantially before the pediatric. The drug is quite potent, even as monotherapy, but rapidly selects for resistant virus.

Antiviral effects

A single point mutation, at codon 103 or at codon 181 of RT, leads to high level NVP resistance [15] (see Chapter 14). Codons Y188L and V106A can also decrease NVP sensitivity. Used as monotherapy, almost complete drug resistance can be seen consistently after as little as 4 to 6 weeks, and appreciable resistance can be found in some patients following even a single dose. When NVP is part of a combination, the drug has activity similar to PI's, although clinically the rapid development of resistance can still be significant. It has been studied as a component of a combination regimen in the treatment of newborns, and in that context can produce long-lasting viral suppression [16].

Pharmacokinetics

The pharmacokinetics of NVP are complex. The drug is lipophilic and distributes into body tissues well. NVP administration auto-induces its metabolism, so that the same dose given over time leads to a decreasing serum concentration. The change in clearance is approximately 1.5–2-fold. Because the induction of metabolism plateaus over time, NVP is given once per day for the first 14 days, then twice daily dosing is initiated. The adult serum half-life is approximately 25 hours. In neonates, hepatic immaturity means NVP metabolism is very slow, and a single oral dose can produce several days at a therapeutic concentration. This effect of NVP, combined with its potency, low cost, and the fact that NVP crosses the placenta well, are the reasons a two-dose NVP regimen (one maternal dose plus one newborn dose) were evaluated for perinatal prophylaxis.

Adverse effects

NVP is associated with two primary adverse effects. First, early after initiation of therapy, hepatitis and/or elevated hepatic transaminases can develop. The other major side effect is rash, which occurs in approximately 8% of children. NVP rash begins as a macular-papular eruption, most often within 5 weeks of starting therapy. In most cases the rash evolves to include fever and malaise. NVP should be stopped if rash occurs because the exanthem can evolve to severe Stevens–Johnson syndrome.

Delavirdine (DLV)

Overview

Delavirdine (DLV, Rescriptor – Pfizer) has no liquid formulation, and there are almost no data about its use in children. It is dosed three times per day and there is a high-level of cross-resistance with NVP. The major side effect, rash, is less severe than that of NVP. Since there is no liquid formulation and since it offers no apparent benefit over the other available NNRTIs, it is not widely used in pediatrics.

Antiviral effects

DLV is similar to other NNRTIs in potency. The resistance pattern varies slightly, although the key sites appear to be RT amino acid mutations K103N and Y181C (in common with other NNRTIs), along with Y188L, P236L, and V106A. DLV has been evaluated in combination with NRTIs, which can delay the development of DLV resistance. However, some investigators feel the benefits of DLV are less than the other NNRTIs.

Pharmacokinetics

DLV has not been studied in children. Dosing in adults is every 8 hours. The drug is hepatically excreted. DLV inhibits the cytochrome P450 system, in contrast to NVP, and so tends to increase PI concentrations. Systemic exposure to ritonavir, for example, is increased by 70%.

Adverse effects

The main adverse effect of DLV is rash. The rash is milder than that seen with NVP, and most cases occurs within the first month on treatment. The rash is generalized, maculopapular, and can be pruritic.

Efavirenz

Overview

Efavirenz (EFV, Sustiva – Bristol Myers Squibb; outside the USA: Stocrin – Merck) was FDA approved for adults and children older than 3 years in September 1998. Solid and liquid formulations exist, but only the solid formulation has been approved and is available in the USA. Liquid efavirenz (Stocrin) is available in certain countries outside the USA. Efavirenz has a long half-life, which allows once a day administration. Because of its activity and because of concerns about the metabolic side effects of the PIs, efavirenz has become an increasingly widely used component of initial highly active antiretroviral therapy regimens [17, 18].

Antiviral effects

Efavirenz has activity similar to other NNRTIs. The resistance pattern is also similar to other NNRTIs, since mutation K103N in the RT gene produces a nearly 20-fold decrease in susceptibility. Studies indicate that efavirenz may sometimes retain effectiveness in the face of the Y181C RT mutation that affects most NNRTIs, as well as the P236L delavirdine-associated mutation, but the spectrum of other mutations in RT apparently influences the degree of resistance when the Y181C mutation is present. Other resistance substitutions have been seen at codons L100I, V108I, Y181C, Y188L, G190S, and P225H.

Pharmacokinetics

Efavirenz is excreted hepatically. The drug induces cytochrome P-450 isoform CYP 3A4, which may decrease PI concentrations. The half-life is long, 40–55 hours, allowing daily dosing. There is good CNS penetration. Efavirenz decreases the levels of saquinavir, to a degree that the drugs should generally not be used together, although it may be possible to use SQV boosted by ritonavir.

Adverse effects

The most common EFV-related problems are rash, dizziness, and other minor CNS abnormalities. Patients also sometimes report central nervous system side effects, including dizziness, impaired concentration, somnolence, hallucinations, and vivid dreams. The impact of these side effects may be less when the drug is given at bedtime, as recommended. Rash, most often a maculopapular eruption, occurred in 30%–40% of children, with 7% reporting severe rash. The rash usually resolves with continued treatment. However, the most problematic toxicity concern is in pregnant women. While efavirenz has not yet been documented to cause birth defects in humans, 3 of 20 pregnant monkeys dosed with efavirenz gave birth to infants with significant birth defects. The three had cleft palate, microphthalmia, and anencephaly with unilateral anophthalmia. It is recommended that women do not use efavirenz during pregnancy, particularly early in gestation, and that birth control be used while a women is on efavirenz.

HIV-protease inhibitors

The HIV structural proteins are initially translated as long preproteins that must be proteolytically cleaved by the viral protease into their viral mature form for infectious virus to be produced (see Chapter 1). The HIV PIs are effective because they can specifically inhibit the HIV protease while not affecting host proteases. Unfortunately, the protease inhibitors can be difficult to use in children. They are relatively hydrophobic and so are not readily made into suspensions or water-based solutions, and require agents such as ethanol, propylene glycol, or vitamin E to help solubilize them in liquid preparations. The PIs taste bad, and they interact with the liver's P450 cytochromes in complex ways. Some protease inhibitors induce certain P450 isoforms, while inhibiting others. Ritonavir, as an example, is a relatively broad inhibitor of the P450 enzyme system and it induces its own metabolism. Ritonavir's complicated pharmacokinetic interactions complicate the use of many other drugs.

Multiprotease inhibitor resistance has been demonstrated as mutations accumulate at L10F/I/R/V, M46I/L, I54V/M/L, V82A/F/T/S, I84V, and L90M. In addition, each PI has specific, associated mutations. Use of any PI begins the progression toward multidrug resistance, although some like nelfinavir seem less likely to induce multidrug resistance.

Amprenavir (APV)

Overview

Amprenavir (APV, Agenerase – GlaxoSmithKline) has a relatively unique resistance pattern, which makes it a candidate to use in combination with other protease inhibitors. There are both capsule and liquid formulations. The drug is approved by the FDA for adults and for children 4 years old and older.

Antiviral effects

APV has a potent antiviral effect, similar to other protease inhibitors [19]. When used as monotherapy, the predominant resistance mutation selected is I50V. In standard combination therapy, mutations are selected include V32I, M46I/L, I47V, I54L/M, and I84V. APV has been evaluated in combination with other PIs, and there appear to be enough differences in its resistance pattern so that using APV with other PIs can sometimes be beneficial in patients previously treated with other PIs.

Pharmacokinetics

APV is cleared by the cytochrome P450 system, which it also inhibits. However, APV does not appear to induce or inhibit its own metabolism. Specifically, APV inhibits the CYP3A4 isoform of the cytochrome P450 system, the most common isoform. The plasma half-life is somewhat variable, but is approximately 7 hours, which is very suitable for twice daily dosing. The liquid form of APV currently contains propylene glycol and large quantities of vitamin E and is not suitable for children under the age of 4 years.

Adverse effects

The most common adverse effects with APV are gastrointestinal. Some patients have headache, malaise, or fatigue. There may be some cutaneous reactions. APV is related to sulfonamides, so should be used with caution in patients with severe sulfa allergy.

Indinavir (IDV)

Clinical overview

Indinavir (IDV, Crixivan – Merck) is widely used to treat adult patients, but pediatric experience is very limited. IDV is potent, has a similar resistance pattern to ritonavir, and produces several adverse effects. Although pediatric studies are not complete, it appears IDV will be administered every 8 hours in children, and should be given on an empty stomach. The medication is only soluble at an acid pH, so food in the stomach buffers the pH and makes the IDV less available. The every-8-hour dosing, the need for an empty stomach, and the lack of an approved liquid formulation, make the drug relatively unappealing for pediatric use, especially in young children.

Like the other protease inhibitors, IDV has interactions with numerous other medications (See Chapter 12). The extent of these interactions is somewhat less than with RTV, which makes drug interactions somewhat easier to manage.

Antiviral effects

IDV is a potent agent, comparable to RTV. The pattern of mutations seen is almost identical to that of RTV, and there is a high degree of cross-resistance. It was in the initial trials of IND that it was learned that low doses of the agent allowed the evolution of PI-resistant quasi-species. When patients were subsequently switched to higher doses of IND, no antiviral effect was seen due to the existence of mutations that had evolved at the lower dose. Thus, subtherapeutic dosing, either by mis-prescription or erratic compliance, will allow permanent PI resistance to occur.

Pharmacokinetics

IND is only soluble at low pH. As a result, it needs to be taken on an empty stomach. Once absorbed, it is carried on plasma proteins and metabolized by glucuronidation and the cytochrome P450 system. Some IND is excreted through the kidneys. Because of urine's neutral pH, the IND can precipitate and produce kidney stones. IND has interactions in both directions with drugs that affect the cytochrome P450 system. It inhibits the metabolism of many drugs, and its many interactions are reviewed in Chapter 12.

Adverse effects

Because of its solubility characteristics, IDV can form crystals in the kidney after filtration through the glomerulus. These crystals can agglomerate into small kidney stones. In order to minimize the formation of IDV stones, patients treated with IDV should drink large amounts of water or other fluids. The proportion of children who will have stones is not yet known, although some studies have suggested a higher peak IDV plasma level after oral dosing in children, which might lead to more stone formation.

Other side effects of IDV include: hyperbilirubinemia, which occurs in 5%–10% of patients; nausea; abdominal pain; headache; and rarely diabetes. As with the other protease inhibitors, some adult and pediatric patients exhibit a pattern of fat redistribution and dyslipidemias in association with IDV.

Lopinavir plus ritonavir (LPV/r)

Clinical overview

Lopinavir (LPV, – Abbott) is available only in a fixed ratio combination with ritonavir (LPV/r, Kaletra) [20]. LPV/r is probably the most potent of the PIs. LPV by itself has a very short half-life, so the RTV is co-administered to inhibit LPV metabolism by the cytochrome P450 enzyme system. The combination can be given every 12 hours. Liquid Kaletra is, like liquid ritonavir, a bad tasting solution with 42% ethanol. There is significant debate among clinicians concerning LPV/r's optimal role in antiretroviral therapy. Some studies suggest that it is more potent and produces a more durable virologic response than other available PIs, leading some clinicians to suggest that it be used for initial therapy. Other clinicians note that LPV requires a somewhat different spectrum of resistance mutations than the other PIs, so that LPV/r can often be used to good effect in a second line "salvage" treatment regimen, and suggest that other PIs be used for initial treatment and that LPV/r be held in reserve. LPV/r is FDA approved for children 6 months of age and older.

Antiviral effects

Kaletra is probably the most potent PI currently licensed. There are 11 mutations which have been linked to resistance: L10F/I/R/V, K20M/R, L24I, M46I/L, F53L, I54V/L, L63P, A71V/T, V82A/F/T/S, I84V, and L90M. The presence of six to eight mutations produces high level resistance and is associated with clinical failure.

Pharmacokinetics

LPV/r can be dosed every 12 hours, and is available as either a capsule or liquid. Attention must be paid to drug–drug interactions, because the ritonavir component, in particular, inhibits the cytochrome P450 system resulting in extensive drug interactions. In addition, Kaletra liquid is 42.4% ethanol. LPV/r should be taken with food, both to enhance absorption and improve tolerance.

Adverse effects

The most common adverse experiences are gastrointestinal upset and diarrhea. As with other PIs, triglyceride levels and elevated cholesterol are fairly common. Pancreatitis has been rarely reported in association with LPV/r. Exacerbation or new onset of diabetes mellitus has also been associated with LPV/r.

Nelfinavir (NLV)

Clinical overview

Nelfinavir (NLV, Viracept, –Agouron/Pfizer) is a less convenient drug to administer than ritonavir, but has fewer adverse reactions. The medication is available in capsules and a granular powder. The powder is somewhat bulky and there are sufficient questions about its bioavailability that many centers prefer to use the capsules dispersed in a solution like milk or formula.

Antiviral effects

NLV is similar to other protease inhibitors in its antiviral effect [21]. Resistance to NLV requires a different set of resistance mutations than ritonavir or indinavir. The most important mutation is D30N, which was found in 56% of patients who received NLV monotherapy by 12 to 16 weeks. There is marked cross-resistance between NLV and the other protease inhibitors, although patients who fail NLV and have only low-level resistance may respond to other protease inhibitors or PI combinations. HIV with high level NLV resistance is also resistant to other PIs. For these HIVs with high level resistance, 65%–80% of isolates with more than tenfold resistance to NLV also had more than a fourfold increase in resistance to other PIs [22]. HIV that is resistant to other PIs usually has significant resistance to NLV, so treatment with NLV offers little benefit if a patient has failed therapy with another PI.

Pharmacokinetics

NLV is hepatically metabolized by multiple cytochrome P450 isoforms, including CYP3A. The adult plasma half-life is 3.5 to 5 hours. The drug is highly protein bound, and relatively little is cleared through the kidneys. Most of the drug is excreted through the GI tract and feces. The standard dosage interval is every 8–12 hours. The granular powder is difficult for most children to take, and many centers use a dispersed capsule if the correct dosage can be achieved.

Adverse effects

NLV has a tolerable level of adverse drug effects. The most common adverse effect is diarrhea, which is generally manageable with symptomatic measures. Some children may, however, be unable to tolerate NLV due to diarrhea. Less common problems include tiredness, abdominal pains, and rashes. Diabetes can occur rarely, as it does with all protease inhibitors.

Ritonavir (RTV)

Clinical overview

Ritonavir (RTV, Norvir, –Abbott) was the first PI FDA-approved for children. It is available in both a liquid formulation and gel-caps. The liquid has a bad taste and contains 43% ethanol. Ritonavir is potent, but because of significant side affects and drug interactions, needs to be used with care.

Antiviral effects

RTV is a potent antiretroviral agent, and demonstrates good antiviral effects when used as part of a combination antiretroviral regimen [23]; it has a relatively complex pattern of resistance mutations. The mutations conferring resistance to RTV are, however, almost identical with those to conferring resistance to indinavir, so patients who are failing therapy with one drug are unlikely to benefit from a switch to the other. The main mutations associated with RTV resistance have been at protease codons 82, 84, and 90. Some patients with high-level resistance to nelfinavir (NLV) will also be refractory to RTV, although it depends on which anti-NLV mutations are present.

Pharmacokinetics

The pharmacokinetics of RTV are complicated by its effect on hepatic enzymes. RTV is hepatically metabolized by the cytochrome P450 system. Complicating its clearance, RTV generally inhibits P450, but induces its own metabolism. RTV is begun at half the normal dose, then increased after a period of induction. Because of the induction of metabolism, this strategy of a low-dose moving to a higher one will yield drug concentrations that are fairly constant. RTV metabolism appears to be saturable, so that increasing doses beyond some threshold level may produce higher than expected levels.

RTV is well absorbed orally, regardless of food. The half-life is 3 to 4 hours. There are many interactions with other medications that can affect the metabolism of the RTV as well as the other compounds. These important interactions are reviewed in Chapter 12.

Adverse effects

RTV is associated with many problematic side effects. Nausea and vomiting are produced both by the RTV itself, and by the ethanol solvent. In some children the nausea becomes chronic and does not decrease with time. RTV can also produce diarrhea, anorexia, headaches, circumoral paresthesias, and elevated hepatic transaminases. In rare circumstances, it may produce diabetes. In regard to laboratory tests, hypercholesterolemia and hypertriglyceridemia are both common.

Care should be taken in coadministering any drug with RTV. There is a long list of absolute and relative contraindications, including many drugs commonly used in HIV disease (see Chapter 12). The common thread is clearance by the cytochrome P450 enzyme system.

Saquinavir (SQV)
Clinical overview

There is less information about pediatric use of saquinavir (SQV, Invirase (hard gel capsule) or Fortivase (soft-gel capsule – see below)–Roche) than other protease inhibitors, primarily because the only approved formuation are adult-sized capsules [24]. SQV is most often used in combination with ritonavir. This combination is rational both because SQV has a distinct resistance pattern, and because RTV increases serum SQV levels. Some patients who have failed NLV may respond to the combination of RTV and SQV, although they will do best if new NRTIs are introduced at the same time.

Although there is no pediatric dose for SQV yet, it seems probable the dosing interval will be every 8 hours. In most cases it will be given in combination with RTV. The adult capsules are relatively large and several must be taken at each dosing interval. The drug interactions of SQV are very much like the other PIs, although are less significant than those of RTV.

Antiviral effects

While some mutations that confer resistance to the other PIs also confer resistance to SQV, for example L10R/V, V82A, I84V, and L90M, the SQV resistance pattern also has some unique features. The key mutations conferring resistance to SQV are G48V and L90M. In its soft-gel preparation, it is probably similar to other PIs in potency.

Pharmacokinetics

SQV is administered as a soft-gel capsule (Fortivase). The previous formulation (Invirase) was not adequately bioavailable (less than 5% absorbed). The soft-gel capsule is enjoying wider use than the hard-gel capsule. However, the levels of SQV and the clinical effects are much improved when the hard-gel capsule is administered together with ritonavir. While absorption of the soft gel capsules in children is similar to adults, children appear to clear oral SQV somewhat more rapidly, and a higher mg/kg dose is required [24]. Food increases SQV absorption in the soft-gel formulation. SQV is cleared almost entirely by cytochrome P450 CYP3A4. The plasma half-life is 1.6 hours, and the standard dosing interval is every eight hours. Concomitant NLV, IND, or RTV therapy increase SQV levels by inhibiting hepatic metabolism (approximately 4-fold, 6-fold, and 20-fold, respectively). RTV can, in fact, increase the serum half-life of SQV so that only twice daily dosing is required. SQV does not penetrate well into the CSF.

Adverse effects

SQV is generally well tolerated. The most common adverse experiences are diarrhea, abdominal pain, headache, and nausea. Diabetes may rarely occur. Photosensitivity can occur with SQV, so sunscreen and protective clothing are suggested.

Atazanavir (ATZ)

Clinical overview

ATZ is a protease inhibitor that has been FDA approved for adults. It has two advantages in adults: (i) once daily dosing; (ii) minimal changes in lipid concentrations, unlike most of the other protease inhibitors. However, ATZ appears to have a shorter half-life in children and adolescents, which means that to achieve once daily dosing, RTV boosting is required. RTV boosting then negates atazanavir's advantages in causing dyslipidemia. Cross-resistance between ATZ and other PIs is common, so the drug does not offer much promise in second line or salvage regimens.

Antiviral effects

The primary mutation isolated from patients failing ATZ therapy has been I50L, often in combination with A71V. Resistance is also associated with I84V, L90M, A71V/T, N88S/D, and M46I (Reyataz package insert).

Pharmacokinetics

Pharmacokinetic studies of ATZ in children are ongoing. Determining a correct dose has not been as easy as simply extrapolating from adult regimens, and to obtain a once daily regimen in children has required RTV boosting. ATZ has many pharmacokinetic interactions because it is an inhibitor of CYP3A and UGT1A1, a pattern typical of protease inhibitors. It interacts with antacids, including proton pump inhibitors like omeprazole, leading to decreased absorption of ATZ. Stomach acid neutralizing agents should not be used with ATZ. Concomitant administration of ATZ and tenofovir lead to significant decreases in ATZ concentrations (~40% in Cmin and ~25% in AUC). If for some special reason this combination must be used, then ATZ should be boosted with ritonavir.

Adverse effects

ATZ produces total hyperbilirubinemia in 35%–50% of patients. In roughly 10% of patients, this effect will be severe enough to produce jaundice and scleral icterus. As a result, because of concerns about kernicterus, ATZ is contraindicated in children less than 3 months old. Other adverse effects are similar to other PIs and NNRTIs.

Fusion inhibitors
Enfuvirtide (ENF, T-20)
Overview

Enfuvirtide (ENF, Fuzeon – Trimeris/Roche) is the first in a novel category of antiretroviral drugs, the fusion inhibitors. ENF is a 36-amino acid peptide that is homologous to a portion of the viral gp41 envelope glycoprotein. It acts by mimicking the native viral portion of gp41, complexing with the virus gp41 and blocking the conformational changes in that molecule that allow fusion of the virus's lipid bilayer and the cell membrane (See Chapter 1). The limitations to ENF include its expense and the fact that it must be administered through injection. The drug is also very expensive.

Antiviral effects

ENF acts to block viral fusion with the host cell membrane. Resistance mutations occur in the gp41 envelope gene, primarily in the region of the first heptide repeat (HR-1). Several candidate resistance mutations have been noted: G36D/S, I37V, V38A/M, Q39R, N42T, N43D. Resistance appears to develop relatively rapidly if ENF is used as monotherapy. ENF has some activity in patients with long histories of antiretroviral therapy and who have virus that is resistant to other antiretroviral drugs [25].

Pharmacokinetics

ENF is a synthetic peptide, and administration of the active form requires subcutaneous injection on an every-12-hour schedule. It does not interact with, or alter, the metabolism of most other antiretroviral drugs.

Adverse effects

By far the most common adverse effect is the generation of injection site reactions.

Combination antiretroviral regimens

Antiretroviral drugs are virtually always given in combinations. While monotherapy with several drugs in clinical trials has demonstrated significant clinical benefit, single drug regimens yield only limited decreases in plasma HIV RNA, modest increases in CD4+ lymphocyte numbers, and lead to rapid emergence of drug resistance. As a result, multidrug regimens, highly active antiretroviral therapy, are standard. Virtually all first-line combination regimens begin with an NRTI "backbone." One of the greatest limitations in current therapeutic strategies is that there are a limited number of NRTIs, and cross-resistance is probably more of a problem than was originally believed. For example, there are currently only two thymidine-derived NRTIs, ZDV and d4T, and one or the other will form a component of most regimens. However, these two drugs have a considerable degree of cross-resistance. Tenofovir may be another option for adults, but experience in pediatrics is currently limited, and it may present particular problems for pediatrics. ZDV and D4T should not be used simultaneously in the same regimen, since both drugs require phosphorylation by the same kinase and will compete with each other for the first phosphorylation step.

After starting with a thymidine-derived NRTI, most combinations add 3TC or DDI. The combination of DDI and D4T has a higher rate of adverse side effects than other combinations, including metabolic problems such as lactic acidosis, and pancreatitis, and so is a combination currently viewed with disfavor. The problems with lactic acidosis are particularly frequent in pregnant women; the combination of D4T and DDI is contraindicated during pregnancy.

The other available nucleoside, abacavir, can be used in combination with both ZDV and 3TC, or simply with 3TC. It appears to be the most potent of the nucleosides, particularly when used in a first-line regimen. ABC is less effective as second-line therapy.

The convenience of fixed-ratio tablets makes some combinations more appealing in children large enough to take the tablets. The fixed dose combination of ZDV and 3TC as Combivir (Glaxo SmithKline), and ABC, ZDV, and 3TC as Trizavir (Glaxo SmithKline), both of which are dosed twice a day, offer some advantages in decreasing pill burden and potentially improving adherence. Trizivir used alone, in particular, has garnered considerable interest from clinicians caring for adolescents because of its low pill burden and the increased potential for adherence. However, recent results indicate that Trizivir alone is less effective than Trizivir plus a PI, or Combivir plus a PI, so Trizivir used alone will probably be a less favored in the future.

After the nucleoside backbone has been chosen, a third and sometimes a fourth drug will be added, depending on the patient's clinical details, prior antiretroviral therapy, resistance testing, if available, the patient's age, and adherence considerations. Among the protease inhibitors, there is no clear choice for first-line therapy. NLV is often given because of its relatively good tolerability, and because second-line PI regimens are somewhat easier to construct after NLV failure than after other PIs. LPV/r is probably the most potent option, but its taste and the ethanol content of the liquid preparation are obstacles for many children. The NNRTIs, either NVP (for young children) or EFV (in older children), are convenient and viable options for components of first-line therapy, as long as the family appears to be likely to be medication adherent. Because high-level resistance develops rapidly when the currently available NNRTIs are used alone, many clinicians would not construct an antiretroviral combination therapeutic regimen using the NNRTIs if there are doubts about the ability of the family to be strictly adherent.

The decisions regarding initial therapy cannot be made casually. Many factors, particularly a family's ability to adhere to complex medical regimens, need to be considered. Erratic compliance with any antiretroviral drug is likely to select resistant virus that limits the future effectiveness of other drugs in the same class. Thus, care must be taken in selecting the regimen, including information like the family's daily schedule, their history of medical compliance, school attendance and whether the school system knows the child's diagnosis. These issues will be considered further in Chapter 15.

In selecting a salvage therapy for children failing their initial regimen, the choice will usually include the other thymidine-derived NRTI (ZDV or D4T) or possibly TDF, an alternate non-thymidine NRTI (3TC or ddI), and one or two drugs from among the PIs and NNRTIs. As discussed above, even if the patient had been previously treated with 3TC, many clinicians would continue to treat with 3TC because of its ability to hypersensitize to other NNRTIs (e.g., AZT, TDF). The choice will depend on the patient's prior experience and resistance testing. Once a patient has documented resistance to an antiretroviral, they will maintain "archived" reservoirs of virus resistant to that agent for life, and the resistant species will rapidly reappear if therapy with that antiretroviral is reinstituted (see also Chapter 1). However, antiretroviral resistant virus is less "fit," and in some ways less pathogenic, than the wild-type virus, so even after viral breakthrough has occurred there continues to be an advantage to using an antiretroviral regimen. This advantage must be weighed against the ongoing selection of resistance while drugs are used in the face of ongoing replication.

There are relatively limited therapeutic options currently available for children. As a result, there is a finite number of effective changes in antiretroviral regimens available, probably no more than three regimens *in toto* using currently available drugs. Other regimens will have limited benefit, with either incomplete suppression or a short period of complete suppression. Regimen switches should not be made casually, and careful consideration should be given for the clinical need to change, taking into account factors like adherence, symptoms, CD4+ lymphocyte count changes, and viral load. The development of new antiretroviral agents with new resistance patterns and new mechanisms of action offer the promise of more effective and durable antiretroviral regimens with greater tolerability.

REFERENCES

1. Fischl, M. A., Richman, D. D., Grieco, M. H. *et al.* The efficacy of azidothymidine (AZT) in the treatment of patients with AIDS and AIDS-related complex. A double-blind, placebo-controlled trial. *N. Engl. J. Med.* 1987;**317**(4):185–191.

2. McKinney, R. E., Jr., Maha, M. A., Connor, E. M. *et al.* A multicenter trial of oral zidovudine in children with advanced human immunodeficiency virus disease. The Protocol 043 Study Group. *N. Engl. J. Med.* 1991;**324**(15):1018–1025.

3. Butler, K. M., Husson, R. N., Balis, F. M. *et al.* Dideoxyinosine in children with symptomatic human immunodeficiency virus infection. *N. Engl. J. Med.* 1991;**324**(3):137–144.

4. Mueller, B. U., Butler, K. M., Stocker, V. L. *et al.* Clinical and pharmacokinetic evaluation of long-term therapy with didanosine in children with HIV infection. *Pediatrics* 1994;**94**(5):724–731.

5. Englund, J. A., Baker, C. J., Raskino, C. *et al.* Zidovudine, didanosine, or both as the initial treatment for symptomatic HIV-infected children. AIDS Clinical Trials Group (ACTG) Study 152 Team. *N. Engl. J. Med.* 1997;**336**(24):1704–1712.

6. Kline, M. W., Fletcher, C. V., Federici, M. E. *et al.* Combination therapy with stavudine and didanosine in children with advanced human immunodeficiency virus infection: pharmacokinetic properties, safety, and immunologic and virologic effects. *Pediatrics* 1996;**97**(6 Pt 1):886–890.

7. Kline, M. W., Van Dyke, R. B., Lindsey, J. C. *et al.* A randomized comparative trial of stavudine (d4T) versus zidovudine (ZDV, AZT) in children with human immunodeficiency virus infection. AIDS Clinical Trials Group 240 Team. *Pediatrics* 1998;**101**(2):214–220.

8. McKinney, R. E., Jr., Johnson, G. M., Stanley, K. *et al.* A randomized study of combined zidovudine-lamivudine versus didanosine monotherapy in children with symptomatic therapy-naive HIV-1 infection. The Pediatric AIDS Clinical Trials Group Protocol 300 Study Team. *J. Pediatr.* 1998;**133**(4):500–508.

9. Bakshi, S. S., Britto, P., Capparelli, E. *et al.* Evaluation of pharmacokinetics, safety, tolerance, and activity of combination of zalcitabine and zidovudine in stable, zidovudine-treated pediatric patients with human immunodeficiency virus infection. AIDS Clinical Trials Group Protocol 190 Team. *J. Infect. Dis.* 1997;**175**(5):1039–1050.

10. Spector, S. A., Blanchard, S., Wara, D. W. *et al.* Comparative trial of two dosages of zalcitabine in zidovudine-experienced children with advanced human immunodeficiency

virus disease. Pediatric AIDS Clinical Trials Group. *Pediatr. Infect. Dis. J.* 1997;**16**(6):623–626.

11. Kline, M. W., Blanchard, S., Fletcher, C. V. *et al.* A phase I study of abacavir (1592U89) alone and in combination with other antiretroviral agents in infants and children with human immunodeficiency virus infection. AIDS Clinical Trials Group 330 Team. *Pediatrics* 1999;**103**(4):e47.

12. Gibb, D., Giaquinto, C., Walker, A. *et al. Three year follow-up of the PENTA 5 trial.* (Abstract 874). In *10th Annual Conference on Retroviruses and Opportunistic Infections*; 2003; Boston, MA.

13. Barditch-Crovo, P., Deeks, S. G., Collier, A. *et al.* Phase i/ii trial of the pharmacokinetics, safety, and antiretroviral activity of tenofovir disoproxil fumarate in human immunodeficiency virus-infected adults. *Antimicrob. Agents Chemother.* 2001;**45**(10):2733–2739.

14. Saez-Llorens, X., Violari, A., Ndiweni, D. *et al.* Once-daily emtricitabine in HIV-infected pediatric patients with other antiretroviral agents. In *10th Conference on Retroviruses and Opportunistic Infections*; 2003; Boston, MA.

15. de Jong, M. D., Vella, S., Carr, A. *et al.* High-dose nevirapine in previously untreated human immunodeficiency virus type 1-infected persons does not result in sustained suppression of viral replication. *J. Infect. Dis.* 1997;**175**(4):966–970.

16. Luzuriaga, K., Bryson, Y., Krogstad, P. *et al.* Combination treatment with zidovudine, didanosine, and nevirapine in infants with human immunodeficiency virus type 1 infection. *N. Engl. J. Med.* 1997;**336**(19):1343–1349.

17. Starr, S. E., Fletcher, C. V., Spector, S. A. *et al.* Combination therapy with efavirenz, nelfinavir, and nucleoside reverse-transcriptase inhibitors in children infected with human immunodeficiency virus type 1. Pediatric AIDS Clinical Trials Group 382 Team. *N. Engl. J. Med.* 1999;**341**(25):1874–1881.

18. McKinney, R. E., Rathore, M., Jankelevich, S., *PACTG 1021:* An ongoing phase I/II study of once-daily emtricitabine, didanosine, and efavirenz in therapy-naive or minimally treated patients. (Abstract 373). In *10th Annual Conference on Retroviruses and Opportunistic Infections*; 2003; Boston, MA.

19. Yogev, R., Church, J., Flynn, P. M. *et al.* Pediatric trial of combination therapy including the protease inhibitor amprenavir (APV). (Abstract 430). In *6th Conference on Retroviruses and Opportunistic Infections*; 1999; Chicago, IL.

20. Abbott Laboratories. Kaletra (lopinavir/r) package insert. 2002.

21. Krogstad, P., Wiznia, A., Luzuriaga, K. *et al.* Treatment of human immunodeficiency virus 1-infected infants and children with the protease inhibitor nelfinavir mesylate. *Clin. Infect. Dis.* 1999;**28**(5):1109–1118.

22. Hertogs, K., Mellors, J. W., Schel, P. *et al.* Patterns of cross-resistance among protease inhibitors in 483 HIV-1 isolates. (Abstract 395). In *5th Annual Conference on Retroviruses and Opportunistic Infections*; 1998; Chicago, IL.

23. Nachman, S. A., Stanley, K., Yogev, R. *et al.* Nucleoside analogs plus ritonavir in stable antiretroviral therapy-experienced HIV-infected children: a randomized controlled trial. Pediatric AIDS Clinical Trials Group 338 Study Team. *J. Am. Med. Assoc.* 2000;**283**(4):492–498.

24. Kline, M. W., Brundage, R. C., Fletcher, C. V. *et al.* Combination therapy with saquinavir soft gelatin capsules in children with human immunodeficiency virus infection. *Pediatr. Infect. Dis. J.* 2001;**20**(7):666–671.

25. Delfraissy, J., Montaner, J., Eron, J. J. *et al.* Summary of pooled efficacy and safety analyses of enuvirtide (ENF) treatment for 24 weeks in TORO 1 and TORO 2 phase III trials in highly antiretroviral (ARV) treatment-experienced patients. (Abstract 568). 2003; Boston, MA.

12 Antiretroviral drug Interactions

Thomas N. Kakuda, Pharm.D.

Department of Medical Affairs, Hoffman LaRoche, Nutley, NJ

Courtney V. Fletcher, Pharm.D.

University of Colorado Health Sciences Center, Denver, CO

Treatment of HIV-infected patients requires polypharmacy, during which drug interactions can occur. Pharmacokinetic interactions are those that affect the absorption, distribution, metabolism, or excretion of a drug. Pharmacodynamic interactions produce antagonistic, additive, or synergistic effects. Interactions can be adverse or beneficial. This chapter provides a framework for understanding HIV-related drug interactions through the principles of pharmacology.

Pharmacokinetic drug interactions

Absorption

Fasting, gastric pH, and enteric P-glycoprotein (PGP) expression all can affect absorption. Table 12.1 delineates drug–food interactions and lists antiretroviral drugs that may be administered without regard to food. Antacids (including the buffer in older formulations of didanosine), H_2-receptor antagonists, and proton pump inhibitors increase gastric pH, impairing the bioavailability of drugs that require low pH for optimal absorption (e.g., delavirdine, indinavir, itraconazole, ketoconazole). This interaction usually can be avoided by administrating the gastric pH-raising agent 1 to 2 hours later [1–3]. Didanosine is much better absorbed in an alkaline environment because it is acid labile. The original formulation of didanosine included a buffer (calcium carbonate and magnesium hydroxide in tablets or citrate-phosphate in sachets) or had to be reconstituted in antacid. The buffer in didanosine does not affect dapsone absorption but significantly decreases ciprofloxacin absorption [4, 5]. Didanosine or antacids do not interfere with nevirapine. The new formulation of didanosine (Videx® EC) does not have significant interactions with ciprofloxacin, indinavir, or azole antifungals [6, 7]. Drug absorption also can be affected by transporters in the gut. For example, PGP expression in the GI tract could account for the poor bioavailability of saquinavir and, possibly, other protease inhibitors (PIs) [8].

Handbook of Pediatric HIV Care, ed. Steven L. Zeichner and Jennifer S. Read.
Published by Cambridge University Press. © Cambridge University Press 2006.

Table 12.1. Drug-food interactions

Drugs best administered with food
  albendazole
  amiodarone
  atazanavir
  atovaquone
  carbamazepine
  erythromycin ethylsuccinate
  hydralazine
  hydrochlorothiazide
  itraconazole capsules[a]
  lithium citrate
  lopinavir/ritonavir
  nelfinavir[a]
  para-aminosalicylic acid[b]
  propranolol
  rifabutin
  ritonavir
  saquinavir[a] **and saquinavir mesylate**[a]
  tenofovir
  tipranavir/ritonavir[a]

Drugs best administered on an empty stomach (1 hour prior to the meal or 2 hours after)
  ampicillin
  azithromycin
  didanosine (all formulations)
  efavirenz[c]
  indinavir (without ritonavir)
  itraconazole solution
  penicillin VK
  rifampin

Antiretroviral drugs that may be administered without regard to food
  abacavir
  amprenavir and fosamorenavir
  delavirdine/emtricitabine
  indinavir/ritonavir
  lamivudine
  nevirapine
  stavudine
  zidovudine

Drugs appearing in **bold** are those likely to be prescribed to an HIV-infected patient.

[a] Absorption is better with a fatty meal.

[b] Absorption is better when sprinkled on acidic food (apple sauce or yogurt) or mixed with juice.

[c] Coadministration with food may increase efavirenz plasma concentrations and incidence of CNS side effects.

Distribution

Drug distribution in the body depends upon binding to plasma proteins and tissues. Albumin or α_1-acid glycoprotein (α_1-AGP, orosomucoid) are the two plasma proteins that bind most drugs. PIs bind preferentially to α_1-AGP. The free or unbound fraction of drug typically exerts the pharmacologic effect. Most PIs are highly protein bound (90–99%) except indinavir ($\sim$60%) [9]. Enfuvirtide (T-20), a fusion inhibitor, also is highly protein bound. The non-nucleoside reverse transcriptase inhibitors (NNRTIs) efavirenz and delavirdine are highly protein bound (98–99%); nevirapine is only moderately ($\sim$60%) bound [10]. Nucleoside and nucleotide reverse transcriptase inhibitors (NRTIs) have negligible protein binding (<50%). When two or more drugs exhibiting extensive protein binding are given concomitantly, one drug can displace the other from the binding site; consequently, the unbound drug may exert a larger pharmacological effect. This interaction can affect both drugs. Protein binding displacement generally is clinically insignificant because a dynamic equilibrium exists between unbound drug in the plasma and the extravascular region. Highly protein bound drugs (>70%) can exhibit a significant displacement interaction if given intravenously, if eliminated primarily by hepatic metabolism (i.e. has a high extraction ratio) and have a narrow therapeutic index. Such drugs include alfentanil, buprenorphine, fentanyl, hydralazine, lidocaine, midazolam, or verapamil. In these instances, close monitoring of the patient is warranted [11]. None of the current antiretroviral drugs, including enfuvirtide, appear to have significant protein binding interactions.

Metabolism

The liver is the primary organ for biotransformation of endogenous and exogenous chemicals, converting lipophilic substances to more water-soluble metabolites, facilitating elimination. Biotransformation often involves two sequential steps: phase I reactions (oxidation, reduction, or hydrolysis) and phase II reactions (conjugation). The cytochrome P-450 enzyme system (CYP450) primarily mediates phase I reactions. CYP450 consists of several isozymes, six of which mediate most drug metabolism: CYP 1A2, 2C9/10, 2C19, 2D6, 2E1, 3A. These isozymes are present to varying degrees based on age, ethnicity, and other factors [12–14]. Table 12.2 summarizes selected CYP450 substrates, inhibitors, and inducers; information regarding population polymorphisms and age-specific issues is included where known. Clinicians can use this table to predict relevant drug interactions by determining which drugs decrease or increase CYP450 activity (inhibitors or inducers, respectively) and drugs that might be affected by these changes (substrates). Enfuvirtide and NRTIs do not significantly affect CYP450 activity, therefore metabolic drug interactions are less likely to occur with these agents. Delavirdine and the PIs, with the exception of tipranavir, inhibit CYP 3A to varying degrees, with ritonavir being the most potent [15, 16]. Because many drugs are substrates of the CYP3A isozyme, concomitant administration with a PI or delavirdine can increase plasma substrate concentrations. Increased concentrations

Table 12.2. Select cytochrome P-450 subfamily substrates, inhibitors, and inducers

---

CYP1A2

Substrates

acetaminophen, alprazolam, amitriptyline, clomipramine, desipramine, exogenous steroids, haloperidol, imipramine, propranolol, **tenofovir**, theophylline, thioridazine

Inhibitors

azithromycin, erythromycin, fluoroquinolones, grapefruit juice, **isoniazid, ketoconazole**

Inducers

charcoal in food, cigarette smoke, phenobarbital, phenytoin, **rifampin**, **ritonavir**

Note

Activity in neonates is very low but matures to adult activity approximately 120 days after birth. Expression of this gene may be polymorphic.

CYP2C9/10

Substrates

diazepam, ibuprofen, naproxen, phenytoin

Inhibitors

amiodarone, chloramphenicol, cimetidine, **fluconazole, isoniazid, metronidazole, miconazole**, omeprazole, **ritonavir, sulfamethoxazole**

Inducers

rifampin

Note

Infants of 1–6 months have activity comparable with adults. Children 3–6 years old have significantly greater activity but become comparable with adult activity after puberty.

CYP2C19

Substrates

diazepam, imipramine, S-mephenytoin, propranolol

Inhibitors

ketoconazole

Note

3–5% of Caucasians, and 20% of Orientals have reduced expression of this gene (poor metabolizers)

CYP2D6 (debrisoquine/sparteine hydroxylase)

Substrates

amitriptyline, chlorpromazine, clomipramine, codeine, desipramine, dextromethorphan, haloperidol[a], hydrocodone, imipramine, **indinavir**, meperidine, metoprolol, morphine, nortriptyline, oxycodone, propranolol, **ritonavir**, **saquinavir**, thioridazine[a], timolol, tramadol, trazodone

Inhibitors

amiodarone, cimetidine, clomipramine, desipramine, haloperidol, quinidine, **ritonavir**

Table 12.2. (*cont.*)

Note

Pregnancy increases CYP2D6 activity [25]. Neonates and infants less than 28 days old have at most 20% of adult activity and therefore should be considered poor metabolizers. Activity comparable with adults occurs by 10 years of age or sooner. 5%–10% of Caucasians, 2% of Blacks, and 1–2% of Orientals have reduced expression of this gene (poor metabolizers)

CYP2E1

Substrates

acetaminophen, ethanol, halothane, isoflurane, **isoniazid**, theophylline

Inhibitors

  isoniazid

Inducers

  ethanol

CYP3A

Substrates

  acetaminophen, alfentanil, alprazolam, amitriptyline[a], **amprenavir**, astemizole, benzphetamine, cannabinoids, carbamazepine, cisapride, chlorpromazine, **clarithromycin**, clindamycin, clonazepam, clorazepate, cocaine, corticosteroids, cyclophosphamide, cyclosporine, **dapsone**, desipramine, dextromethorphan, diazepam, diltiazem, docetaxol, dronabinol, **efavirenz**, ergotamine, erythromycin, estazolam, estrogens, ethosuximide, etoposide, fentanyl, fexofenadine, flurazepam, ifosfamide, imipramine, **indinavir**, itraconazole, ketoconazole, lansoprazole, lidocaine, **lopinavir**, meperidine, miconazole, midazolam, nefazodone, **nevirapine**, nifedipine, nortriptyline, ondansetron, oral contraceptives, paclitaxel, phenobarbital, phenytoin, quinidine, quinine, **rifampin**, **rifabutin**, **ritonavir**, **saquinavir**, tacrolimus, terfenadine, testosterone, triazolam, trimethoprim, verapamil, zileuton

Inhibitors

  amiodarone, **amprenavir**, **azithromycin**, cimetidine, **clarithromycin**, clotrimazole, cyclosporine, **delavirdine**, diltiazem, econazole, **erythromycin**, **fluconazole**, grapefruit juice, **indinavir**, **isoniazid**, **itraconazole**, **ketoconazole**, **metronidazole**, miconazole, norfloxacin, propoxyphene, quinine, **ritonavir**, **saquinavir**, troleandomycin, verapamil, zafirlukast

Inducers

  carbamazepine, dexamethasone, **efavirenz**, ethosuximide, **nevirapine**, **rifabutin**, **rifampin**, phenobarbital, phenytoin, **tipranavir**, troglitazone

Note

High levels of CYP3A are present during embryogenesis. CYP3A4 activity is greater in infants and children compared with adults. Expression of this gene may be polymorphic.

Drugs appearing in **bold** are those likely to be prescribed to an HIV-infected patient.
[a] indicates a minor metabolic pathway for this drug.

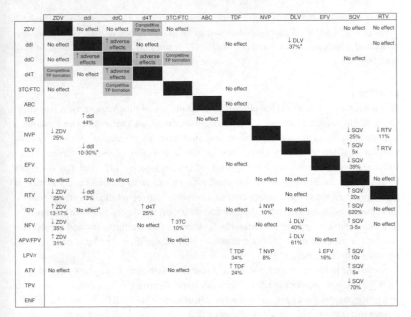

Fig. 12.1. Antiretroviral drug interactions: effect of drug on area-under-the-curve (AUC)
[a] administer didonosine 1–2 hours later.

can lead to toxicity (in which case the combination should be avoided) or it can be therapeutically useful. Ritonavir boosted regimens (e.g., lopinavir/ritonavir) represent an advantageous use of the interaction [9, 15].

Some drugs can induce drug metabolism. Rifampin is a potent inducer of CYP3A and 2C9/10 and increases drug metabolism, including that of PIs. Because of this interaction, PI therapy may be deferred for the duration of rifampin therapy, or rifabutin substituted (if treating MAC) [17]. Efavirenz, nevirapine, tipranavir and certain anticonvulsants also are CYP3A inducers. Receipt of efavirenz or nevirapine is associated with decreased plasma concentrations of some PIs [10]. Dose adjustment of the PI or adding ritonavir may be required. Lastly, some drugs may exhibit both inhibition and induction properties. Figure 12.1 represents the pharmacokinetic interactions among currently available antiretroviral drugs. Conjugation (phase II) reactions increase the water solubility of metabolites, thereby facilitating excretion. Transferases, including uridine diphosphoglucuronyltransferase (UDPGT) and N-acetyl transferase (NAT), mediate Phase II. UDPGT conjugates glucuronic acid with bilirubin, zidovudine, and its metabolite 3′-amino-3′deoxythymidine. Atovaquone and fluconazole (doses >200 mg/day) inhibit UDPGT causing decreased zidovudine clearance [3, 18]. Inhibition of

UDPGT by atazanavir and indinavir also can cause hyperbilirubinemia seen with these drugs [19]. Inhibition of glucuronidation may be more serious in infants than adolescents and adults since adult activity of UDPGT is not achieved until 6–18 months of age [14].

Excretion

Two processes can affect renal elimination: inhibition of tubular secretion and alterations in glomerular filtration. Cimetidine, probenecid, and trimethoprim are known inhibitors of renal tubular secretion and may lead to increased plasma concentrations of drugs primarily eliminated by this route. For example, trimethoprim-sulfamethoxazole increases the exposure of lamivudine by 44%, but has no effect on indinavir [20, 21]. Probenecid is used with cidofovir to reduce the incidence of nephrotoxicity. However, probenecid can interact negatively with zidovudine; zidovudine should be discontinued or dose-reduced 50% on the day of cidofovir administration. Ganciclovir competes for renal tubular secretion with didanosine and zidovudine and increases their plasma concentrations; this interaction may be more clinically significant for didanosine [22].

Alterations in kidney function can occur from renal disease or may be drug-induced. All NRTIs except zidovudine have significant renal elimination. Concomitant use with a nephrotoxic drug may require a dosage adjustment of the NRTI, as would administration to a patient with renal insufficiency [23].

Pharmacodynamic drug interactions

Pharmacodynamic interactions occur when two drugs share similar mechanisms of action. These interactions may be additive, synergistic, or antagonistic. The NRTIs are often used in combination because of their additive or synergistic interaction. However, not all combinations of NRTIs are feasible. For example, stavudine and zidovudine are antagonistic because they are both thymidine analogues and share a common activation pathway. In contrast, lamivudine is a cytosine analogue, and a different set of kinases mediate its initial phosphorylation; thus lamivudine can be coadministered with either zidovudine or stavudine. Lamivudine, however, should not be given with emtricitabine or zalcitabine, both cytosine analogues, because of the potential for intracellular phosphorylation competition [24]. Other similar potential interactions include amdoxovir and abacavir, both guanosine derivatives and tenofovir and didanosine, both adenosine analogues. Further studies of these and other intracellular NRTI interactions are needed. Tenofovir increases plasma didanosine concentrations by approximately 44%, which may be sufficient to increase the likelihood of adverse reactions.

Pharmacodynamic interactions also can occur when drugs produce similar side effects. Common side effects of antiretrovirals are categorized in Table 12.3; drugs that

Table 12.3. Drugs with overlapping toxicities

Crystalluria	Hematologic	Hyperglycemia	Pancreatitis
acyclovir[a]	α-interferon	*corticosteroids*	alcohol
Ganciclovir	amphotericin	**didanosine**	*aminosalicylates*
indinavir	cidofovir	megesterol	calcium
sulfonamides	dapsone	pentamidine	**didanosine**
	doxorubicin	*protease inhibitors*	**lamivudine**[b]
Dermatologic	flucytosine		pentamidine
α-interferon	ganciclovir	**Hyperlipidemia**	valproic acid
abacavir	interleukin-2	α-interferon	
amprenavir	pentamidine	β-*antagonists*	**Peripheral neuropathy**
bleomycin	pyrimethamine	*corticosteroids*	cidofovir
delavirdine	sulfadiazine	cyclosporine	dapsone
efavirenz	TMP-SMX	**efavirenz**	**didanosine**
indinavir	**zidovudine**	*protease inhibitors*	ethambutol
interleukin-2		*thiazide diuretics*	ethionamide
nevirapine	**Hyperbilirubinemia**		isoniazid
TMP-SMX	**atazanavir**	**Hyperuricemia**	metronidazole
	cyclosporine	cyclosporine	phenytoin
Gastrointestinal (N/V)	dapsone	**didanosine**	**stavudine**
adefovir	**indinavir**	**ritonavir**	thalidomide
α-interferon	interleukin-2		TMP-SMX
doxorubicin	interleukin-6	**Nephrotoxicity**	**zalcitabine**
foscarnet	lithium	adefovir	
ganciclovir	methotrexate[a]	*aminoglycosides*	**Uveitis**
interleukin-2	octreotide	amphotericin	ethambutol
probenecid	pancuronium	cidofovir	**indinavir**
ritonavir		foscarnet	rifabutin
zidovudine		ganciclovir	*sulfonamides*
		interleukin-2	terbenafine
		pentamidine	
		tenofovir	

Abbreviations: N/V, nausea and vomiting; TMP-SMX, trimethoprim-sulfamethoxazole
Drugs appearing in **bold** are those likely to be prescribed to an HIV-infected patient
Italics represent pharmacological classes.
[a] at higher doses.
[b] primarily in children.

produce similar side effects are also presented. The use of two or more drugs with common adverse effects is likely to increase the probability of or the intensity with which the side effect occurs. Clinically significant interactions with commonly prescribed HIV medications are summarized in Table 12.3. Suggestions for avoiding select interactions

Table 12.4. Clinically significant drug interactions with commonly prescribed HIV/AIDS medications

HIV/AIDS drug	Interaction with	Comments
Antiretrovirals		
Zidovudine	Atovaquone	Zidovudine AUC ↑ 31%; may require dose adjustment.
	Cidofovir	Hold zidovudine on day of infusion (see probenecid).
	Fluconazole	Zidovudine AUC ↑ 74%; may require dose adjustment.
	Ganciclovir	Consider holding zidovudine during induction therapy to avoid neutropenia.
	Nelfinavir	Zidovudine AUC ↓ 35%; may require dose adjustment.
	Probenecid	Zidovudine AUC ↑ 106%; may require dose adjustment.
	Rifampin	Zidovudine AUC ↓ 47%; may require dose adjustment.
	Stavudine	Contraindicated due to competitive phosphorylation (see text).
	Valproic acid	Zidovudine AUC ↑ 80%; may require dose adjustment.
	Miscellaneous	See Table 12.3, drugs that may cause gastrointestinal or hematologic side effects.
Didanosine	Allopurinol	Didanosine AUC ↑ ~4-fold; coadministration is not recommended.
	Delavirdine	Separate administration by at least 1–2 hours if using Videx or consider Videx EC (see text).
	Ganciclovir	Didanosine AUC ↑ 111%; may require dose adjustment.
	Hydroxyurea	↑ risk of adverse effects.
	Indinavir	Separate administration by at least 1–2 hours if using Videx or consider Videx EC (see text).
	Itraconazole[a]	Separate administration by at least 1–2 hours if using Videx or consider Videx EC (see text).
	Ketoconazole	Separate administration by at least 1–2 hours if using Videx or consider Videx EC (see text).
	Fluoroquinolones	Separate administration by at least 1–2 hours if using Videx or consider Videx EC (see text).
	Ribavirin	Phosphorylation increased in vitro >50%, ↑ risk of adverse effects.
	Tetracycline	Separate administration by at least 1–2 hours if using Videx or consider Videx EC (see text), doxycycline, or minocycline.
	Tenofovir	Didanosine AUC ↑ 44%; may require dose adjustment.
	Miscellaneous	See Table 12.3, drugs that may cause hyperglycemia, hyperuricemia, pancreatitis, and peripheral neuropathy.

Table 12.4. (cont.)

Zalcitabine	*Aminoglycosides*	↑ risk of peripheral neuropathy due to ↑concentrations from renal impairment.
	Amphotericin	↑ risk of peripheral neuropathy from renal impairment.
	Antacids[e]	↓ zalcitabine absorption; separate administration by at least 2 hours.
	Cimetidine	Zalcitabine AUC ↑ 36%; may require dose adjustment.
	Doxorubicin	Phosphorylation inhibited in vitro >50%, clinical significance unknown.
	Foscarnet	↑ risk of peripheral neuropathy from renal impairment.
	Lamivudine	Contraindicated due to competitive phosphorylation (see text).
	Probenecid	↑ zalcitabine plasma conc.; may require dose adjustment.
	Miscellaneous	See Table 12.3, drugs that may cause peripheral neuropathy.
Stavudine	Indinavir	Stavudine AUC ↑ 25%.
	Zidovudine	Contraindicated due to competitive phosphorylation (see text)
	Miscellaneous	See Table 12.3, drugs that may cause peripheral neuropathy.
Lamivudine	Zalcitabine	Contraindicated due to competitive phosphorylation (see text).
	TMP-SMX	Lamivudine AUC ↑ 44%.
	Miscellaneous	See Table 12.3, drugs that may cause pancreatitis.
Abacavir	Amdoxovir	Potential contraindication due to competitive phosphorylation.
	Amprenavir	Amprenavir AUC ↑ 29%; no dose adjustment recommended.
	Miscellaneous	See Table 12.3, drugs that may cause dermatologic side effects.
Tenofovir	Didanosine	Didanosine AUC ↑ 44%; may require dose adjustment.
	Lopinavir/ ritonavir	Tenofovir AUC ↑ 34%; may require dose adjustment.
	Miscellaneous	See Table 12.3, drugs that may cause nephrotoxicity.
Nevirapine	Ketoconazole	Ketoconazole AUC ↓ 63%, ↑ nevirapine plasma conc.; coadministration is not recommended.
	Oral contraceptives	Potential ↓ in estrogen plasma conc.; advise patient about alternative birth control methods.
	Phenytoin	↓ phenytoin plasma conc.; adjust dose based on phenytoin levels or response.
	Protease inhibitors	↓ protease inhibitor plasma conc.; may require dose adjustment.

(cont.)

Table 12.4. (*cont.*)

	Rifamycins	↓ nevirapine plasma conc.; may require dose adjustment.
	Miscellaneous	See Table 12.3, drugs that may cause gastrointestinal or dermatologic side effects.
Delavirdine	*Antacids*[e]	Delavirdine AUC ↓ 41%; separate administration by at least 2 hours (see text).
	Barbiturates	↓ delavirdine plasma conc.; consider an alternative anticonvulsant or antiretroviral.
	Astemizole	Contraindictated due to potential cardiotoxicity, consider loratidine.
	Ca²⁺ channel antagonists	May ↑ potential for arrhythmia.
	Carbamazepine	↓ delavirdine plasma conc.; consider an alternative anticonvulsant or antiretroviral.
	Cisapride	Contraindicated due to potential cardiotoxicity.
	Clarithromycin	Clarithromycin AUC ↑ 100%, 14-OH clarithromycin AUC ↓ 75%, delavirdine AUC ↑ 44%; consider azithromycin.
	Ergot derivatives	May ↑ potential for ergotism.
	Fluoxetine	↑ delavirdine plasma conc.; may require dose adjustment.
	H₂-antagonists	Avoid (see text).
	Indinavir	Indinavir AUC ↑ 40%; dose combinations typically used in adults include IDV/DLV 400–600/400 tid or 800–1200/600 bid.
	Ketoconazole	↑ delavirdine plasma conc.; may require dose adjustment.
	Phenytoin	↓ delavirdine plasma conc.; consider an alternative anticonvulsant or antiretroviral.
	Proton pump inhibitors	Avoid (see text).
	Rifabutin	Delavirdine AUC ↓ 80%, rifabutin AUC ↑ 100%; coadministration is not recommended.
	Rifampin	Delavirdine AUC ↓ 96%; coadministration is not recommended.
	Saquinavir	Saquinavir AUC ↑ ~5-fold; dose adjustment recommended.
	Miscellaneous	See Table 12.3, drugs that may cause dermatologic side effects.
Efavirenz	Clarithromycin	Clarithromycin AUC ↓ 39%, 14-OH clarithromycin AUC ↑ 34%; consider azithromycin.
	Oral contraceptives	↑ ethinyl estradiol plasma conc., does not require any adjustment.
	Indinavir	Indinavir AUC ↓ 31%; dose adjustment recommended.

Table 12.4. (*cont.*)

	Rifabutin	Rifabutin AUC ↓ 38%; coadministration is not recommended.
	Saquinavir	Saquinavir AUC ↓ 62%; coadministration is not recommended.
	Miscellaneous	See Table 12.3, drugs that may cause dermatologic side effects and hyperlipidemia.
Protease inhibitors	Astemizole	Contraindictated due to potential cardiotoxicity, consider loratidine.
	Barbiturates	↓ *protease inhibitor* plasma conc., may require dose adjustment.
	Benzodiazepines	Use lorazepam or temazepam; midazolam and triazolam are contraindicated.
	Cisapride	Contraindictated due to potential cardiotoxicity.
	Delavirdine	↑ *protease inhibitor* plasma conc., may require dose adjustment.
	Ergot derivatives	Contraindicated due to ↑ potential for ergotism.
	Nevirapine	↓ *protease inhibitor* plasma conc., may require dose adjustment.
	Phenytoin	↓ *protease inhibitor* plasma conc., may require dose adjustment.
	Rifabutin	Avoid with saquinavir or ritonavir, ↓ rifabutin dose by 50% with indinavir or nelfinavir.
	Rifampin	Contraindicated (see text).
	Miscellaneous	See Table 12.3, drugs that may cause hyperglycemia and hyperlipidemia.
Saquinavir	Amprenavir	Amprenavir AUC ↓ 32%; may require dose adjustment.
	Clarithromycin	Saquinavir AUC ↑ 177%, clarithromycin AUC ↑ 45%; may require dose adjustment.
	Delavirdine	Saquinavir AUC ↑ ~fivefold; may require dose adjustment.
	Efavirenz	Saquinavir AUC ↓ 62%; coadministration is not recommended.
	Indinavir	Saquinavir AUC ↑ 364–620%; may require dose adjustment.
	Ketoconazole	Saquinavir AUC ↑ 30%, ketoconazole AUC ↑ 44%; may require dose adjustment.
	Nelfinavir	Saquinavir AUC ↑ 392%; may require dose adjustment.
	Oral contraceptives	Interaction unknown, suggest alternative birth control methods until further studies can be made.
	Ranitidine	Saquinavir AUC ↑ 67%; may require dose adjustment.
	Ritonavir	Saquinavir AUC ↑ 1587%; dose combinations typically used in adults include SQV/RTV 400/400 bid, 1000/100 bid, and 1600/100 qd.

(*cont.*)

Table 12.4. (cont.)

	Miscellaneous	See Table 12.3, drugs that may cause hyperglycemia and hyperlipidemia.
Amprenavir	Abacavir	Amprenavir AUC ↑ 29%; no dose adjustment recommended.
	Indinavir	Amprenavir AUC ↑ 33%; may require dose adjustment.
	Ketoconazole	Amprenavir AUC ↑ 31%; may require dose adjustment.
	Lopinavir/ ritonavir	Amprenavir AUC ↑ 72%, lopinavir AUC ↓ 35%, dose combinations typically used in adults include APV/LPV/RTV 750/400/100 BID and 750/533/133 bid.
	Saquinavir	Amprenavir AUC ↓ 32%; may require dose adjustment.
	Ritonavir	Amprenavir AUC ↑ 62–64%; dose combinations typically used in adults include APV/RTV 600/100 BID and 1200/200 QD.
	Miscellaneous	See Table 12.3, drugs that may cause dermatologic side effects, hyperglycemia, and hyperlipidemia.
Indinavir	Amprenavir	Amprenavir AUC ↑ 33%; may require dose adjustment.
	Antacids	Separate administration by at least 2 hours (see text).
	Atazanavir	↑ risk of hyperbilirubinemia (see text).
	Clarithromycin	Indinavir AUC ↑ 29%, clarithromycin AUC ↑ 53%; may require dose adjustment.
	Delavirdine	Indinavir AUC ↑ 40%; dose combinations typically used in adults include IDV/DLV 400–600/400 tid or 800–1200/600 bid.
	Didanosine	Separate administration by at least 1–2 hours if using Videx or consider Videx EC (see text).
	Efavirenz	Indinavir AUC ↓ 31%; recommend indinavir 1000mg TID.
	H_2-antagonists	Avoid (see text).
	Ketoconazole	↑ indinavir plasma conc.; may require dose adjustment.
	Nelfinavir	Indinavir AUC ↑ 51%, nelfinavir AUC ↑ 83%; may require dose adjustment.
	Oral contraceptives	Ethinyl estradiol AUC ↑ 24%, norethindrone AUC ↑ 26%; no dose adjustment recommended.
	Proton pump inhibitors	Avoid (see text).
	Ritonavir	Indinavir AUC ↑ 3-5-fold; dose combinations typically used in adults include IDV/RTV 400/400 BID and 800/100–200 BID.

Table 12.4. (*cont.*)

	Saquinavir	Saquinavir AUC ↑ 364–620%; may require dose adjustment.
	Stavudine	Stavudine AUC ↑ 25%; may require dose adjustment.
	Miscellaneous	See Table 12.3, drugs that may cause crystalluria, dermatologic side effects, hyperbilirubinemia, hyperglycemia, hyperlipidemia, nephrotoxicity, and uveitis.
Ritonavir	Amprenavir	Amprenavir AUC ↑ 62%–64%; dose combinations typically used in adults include APV/RTV 600/100 bid and 1200/200 qd.
	Analgesics	Use acetaminophen, aspirin, or oxycodone.
	Antiarrhythmics[c]	Contraindicated.
	Clarithromycin	Clarithromycin AUC ↑ 77%, 14-OH clarithromycin AUC ↓ 100%; consider azithromycin.
	Cycloserine	Avoid ritonavir solution due to alcohol content, may ↑ potential for seizures.
	Desipramine	Desipramine AUC ↑ 145%; may require dose adjustment.
	Indinavir	Indinavir AUC ↑ 3–5-fold; dose combinations typically used in adults include IDV/RTV 400/400 bid and 800/100–200 bid.
	Ketoconazole	Ketoconazole AUC ↑ 3.4-fold; may require dose adjustment.
	Loperamide	Loperamide AUC ↑ 145%; may require dose adjustment.
	Meperidine	Meperidine AUC ↓ 62%, normeperidine AUC ↑ 47%; consider alternative analgesic.
	Metronidazole	Avoid ritonavir solution due to alcohol content, may cause a "disulfiram-like" reaction.
	Nelfinavir	Nelfinavir AUC ↑ 152%; may require dose adjustment.
	Oral contraceptives	Ethinyl estradiol AUC ↓ 40%; advise patient about alternative birth control methods.
	Saquinavir	Saquinavir AUC ↑ 1587%; dose combinations typically used in adults include SQV/RTV 400/400 bid, 1000/100 bid and 1600/100 qd.
	Theophylline	Theophylline AUC ↓ 43%; adjust dose based on theophylline levels or response.
	Miscellaneous	See Table 12.3, drugs that may cause gastrointestinal side effects, hyperglycemia, hyperlipidemia, and hyperuricemia.
Nelfinavir	Indinavir	Indinavir AUC ↑ 51%, nelfinavir AUC ↑ 83%; may require dose adjustment.
	Ketoconazole	Nelfinavir AUC ↑ 35%; may require dose adjustment.
	Oral contraceptives	Ethinyl estradiol AUC ↓ 47%, norethindrone AUC ↓ 18%; advise patient about alternative birth control methods.

(*cont.*)

Table 12.4. (*cont.*)

	Ritonavir	Nelfinavir AUC ↑ 152%; may require dose adjustment.
	Saquinavir	Saquinavir AUC ↑ 392%; may require dose adjustment.
	Zidovudine	Zidovudine AUC ↓ 35%; may require dose adjustment.
	Miscellaneous	See Table 12.3, drugs that may cause hyperglycemia and hyperlipidemia.
Lopinavir/ ritonavir	Amprenavir	Amprenavir AUC ↑ 72%, lopinavir AUC ↓ 35%, dose combinations typically used in adults include APV/LPV/RTV 750/400/100 bid or 750/533/133 bid.
	Atovaquone	↓ atovaquone plasma conc.; may require dose adjustment.
	Clarithromycin	Reduce clarithromycin dose 50% if CL_{CR} 30–60 ml/min or 75% if CL_{CR} <30 ml/min.
	Dexamethasone	↓ lopinavir plasma conc.; may require dose adjustment.
	Itraconazole	↑ itraconazole plasma conc.; doses >200 mg/day not recommended.
	Ketoconazole	Ketoconazole AUC ↑ ~3-fold; doses >200 mg/day not recommended.
	Metronidazole	Avoid lopinavir/ritonavir solution due to alcohol content, may cause a "disulfiram-like" reaction.
	Oral contraceptives	Ethinyl estradiol AUC ↓ 42%, norethindrone AUC ↓ 17%; advise patient about alternative birth control methods.
	Ritonavir	Lopinavir AUC ↑ 46%.
	Tenofovir	Tenofovir AUC ↑ 34%; may require dose adjustment.
	Miscellaneous	See Table 12.3, drugs that may cause hyperglycemia and hyperlipidemia.
Other antivirals		
Acyclovir	*Miscellaneous*	See Table 12.3, drugs that may cause crystalluria and nephrotoxicity.
Foscarnet	*Miscellaneous*	See Table 12.3, drugs that may cause gastrointestinal side effects and peripheral neuropathy.
Ganciclovir	Imipenam	Contraindicated due to potential seizures.
	Didanosine	Didanosine AUC ↑ 111%; may require dose adjustment.
	Probenecid	Ganciclovir AUC ↓ 53%; may require dose adjustment.

Table 12.4. (*cont.*)

	Zidovudine	Consider holding zidovudine during induction therapy to avoid neutropenia.
	Miscellaneous	See Table 12.3, drugs that may cause gastrointestinal and hematologic side effects.
Cidofovir	Zidovudine	Hold zidovudine on day of infusion (see probenecid).
	Miscellaneous	See Table 12.3, drugs that may cause nephrotoxicity.
Anti-fungals		
Amphotericin	*Miscellaneous*	See Table 12.3, drugs that may cause hematologic side effects and nephrotoxicity.
Azoles[d]	Astemizole	Contraindicated due to potential cardiotoxicity.
	Cisapride	Contraindicated due to potential cardiotoxicity.
	Rifampin	↓ azole plasma conc.; may require dose adjustment.
	Sulfonylureas	↓ *sulfonylurea* plasma conc.; may require dose adjustment.
	Trimetrexate	↑ trimetrexate plasma conc.; may require dose adjustment.
	Warfarin	↑ INR, may require dose adjustment.
Ketoconazole	Amprenavir	Amprenavir AUC ↑ 31%; may require dose adjustment.
	Antacids[e]	Separate administration by at least 2 hours (see text)
	Delavirdine	↑ delavirdine plasma conc.; may require dose adjustment.
	Indinavir	↑ indinavir plasma conc.; may require dose adjustment.
	Isoniazid	↓ ketoconazole plasma conc.; may require dose adjustment.
	H₂-antagonists	Avoid, consider fluconazole.
	Isoniazid	↓ ketaconazole plasma conc.; may require dose adjustment.
	Lopinavir/ ritonavir	Ketoconazole AUC ↑ ~3-fold; doses >200 mg/day not recommended.
	Nelfinavir	Nelfinavir AUC ↑ 35%; may require dose adjustment.
	Nevirapine	Ketoconazole AUC ↓ 63%; ↑ nevirapine plasma conc., coadministration is not recommended.
	Proton pump inhibitors	Avoid, consider fluconazole.
	Ritonavir	Ketoconazole AUC ↑ 3.4-fold; may require dose adjustment.
	Saquinavir	Saquinavir AUC ↑ 30%, ketoconazole AUC ↑ 44%; may require dose adjustment.

(cont.)

Table 12.4. (*cont.*)

Fluconazole	Clarithromycin	Clarithromycin AUC ↑ 33%; may require dose adjustment.
	Rifabutin	↑ rifabutin plasma conc.; may require dose adjustment.
	Theophylline	↑ theophylline plasma conc., adjust dose based on theophylline levels.
	Zidovudine	Zidovudine AUC ↑ 74%; may require dose adjustment.
Itraconazole	*Antacids*[e]	Separate administration by at least 2 hours (see text).
	H₂-antagonists	Avoid, consider fluconazole.
	Lopinavir/ ritonavir	↑ itraconazole plasma conc.; doses >200 mg/day not recommended.
	Proton pump inhibitors	Avoid, consider fluconazole.
	Rifabutin	↓ itraconazole plasma conc.; may require dose adjustment.

Anti-tuberculosis

Isoniazid	*Antacids*[e]	Separate administration by at least 2 hours.
	Carbamazepine	↑ carbamazepine plasma conc.; adjust dose based on carbamazepine levels or response.
	Ketoconazole	↓ ketaconazole plasma conc.; may require dose adjustment.
	Phenytoin	↑ phenytoin plasma conc.; adjust dose based on phenytoin levels or response.
	Miscellaneous	See Table 12.3, drugs that may cause peripheral neuropathy.
Rifampin	Atovaquone	↓ atovaquone plasma conc., ↑ rifampin plasma conc.; avoid.
	Azoles[d]	↑ *azole* plasma conc.; may require dose adjustment.
	Dapsone	↓ dapsone plasma conc.; avoid.
	Delavirdine	Delavirdine AUC ↓ 96%; coadministration is not recommended.
	Phenytoin	↓ phenytoin plasma conc.; adjust dose based on phenytoin levels or response.
	Protease inhibitors	Contraindicated.
	Zidovudine	Zidovudine AUC ↓ 47%; may require dose adjustment.
Rifabutin	Delavirdine	Delavirdine AUC ↓ 80%, rifabutin AUC ↑ 100%; coadministration is not recommended.
	Efavirenz	Rifabutin AUC ↓ 38%; coadministration is not recommended.

Table 12.4. (cont.)

	Fluconazole	↑ rifabutin plasma conc.; may require dose adjustment.
	Itraconazole	↓ itraconazole plasma conc.; may require dose adjustment.
	Protease inhibitors	Avoid with saquinavir or ritonavir, ↓ rifabutin dose by 50% with indinavir or nelfinavir.
	Saquinavir	Rifabutin AUC ↑ 193%; may require dose adjustment.
Ethambutol	*Antacids*[e]	Separate administration by at least 2 hours.
	Miscellaneous	See Table 12.3, drugs that may cause peripheral neuropathy and uveitis.
Capreomycin	*Aminoglycosides*	May ↑ potential for respiratory distress.
	Non-depolarizing neuromuscular antagonist	Enhanced neuromuscular blockade.
Clarithromycin	Astemizole	Contraindicated due to potential cardiotoxicity; consider azithromycin or loratidine.
	Carbamazepine	↑ carbamazepine plasma conc.; adjust dose based on carbamazepine levels or response.
	Cisapride	Contraindicated due to potential cardiotoxicity; consider azithromycin or metoclopramide.
	Ergot derivatives	May ↑ potential for ergotism; consider azithromycin.
	Fluconazole	Clarithromycin AUC ↑ 33%; may require dose adjustment.
	Indinavir	Indinavir AUC ↑ 29%, clarithromycin AUC ↑ 53%; may require dose adjustment.
	Lopinavir/ ritonavir	Reduce clarithromycin dose 50% if CL_{CR} 30–60 mL/min or 75% if CL_{CR} <30 mL/min.
	Ritonavir	Clarithromycin AUC ↑ 77%, 14-OH clarithromycin AUC ↓ 100%; consider azithromycin.
	Saquinavir	Saquinavir AUC ↑ 177%, clarithromycin AUC ↑ 45%; may require dose adjustment.
	Theophylline	↑ theophylline plasma conc.; adjust dose based on theophylline levels or response.
Clofazimine	Phenytoin	↓ phenytoin plasma conc.; adjust dose based on phenytoin levels or response.
Cycloserine	Ritonavir[d]	Avoid ritonavir solution due to alcohol content, may ↑ potential for seizures.

(*cont.*)

Table 12.4. (*cont.*)

Other anti-infectives

Atovaquone	Lopinavir/ ritonavir	↓ atovaquone plasma conc.; may require dose adjustment.
	Rifampin	↓ atovaquone plasma conc., ↑ rifampin plasma conc.; avoid.
	Zidovudine	Zidovudine AUC ↑ 31%; may require dose adjustment
Clindamycin	Erythromycin	Contraindicated due to antagonism.
	Non-depolarizing neuromuscular antagonist	Enhanced neuromuscular blockade.
Dapsone	Probenecid	↑ dapsone plasma conc.; may require dose adjustment.
	Pyrimethamine	↑ potential for bone marrow suppression.
	Rifampin	↓ dapsone plasma conc.; avoid.
	Trimethoprim	↑ dapsone plasma conc., ↑ trimethoprim plasma conc.; may require dose adjustment.
	Miscellaneous	See Table 12.3, drugs that may cause hyperbilirubinemia.
Erythromycin	Astemizole	Contraindictated due to potential cardiotoxicity; consider loratidine.
	Cisapride	Contraindictated due to potential cardiotoxicity.
Pentamidine	*Miscellaneous*	See Table 12.3, drugs that may cause hematologic side effects, hyperglycemia, nephrotoxicity, and pancreatitis.
TMP/SMX	Dapsone	↑ dapsone plasma conc., ↑ trimethoprim plasma conc.; may require dose adjustment.
	Lamivudine	Lamivudine AUC ↑ 44%; may require dose adjustment.
	Phenytoin	↑ phenytoin plasma conc.; adjust dose based on phenytoin levels.
	Sulfonylureas	↑ sulfonylurea plasma conc.; may require dose adjustment.
	Warfarin	↑ INR; may require dose adjustment.
	Miscellaneous	See Table 12.3, drugs that may cause crystalluria, hematologic side effects, peripheral neuropathy, and uveitis.
Trimetrexate	*Azoles*[a]	↑ trimetrexate plasma conc.; may require dose adjustment.

Miscellaneous

Megesterol	*Miscellaneous*	See Table 12.3, drugs that may cause hyperglycemia.

Table 12.4. (*cont.*)

Probenecid	Dapsone	↑ dapsone plasma conc.; may require dose adjustment.
	Ganciclovir	Ganciclovir AUC ↓ 53%; may require dose adjustment.
	Zidovudine	Zidovudine AUC ↑ 106%; may require dose adjustment.
	Miscellaneous	See Table 12.3, drugs that may cause gastrointestinal side effects.
Somatropin	*Miscellaneous*	See Table 12.3, drugs that may cause pancreatitis.
Thalidomide	*Miscellaneous*	See Table 12.3, drugs that may cause peripheral neuropathy.

Italics represent pharmacological classes.

Abbreviations: AUC, area-under-the-curve; conc, concentration(s); INR, international normalized ratio

[a] applies only to capsule formulation.

[b] applies only to solution formulation.

[c] antiarrhythmics that may interact include amiodarone, disopyramide, encainide, flecainide, lidocaine, mexilitine, propafenone, and quinidine.

[d] *azoles* that may interact include fluconazole, itraconazole, and ketoconazole.

[e] *antacids* include buffer didanosine and sucralfate.

are provided; many of the strategies rely on using an alternative non-interacting drug or dose adjustment.

Conclusions

Pharmacokinetic interactions can result in a change in systemic concentrations through changes in absorption, distribution, metabolism, or excretion. Alterations in systemic concentrations can result in beneficial or undesired therapeutic responses. Drug effects also can be modified by pharmacodynamic drug interactions (additive, antagonistic, or synergistic). Knowledge of the pharmacologic profile of the agents enables clinicians to predict drugs interactions and their likely outcomes.

Acknowledgments

Grant Support: RO1 AI33835, UO1 AI41089, and UO1 AI38858 from the National Institute of Allergy and Infectious Diseases

REFERENCES

1. Morse, G. D., Fischl, M. A., Shelton, M. J., Cox, S. R., Driver, M. DeRemer, M., Single-dose pharmacokinetics of delavirdine mesylate and didanosine in patients with human immunodeficiency virus infection. *Antimicrob Agents Chemother*. 1997;**41**(1):169–174.

2. Shelton, M. J., Mei, H., Hewitt, R. G., DeFrancesco, R. If taken 1 hour before indinavir (IDV), didanosine does not affect IDV exposure, despite persistent buffering effects. *Antimicrob. Agents Chemother.* 2001;**45**(1):298–300.

3. Lomaestro, B. M., Piatek, M. A. Update on drug interactions with azole antifungal agents. *Ann. Pharmacother.* 1998;**32**:915–928.

4. Sahai, J., Garber, G., Gallicano, K., Oliveras, L., Cameron, D. W. Effects of the antacids in didanosine tablets on dapsone pharmacokinetics. *Ann. Intern. Med.* 1995;**123**(8):584–587.

5. Knupp, C. A., Barbhaiya, R. H. A multiple-dose pharmacokinetic interaction study between didanosine (Videx) and ciprofloxacin (Cipro) in male subjects seropositive for HIV but asymptomatic. *Biopharm. Drug Dispos.* 1997;**18**(1):65–77.

6. Damle, B. D., Mummaneni, V., Kaul, S., Knupp, C. Lack of effect of simultaneously administered didanosine encapsulated enteric bead formulation (Videx EC) on oral absorption of indinavir, ketoconazole, or ciprofloxacin. *Antimicrob. Agents Chemother.* 2002;**46**(2):385–391.

7. Damle, B. D., Hess, H., Kaul, S., Knupp, C. Absence of clinically relevant drug interactions following simultaneous administration of didanosine-encapsulated, enteric-coated bead formulation with either itraconazole or fluconazole. *Biopharm. Drug Dispos.* 2002;**23**(2):59–66.

8. Huisman, M. T., Smit, J. W., Schinkel, A. H.. Significance of P-glycoprotein for the pharmacology and clinical use of HIV protease inhibitors. *AIDS* 2000;**14**:237–242.

9. Acosta, E.P. Pharmacokinetic enhancement of protease inhibitors. *J. Acquir. Immune Defic. Syndr.* 2002;**29**:S11–S18.

10. Smith, P. F., DiCenzo, R., Morse, G. D. Clinical pharmacokinetics of non-nucleoside reverse transcriptase inhibitors. *Clin. Pharmacokinet.* 2001;**40**(12):893–906.

11. Sansom, L, Evans, A.M. What is the true clinical significance of plasma protein binding displacement interactions? *Drug Saf.* 1995;**12**(4):227–233.

12. Leeder, J. S., Kearns, G. L. Pharmacogenetics in pediatrics: implications for practice. *Pediatr. Clin. North Am.* 1997;**44**:55–77.

13. de Wildt, S. N., Kearns, G. L., Leeder, J. S., van den Anker, J. N. Cytochrome P450 3A: ontogeny and drug disposition. *Clin. Pharmacokinet.* 1999;**37**(6):485–505.

14. de Wildt, S. N., Kearns, G. L., Leeder, J. S., van den Anker, J. N. Glucuronidation in humans: pharmacogenetic and developmental aspects. *Clin. Pharmacokinet.* 1999;**36**(6):439–452.

15. Rathbun, R. C., Rossi, D. R. Low-dose ritonavir for protease inhibitor pharmacokinetic enhancement. *Ann. Pharmacother.* 2002;**36**:702–706.

16. Tran, J. Q., Gerber, J. G., Kerr, B. M. Delavirdine: clinical pharmacokinetics and drug interactions. *Clin. Pharmacokinet.* 2001;**40**(3):207–226.

17. Burman, W. J., Gallicano, K., Peloquin, C. Therapeutic implications of drug interactions in the treatment of human immunodeficiency virus–related tuberculosis. *Clin. Infect. Dis.* 1999;**28**:419–430.

18. Lee, B. L., Tauber, M. G., Sadler, B., Goldstein, D., Chambers, H. F. Atovaquone inhibits the glucuronidation and increases the plasma concentrations of zidovudine. *Clin. Pharmacol. Ther.* 1996;**59**:14–21.

19. Zucker, S. D., Qin, X., Rouster, S. D. *et al.* Mechanism of indinavir-induced hyperbilirubinemia. *Proc. Natl Acad. Sci.* 2001;**98**(22):12671–12676.

20. Moore, K. H. P, Yuen, G. J., Raasch, R. H. *et al.* Pharmacokinetics of lamivudine administered alone and with trimethoprim-sulfamethoxazole. *Clin. Pharmacol. Ther.* 1996;**59**:550–558.

21. Sturgill, M. G., Seibold, J. R., Boruchoff, S. E., Yeh, K. C., Haddix, H., Deutsch, P. Trimethoprim/sulfamethoxazole does not affect the steady-state disposition of indinavir. *J. Clin. Pharmacol.* 1999;**39**:1077–1084.

22. Cimoch, P. J., Lavelle, J., Pollard, R. *et al.* Pharmacokinetics of oral ganciclovir alone and in combination with zidovudine, didanosine, and probenecid in HIV-infected subjects. *J. Acquir. Immune Defic. Syndr.* 1998;**17**:227–234.

23. Jayasekara, D., Aweeka, F. T., Rodriguez, R., Kalayjian, R. C., Humphreys, M. H., Gambertoglio, J. G. Antiviral therapy for HIV patients with renal insufficiency. *J. Acquir. Immune Defic. Syndr.* 1999;**21**:384–395.

24. Stein, D. S., Moore, K. H. P. Phosphorylation of nucleoside analog antiretrovirals: a review for clinicians. *Pharmacotherapy* 2001;**21**(1):11–34.

13 Metabolic complications of antiretroviral therapy in children

Carol J. Worrell, M.D.

HIV and AIDS Malignancy Branch, National Cancer Institute, Bethesda, MD

Introduction

The introduction of highly active antiretroviral therapy (HAART) has revolutionized the care of HIV-1 infected children and adults in the developed world. However, unforeseen toxicities attributable to the use of HAART continue to emerge. Pediatricians who care for HIV-infected children and adolescents increasingly face a population that has had extensive and prolonged exposure to HAART. These toxicities have been described extensively in the adult literature yet the definitions of particular syndromes, their etiology, prevalence, diagnosis, and management remain unclear. The consequences of these changes for the overall health of the patients are also uncertain. The pediatric data are quite limited. The available information suggests that the manifestations of these toxicities in HIV-infected children can be subtle and may vary with developmental stage. Younger children may have different presentations than adults. Metabolic complications have been reported in association with the use of nucleoside reverse transcriptase inhibitors (NRTIs) and protease inhibitors (PIs). Non-nucleoside reverse transcriptase inhibitors (NNRTIs) have not been directly implicated. There may be significant intraclass variability, with respect to individual drug effects. The complications discussed in this chapter will include the fat redistribution syndrome, abnormalities in lipid and glucose metabolism, and hyperlactatemia and lactic acidosis.

Fat redistribution syndrome, lipid abnormalities, and insulin resistance

Background

This constellation of clinical and laboratory abnormalities is often referred to as the lipodystrophy syndrome, but a uniform case definition of lipodystrophy in the context of HIV infection does not yet exist. Although originally associated with the

Handbook of Pediatric HIV Care, ed. Steven L. Zeichner and Jennifer S. Read.
Published by Cambridge University Press. © Cambridge University Press 2006.

382

introduction of protease inhibitors, it appears that multiple factors may contribute to the development of these abnormalities. Host-related factors that have consistently been associated with these changes include older age and Caucasian race, each of which is associated with an increased risk of subcutaneous fat wasting [1–4]. Non-Caucasian race and female gender may be associated with an increased tendency to develop central obesity as opposed to peripheral fat wasting [1, 5]. There is also some evidence to suggest that dysregulation of inflammatory responses, particularly when they lead to elevated levels of tumor necrosis factor alpha (TNFα), may contribute to the altered fat distribution and metabolic abnormalities associated with HAART [6].

Alterations in body fat distribution have been shown to predate the HAART era and may be associated with HIV infection itself. Kotler *et al.* documented alterations in the distribution of fat in HIV-infected patients consisting of increased visceral and decreased subcutaneous fat content regardless of treatment status (i.e., untreated, treated with a non-PI-containing antiretroviral regimen, or treated with a PI-containing antiretroviral regimen) [7]. Alterations in lipid metabolism during HIV infection have also been well documented prior to HAART. AIDS itself is associated with elevated levels of plasma triglycerides, very low density lipoprotein (VLDL) and free fatty acids (FFA), and decreased levels of cholesterol, high density lipoproteins (HDL), and low density lipoproteins (LDL) [8]. Duration of HIV infection, HIV RNA at baseline, and HIV RNA response to HAART have all been associated with the development of lipodystrophy [2–4]. CD4 count at baseline and CD4 response to therapy have been less consistently associated with these changes.

Although the first reports of lipodystrophy occurred with the introduction of PI therapy, several studies have documented the occurrence of fat redistribution in patients treated with NRTIs alone [2–4, 9]. PIs and NRTIs are believed to exert their effects on fat distribution and lipid metabolism by different mechanisms, and may act synergistically when used in combination [1]. Several studies have suggested that the addition of PI therapy to NRTI therapy may accelerate the progression of symptoms already present in patients who had been receiving therapy with NRTIs alone [2, 10–12]. Drug-related factors will be discussed in more detail below.

Many of the descriptions of HIV-associated lipodystrophy were compiled using sub-optimal study designs. It appears that lipodystrophy in the setting of HIV infection is likely to be a progressive, cumulative process with multiple factors contributing to its pathogenesis. Most studies have been cross-sectional in design with the result that the relative contribution of drugs in use at the time of study may be overestimated and associated with outcomes that actually represent cumulative effects [1]. The lack of a uniform case definition has meant that there is significant heterogeneity in the way different investigators characterize lipodystrophy, and therefore significant variability in the characteristics of the patients chosen for study. Lipodystrophy has been defined in some studies as a syndrome that includes dyslipidemia and/or altered glucose metabolism, and in others as a syndrome that consists of fat redistribution (also not consistently defined) without other associated metabolic changes. In addition, there are no uniform criteria to assess the severity of the changes.

Wide variations exist in the use of terminology and diagnostic methodology among studies. Diverse criteria have been used for diagnosis and have included one or more of the following: self-report; physician report; anthropometric measurements (skin-fold thickness, waist to hip ratio, etc.); bioelectrical impedance analysis (BIA); dual-energy X-ray absorptiometry (DEXA); computerized tomography (CT); and magnetic resonance imaging (MRI).

One result of the heterogeneity in definitions and methodologies is the wide variation in estimates of the prevalence and cumulative incidence of lipodystrophy among antiretroviral users between cross-sectional studies, which range from 3% to 83% [4, 13–15].

Fat redistribution syndrome

Fat redistribution syndrome (FRS) is characterized by altered body habitus due to lipoatrophy, lipohypertrophy, or a combination of both [16]. The hallmarks of the alterations in body shape are the loss of subcutaneous fat from the face, limbs, or buttocks (lipoatrophy) and the increase of fat deposition centrally, with increased abdominal girth due to visceral fat accumulation, breast enlargement, dorsocervical fat accumulation ("buffalo hump"), and the development of lipomas (lipohypertrophy) [11, 16–18]. The overall appearance is of peripheral wasting and central obesity; it is not always associated with a change in weight. These phenotypic changes can occur independently of dyslipidemia and altered glucose metabolism [4].

Other disease processes are associated with alterations in body fat distribution, including Cushing's syndrome, growth hormone deficiency, hypothyroidism, and testosterone deficiency. Most studies have not demonstrated an association between FRS and these other disease processes.

Several trials have documented the occurrence of FRS in HIV-infected pediatric patients, and estimates of the incidence of FRS in HIV-infected children on antiretroviral therapy range from 18% to 33% [19–23]. All three forms of FRS (lipoatrophy, lipohypertrophy, and the combined form) have been described in HIV-infected children. In a cross-sectional study of 39 HIV-infected children on stable antiretroviral regimens for more than 12 months, Jaquet *et al.* observed an overall incidence of FRS of 33.3% [21]. The presence of lipoatrophy and/or lipohypertrophy was determined by clinical characteristics and anthropometric measurements. Twenty percent of the children with FRS had truncal lipohypertrophy, 8% had peripheral lipoatrophy, and 5% had the combined form of FRS. The combined form of FRS was observed only in adolescents and the changes were more severe than those seen in prepubertal children.

Fat redistribution may not always be clinically apparent in prepubertal children. Arpadi *et al.* followed 28 HIV-infected children in a longitudinal observational study of body composition, and found that eight children (29%) had lipodystrophy, defined as the combined form (truncal fat accumulation plus extremity lipoatrophy) by DEXA scanning. Only one of these children had been identified clinically [20].

Abnormalities in lipid and glucose metabolism

Lipoatrophy and lipohypertrophy can contribute to disorders of carbohydrate and lipid metabolism in several ways. Adipocytes function both as storage depots for fat and as endocrine cells which secrete several molecules that influence insulin sensitivity and energy balance, blood pressure control, and coagulation. These molecules include leptin and Acrp30 (adiponectin), which are insulin sensitizers, as well as TNF-α and IL-6, which are insulin antagonists [24]. Loss of adipocytes leads to excess calories being diverted away from their normal storage areas, resulting in dyslipidemia and lipid accumulation (in the form of triglycerides) in tissues such as the liver, muscle, and pancreatic β cells [24].

The anatomic distribution of adipose tissue into visceral (as opposed to subcutaneous) depots is known to be a strong and independent predictor of adverse outcomes such as coronary artery disease and diabetes in the non-HIV-infected population [25]. Enlargement of visceral abdominal adipose tissue depots is a major component of the lipohypertrophy that is seen in HIV-infected patients. Accumulation of visceral abdominal adipose tissue has been associated with glucose intolerance, hyperinsulinemia, and hypertriglyceridemia, and a very high rate of premature coronary artery disease, although the mechanisms behind these associations remain unclear [24–26].

Dyslipidemia and insulin resistance have most often been reported in association with PI therapy. Hadigan *et al.* have also demonstrated significant fasting hyperinsulinemia and hypertriglyceridemia associated with truncal adiposity in HIV-infected women who had not been treated with PIs [5]. Mild to moderate elevations in triglyceride levels have been documented in other studies of PI-naïve, NRTI-treated patients [5, 16].

PI therapy has been associated with increases in LDL cholesterol and triglyceride levels, and decreases in HDL cholesterol levels [16]. With respect to glucose metabolism, PI therapy has been associated with the following spectrum of abnormalities in the adult literature: hyperglycemia (usually asymptomatic), impaired glucose tolerance, insulin resistance, new onset non-insulin-dependent diabetes mellitus, increases in insulin requirements of patients with pre-existing insulin-dependent diabetes mellitus, and, rarely, diabetic ketoacidosis [14, 16]. Insulin resistance may occur in as many as 40% of patients treated with PIs, while rates of hyperglycemia and diabetes are considerably lower [3%–17% and 1%–6%, respectively) [27, 28].

Dyslipidemia and abnormalities of glucose metabolism have been demonstrated in pediatric patients receiving antiretroviral therapy [19, 22, 29, 30]. In a cross-sectional study of 29 HIV-infected children described earlier, hypertriglyceridemia was documented in 41%, hypercholesterolemia in 41%, and a combination of both in 24% [22].

None of the patients had abnormal fasting glucose levels. Insulin and C-peptide levels were not measured in this study.

A cross-sectional evaluation of forty HIV-infected children by Amaya, et al., revealed hypercholesterolemia in 68%, hypertriglyceridemia in 28%, and insulin resistance in 8% [19]. Insulin resistance was defined as an abnormally elevated fasting insulin or C-peptide level with a normal serum glucose level. Fasting serum glucose levels were normal for children. The mean age of the children with insulin resistance was significantly higher than that of the unaffected group ($P = 0.007$).

PI-associated effects

The effects of individual PIs on lipid metabolism are fairly similar with the exception of ritonavir, which appears to cause a higher degree of hypertriglyceridemia than other PIs [31, 32]. PI therapy has also been associated with changes in body habitus [4, 12–15, 33]. Both the risk of fat wasting and the probability of intra-abdominal fat accumulation increase with the duration of PI therapy [1, 2, 14, 15, 28]. While all PIs have been implicated in the development of FRS, few prospective studies have been carried out to determine the relative effects of individual PIs [11].

The pathogenesis of PI-associated metabolic changes is unknown. Several hypotheses have been proposed that involve the interaction of PIs with various proteins involved in adipocyte function and differentiation, lipid handling, and glucose transport. In vitro and in vivo studies investigating the mechanisms underlying the adverse effects associated with PIs are currently under way.

NRTI-associated effects

NRTI use has been independently associated with the development of FRS and, in particular, with the development of lipoatrophy [2–4, 9]. The probability of developing lipoatrophy increases with the duration of NRTI therapy [2]. Among the NRTIs, stavudine has been the most widely implicated in the development of FRS [1, 3].

NRTI-associated fat redistribution is believed to occur as a result of tissue-specific mitochondrial toxicity. Clinical manifestations that have been attributed to NRTI-related mitochondrial toxicity include lipoatrophy, myopathy, cardiomyopathy, peripheral neuropathy, pancreatitis, hepatic steatosis and lactic acidosis, anemia, and proximal renal tubular dysfunction (associated with adefovir therapy). Nucleoside analogues such as the NRTIs are known to inhibit DNA polymerase γ, the polymerase responsible for mitochondrial DNA replication [2, 27, 34, 35]. The main function of mitochondria is to generate energy for the cell in the form of adenosine triphosphate (ATP). Agents that are toxic to mitochondria lead to impaired ATP synthesis. The oxidative phosphorylation system generates energy by using intracellular fatty acids and glucose as fuel. Impairment of the system leads to the intracellular accumulation of fat (in the form of free fatty acids and triglycerides) and lactate [34, 35].

Diagnosis
Fat redistribution
Anthropometric measurements
Measurements of simple body circumferences over time (i.e., abdominal circumference, waist to hip ratios, limb circumference) can be useful by indicating that a significant change may be occurring, but cannot accurately determine its nature (i.e., loss of fat mass vs. loss of lean body mass). Skinfold measurements using calipers can be imprecise and are very operator-dependent. They should be collected under highly standardized conditions [1].

Dual energy X-ray absorptiometry (DEXA)
This gives a two-dimensional image that is very reliable for measuring limb fat and total body fat, but cannot distinguish subcutaneous abdominal fat from visceral fat [11]. Comparisons between different machines within the same or at different institutions require standardization of calibration.

Single cut CT or MRI
This produces three-dimensional images that can distinguish between subcutaneous and visceral fat compartments. Single cut CT or MRI scans at L4 can be used to analyze abdominal fat, and can be used in combination with DEXA scans to more fully characterize changes in fat distribution [1, 11, 16, 18]. Single cut scans of the mid-thigh and/or the arm have been used to characterize peripheral fat content. Standardization of calibration is required when comparing results from different machines.

Whole body CT or MRI
This can also be utilized but is impractical due to its cost and the lack of standardization of measures for whole body fat changes.

Dyslipidemia
Dyslipidemia is diagnosed by a fasting lipid profile. This should include total cholesterol, HDL cholesterol, and triglycerides. LDL cholesterol is calculated from these values, except when the triglyceride level exceeds 400 mg/dl, at which point the calculated value becomes unreliable [36]. In this event, decisions may be based on the direct measurement of LDL (not uniformly available and generally expensive), or on the calculation of non-HDL cholesterol using the formula: non-HDL cholesterol = total cholesterol − HDL cholesterol [37].

There are currently no recommendations for the monitoring of either dyslipidemia or abnormalities in glucose metabolism (discussed below) for pediatric patients with HIV infection. The Adult AIDS Clinical Trials Group recommends obtaining fasting lipid profiles before the initiation of HAART; this should be repeated after 3 months of therapy and if normal, once yearly or with any change in antiretroviral regimen [18, 37].

Abnormalities of glucose metabolism

Monitoring for abnormalities of glucose metabolism essentially involves monitoring for changes associated with non-insulin-dependent diabetes mellitus. These include evidence of insulin resistance (high fasting plasma insulin and C-peptide levels), suggestive evidence of insulin resistance such as impaired fasting glucose (a level of 110–125 mg/dl), impaired glucose tolerance (a serum glucose level between 140–199 mg/dl two hours after a 75-gram oral glucose load), or evidence of frank diabetes mellitus (fasting glucose ≥ 126 mg/dl or 2-hour glucose level after a glucose challenge of ≥ 200 mg/dl) [11, 37].

It should be kept in mind that fasting glucose can be normal in the setting of insulin resistance, so that this test alone may not be sufficient to determine the presence of abnormalities in glucose metabolism. An evaluation should probably be performed of all children who are starting PI-based HAART, as well as those with significant dyslipidemia and/or body habitus changes. A 2-hour oral glucose tolerance test should be obtained when evidence of a significant disturbance of glucose homeostasis is observed.

Management

There are currently no recommendations for the management of FRS, dyslipidemia, or abnormalities of glucose metabolism for pediatric patients with HIV infection. Recommendations for the management of dyslipidemia in otherwise healthy children consist primarily of dietary and lifestyle interventions. Pilot studies in HIV-infected adults with metabolic changes and/or FRS have shown improvement in lipid profiles, insulin sensitivity, and body habitus after the institution of dietary changes and exercise regimens [38, 39]. In HIV-uninfected children bile acid sequestrants are the first line of therapy when pharmacologic agents are used. These drugs may potentially interfere with absorption of antiretroviral drugs and are quite unpalatable [40, 41].

Lipid-lowering agents and insulin-sensitizing agents are being studied in HIV-infected adults but have significant safety issues, including potential interactions with PIs via the cytochrome P-450 system.

Treatment with recombinant human growth hormone has been associated with reductions in total and visceral fat in adult patients with FRS; however, many patients developed glucose intolerance on therapy and the benefits appear to be short-lived, with recurrence of fat accumulation when therapy is stopped [16, 37].

The potential for changes in antiretroviral therapy to reverse metabolic and body habitus changes associated with HAART has been examined in adults in several small studies that have yielded mixed results [42–44]. The substitution of nevirapine for a PI in HAART regimens in NNRTI-naïve patients appears to be associated with improvement of the lipid profile (and with maintenance of virologic and immunologic gains from PI-based HAART), and may also lead to some improvement in morphologic changes, but the evidence for the latter effect is less compelling [42, 43]. Studies of regimens containing efavirenz have not shown a consistent benefit. Other strategies have focused on abacavir as either a substitute for a PI in HAART regimens on which patients have achieved virologic suppression, or as an NRTI substitute in regimens containing stavudine or zidovudine. Small but significant improvements have been seen after abacavir substitution in both settings with respect to lipoatrophy, lipid abnormalities, and insulin sensitivity [44]. The ability to maintain virologic suppression and immunologic gains in the long term with a triple NRTI regimen remains a concern, as does the effectiveness of abacavir in the setting of the NRTI-experienced patient [36, 45].

Hyperlactatemia and lactic acidosis

Another proposed consequence of mitochondrial toxicity related to treatment with NRTIs is a spectrum of abnormalities characterized by disturbances in lactate homeostasis. The spectrum of disease ranges from asymptomatic hyperlactatemia to lactic acidosis with hepatic steatosis and its accompanying high mortality rate. This latter complication fortunately appears to be quite rare, perhaps occurring in less than 1% of patients; however, its precise incidence is difficult to ascertain as most cases have been reported as isolated events rather than in the context of whole populations of patients [16, 46].

The pediatric data in this area is even more limited than the data available regarding fat redistribution and abnormalities of lipid and glucose metabolism and primarily consists of uncontrolled case series and isolated case reports.

Background

The proposed mechanism of mitochondrial damage by NRTIs is outlined above. Impairment of oxidative phosphorylation leads to the synthesis of ATP via anaerobic glycolysis, resulting in an excess production of lactate in the cell that eventually enters the systemic circulation. The liver, and, to a lesser extent, the kidneys have the ability to markedly increase their level of lactate clearance under conditions of lactate excess [46]. A combination of increased production in many tissues and decreased clearance may be required for a patient to develop fulminant lactic acidosis. Sustained production of ATP by anaerobic glycolysis results in the production of organic acids and is believed to lead to a drop in pH, thereby compromising hepatic and renal function and diminishing clearance of lactate from the systemic circulation [37].

Mitochondrial dysfunction can result in a broad spectrum of abnormalities, and multiorgan system dysfunction with broad phenotypic variation is characteristic. Findings can include varying combinations of hyperlactatemia, myopathy, cardiomyopathy, hepatopathy, encephalopathy, peripheral neuropathy, and pancreatitis [47, 48].

Asymptomatic (compensated) hyperlactatemia

This type of clinical (or sub-clinical) presentation consists of mild to moderate elevations of venous lactate levels which can occur on a chronic or an intermittent basis and may be common in adult patients treated with HAART regimens that include NRTIs [46, 49]. In a prospective, longitudinal study of 349 HIV-infected adults, the presence of mild to moderate elevations in lactate was not associated with progression to symptomatic hyperlactatemia or fulminant lactic acidosis [49]. Other studies in adults have estimated the incidence of mild to moderate hyperlactatemia at between 8 and 35% [50, 51].

A small prospective study by Giaquinto *et al.* reported asymptomatic, transient elevations in venous lactate levels on at least one occasion in 17 (85%) of 20 infants who had been exposed to NRTIs in utero and to zidovudine during delivery and for 6 weeks after birth [52]. The same group reported mild, asymptomatic elevations of lactate levels in 3 (8%) of 29 HIV-infected children ranging in age from 5 months to 17 years who were being treated with at least one NRTI.

Symptomatic hyperlactatemia

This syndrome has not yet been described in children. The presentation described in adults consists of hyperlactatemia in the setting of non-specific symptoms – abdominal pain, nausea, abdominal distention, fatigue, exercise-induced dyspnea, and abnormal liver function tests – which may ultimately progress to fulminant lactic acidosis [46, 53, 54]. Tachycardia, weight loss, or peripheral neuropathy may also be present [53]. Most patients show symptomatic improvement after cessation of antiretroviral therapy. Lactate levels may increase initially after cessation of antiretrovirals and may take weeks to months to normalize. Hepatic steatosis is usually present and micro- and macrovesicular steatosis may be seen on liver biopsy [54]. Some patients may tolerate re-challenge with an NRTI [46].

Decompensated lactic acidosis

The presentation of lactic acidosis associated with NRTI therapy is much more severe than that of symptomatic hyperlactatemia. Non-specific gastrointestinal complaints are predominant and may consist of nausea, vomiting, abdominal pain, distention, tender hepatomegaly, fatigue, malaise, and prostration [46]. There may be concurrent pancreatitis, neuropathy, and elevated creatine kinase. Fulminant metabolic acidosis develops rapidly, leading to arrhythmias and organ failure [46]. In adults, this syndrome appears to be significantly associated with age, female gender, obesity, pre-existing liver disease (e.g., chronic hepatitis B or C), and the use of stavudine [37,

46, 53, 54]. This syndrome has also been described in HIV-infected pediatric patients (including an infant, a toddler, and an adolescent) in isolated case reports [55–57].

Delayed manifestations of mitochondrial toxicity

The presentations described above all involve patients who were receiving therapy with NRTIs at the time abnormalities were detected, and all of the patients responded to withdrawal of NRTI therapy. Another presentation of fulminant disease, believed to be due to NRTI-related mitochondrial dysfunction, has been described in HIV-uninfected, NRTI-exposed children that manifests itself months after the exposure has ceased. Blanche *et al.* described eight children with persistent mitochondrial dysfunction after perinatal exposure to NRTIs [58, 59]. The mothers had received either zidovudine alone or, as part of a separate study, zidovudine plus lamivudine, beginning at 32 weeks' gestation and continuing through delivery. The infants then continued the same regimen their mothers had received for the first 6 weeks of life. None of the children were identified while still receiving NRTI prophylaxis, with the earliest signs and symptoms beginning at four months of age. There was considerable phenotypic variation among the affected children, who ranged from asymptomatic with persistent biochemical abnormalities to floridly symptomatic with signs and symptoms consistent with what has been described in inherited mitochondrial disorders. Two of the children died. Five had persistently elevated blood lactate concentrations. Upon examination of enzyme activity in skeletal muscle mitochondria, all of the children were found to have decreased activity in respiratory-chain complexes I, IV, or both. No substantial decrease in mitochondrial DNA content was observed in the two patients who were most severely affected or in the one other patient in which this was examined. Large deletions or duplications of mitochondrial DNA were not seen in any patient, and none of the mutations associated with the currently characterized mitochondrial diseases was found.

This level of mitochondrial disease (8/1,754) far exceeds the estimated background prevalence of mitochondrial disease of 1/3000 to 1/4000 in the general population [47]. Four of the women were of African origin (not further specified), one was from North Africa, and 3 were European. Zidovudine dosing was 500 mg per day for the mothers, and 8 mg/kg per day for the infants. Lamivudine was given at doses of 300 mg per day for the mothers, and 4 mg/kg per day for the infants. In the zidovudine/lamivudine group, mean prenatal exposure to NRTIs was 17.2 weeks (range 0–40) and mean postnatal exposure was 5.2 weeks (range 2–6 weeks).

As a result of these observations, several large databases including over 23 000 children with perinatal exposure to HIV who were uninfected or of indeterminate status have been examined retrospectively for evidence of mitochondrial diseases [60]. None have found evidence suggestive of mitochondrial dysfunction or metabolic disease; however, the majority of the reviews focused on causes of death and may have missed less severe presentations [60]. Nevertheless, two large studies have looked specifically for signs and symptoms that could be associated with mitochondrial/metabolic complications and have not found evidence of them [60].

Diagnosis and management

Diagnosis is based on clinical signs and symptoms and requires a high index of suspicion. Routine monitoring of lactate levels has not been shown to be of benefit and is not recommended [37, 49, 51]. Lactate levels should always be obtained under standardized conditions and with the patient at rest, and should be confirmed if abnormal. When lactate levels are obtained based on clinical suspicion, levels of 2–5 mmol/l are considered mild-moderate, and levels >5 mmol/l are considered indicative of severe acidemia [16, 51]. Antiretrovirals should be held for lactate levels >5 mmol/l and other causes of associated clinical findings (e.g., myopathy, neuropathy, transaminitis) should be excluded while a diagnosis of NRTI-related mitochondrial toxicity is pursued.

Multisystem disease is almost always present in the symptomatic forms of hyperlactatemia. Specific diagnostic studies (e.g., electrocardiogram, echocardiography, abdominal CT, MRI of the brain, liver biopsy, muscle biopsy, etc.) should be obtained according to the presenting symptoms. Biochemical studies specifically looking for mitochondrial failure should be obtained in consultation with a neurologist and include: blood and CSF lactate; skin biopsy for fibroblast culture and biochemical studies; muscle biopsy for histology, mitochondrial DNA studies, respiratory-chain enzyme activity, and electron microscopy [47].

In addition to early detection and discontinuation of antiretrovirals in severe cases, further treatment is supportive. Treatment options that are based on the treatment of inherited mitochondrial disease and whose use has been reported anecdotally in NRTI-related lactic acidosis include respiratory chain co-factors, antioxidants, and nutrients; riboflavin, thiamine, L-carnitine, coenzyme Q 10, vitamins C, E, and A, and idebenone (an analogue of coenzyme Q 10) [16, 37]. No firm dosing recommendations exist for any of these agents in this setting.

Conclusions

Long-term metabolic complications due to antretroviral therapy occur in children as well as in adults. Developmental stage appears to play a significant role in determining their presentation, which in younger children can be quite distinct from that seen in adults. NRTIs and PIs can contribute to changes in fat distribution and alterations of lipid and glucose metabolism independently, however the greatest impact appears to occur when they are used in combination. Current data do not suggest that PIs contribute to mitochondrial toxicity and the development of hyperlactatemia and lactic acidosis. The effects described are cumulative and progressive, yet both the pediatric and the adult literature consist largely of cross-sectional studies, uncontrolled case series, and isolated case reports. The overall effect is that a reading of the literature raises as many questions as it answers. Well-designed prospective, longitudinal studies are needed but will remain difficult to design as long as consensus regarding the definitions of particular syndromes remains elusive.

REFERENCES

1. John, M., Nolan, D., Mallal, S. Antiretroviral therapy and the lipodystrophy syndrome. *Antiviral Ther.* 2001;**6**(1):9–20.
2. Mallal, S. A., John, M., Moore, C. B., James, I. R., McKinnon, E. J. Contribution of nucleoside analogue reverse transcriptase inhibitors to subcutaneous fat wasting in patients with HIV infection. *AIDS* 2000;**14**(10):1309–1316.
3. Chene, G., Angelini, E., Cotte, L. *et al.* Role of long-term nucleoside-analogue therapy in lipodystrophy and metabolic disorders in human immunodeficiency virus-infected patients. *Clin. Infect. Dis.* 2002;**34**(5):649–657.
4. Gervasoni, C., Ridolfo, A. L., Trifiro, G. *et al.* Redistribution of body fat in HIV-infected women undergoing combined antiretroviral therapy. *AIDS* 1999;**13**(4):465–471.
5. Hadigan, C., Miller, K., Corcoran, C., Anderson, E., Basgoz, N., Grinspoon, S. Fasting hyperinsulinemia and changes in regional body composition in human immunodeficiency virus-infected women. *J. Clin. Endocrinol. Metab.* 1999;**84**(6):1932–1937.
6. Ledru, E., Christeff, N., Patey, O., de Truchis, P., Melchior, J. C., Gougeon, M. L. Alteration of tumor necrosis factor-alpha T-cell homeostasis following potent antiretroviral therapy: contribution to the development of human immunodeficiency virus-associated lipodystrophy syndrome. *Blood* 2000;**95**(10):3191–3198.
7. Kotler, D. P., Rosenbaum, K., Wang, J., Pierson, R. N. Studies of body composition and fat distribution in HIV-infected and control subjects. *J. Acquir Immune. Defic. Syndr. Hum. Retrovirol.* 1999;**20**(3):228–237.
8. Grunfeld, C., Pang, M., Doerrler, W., Shigenaga, J. K., Jensen, P., Feingold, K. R. Lipids, lipoproteins, triglyceride clearance, and cytokines in human immunodeficiency virus infection and the acquired immunodeficiency syndrome. *J. Clin. Endocrinol. Metab.* 1992;**74**(5):1045–1052.
9. Saint-Marc, T., Partisani, M., Poizot-Martin, I. *et al.* A syndrome of peripheral fat wasting (lipodystrophy) in patients receiving long-term nucleoside analogue therapy. *AIDS* 1999;**13**(13):1659–1667.
10. Hadigan, C., Corcoran, C., Stanley, T., Piecuch, S., Klibanski, A., Grinspoon, S. Fasting hyperinsulinemia in human immunodeficiency virus-infected men: relationship to body composition, gonadal function, and protease inhibitor use. *J. Clin. Endocrinol. Metab.* 2000;**85**(1):35–41.
11. Jain, R. G., Furfine, E. S., Pedneault, L., White, A. J., Lenhard, J. M. Metabolic complications associated with antiretroviral therapy. *Antiviral Res.* 2001;**51**(3):151–177.
12. van der Valk, M., Gisolf, E. H., Reiss, P. *et al.* Increased risk of lipodystrophy when nucleoside analogue reverse transcriptase inhibitors are included with protease inhibitors in the treatment of HIV-1 infection. *AIDS* 2001;**15**(7):847–855.
13. Dong, K. L., Bausserman, L. L., Flynn, M. M. *et al.* Changes in body habitus and serum lipid abnormalities in HIV-positive women on highly active antiretroviral therapy (HAART). *J. Acquir. Immune Defic. Syndr.* 1999;**21**(2):107–113.

14. Carr, A., Samaras, K., Burton, S. *et al.* A syndrome of peripheral lipodystrophy, hyperlipidaemia and insulin resistance in patients receiving HIV protease inhibitors. *AIDS* 1998;**12**(7):F51–F58.

15. Carr, A., Samaras, K., Thorisdottir, A., Kaufmann, G. R., Chisholm, D. J., Cooper, D. A. Diagnosis, prediction, and natural course of HIV-1 protease-inhibitor-associated lipodystrophy, hyperlipidaemia, and diabetes mellitus: a cohort study. *Lancet* 1999;**353**(9170):2093–2999.

16. Herman, J., Easterbrook, P. The metabolic toxicities of antiretroviral therapy. *Int. J. STD AIDS* 2001;**12**:555–564.

17. Qaqish, R., Rublein, J., Wohl, D. HIV-associated lipodystrophy syndrome. *Pharmacotherapy* 2000;**20**(1):13–22.

18. Wanke, C. A., Falutz, J. M., Shevitz, A., Phair, J. P., Kotler, D. P. Clinical evaluation and management of metabolic and morphologic abnormalities associated with human immunodeficiency virus. *Clin. Infect. Dis.* 2002;**34**(2):248–259.

19. Amaya, R., Kozinetz, C., McMeans, A., Schwarzwald, H., Kline, M. Lipodystrophy syndrome in human imunnodeficiency virus-infected children. *Pediatr. Infect. Dis. J.* 2002;**21**(5):405–410.

20. Arpadi, S. M., Cuff, P. A., Horlick, M., Wang, J., Kotler, D. P. Lipodystrophy in HIV-infected children is associated with high viral load and low CD4+ -lymphocyte count and CD4+ -lymphocyte percentage at baseline and use of protease inhibitors and stavudine. *J. Acquir. Immune Defic. Syndr.* 2001;**27**(1):30–34.

21. Jaquet, D., Levine, M., Ortega-Rodriguez, E. *et al.* Clinical and metabolic presentation of the lipodystrophic syndrome in HIV-infected children. *AIDS* 2000;**14**(14):2123–2128.

22. Meneilly, G., Forbes, J., Peabody, D., Remple, V., Burdge, D. Metabolic and body composition changes in HIV-infected children on antiretroviral therapy. In *Eighth Conference on Retroviruses and Opportunistic Infections*; 2001; February 4–8, 2001; Chicago, Illinois.

23. Brambilla, P., Bricalli, D., Sala, N. *et al.* Highly active antiretroviral-treated HIV-infected children show fat distribution changes even in absence of lipodystrophy. *AIDS* 2001;**15**(18):2415–2422.

24. Savage, D. B. Leptin: a novel therapeutic role in lipodystrophy. *J. Clin. Invest.* 2002;**109**:1285–1286.

25. Montague, C. T., O'Rahilly, S. The perils of portliness: causes and consequences of visceral adiposity. *Diabetes* 2000;**49**(6):883–888.

26. Flier, J. Obesity. In Braunwald, E. *et al.*, ed. *Harrison's Principles of Internal Medicine*. 15th edn. McGraw-Hill Companies, 2001.

27. Powderly, W. G., Long-term exposure to lifelong therapies. *J. Acquir. Immune Defic. Syndr.* 2002;**29** Suppl 1:S28–S40.

28. Mulligan, K., Grunfeld, C., Tai, V. W. *et al.* Hyperlipidemia and insulin resistance are induced by protease inhibitors independent of changes in body composition in patients with HIV infection. *J. Acquir. Immune Defic. Syndr.* 2000;**23**(1):35–43.

29. Melvin, A. J., Lennon, S., Mohan, K. M., Purnell, J. Q. Metabolic abnormalities in HIV type 1-infected children treated and not treated with protease inhibitors. *AIDS Res. Hum. Retroviruses* 2001;**17**(12):1117–1123.

30. Arpadi, S. M., Cuff, P. A., Horlick, M., Kotler, D. P. Visceral obesity, hypertriglyceridemia and hypercortisolism in a boy with perinatally acquired HIV infection receiving protease inhibitor-containing antiviral treatment. *AIDS* 1999;**13**(16):2312–2313.

31. Tsiodras, S., Mantzoros, C., Hammer, S., Samore, M. Effects of protease inhibitors on hyperglycemia, hyperlipidemia, and lipodystrophy: a 5-year cohort study. *Arch. Intern. Med.* 2000;**160**(13):2050–2056.

32. Cheseaux, J. J., Jotterand, V., Aebi, C. *et al.* Hyperlipidemia in HIV-infected children treated with protease inhibitors: relevance for cardiovascular diseases. *J. Acquir. Immune Defic. Syndr.* 2002;**30**(3):288–293.

33. Carr, A., Samaras, K., Chisholm, D. J., Cooper, D. A. Pathogenesis of HIV-1-protease inhibitor-associated peripheral lipodystrophy, hyperlipidaemia, and insulin resistance. *Lancet* 1998;**351**(9119):1881–1883.

34. Brinkman, K., ter Hofstede, H. J., Burger, D. M., Smeitink, J. A., Koopmans, P. P. Adverse effects of reverse transcriptase inhibitors: mitochondrial toxicity as common pathway. *AIDS* 1998;**12**(14):1735–17244.

35. Kakuda, T. N., Pharmacology of nucleoside and nucleotide reverse transcriptase inhibitor-induced mitochondrial toxicity. *Clin. Ther.* 2000;**22**(6):685–708.

36. Dube, M. P., Sprecher, D., Henry, W. K. *et al.* Preliminary guidelines for the evaluation and management of dyslipidemia in adults infected with human immunodeficiency virus and receiving antiretroviral therapy: recommendations of the Adult AIDS Clinical Trial Group Cardiovascular Disease Focus Group. *Clin. Infect. Dis.* 2000;**31**(5):1216–1224.

37. The Adult AIDS Clinical Trials Group. *AACTG Metabolic Complications Guides*. Adult AIDS Clinical Trials Group; 2002.

38. Roubenoff, R., Weiss, L., McDermott, A. *et al.* A pilot study of exercise training to reduce trunk fat in adults with HIV-associated fat redistribution. *AIDS* 1999;**13**(11):1373–1375.

39. Jones, S. P., Doran, D. A., Leatt, P. B., Maher, B., Pirmohamed, M. Short-term exercise training improves body composition and hyperlipidaemia in HIV-positive individuals with lipodystrophy. *AIDS* 2001;**15**(15):2049–2051.

40. American Academy of Pediatrics. Committee on Nutrition. "Cholesterol in childhood". *Pediatrics* 1998;**101**(1 Pt 1):141–147.

41. Wedekind, C. A., Pugatch, D. Lipodystrophy syndrome in children infected with human immunodeficiency virus. *Pharmacotherapy* 2001;**21**(7):861–866.

42. Barreiro, P., Soriano, V., Blanco, F., Casimiro, C., de la Cruz, J. J., Gonzalez-Lahoz, J. Risks and benefits of replacing protease inhibitors by nevirapine in HIV-infected subjects under long-term successful triple combination therapy. *AIDS* 2000;**14**(7):807–812.

43. Martinez, E., Conget, I., Lozano, L., Casamitjana, R., Gatell, J. M. Reversion of metabolic abnormalities after switching from HIV-1 protease inhibitors to nevirapine. *AIDS* 1999;**13**(7):805–810.

44. Carr, A., Workman, C., Smith, D. E. *et al.* Abacavir substitution for nucleoside analogs in patients with HIV lipoatrophy: a randomized trial. *J. Am. Med. Assoc.* 2002;**288**(2):207–215.

45. Currier, J. S., Metabolic complications of Antiretroviral Therapy and HIV Infection. In *Medscape HIV/AIDS Annual Update 2001* edn. Medscape; 2001.

46. John, M., Mallal, S. A. Hyperlactatemia syndromes in people with HIV infection. *Curr. Opin. Infect. Dis.* 2002;**15**:23–29.

47. Haas, R. H., A comparison of genetic mitochondrial disease and nucleoside analogue toxicity. Does fetal nucleoside toxicity underlie reports of mitochondrial disease in infants born to women treated for HIV infection? *Ann. N. Y. Acad. Sci.* 2000;**918**:247–261.

48. Vu, T. H., Sciacco, M., Tanji, K. *et al.* Clinical manifestations of mitochondrial DNA depletion. *Neurology* 1998;**50**(6):1783–1790.

49. John, M., Moore, C. B., James, I. R. *et al.* Chronic hyperlactatemia in HIV-infected patients taking antiretroviral therapy. *AIDS* 2001;**15**(6):717–723.

50. Boubaker, K., Flepp, M., Sudre, P. *et al.* Hyperlactatemia and antiretroviral therapy: the Swiss HIV Cohort Study. *Clin. Infect. Dis.* 2001;**33**(11):1931–1937.

51. Brinkman, K., Management of hyperlactatemia: no need for routine lactate measurements. *AIDS* 2001;**15**(6):795–797.

52. Giaquinto, C., De Romeo, A., Giacomet, V. *et al.* Lactic acid levels in children perinatally treated with antiretroviral agents to prevent HIV transmission. *AIDS* 2001;**15**(8):1074–1075.

53. Gerard, Y., Maulin, L., Yazdanpanah, Y. *et al.* Symptomatic hyperlactataemia: an emerging complication of antiretroviral therapy. *AIDS* 2000;**14**(17):2723–2730.

54. Lonergan, J. T., Behling, C., Pfander, H., Hassanein, T. I., Mathews, W. C. Hyperlactatemia and hepatic abnormalities in 10 human immunodeficiency virus-infected patients receiving nucleoside analogue combination regimens. *Clin. Infect. Dis.* 2000;**31**(1):162–166.

55. Scalfaro, P., Chesaux, J. J., Buchwalder, P. A., Biollaz, J., Micheli, J. L. Severe transient neonatal lactic acidosis during prophylactic zidovudine treatment. *Intens. Care Med.* 1998;**24**(3):247–250.

56. Miller, K. D., Cameron, M., Wood, L. V., Dalakas, M. C., Kovacs, J. A. Lactic acidosis and hepatic steatosis associated with use of stavudine: report of four cases. *Ann. Intern. Med.* 2000;**133**(3):192–196.

57. Church, J. A., Mitchell, W. G., Gonzalez-Gomez, I. *et al.* Mitochondrial DNA depletion, near-fatal metabolic acidosis, and liver failure in an HIV-infected child treated with combination antiretroviral therapy. *J. Pediatr.* 2001;**138**(5):748–751.

58. Blanche, S., Tardieu, M., Rustin, P. *et al.* Persistent mitochondrial dysfunction and perinatal exposure to antiretroviral nucleoside analogues. *Lancet* 1999;**354**(9184):1084–1089.

59. Mandelbrot, L., Landreau-Mascaro, A., Rekacewicz, C. *et al.* Lamivudine-zidovudine combination for prevention of maternal–infant transmission of HIV-1. *J. Am. Mid. Assoc.* 2001;**285**(16):2083–2093.

60. The Perinatal Safety Review Working Group. Nucleoside exposure in the children of HIV-infected women receiving antiretroviral drugs: abscence of clear evidence for mitochondrial disease in children who died before 5 years of age in five United States cohorts. *J. Acquir. Immune Defic. Syndr.* 2000;**25**:261–268.

14 HIV drug resistance

Frank Maldarelli, M.D., Ph.D.

HIV-1 Drug Resistance Program, National Cancer Institute, National Institutes of Health, Bethesda, MD

Introduction

One of the most challenging limitations of antiretroviral therapy is the emergence of drug resistant mutants of HIV, which occurs in 30%–40% of treated patients. For the individual, drug resistance renders antiretroviral therapy much less effective, resulting in the return of HIV viremia and disease progression. Resistant variants are transmitted when new HIV infections occur, and spread of resistant HIV to newly infected individuals is a growing public health concern. The benefits of HIV resistance testing have been reported in several clinical trials; resistance testing is recommended in certain clinical situations in adult populations. Many questions remain however, and methods to study and analyze HIV drug resistance continue to evolve. Several excellent reviews on HIV drug resistance testing have recently been published [1–8].

Collections of drug resistance mutations are often depicted in tables (see Tables 14.1 and 14.2); such tables, although useful, do not depict degrees of resistance or complexities of interactions among mutations. Online compendia of mutations, frequently updated (e.g., hivdb.stanford.edu, hiv-web.lanl.gov (a sequence compendium of utility for researchers), www.hivresistanceweb.com, www.iasusa.org/resistance_mutations/index.html) provide additional information concerning antiretroviral resistance mutations.

Mechanisms of drug resistance

Studies of HIV replication suggest that HIV populations in vivo are characterized by high genetic diversity; as a result it is likely that some HIV drug resistance mutations are present even prior to the initiation of antiviral therapy. Initiation of antiretrovirals serves to suppress sensitive HIV and permit growth of resistant virus. The lack of complete inhibition of HIV expression even under maximal currently accepted antiviral regimens allows additional evolution of drug resistance to take place during therapy.

Handbook of Pediatric HIV Care, ed. Steven L. Zeichner and Jennifer S. Read.
Published by Cambridge University Press. © Cambridge University Press 2006.

Table 14.1. The figure lists the principal amino acids conferring resistance to the HIV reverse transcriptase inhibitors, and shows the mutations that are included in the nucleoside analogue (NAMS) group of mutations, and the 69 insertion and Q151M multiple resistance complexes. Mutations that confer high-level resistance are indicated by black boxes. "Secondary" mutations are shown in gray. They do not confer significant resistance themselves, but further decrease sensitivity to the drugs when primary mutations are present. See text for details.

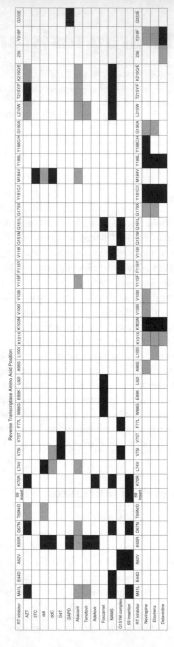

Table 14.2. The figure lists the principal amino acids conferring resistance to the HIV protease inhibitors. Mutations that confer high level resistance (decreased sensitivity to the drug by three- to five-fold or more) are indicated by black boxes. "Secondary" mutations are shown in gray. They do not confer significant resistance themselves, but further decrease sensitivity to the drugs when primary mutations are present. See text for details.

Protease Amino Acid Position

Protease Flap domain (spanning M46I – L63P*)

Inhibitor	L10F/I/V	K20M/R*	L24I	D30N	V32I	L33F/V*	M36I	R41T	M46I	I47V	G48V	I50V	I50L	F53L	I54V/T/M/L	L63P*	A71V/T	G73S	V77I*	V82A	V82S/F/T	I84V	N88D	N88S	L90M	T91S
Indinavir																										
Ritonavir																										
Saquinavir																										
Nelfinavir																										
Amprenavir																										
Atazanavir																										
Lopinavir																										

Nucleoside and nucleotide reverse transcriptase inhibitors

Reverse transcriptase (RT) is the target of many antiretrovirals. RT is a viral enzyme that catalyzes "reverse transcription," the synthesis of a full length DNA copy of the viral genome (provirus) from virion-encapsidated mRNA (Fig. 14.1). It is structurally similar to a variety of DNA polymerases and contains "palm," "fingers," and "thumb" domains (Fig. 14.2). To produce the provirus, RT must carry out a series of reactions, including the synthesis of a DNA copy of the viral genomic RNA (RNA-dependent DNA polymerization), RNase H activity (the degradation of the RNA in an molecule composed of RNA and DNA), and the synthesis of the complementary DNA strand to produce the double-stranded DNA provirus (DNA-dependent DNA polymerization). HIV RT can catalyze the removal of an incorporated nucleotide in an excision mechanism. NRTIs act as chain terminators of reverse transcription, as they are incorporated into growing DNA strands, but prevent additional incorporation of nucleosides. The collection of mutations conferring resistance to NRTIs has been confusing and the mechanisms of resistance have remained difficult to characterize; for NRTIs, two general mechanisms conferring drug resistance are evident, mechanisms that enhance excision, and steric hindrance mechanisms. HIV RT can catalyze the removal of an incorporated nucleotide in an excision mechanism. Mutations that enhance this function cause resistance by enabling the RT to remove the otherwise lethal chain terminating nucleotide analogues more efficiently. Resistance mutations that act through steric mechanisms block the drugs from binding to RT. For NNRTIs, mutations inhibit binding of drug to the enzyme. The convention for denoting resistance mutations uses the single letter amino acid code that occurs in the wild-type enzyme followed by the amino acid position of the mutation, followed by the single letter amino acid code for the mutant, e.g., M184V refers to a methionine (M) in the wild type that is changed to valine (V) in the mutant at amino acid position 184 of reverse transcriptase. If alternative amino acids are present, a forward slash is utilized: T215Y/F indicates either a tyrosine or phenylalanine resistance mutation occurs at position 215. Key resistance mechanisms and some associated mutations follow.

NRTI resistance due to excision mechanisms
Nucleoside associated mutations (NAMs)
Therapy with a number of NRTIs resulted in emergence of a suite of mutations in RT, conferring a variable degree of resistance to the NRTIs. These RT nucleoside-associated mutations (TAMs), sometimes called "thymidine analogue mutations" (or TAMS) because they were initially noted to confer resistance to the thymidine analogue RTIs, such as zidovudine, include M41L, D67N, K70R, L210W, T215Y/F, and K219Q/E. The mechanism through which NAMs confer resistance has been unclear, as these mutants do not appear to inhibit NRTI-triphosphate incorporation, as would be expected for a mutation that altered the ability of the NRTIs to interact with RT and be incorporated into the growing cDNA. Instead, several groups demonstrated

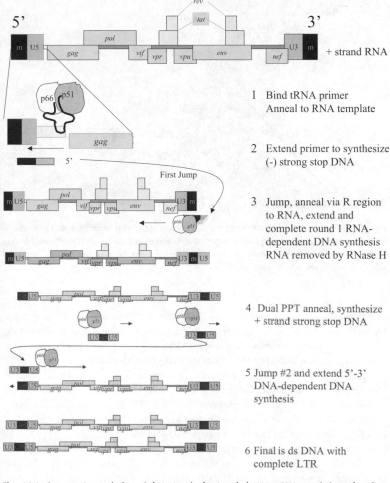

5' **3'**

1. Bind tRNA primer
   Anneal to RNA template

2. Extend primer to synthesize (−) strong stop DNA

   First Jump

3. Jump, anneal via R region to RNA, extend and complete round 1 RNA-dependent DNA synthesis RNA removed by RNase H

4. Dual PPT anneal, synthesize + strand strong stop DNA

5. Jump #2 and extend 5'-3' DNA-dependent DNA synthesis

6. Final is ds DNA with complete LTR

Fig. 14.1. Reverse transcription. Substrate single-stranded HIV mRNA consisting of coding sequences and distinct end structures (unique 5′ (U5) regions, unique 3′ regions (U3), and common repeat (R) sequences) is converted into double-stranded proviral DNA with identical long terminal repeat (U3-R-U5) structures at 5′ and 3′ ends.

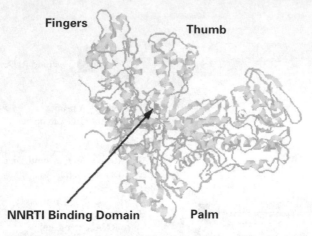

Fingers · **Thumb**

NNRTI Binding Domain · **Palm**

Fig. 14.2. HIV reverse transcriptase X-ray crystal structure of HIV RT heterodimer with p66 subunit and p51 subunit demonstrating typical fingers, palm, and thumb domains; crystallographic data of Ding and coworkers was displayed using RASMOL and the NCBI Entrez suite of structural information at www.ncbi.nlm.nih.gov.

that RT containing TAMs could remove zidovudine (ZDV) incorporated into cDNA at higher than wild-type levels via an excision mechanism. Excision is an energy-requiring reaction, with either pyrophosphate alone or ATP representing the energy donor. Intracellularly, it is likely that ATP functions as the pyrophosphate donor. The putative ATP binding domain within RT is in close proximity to amino acids 67, 70, 210, 215 and 219. One suggestion is that TAMS facilitate binding of ATP, which results in more effective excision of NRTIs. The mutant RT can thus excise the NRTI from the cDNA at increased levels, so that the NRTI no longer terminates the growing cDNA chain and synthesis of the cDNA can continue, producing a functional provirus.

A group of mutations conferring high level resistance to the NRTIs, the 69/70 insertion mutations (or 69/70 ins), consists of an insertion of a variable number of amino acids between amino acids 69 and 70 and is associated with a series of additional mutations (M41L, A62V, D67N, and K70R) [9, 10]. The insertion mutants also appear to act through excision mechanisms [11–13] and result in high level resistance to all NRTIs. The presence of these mutations in a patient's virus severely limits the clinical utility of the NRTI.

NRTI resistance due to steric and positional effects

While the NAMs and the 69/70 insertion mutations act by enhancing the ability of RT to excise NRTIs incorporated into cDNA, other NRTI mutations act by blocking access of the NRTI-triphosphates to RT. A number of HIV drug resistance mutations are localized near the active site of RT and these mutations may enable RT to exclude the triphosphosphorylated drug, while permitting incorporation of the natural deoxynucleotide triphosphates (dNTPs). Mutations may act directly by altering the shape of RT's active site or the region surrounding the active site, or by changing the orientation of the incoming nucleotide with respect to the template. M184V confers strong resistance to lamivudine (3TC) and zalcitabine (ddC) and is observed within weeks after 3TC monotherapy. A combination of crystallographic and enzymatic studies have suggested that replacement of methionine with isoleucine at position 184 prevents 3TC and ddC from gaining access to the enzyme active site [14, 15]; a second 184 mutant, M184V, appears to act in similar fashion [15]. M184I emerges after 3TC therapy, often before M184V becomes apparent, but is quickly replaced by M184V. It has been suggested that both mutants exist prior to the initiation of therapy, within the large numbers of viruses present within a patient (see Chapter 1) to 3TC therapy and that these mutants are then rapidly selected for once therapy begins. M184I is actually more prevalent than M184V among the viral population prior to the start of treatment, but M184V confers greater resistance to 3TC, becoming the dominant mutant with prolonged therapy [16].

A group of mutations characterized by the presence of Q151M and including A62V, V75I, F77L, and F116Y emerged in early studies of alternating ZDV/ddI monotherapy. Q151 lies in the part of RT near the incoming nucleotide, and steric interference of incoming dideoxy NRTIs has been suggested as the mechanism by which this suite of mutations results in high level resistance to all NRTIs [17, 18]. Fortunately, the Q151M complex comprises a relatively small proportion of resistant viruses [19].

Non-nucleoside reverse transcriptase inhibitors

The non-nucleoside reverse transcriptase inhibitors (NNRTIs) are a group of chemically diverse compounds that inhibit cDNA synthesis but, unlike the NRTIs, do not directly compete with the native dNTPs. Incubation of an NNRTI with RT results in spatial rearrangement of a series of RT residues into a hydrophobic domain or "pocket" that binds NNRTI molecules within the palm at the base of the thumb domain (Fig. 14.2). Once bound, the NNRTIs block RT activity by disrupting the molecular configuration of the active site, preventing polymerization. Mutations in RT that change the spatial characteristics of NNRTI binding region, or entry to the pocket to which the NNRTIs bind, result in drug resistance. Such mutations cluster in specific domains within the reverse transcriptase (amino acids 100–110, 180–190, 225–235) corresponding to the boundaries of the pocket that forms upon incubation with NNRTIs. Even though the NNRTIs have different chemical structures, they all bind to the same site in RT, so mutations that confer resistance to one NNRTI also confer resistance to the others. One potent mutation conferring cross-resistance to NNRTIs is the lysine to arginine

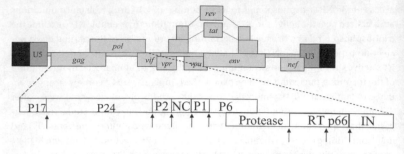

Fig. 14.3. HIV genomic organization with *gag/pol* detail. Arrows indicate sites of cleavage by HIV protease.

mutation at position 103 (K103N), a mutation which prevents effective drug binding [20]; other mutations conferring cross resistance to NNRTIs include mutations at position 181 (Y1811C/I and 188 (Y188L/C/H). Additional mutations and polymorphisms that may play a role in HIV drug resistance continue to be identified.

Protease inhibitors

The HIV protease is a 99-amino acid aspartyl protease that carries out proteolytic processing of the HIV gag and gag/pol polyprotein precursor, an essential maturational step in the HIV life cycle [21] (Fig. 14.3, and Chapter 1); protease is part of the Gag/Pol polyprotein, and so the initial processing events take place while protease is still part of the precursor. In the absence of protease activity, when the enzyme is inhibited by the PIs, the polyprotein precursors are not processed and the virion does not assume its mature, infectious form.

Protease is active as a homodimer and has two-fold symmetry (Fig. 14.4); lack of protease activity may result in non-infectious virions or severely impair or abolish virus morphogenesis [22, 23]. Analyses of crystallographic data have identified critical structural regions of protease in addition to the active site itself, including an adjacent "flap" domain [24, 25], and the monomer–monomer interface [26]. Inhibitors of HIV-1 protease are small peptide-like drugs that occupy the protease active site and inhibit enzymatic activity.

Mutation patterns for protease inhibitors are often complex. Certain "primary" mutations confer a modest degree of drug resistance to individual protease inhibitors decreasing sensitivity to the drugs by about three- to fivefold. Certain mutations are specific for individual proteases, notably D30N, which confers resistance to nelfinavir. Other primary mutations exhibit cross-resistance such as V82A (reduces sensitivity to both indinavir and ritonavir) or L90M (reduced sensitivity to saquinavir and nelfinavir). Additional, "secondary" mutations do not confer significant resistance themselves, but

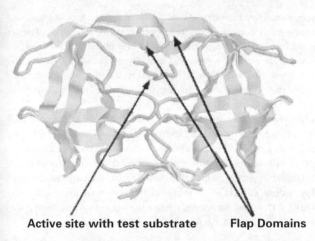

Active site with test substrate   **Flap Domains**

Fig. 14.4. HIV protease. Crystallographic data of protease homodimer with monomers in red and blue. Active site location of Asp25 and position of flap domains are indicated. Data [25] were rendered as described in Fig. 14.2.

further decrease sensitivity to the drugs when primary mutations are present. Primary mutations are relatively specific for individual protease inhibitors, but secondary mutations may confer resistance to many protease inhibitors. Thus, the effectiveness of a second PI-containing regimen after the failure of an initial PI-containing regimen may be compromised to some degree if secondary mutations are present. HIV that is significantly resistant to one PI is often broadly cross-resistant to others [27–29].

In addition to resistance mutations occurring within the protease gene proper, additional mutations at protease cleavage sites within Gag and Gag/Pol polyproteins can confer resistance to the PIs. These mutations presumably increase the susceptibility of the polyprotein to cleavage by protease, so that inhibition of the enzyme by the PIs is less effective [30–33]. Comparatively little data are available regarding the relative contributions of cleavage site mutations to the development of clinical resistance.

Fusion inhibitors

HIV fusion inhibitors are new antiretrovirals that block fusion of the lipid envelopes of HIV and the host cell membranes. Fusion is mediated by the gp41 glycoprotein of HIV, and fusion inhibitors can inhibit HIV replication [34]. The recently FDA-approved enfuvirtide (T-20, Fuzeon) and T-1249 are peptides that include a short part of the gp41 amino acid sequence. They bind to gp41 and prevent it from forming the "six helix" bundle required to bring the virion envelope together with the host cell plasma membrane to promote fusion. Following exposure to fusion inhibitor monotherapy, resistant viruses may emerge within 2 weeks, and mutations in at least three amino acids have been associated with resistance [35]. Commercial genotyping assays are under development for this region of *env* to detect the presence of mutations that confer resistance to this class of drugs.

Some mutations that confer resistance to one antiretroviral drug can increase the sensitivity of the virus to another drug. Perhaps the best example of this phenomenon is the M184V mutation that confers high level resistance to 3TC. When this mutation is present together with TAMS, the virus shows increased susceptibility to ZDV, D4T, and perhaps tenofovir. In patients with complicated resistance patterns and few antiretroviral therapy options, clinicians sometimes elect to continue treatment with 3TC, together with ZDV, D4T, or tenofovir, even when a patient's virus has the M184V mutation, hoping to maintain the higher sensitivity to the other NRTIs.

HIV drug resistance assays

A variety of HIV drug resistance assays are available for clinical use, but are generally divided into assays that determine either genotypic or phenotypic resistance. All commercial resistance assays use plasma as starting material.

Genotyping assays

Genotyping assays determine the nucleic acid sequence of portions of the HIV genome relevant to drug resistance. The most straightforward method involves direct nucleic acid sequencing, and comparing the sequence to standard wild-type HIV to identify changes corresponding to drug resistance. Genotypic assays typically determine the sequence of DNA ("cDNA") that is produced from plasma viral genomic RNA following in vitro reverse transcription and PCR amplification, followed by highly automated DNA sequencing. As described above, HIV populations are genetically highly diverse and there is no single sequence for all viruses; the results of genotyping assays represent, in general, the most common sequence and only variants composing 20%–25% or more of the population or more will be represented in the final analysis. This has significant clinical implications because minority, resistant viral species may exist within a patient and these resistant species may not be detected through viral genotypic assays. This is particularly true for highly experienced patients who are no longer receiving certain antiretrovirals. These patients may harbor minority resistant "archived" viral species that are not detected by viral genotyping, but which can re-emerge when treatment with certain drugs is resumed.

Assays commercially are available, either as a service (Virco/Johnson and Johnson; Virologic) or as kits (TruGene, Visible Genetics) and have a number of similarities. The viral load necessary to detect mutations is a function of the ability to synthesize cDNA;

1000 copies HIV RNA/ml are generally required. Samples with between 1000 and 5000 copies/ml are occasionally difficult to amplify and amplification sometimes succeeds with lower viral loads. The TrueGene kit produced by Visible Genetics has been used with pediatric samples [36]; genotypic results were obtained from samples with viral loads <1000 and with small volumes (<0.5 ml) and genotypes were obtained on 98% of samples. Turnaround time for services is of the order of 1–2 weeks.

Phenotyping

Assessing resistance from a series of complex mutational patterns is often difficult, and phenotyping provides a functional evaluation of drug susceptibility using an in vitro assay of HIV replication. Two assays are commercially available [37, 38] (Fig. 14.5). HIV protease and RT sequences are amplified from patient material via reverse transcription and PCR. The PCR product is introduced into a recombinant molecular clone of HIV [39]. The recombinant HIV is transfected into cells capable of producing HIV virions. The virions contain the RT or protease gene from the patient and are subsequently used to inoculate cultures of susceptible cells (Fig. 14.5(b)). Parallel cultures are inoculated with wild-type HIV; infections are carried out in the presence of increasing concentrations of antiviral agents, and the growth of the virus in the different drug concentrations permits an estimate of the degree of resistance of the patient's virus. The relationship between drug concentration and virus inhibition is not a simple linear dose response curve (see Fig. 14.5C). Results are typically reported as the concentration of drug that inhibits virus replication by 50% (IC50). Comparison of this value to the IC50 obtained for a standard laboratory strain shows by what fold a patient's virus is resistant to a particular drug compared to a wild-type virus.

Increases in IC50 are associated with drug resistance, but the degree of virologic resistance associated with clinical drug failure is not clear in all circumstances. Establishment of effective cutoffs has been a major effort in development of these assays. For some antiretrovirals, such as efavirenz or 3TC, where single amino acid changes produce high level resistance, large increases in IC50 are noted. In these examples, 50–1000-fold changes may occur, and identifying resistance is straightforward. For some newer agents, such as abacavir [40], or lopinavir/ritonavir [41], phenotypic sensitivity has been prospectively studied in clinical trials, and useful estimates of clinical sensitivity were obtained. In contrast, drugs such as ddI or D4T have a more restricted dynamic range in phenotyping assays. As a result, cutoffs for D4T or ddI resistance are relatively difficult to assign. One approach has been to evaluate the distribution of drug resistance in isolates from drug-naïve individuals and to assign cutoffs at IC50 levels several standard deviations beyond the mean drug naïve level [42].

The two commercial phenotyping assays have been compared directly, with remarkably concordant results [43]. Improvements in interpretation algorithms and additions to the databases will undoubtedly continue to improve overall interpretation and consistency.

A. Virus Preparation

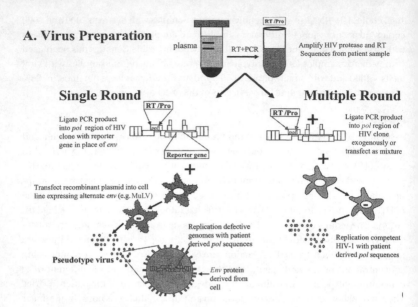

plasma → RT+PCR → RT /Pro — Amplify HIV protease and RT Sequences from patient sample

Single Round

Ligate PCR product into *pol* region of HIV clone with reporter gene in place of *env*

Reporter gene

+

Transfect recombinant plasmid into cell line expressing alternate *env* (e.g. MuLV)

Pseudotype virus

Replication defective genomes with patient derived *pol* sequences

Env protein derived from cell

Multiple Round

Ligate PCR product into *pol* region of HIV clone exogenously or transfect as mixture

+

Replication competent HIV-1 with patient derived *pol* sequences

B. Virus Inoculation

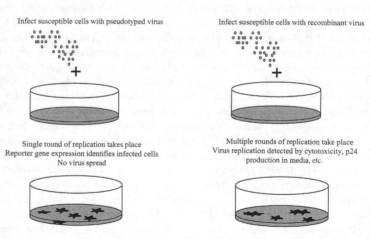

Infect susceptible cells with pseudotyped virus

Infect susceptible cells with recombinant virus

Single round of replication takes place
Reporter gene expression identifies infected cells
No virus spread

Multiple rounds of replication take place
Virus replication detected by cytotoxicity, p24 production in media, etc.

Fig. 14.5. Comparison of HIV single round and multiple round phenotyping assays.

C. Quantitating resistance

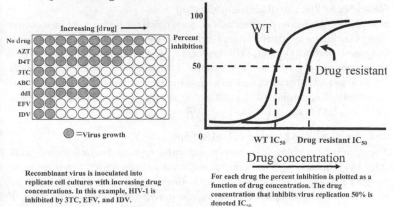

Recombinant virus is inoculated into replicate cell cultures with increasing drug concentrations. In this example, HIV-1 is inhibited by 3TC, EFV, and IDV.

For each drug the percent inhibition is plotted as a function of drug concentration. The drug concentration that inhibits virus replication 50% is denoted IC_{50}.

Fig. 14.5. (*cont.*)

Evidence base for the use of drug resistance assays in clinical management of HIV infection

Several randomized, prospective studies (GART, VIRADAPT, ARGENTA, VIRA3001) have investigated the utility of resistance testing in management of antiretroviral therapy. The specific benefit of additional "expert" advice was not evaluated in these trials but was specifically investigated in HAVANA [44], where genotyping was found to be superior to no genotyping, even in the absence of expert advice, using only an algorithm to interpret the genotype. Expert advice was beneficial even in the absence of genotyping. The durations of these studies were relatively short, 12–24 wks, and the durability of the benefit due to resistance testing beyond one year has not been studied. Many of the studies were performed prior to the widespread use of ultra-sensitive assays capable of detecting viral loads down to 50 copies/ml limit assays and instead used suppression of viral load to below 400 copies/ml or 500 copies/ml as the measure of success; it is not clear whether all successful treatments reached the more stringent measure of suppression. Several trials have not demonstrated benefit of resistance testing [45, 46], but some patients in these studies may have had such extensive prior experience with antiretroviral therapy and had virus that was so resistant that few would be expected to have an excellent response to a new therapy.

A meta-analysis of several genotyping studies [47] concluded that genotyping can be beneficial, at least over the course of a few months. None of these studies specifically studied pediatric patients. A randomized trial of resistance testing in pediatric populations (PERA, PENTA-8) has been initiated in Europe (www.ctu.mrc.ac.uk/penta/pera.htm).

Use of resistance testing in clinical practice

Guidelines for the use of resistance testing

Several sets of guidelines recommend the use of resistance testing in defined circumstances, including the DHHS/Kaiser Guidelines (www.aidsinfo.nih.gov) and the IAS and Euro Guidelines Group for HIV Resistance [48, 49]. Resistance testing has been recommended in first regimen and multiple regimen failures. Resistance testing for newly diagnosed patients infected in geographic areas with high resistance has been recommended or considered; specific testing of pregnant women has been recommended by IAS but not by DHHS.

Resistance testing – practical considerations

Practitioners contemplating the use of resistance testing must choose among the available assays. Genotyping represents the less expensive alternative, but phenotyping may be particularly useful when a patient is infected with a virus that has a complex genotype, and genotyping and phenotying may provide complementary information. Resistance testing represents just one aspect of the clinical evaluation of HIV-infected patients, and testing is useless without an accurate and comprehensive history and physical examination. Graphs detailing drug history and adherence, viral load, and CD4+ lymphocyte counts over time are extremely useful in understanding the results of any drug resistance testing. Several points regarding interpretation of resistance testing in clinical settings bear enumerating.

- Genotyping results report the presence of drug resistance mutations, sensitivity is inferred but not guaranteed.
- Phenotyping results may indicate sensitivity, but cutoffs have not been clinically determined for all antiretrovirals. Increases in IC50 values of 1.8-fold or more have been associated with resistance.
- Phenotyping cutoffs for certain drugs have been adjusted (ddI, D4T) since the assays were introduced; results of phenotypic assays prior to adjustment may suggest drug sensitivity when resistance is present.
- A patient's virus may continue to evolve, particularly when treatment continues with high viral loads. Resistance results obtained at one time may not reflect the viral genotype or phenotype at subsequent times. Results are time sensitive, and relate to the current regimen, but there is no specific "expiration date" for individual drugs or for the assay as a whole.
- Additional mutations may be present but not evident because the patient is not currently taking a particular drug at the time the test was performed.
- The presence of mutations conferring resistance to NNRTIs generally precludes their use in any future regimen. High level resistance resulting from K103N suggests little utilty of continuing NNRTI therapy.
- The presence of Q151M complex or 69 insertion mutants results in high level cross-resistance to NRTIs. Construction of salvage regimens should be adjusted accordingly, anticipating little or no antiviral contribution from NRTIs.

- The presence of M184V confers high level resistance to lamivudine, but increases activity of AZT, D4T, and perhaps tenofovir in the presence of NAMs. Continued therapy with lamivudine maintains M184V and may help preserve some degree of activity in complex resistance profiles including NAMs. Lamivudine has a favorable toxicity and drug interaction profile; including this agent in salvage regimens carries little negative consequence and may provide a degree of indirect antiviral activity.

Results of HIV drug resistance tests represent one aspect of the evaluation of the patient with drug-resistant HIV. The successful construction of salvage regimens cannot be dictated simply by genotypes or phenotypes, but must include consideration of prior therapy, patient tolerability, etc. In a final analysis, the best drug regimens are those constructed in cooperation with the patient and the health care team.

REFERENCES

1. Van Houtte, M., Update on resistance testing. *J. HIV Ther.*, 2001;**6**(3):61–64.
2. Geretti, A. M., Easterbrook, P. Antiretroviral resistance in clinical practice. *Int. J. STD AIDS*, 2001;**12**(3):145–153.
3. Hanna, G. Aquila, R. T. Clinical use of genotypic and phenotypic drug resistance testing to monitor antiretroviral chemotherapy. *Clin. Infect. Dis.*, 2001; **32**(5): 774–782.
4. Rice, H. L., Zolopa, A. R. HIV drug resistance testing: an update for the clinician. *AIDS Clin. Care*, 2001;**13**(10): 89–91, 94–96, 100.
5. Schmidt, B., Walter, H., Zeitler, N., Karn, K. Genotypic drug resistance interpretation systems – the cutting edge of antiretroviral therapy. *AIDS Rev*, 2002; **4**(3): 148–156.
6. Shafer, R. W. Genotypic testing for human immunodeficiency virus type 1 drug resistance. *Clin. Microbiol. Rev.*, 2002; **15**(2):247–277.
7. Haubrich, R., Demeter, L. International perspectives on antiretroviral resistance. Clinical utility of resistance testing: retrospective and prospective data supporting use and current recommendations. *J. Acquir. Immune Defic. Syndr.*, 2001;**26** Suppl1: S51–S59.
8. Lerma, J. G., Heneine, W. Resistance of human immunodeficiency virus type 1 to reverse transcriptase and protease inhibitors: genotypic and phenotypic testing. *J. Clin. Virol.*, 2001;**21**(3):197–212.
9. Larder, B. A., Bloor, S., Kemp, S. D. *et al.* A family of insertion mutations between codons 67 and 70 of human immunodeficiency virus type 1 reverse transcriptase confer multinucleoside analog resistance. *Antimicrob. Agents Chemother.*, 1999;**43**(8):1961–1967.
10. Lobato, R. L., Kim, E. Y., Kagan, R. M., Merigan, T. C., Genotypic and phenotypic analysis of a novel 15-base insertion occurring between codons 69 and 70 of HIV type 1 reverse transcriptase. *AIDS Res. Hum. Retroviruses*, 2002; **18**(10):733–736.
11. Lennerstrand, J., Stammers, D. K., Larder, B. A. Biochemical mechanism of human immunodeficiency virus type 1 reverse transcriptase resistance to stavudine. *Antimicrob. Agents Chemother.*, 2001; **45**(7):2144–2146.
12. Mas, A., Parera, M., Briones, C. *et al.* Role of a dipeptide insertion between codons 69 and 70 of HIV-1 reverse transcriptase in the mechanism of ZDV resistance. *Embo. J*, 2000; **19**(21):5752–5761.

13. Boyer, P. L., Sarafianos, S. G., Arnold, E., Hughes, S. H. Nucleoside analog resistance caused by insertions in the fingers of human immunodeficiency virus type 1 reverse transcriptase involves ATP-mediated excision. *J. Virol.*, 2002; **76**(18):9143–9151.

14. Gao, H. Q., Boyer, P. L., Sarafianos, S. G., Arnold, E., Hughes, S. H. The role of steric hindrance in 3TC resistance of human immunodeficiency virus type-1 reverse transcriptase. *J. Mol. Biol.*, 2000; **300**(2):403–418.

15. Sarafianos, S. G., Das, K., Clark, A. D., Jr. *et al.* Lamivudine (3TC) resistance in HIV-1 reverse transcriptase involves steric hindrance with beta-branched amino acids. *Proc. Natl Acad. Sci. USA*, 1999; **96**(18):10027–10032.

16. Frost, S. D., Nijhuis, M., Schuurman, R., Boucher, C. A., Brown, A. J. Evolution of lamivudine resistance in human immunodeficiency virus type 1-infected individuals: the relative roles of drift and selection. *J. Virol.*, 2000; **74**(14):6262–6268.

17. Ray, A. S., Basavapathruni, A., Anderson, K. S. Mechanistic studies to understand the progressive development of resistance in human immunodeficiency virus type 1 reverse transcriptase to abacavir. *J. Biol. Chem.*, 2002; **277**(43):40479–40490.

18. Huang, H., Chopra, R., Verdine, G. L., Harrison, S. C. Structure of a covalently trapped catalytic complex of HIV-1 reverse transcriptase: implications for drug resistance. *Science*, 1998; **282**(5394):1669–1675.

19. Schmit, J. C., Ruiz, L., Stuyver, L. *et al.* Comparison of the LiPA HIV-1 RT test, selective PCR and direct solid phase sequencing for the detection of HIV-1 drug resistance mutations. *J. Virol. Methods*, 1998; **73**(1):77–82.

20. Hsiou, Y., Ding, J., Das, K. *et al.* The Lys103Asn mutation of HIV-1 RT: a novel mechanism of drug resistance. *J. Mol. Biol.*, 2001; **309**(2):437–445.

21. Swanstrom, R., Erona, J. Human immunodeficiency virus type-1 protease inhibitors: therapeutic successes and failures, suppression and resistance. *Pharmacol Ther.*, 2000; **86**(2):145–170.

22. Kaplan, A. H., Zack, J. A., Krigge M. *et al.* Partial inhibition of the human immunodeficiency virus type 1 protease results in aberrant virus assembly and the formation of noninfectious particles. *J. Virol.*, 1993; **67**(7):4050–4055.

23. Rose, R. E., Gong, Y. F., Greytok, J. A. *et al.* Human immunodeficiency virus type 1 viral background plays a major role in development of resistance to protease inhibitors. *Proc. Natl Acad. Sci. USA*, 1996; **93**(4):1648–1653.

24. Scott, W. R., Schiffer, C. A. Curling of flap tips in HIV-1 protease as a mechanism for substrate entry and tolerance of drug resistance. *Structure Fold Des.* 2000; **8**(12):1259–1265.

25. Prabu-Jeyabalan, M., Nalivaika, E., Schiffer, C. A. Substrate shape determines specificity of recognition for HIV-1 protease: analysis of crystal structures of six substrate complexes. *Structure* (Camb), 2002; **10**(3):369–381.

26. Pettit, S. C., Gulnik, S., Everitt, L., Kaplan, A. H. The dimer interfaces of protease and extra-protease domains influence the activation of protease and the specificity of GagPol cleavage. *J. Virol.* 2003; **77**(1):366–374.

27. Hertogs, K., Bloor, S., Kemp, S. D. *et al.* Phenotypic and genotypic analysis of clinical HIV-1 isolates reveals extensive protease inhibitor cross-resistance: a survey of over 6000 samples. *AIDS*, 2000; **14**(9):1203–1210.

28. Shafer, R. W., Winters, M. A., Palmer, S., Merigan, T. C. Multiple concurrent reverse transcriptase and protease mutations and multidrug resistance of HIV-1 isolates from heavily treated patients. *Ann. Intern. Med.*, 1998; **128**(11):906–911.

29. Harrigan, P. R., Larder, B. A. Extent of cross-resistance between agents used to treat human immunodeficiency virus type 1 infection in clinically derived isolates. *Antimicrob. Agents Chemother.*, 2002; **46**(3):909–912.

30. Robinson, L. H., Myers, R. E., Snowden, B. W., Tisdale, M., Blair, E. D. HIV type 1 protease cleavage site mutations and viral fitness: implications for drug susceptibility phenotyping assays. *AIDS Res. Hum. Retroviruses*, 2000; **16**(12):1149–1156.

31. Doyon, L., Croteau, G., Thibeault, D., Poulin, E., Pilote, L., Lamarre, D. Second locus involved in human immunodeficiency virus type 1 resistance to protease inhibitors. *J. Virol.*, 1996; **70**(6):3763–3769.

32. Croteau, G., Doyon, L., Thibeault, D., McKercher, G., Pilote, L., Lamarre, D. Impaired fitness of human immunodeficiency virus type 1 variants with high-level resistance to protease inhibitors. *J. Virol.*, 1997; **71**(2):1089–1096.

33. Zhang, Y. M., Imamichi, H., Imamichi, T. *et al.* Drug resistance during indinavir therapy is caused by mutations in the protease gene and in its Gag substrate cleavage sites. *J. Virol.*, 1997; **71**(9):6662–6670.

34. Kilby, J. M., Hopkins, S., Venetta, T. M. *et al.* Potent suppression of HIV-1 replication in humans by T-20, a peptide inhibitor of gp41-mediated virus entry. *Nat. Med.* 1998; **4**(11):1302–1307.

35. Wei, X., Decker, J. M., Liu, H. *et al.* Emergence of resistant human immunodeficiency virus type 1 in patients receiving fusion inhibitor (T-20) monotherapy. *Antimicrob. Agents Chemother.*, 2002; **46**(6):1896–1905.

36. Cunningham, S., Ank, B., Lewis, D. *et al.* Performance of the applied biosystems ViroSeq human immunodeficiency virus type 1 (HIV-1) genotyping system for sequence-based analysis of HIV-1 in pediatric plasma samples. *J. Clin. Microbiol.*, 2001; **39**(4):1254–1257.

37. Hertogs, K., de Bethune, M. P., Miller, V. *et al.* A rapid method for simultaneous detection of phenotypic resistance to inhibitors of protease and reverse transcriptase in recombinant human immunodeficiency virus type 1 isolates from patients treated with antiretroviral drugs. *Antimicrob. Agents Chemother.*, 1998; **42**(2):269–276.

38. Petropoulos, C. J., Parkin, N. T., Limoli, K. L. *et al.* A novel phenotypic drug susceptibility assay for human immunodeficiency virus type 1. *Antimicrob. Agents Chemother.*, 2000; **44**(4):920–928.

39. Kellam, P., Larder, B. A. Recombinant virus assay: a rapid, phenotypic assay for assessment of drug susceptibility of human immunodeficiency virus type 1 isolates. *Antimicrob. Agents Chemother.*, 1994; **38**(1):23–30.

40. Falloon, J., Ait-Khaled, M., Thomas, D. A. *et al.* HIV-1 genotype and phenotype correlate with virological response to abacavir, amprenavir and efavirenz in treatment-experienced patients. *AIDS*, 2002; **16**(3):387–396.

41. Kempf, D. J., Isaacson, J. D., King, M. S. *et al.* Analysis of the virological response with respect to baseline viral phenotype and genotype in protease inhibitor-experienced HIV-1-infected patients receiving lopinavir/ritonavir therapy. *Antivirals. Ther.*, 2002; **7**(3): 165–174.

42. Harrigan, P. R., Montaner, J. S., Wegner, S. A. *et al.* World-wide variation in HIV-1 phenotypic susceptibility in untreated individuals: biologically relevant values for resistance testing. *AIDS*, 2001; **15**(13):1671–1677.

43. Qari, S. H., Respess, R., Weinstock, H. *et al.* Comparative analysis of two commercial phenotypic assays for drug susceptibility testing of human immunodeficiency virus type 1. *J. Clin. Microbiol.*, 2002; **40**(1):31–35.

44. Tural, C., Ruiz, L., Holtzer, C. *et al.* Clinical utility of HIV-1 genotyping and expert advice: the Havana trial. *AIDS*, 2002; **16**(2):209–218.

45. Meynard, J. L., Vray, M., Morand-Joubert, L. *et al.* Phenotypic or genotypic resistance testing for choosing antiretroviral therapy after treatment failure: a randomized trial. *AIDS*, 2002; **16**(5):727–736.

46. Melnick, J. R., Cameron, M. Snyder, M. *et al.* Impact of phenotypic antiretroviral drug resistance testing on the response to salvage antiretroviral therapy (ART) in heavily experienced patients. *7th Conf. Retroviruses and Opportunistic Infect.*, 2000: Abstract 786.

47. Torre, D., Tambini, R. Antiretroviral drug resistance testing in patients with HIV-1 infection: a meta-analysis study. *HIV Clin. Trials*, 2002; **3**(1):1–8.

48. Vandamme, A. M., Houyez, E., Banhegyi, D. *et al.* Laboratory guidelines for the practical use of HIV drug resistance tests in patient follow-up. *Antiviral Ther.*, 2001; **6**(1):21–39.

49. Hirsch, M. S., Brun-Vezinet, E., D'Aquila, R. T. *et al.* Antiretroviral drug resistance testing in adult HIV-1 infection: recommendations of an International AIDS Society-USA Panel. *J. Am. Med. Assoc.*, 2000; **283**(18):2417–2426.

15 Initiating and changing antiretroviral therapy

Lynne M. Mofenson, M.D. and Leslie K. Serchuck, M.D.

Center for Research for Mothers and Children, National Institute of Child Health & Human Development, National Institutes of Health, Bethesda, MD

Introduction

Guidelines for antiretroviral therapy (ART) in children must incorporate certain unique considerations, including: age-related changes in drug pharmacokinetics; initiation of therapy during primary HIV infection; normal age-related changes in immunologic parameters; pediatric-specific features of the natural history of HIV infection (i.e., virologic parameters during primary infection, rapidity of disease progression, and frequency of central nervous system and growth abnormalities); prior antiretroviral (ARV) exposure of newborns (in utero and neonatal); and pediatric-specific adherence issues (i.e., availability and palatability of drug formulations; relationship of drug administration to food intake in infants; dependence on caregiver for drug administration).

Guidelines for treatment of HIV-infected children often rely on data regarding virologic/immunologic response to drug regimens in adult clinical trials, taking into account the specific considerations in pediatric HIV infection delineated above, and with attention to data from pediatric populations. Guidelines for pediatric ART have been developed in the USA and Europe, and by the World Health Organization. US pediatric ART guidelines [1], as well as adult guidelines (applicable to postpubertal adolescents) [2], are available at http://AIDSInfo.nih.gov. Guidelines for pediatric ART in Europe (http://www.ctu.mrc.ac.uk/PENTA) [3] and in resource-poor settings (http://www.who.int/hiv/pub/prev_care/en/ScalingUp_E.pdf) have been developed. The US pediatric guidelines for ART are the focus of this chapter, and the other guidelines are addressed only briefly. None of these guidelines is intended to supplant the clinical judgment of experienced clinicians. Whenever possible, HIV-infected children should be managed by, or in consultation with, a pediatric HIV specialist.

Handbook of Pediatric HIV Care, ed. Steven L. Zeichner and Jennifer S. Read.
Published by Cambridge University Press. © Cambridge University Press 2006.

Table 15.1. US Public Health Service guidelines for HIV-infected postpubertal adolescents and adults: indications for initiation of antiretroviral therapy

Clinical Category	CD4+ cell count	Plasma HIV RNA	Recommendation
Chronic infection			
Symptomatic	Any value	Any value	Treat
Asymptomatic	CD4+ T-cells <200/mm^3	Any value	Treat
Asymptomatic	CD4+ T-cells >200 but ≤350/mm^3	Any value	Therapy should be offered, with full discussion of risks/benefits with the patient.
Asymptomatic	CD4+ T-cells >350/mm^3	≥100 000 copies/ml	Most clinicians recommend deferring therapy, but some clinicians will treat.
Asymptomatic	CD4+ T-cells >350/mm^3	<100 000 copies/ml	Defer therapy
Acute infection[a]	Any value	Any value	Consider therapy (discuss potential benefits/risks with patient)

Modified from [2].

[a] Acute primary infection or documented seroconversion within the previous 6 months.

When should antiretroviral therapy be started?

Adult Guidelines (applicable to postpubertal adolescents) (Table 15.1)
Chronic infection

Early initiation of highly active antiretroviral therapy (HAART) may help control disease better because: viral replication is easier to block with lower viral loads at the start of therapy; early control of replication may decrease the likelihood of development of ARV drug resistance; and early treatment may preserve immune function. However, delaying treatment may help preserve the maximum number of treatment options and decrease the duration of exposure to ARVs, potentially decreasing the chance that the virus may become resistant or the possibility that the patient may become non-adherent or experience drug-related toxicities.

Current adult guidelines recommend initiation of HAART for symptomatic HIV disease and for those, even if asymptomatic, with CD4+ cell counts <200/mm^3 [2]. For asymptomatic adults with CD4+ cell counts between 200 and 350/mm^3, many experts would offer treatment, although this is still controversial. Some clinicians defer therapy in patients in this category and carefully monitor CD4+ cell counts and plasma HIV RNA levels. For asymptomatic adults with CD4+ cell counts >350/mm^3, aggressive and conservative approaches have been advocated. In the aggressive approach, ART is recommended for those with CD4+ cell counts >350/mm³ if plasma HIV RNA is ≥100 000 copies/ml. In the conservative approach, patients with plasma HIV RNA <100 000 copies/ml are monitored frequently, but not treated.

Acute infection

Therapy for adults with acute HIV infection should be considered, although treatment in such circumstances is based on theoretical considerations, not definitive clinical trial data. During acute infection, viral replication is very high, with widespread viral dissemination. Early treatment of primary infection aims to decrease the number of infected cells, maintain or restore HIV-specific immune responses, preserve immune function, and possibly lower the viral "set point," improving the subsequent course of disease.

Guidelines for infants, children, and prepubertal adolescents (Table 15.2)

Adherence is especially important to consider when initiating therapy in children. It is essential to fully assess and discuss potential adherence problems with the family and to address potential barriers to adherence prior to initiating therapy (see Chapter 7).

HIV-infected infants

Because HIV-infected infants are at particularly high risk for disease progression, and surrogate markers such as CD4+ cell count and plasma HIV RNA levels are less predictive of progression risk in this age group, recommendations for initiation of therapy in infants are more aggressive than those for older children. When ART is administered during infancy, therapy is initiated during primary infection, consistent with adult treatment guidelines concerning acute HIV infection. Early initiation of therapy could theoretically diminish viral dissemination, lead to prolonged virologic suppression, and preserve thymic function, resulting in immune preservation, clinical stability, and normal growth and cognitive development.

ART should be initiated for infants who have HIV-related clinical (CDC Pediatric Clinical Category A, B or C) or immunologic (CDC Pediatric Immune Category 2 or 3) disease, regardless of HIV RNA level. Therapy should be considered for HIV-infected infants who are asymptomatic and have normal immune parameters. Many experts would treat all HIV-infected infants, regardless of clinical, immunologic, or virologic parameters. Other experts would treat all infected infants <6 months old, and would consider clinical and immunologic parameters and assessment of adherence issues for decisions regarding initiation of therapy in infants 6 to 12 months of age.

There are potential problems with early initiation of therapy for infants. Accurate drug pharmacokinetic data may not be available for infants, and it may be difficult for families of infants to assure adherence. Resistance can develop rapidly (particularly

Table 15.2. US Public Health Service guidelines for HIV-infected infants, children and young adolescents: indications for initiation of antiretroviral therapy

Clinical category		CD4+ Cell Percentage	Plasma HIV RNA copy number	Recommendation
Infants				
Symptomatic (Clinical category A, B, or C)	*or*	<25% (Immune category 2 or 3)	Any value[a]	Treat
Asymptomatic (Clinical category N)	*and*	≥25% (Immune category 1)	Any value[a]	Consider Treatment[b]
Children ≥12 months of age				
AIDS (Clinical category C)	*or*	<15% (Immune category 3)	Any value	Treat
Mild–moderate symptoms (Clinical category A or B)	*or*	15–25%[c] (Immune category 2)	≥100 000 copies/ml[d]	Consider treatment
Asymptomatic (Clinical category N)	*and*	>25% (Immune category 1)	<100 000 copies/ml[d]	Many experts would defer therapy and closely monitor clinical, immune and viral parameters

Reference [1].

[a] Plasma HIV RNA levels are higher in HIV-infected infants than older children and adults, and may be difficult to interpret in infants because overall HIV RNA levels are high and there is overlap in RNA levels between infants who have and those who do not have rapid disease progression.

[b] Because HIV infection progresses more rapidly in infants than older children or adults, some experts would treat all HIV-infected infants <6 months or <12 months of age, regardless of clinical, immunologic or virologic parameters.

[c] Many experts would initiate therapy if CD4+ cell percentage is between 15 and 20%, and defer therapy with increased monitoring frequency in children with CD4+ cell percentage 21 to 25%.

[d] There is controversy among pediatric HIV experts regarding the plasma HIV RNA threshold warranting consideration of therapy in children in the absence of clinical or immune abnormalities; some experts would consider initiation of therapy in asymptomatic children if plasma HIV RNA levels were between 50 000 and 100 000 copies/ml.

with high viral replication in infected infants) when drug concentrations are sub-therapeutic, from either incomplete adherence or inadequate dosage. Potential long-term toxicity such as lipodystrophy, dyslipidemia, glucose intolerance, osteopenia, and mitochondrial dysfunction are a concern [4–8]. The risks and benefits of early initiation of therapy should be discussed with the caregiver and adherence addressed before initiating therapy.

HIV-infected children over 12 months of age

Treatment is recommended for all children over 12 months of age with clinical AIDS (Clinical Category C) or severe immune suppression (Immune Category 3), regardless of virologic status. ART should be considered for children who have mild–moderate clinical symptoms (Clinical Categories A or B), moderate immunologic suppression (Immune Category 2), and/or confirmed plasma HIV RNA levels ≥100 000 copies/ml. Many experts would defer treatment in asymptomatic children aged ≥ 12 months with normal immune status in situations in which the risk for clinical disease progression is low (e.g., HIV RNA <100 000 copies/ml) and when other factors (i.e., concern for adherence, safety, and persistence of ARV response) favor postponing treatment.

If therapy is deferred, the clinician should carefully monitor virologic, immunologic and clinical status. Factors that should be considered in deciding when to initiate therapy include: development of clinical symptoms; high or increasing HIV RNA levels; rapidly declining CD4+ lymphocyte count or percentage to values approaching those indicative of severe immune suppression (CDC Pediatric Immune Category 3); and the ability of the caregiver and child to adhere to the prescribed regimen.

European pediatric ART guidelines (Table 15.3)

The primary difference between the USA and European guidelines relates to when to initiate therapy in HIV-infected infants. The difficulties of long-term adherence, problems with data on optimal dosing for infants, and an increasing recognition of the potential for drug toxicity has led to a less aggressive approach to initiation of therapy in the PENTA guidelines [3]. Treatment is recommended for infants with CDC Stage B or C disease or CD4+ cell percentage <25–35%, indicating severe immune suppression. For children aged >12 months, the recommendations are similar to those in the USA.

World Health Organization interim guidelines for resource-limited settings (Table 15.4)

The World Health Organization (WHO) has released guidelines for ARV use in resource-limited settings, with the intent of facilitating the dramatic scale-up that is needed in countries with limited infrastructures and significant resource limitations in order to provide care to millions of infected people. Recognizing that the availability of affordable and accurate laboratory testing is severely constrained in many

Table 15.3. European guidelines for HIV-infected infants, children and young adolescents: indications for initiation of antiretroviral therapy.

Age	Clinical	Immunologic	Comments
<12 months	CDC Stage B or C (AIDS) disease	CD4% < 25–35%	Strongly consider initiation of therapy if viral load > 1 million copies/mL
1–3 years	CDC Stage C disease	CD4% < 20%	Strongly consider initiation of therapy if viral load > 250,000 copies/mL
4–8 years	CDC Stage C disease	CD4% < 15%	Strongly consider initiation of therapy if viral load > 250,000 copies/mL
9–12 years	CDC Stage C disease	CD4% < 15%	Strongly consider initiation of therapy if viral load > 250,000 copies/mL
13–17 years	CDC Stage C disease	CD4 absolute count of 200–350 cells/mm^3	

Reference [3].

Table 15.4. World Health Organization guidelines for HIV-infected infants, children and young adolescents: indications for initiation of antiretroviral therapy in resource-poor settings

CD4+ testing	Age	HIV diagnostic testing	Treatment recommendation
If CD4+ testing is available	<18 months	Positive HIV virologic test[a]	– WHO Pediatric Stage III disease (AIDS), irrespective of CD4+ cell percentage[b] – WHO Pediatric Stage I disease (asymptomatic) or Stage II disease with CD4+ percentage <20%[c]
		HIV virologic testing not available but infant HIV seropositive or born to known HIV-infected mother (Note: HIV antibody test *must* be repeated at age 18 months to obtain definitive diagnosis of HIV infection)	– WHO Pediatric Stage III disease (AIDS) with CD4+ cell percentage <20%
	≥18 months	HIV seropositive	– WHO Pediatric Stage III disease (AIDS) irrespective of CD4+ cell percentage[b] – WHO Pediatric Stage I disease (asymptomatic) or Stage II disease with CD4+ percentage <15%[c]
If CD4+ testing is not available	<18 months	Positive HIV virologic test	– WHO Pediatric Stage III[b]
		HIV virologic testing not available but infant HIV seropositive or born to known HIV-infected mother	– Treatment not recommended[d]
	≥18 months	HIV seropositive	– WHO Pediatric Stage III[b]

Source: http://www.who.int/hiv/pub/prev_care/en/ScalingUp_E.pdf.

[a] HIV DNA PCR or HIV RNA or immune complex dissociated p24 antigen assays.

[b] Initiation of ARVs can also be considered for children who have advanced WHO Pediatric Stage II disease including clinical findings such as severe recurrent or persistent oral candidiasis outside the neonatal period, weight loss, fevers, or recurrent severe bacterial infections, irrespective of CD4+ count.

[c] The rate of decline in CD4+ percentage (if measurement available) should be factored into the decision making.

[d] Many of the clinical symptoms in the WHO Pediatric Stage II and III disease classification are not specific for HIV infection and significantly overlap those seen in children without HIV infection in resource-limited settings; thus, in the absence of virologic testing and CD4+ cell assay availability, HIV-exposed children <18 months of age should generally not be considered for ART regardless of symptoms.

resource-limited countries, these guidelines reflect decision making in situations in which virologic assays and CD4+ cell counts may not be available.

If CD4+ testing is available, the WHO recommends treatment for HIV-infected children <18 months of age if the child has WHO Pediatric Stage III disease (AIDS), or if the child has less advanced clinical disease but a CD4+ percentage <20%. If neither CD4+ nor HIV virologic testing is available, but a child <18 months old is HIV seropositive or was born to an HIV-infected mother, treatment is recommended if the child has AIDS with a CD4+ percentage <20%. *In such situations, HIV antibody testing at age 18 months is required to confirm HIV infection status; ARVs would be continued only in those children with proven infection, as documented by positive HIV antibody.* For children 18 months of age or older who are HIV seropositive, treatment is recommended if the child has AIDS, or if the child has less advanced clinical disease but a CD4+ percentage <15%.

If CD4+ testing is not available, treatment is recommended for children with AIDS (with a positive HIV virologic test if <18 months old or HIV seropositive if 18 months of age or older). Treatment is not recommended in the absence of CD4+ and HIV virologic testing for children less than 18 months of age who are seropositive or who were born to HIV-infected mothers.

What is the recommended initial antiretroviral regimen (Tables 15.5 and 15.6)

Combination therapy is now recommended for all HIV-infected children and adults being treated. Compared to monotherapy, combination therapy yields significantly lower rates of disease progression, a greater and more sustained virologic and immunologic response, and less drug resistance. When using combination therapy, all drugs should be started at the same time or within one to two days of each other. Sequential initiation of drugs increases the possibility that ARV resistance will develop. Monotherapy is no longer recommended, except for ZDV as perinatal transmission prophylaxis in infants of indeterminate infection status during the first six weeks of life. Infants confirmed as HIV-infected while receiving ZDV chemoprophylaxis during the first 6 weeks of life should have ZDV discontinued pending decisions regarding initiation of ART.

Children and prepubertal adolescents

The initial ARV regimen chosen for infected infants theoretically could be influenced by the ARV regimen their mothers may have received during pregnancy. Current US guidelines suggest consideration of resistance testing before initiation of therapy in newly diagnosed infants, particularly if the mother has known or suspected infection with drug-resistant virus [1]. However, there are no definitive data at this time that demonstrate that resistance testing in this setting correlates with greater success of

Table 15.5. US Public Health Service guidelines for HIV-infected infants, children and young adolescents: recommended antiretroviral options for initial therapy

Protease inhibitor-based regimens

Strongly recommended: Two NRTIs[a] *plus* lopinavir/ritonavir *or* nelfinavir *or* ritonavir

Alternative recommendation: Two NRTIs[a] *plus* amprenavir (children ≥4 years old)[b] *or* indinavir

Non-nucleoside reverse transcriptase inhibitor-based regimens

Strongly recommended: Children >3 years: Two NRTIs[a] *plus* efavirenz[c] (with or without nelfinavir)

                                  Children ≤3 years or who can't swallow capsules: Two NRTIs[a] *plus* nevirapine[c]

Alternative recommendation: Two NRTIs[a] *plus* nevirapine[c] (children >3 years)

Nucleoside analogue-based regimens

Strongly recommended: None

Alternative recommendation: Zidovudine *plus* lamivudine *plus* abacavir

Use in special circumstances: Two NRTIs[a]

Regimens that are not recommended

                                  Monotherapy[d]

                                  Certain two NRTI combinations[a]

                                  Two NRTIs *plus* saquinavir soft or hard gel capsule as a sole PI[e]

Insufficient data to recommend

                                  Two NRTIs[a] *plus* delavirdine

                                  Dual PIs, including saquinavir soft or hard gel capsule with low dose ritonavir, with the exception of lopinavir/ritonavir[d]

                                  NRTI *plus* NNRTI *plus* PI[f]

                                  Tenofovir-containing regimens

                                  Enfuvirtide (T-20)-containing regimens

                                  Emtricitabine (FTC)-containing regimens

                                  Atazanavir-containing regimens

                                  Fosamprenavir-containing regimens

Reference [1]

[a] Dual NRTI combination recommendations:

Strongly recommended choices: zidovudine plus lamivudine or didanosine or stavudine plus lamivudine.

Alternative choices: abacavir plus zidovudine or lamivudine; or didanosine plus lamivudine.

Use in special circumstances: stavudine plus didanosine; or zalcitabine plus zidovudine.

Not recommended: zalcitabine plus didanosine, stavudine, or lamivudine; or zidovudine plus stavudine.

Insufficient data: tenofovir- or emtricitabine-containing regimens.

[b] Amprenavir should not be administered to children under age 4 years due to the propylene glycol and vitamin E content of the oral liquid preparation and lack of pharmacokinetic data in this age group.

c Efavirenz is currently available only in capsule form, although a liquid formulation is currently under study to determine appropriate dosage in HIV-infected children under age 3 years; nevirapine would be the preferred NNRTI for children under age 3 years or who require a liquid formulation.

d Except for zidovudine chemoprophylaxis administered to HIV-exposed infants during the first 6 weeks of life to prevent perinatal HIV transmission; if an infant is confirmed as HIV-infected while receiving zidovudine prophylaxis, therapy should either be discontinued or changed to a combination antiretroviral drug regimen.

e With the exception of lopinavir/ritonavir, data on the pharmacokinetics and safety of dual PI combinations (e.g., low dose ritonavir pharmacologic boosting of saquinavir, indinavir, or nelfinavir) are limited, use of dual PIs as a component of initial therapy is not recommended, although such regimens may have utility as secondary treatment regimens for children who have failed initial therapy. Saquinavir soft and hard gel capsule require low dose ritonavir boosting to achieve adequate levels in children, but pharmacokinetic data on appropriate dosing is not yet available.

f With the exception of efavirenz plus nelfinavir plus 1 or 2 NRTIs, which has been studied in HIV-infected children and shown to have virologic and immunologic efficacy in a clinical trial.

NRTI: Nucleoside analogue reverse transcriptase inhibitor.
NNRTI: Non-nucleoside analogue reverse transcriptase inhibitor.
PI: Protease inhibitor

---

initial ART. It will be important to continue to monitor the frequency of perinatal transmission of ARV-resistant HIV isolates because maternal therapy with multiple ARV agents is becoming increasingly common and the prevalence of resistant viral strains in the pediatric HIV-infected population may increase over time [9].

ARV drug regimens are classified as strongly recommended; recommended as alternative; use in special circumstances; not recommended; or insufficient data to make a recommendation [1]. Recommendations on the optimal initial therapy for children are continually being modified as new data become available, new therapies or drug formulations are developed, and late toxicities become recognized.

Choice of dual NRTI backbone

A dual NRTI combination forms the backbone of recommended regimens, and is given with a PI, an NNRTI, or a third NRTI. The strongly recommended dual NRTI combinations for inclusion in the initial therapy regimen in children are: ZDV/lamivudine (3TC), ZDV/didanosine (ddI), and stavudine (d4T)/3TC.

Alternative dual NRTI combinations include ZDV/abacavir (ABC), 3TC/ABC, and ddI/3TC. Although some studies have shown that dual NRTI backbone regimens containing ABC may have similar potency to ZDV/3TC in children [10], ABC has the potential for life-threatening hypersensitivity reactions in about 5% of patients. There is less pediatric experience with ddI/3TC than the other recommended dual NRTIs.

Table 15.6. US Public Health Service Guidelines for HIV-infected postpubertal adolescents and adults: recommended antiretroviral options for initial therapy

Non-nucleoside reverse transcriptase inhibitor-based regimens

Preferred regimens	Efavirenz **plus** (lamivudine **or** emtricitabine[b]) **plus** (zidovudine **or** tenofovir[a]) – *except for pregnant women or women with pregnancy potential*
Alternative regimens	Efavirenz **plus** (lamivudine **or** emtricitabine[b]) **plus** (abacavir **or** didanosine **or** stavudine) – *except for pregnant women or women with pregnancy potential*
	Nevirapine **plus** (lamivudine **or** emtricitabine[b]) **plus** (zidovudine **or** stavudine[a] **or** didanosine **or** abacavir **or** tenofovir) Note: High incidence of symptomatic hepatic events observed in women with CD4+ > 250 cells/mm^3 before therapy and then with CD4 > 400 cells/mm^3 before therapy. Nevirapine should not be initiated in these patients unless benefit clearly outweighs risk.

Protease inhibitor-based regimens

Preferred regimens	Lopinavir/ritonavir **plus** (lamivudine **or** emtricitabine[a]) **plus** (zidovudine[a])
Alternative regimens	Atazanavir **plus** (lamivudine **or** emtricitabine[b]) **plus** (zidovudine **or** stavudine[a] **or** abacavir **or** didanosine) **or** (tenofovir **plus** ritonavir 100 mg/day)
	Fosamprenavir **plus** (lamivudine **or** emtricitabine) **plus** (zidovudine **or** stavudine **or** abacavir **or** tenofovir **or** didanosine)
	Fosamprenane/ ritonavir **plus** (lamivudine) **or** emtricitabine) **plus** (ziduvodine **or** stavudine **or** abacavir **or** tenofovir or didanosine)
	Indinavir/ritonavir[c] **plus** (lamivudine **or** emtricitabine[b]) **plus** (zidovudine **or** stavudine[a] **or** abacavir **or** tenofovir **or** didanosine)
	Lopinavir/ritonavir **plus** (lamivudine **or** emtricitabine[b]) **plus** (stavudine **or** abacavir **or** tenofovir **or** didanosine)
	Nelfinavir[d] **plus** (lamivudine **or** emtricitabine[b]) **plus** (zidovudine **or** stavudine[a] **or** abacavir **or** tenofovir **or** didanosine)
	Saquinavir sgc, hcg or tablets /ritonavir[c] **plus** (lamivudine **or** emtricitabine[b]) **plus** (zidovudine **or** stavudine[a] **or** abacavir **or** tenofovir **or** didanosine)

Nucleoside analogue-based regimen – only when a PI- or NNRTI-based regimen cannot or should not be used as first line therapy

	Abacavir **plus** lamivudine **plus** zidovudine

Modified from [2].

[a] Higher incidence of lipoatrophy, hyperlipidemia, and mitochondrial toxicities reported with stavudine than with other NRTIs.

[b] Long-term efficacy data on emtricitabine used in combination with these regimens is limited or not available.

[c] Low-dose (100–400 mg) ritonavir.

[d] Nelfinavir available in 250-mg or 625-mg tablet.

[e] sgc = soft gel capsule; hgc = hard gel capsule.

NNRTI: Non-nucleoside analogue reverse transcriptase inhibitor.

NRTI: Nucleoside analogue reverse transcriptase inhibitor.

PI: Protease inhibitor.

The dual NRTI combinations d4T/ddI and ZDV/zalcitabine (ddC) are recommended for use only in special circumstances; d4T/ddI-based combination regimens are associated with greater rates of neurotoxicity, hyperlactatemia, and lipodystrophy than ZDV/3TC-based therapies, and ddC is less potent than the other NRTI drugs and has greater toxicity.

Certain dual NRTI drug combinations should not be given. These include ZDV and d4T, due to pharmacologic interactions that can result in potential virologic antagonism, and dual regimens combining ddC with ddI, d4T or 3TC, as pediatric experience with these combinations is limited and there is overlapping neurotoxicity between the drugs. Emtricitabine (FTC) is approved for use in individuals aged 3 months or older. [1]. Therefore, there are insufficient data to recommend use of FTC for initial therapy in children.

Drug regimens (Table 15.5)

Strongly recommended regimens for initial therapy

Based on clinical trials in infected adults and children, the ARV regimens that are strongly recommended for initial therapy in children include the combination of two NRTIs plus one of the recommended PIs, or the combination of two NRTIs plus the NNRTI efavirenz for children over age 3 years (or nevirapine for children 3 years of age or younger or who cannot take capsules).

Lopinavir/ritonavir, nelfinavir and ritonavir are the recommended PIs for use in PI-based regimens in young children because they are available in appropriate formulations (nelfinavir is available in a powder which can be mixed with water or food; lopinavir/ritonavir and ritonavir are available as liquids) and there is experience with these drugs in pediatric populations, with relatively low rates of toxicity [11, 12–15]. Combination therapy with two NRTIs and a potent PI can produce sustained suppression of viral replication to undetectable levels in a substantial proportion of children, although the rate of response may be somewhat less than in adults, particularly for younger children [10–16]. Additionally, longer-term clinical and immunologic benefits have been reported in children receiving these regimens, including improvements in growth, an important measure of response to therapy in children [16–18].

Efavirenz, in combination with two NRTIs with or without nelfinavir, is the strongly recommended NNRTI for NNRTI-based initial therapy of children over age 3 years who can take capsules, based on clinical trial experience in children [19] and because higher rates of toxicity have been observed in clinical trials in adults with nevirapine. However, regimens including efavirenz combined with nelfinavir and NRTIs contain drugs from all three available drug classes and therefore there is the potential for development of resistance to all three classes if virologic failure occurs. In clinical trials in adults, a PI-sparing regimen of efavirenz in combination with dual NRTIs was associated with an excellent virologic and immunologic response comparable to PI-containing regimens, with similar or better tolerability [20]. While there have not been clinical trials of efavirenz as part of a PI-sparing regimen as initial therapy in pediatric patients, it seems reasonable to extrapolate efficacy from the adult data. A liquid formulation of efavirenz is under study in children under age 3 years and is available by expanded access in the USA and other countries [21]. Because efavirenz is only commercially available in a capsule and nevirapine is available in a liquid formulation, nevirapine is the strongly recommended NNRTI for children who require a liquid formulation or who are 3 years or age or younger.

Alternative regimens for initial therapy

The following ARV regimens are recommended as alternatives for initial therapy of children: two NRTIs plus indinavir or amprenavir (the latter only for children 4 years of age or older); the combination of two NRTIs with nevirapine (for children over 3 years of age); or the triple NRTI combination of ZDV/3TC/ABC. Each of these alternative regimens has demonstrated evidence of virologic suppression in some children [18, 22, 23].

However, either experience in the pediatric population is more limited than for the strongly recommended regimens or the extent and durability of suppression less well defined in children. Additionally, for some drugs, although clinical trials in children have demonstrated reasonable virologic response in combination regimens, the potential for serious adverse effects make them less favorable choices for initial therapy at this time. There is no liquid formulation of indinavir, and therefore it can only be used in children who can swallow capsules. Additionally, there has been a high rate of hematuria, sterile leukocytouria, and nephrolithiasis reported in pediatric patients receiving indinavir [18, 24]. Amprenavir liquid formulation cannot be administered to children under age 4 years due to the high concentration of propylene glycol and vitamin E in the liquid preparation.

Serious hepatobiliary toxicity appears more frequent in adult studies with use of nevirapine than efavirenz [25, 26]. No comparative trials of nevirapine and efavirenz have been conducted in children. Because of the potential for higher rates of hepatic toxicity, a nevirapine-based regimen is viewed as an alternative rather than as recommended for NNRTI-based regimens, with the exception of children under age 3 years (for whom no data are available on appropriate dose for efavirenz, the recommended NNRTI) or those who require a liquid formulation (which is not yet available for efavirenz).

Triple NRTI regimens can be considered as alternative regimens as initial therapy when PI- or NNRTI-based regimens cannot be given (for example, due to potential important drug interactions). Data on the efficacy of triple NRTI regimens for treatment of ARV-naïve children is limited; in small observational studies, response rates of 47%–50% have been reported [27–29]. A triple-NRTI regimen avoids the initial use of PIs and NNRTIs and can be administered twice a day in children, which may facilitate adherence. However, the long-term durability of viral load suppression with such a regimen is uncertain, recent data from studies in adult populations suggest an inferior virologic response compared to efavirenz-based regimens [30], and there is a potentially life-threatening hypersensitivity syndrome associated with ABC.

Use in special circumstances for initial therapy

Dual NRTI therapy alone is recommended for initial therapy only in special circumstances. Therapy with two NRTIs alone has been shown to provide clinical, virologic and immunologic benefit in pediatric studies, but the extent and durability of virologic suppression is less than with PI-containing combination regimens [31, 32, 11]. Use of a regimen consisting of two NRTIs alone might be considered as there are concerns regarding the feasibility of adherence to a more complex drug regimen. It is important to note that drug regimens that do not result in sustained viral suppression, such as a dual NRTI regimen, may result in the development of viral resistance to the drugs being used and cross-resistance to other drugs within the same drug class.

Not recommended for initial therapy

ARV regimens not recommended for initial treatment of ARV-naïve children include monotherapy, certain dual NRTI combinations (ZDV plus d4T; and ddC plus ddI, d4T or 3TC), and regimens of two NRTIs plus saquinavir-soft gel capsule or saquinavir-hard gel capsule. These combinations are not recommended either because of pharmacological antagonism, potential overlapping toxicities, or inferior virologic response. There are only limited data on saquinavir in children, and pharmacokinetic studies have found lower than expected plasma drug concentrations [33, 34]. Combining saquinavir with another PI, either nelfinavir or ritonavir, is required in children to increase saquinavir exposure to acceptable levels; however, these regimens have been principally studied in small numbers of ARV-experienced children (not ARV-naïve children), and appropriate dosing of dual PI regimens in pediatric patients is not yet established [33–35].

Insufficient data to recommend for initial therapy

There are insufficient data to recommend several ARV drugs or regimens as initial therapy for ARV-naive children, although they may be useful in children who have failed other regimens. The NNRTI delavirdine has not been studied in HIV-infected children and is not available in a liquid formulation. Dual PI-based regimens (with the exception of lopinavir/ritonavir) have only limited data on appropriate dosing and safety in children; these regimens often use one PI, often ritonavir, to "boost" levels of the other PI to a therapeutic range [36]. There are also minimal pediatric data on regimens containing agents from three drug classes (e.g., NRTI plus an NNRTI plus a PI), with the exception of efavirenz plus nelfinavir and 1 or 2 NRTIs, which has been shown to be effective in HIV-infected children [19]. The reverse transcriptase inhibitors tenofovir and emtricitabine (FTC), and the PIs atazonavir, tipranavir, and fosamprenavir, do not have pediatric pharmacokinetic and safety data currently available and are not available in liquid formulations. Finally, the fusion inhibitor enfuvirtide has been approved for children over age 6 years [37], but requires administration by subcutaneous injection and has only been studied in ARV-experienced children; thus, more data are needed before it would be considered for use as initial therapy in children.

Adults and postpubertal adolescents (Table 15.6)

Regimens recommended for initial therapy for infected adults and adolescents include some ARV drug combinations or agents not yet recommended for initial therapy in children. Low, non-therapeutic doses of ritonavir, a potent liver cytochrome P450 enzyme inhibitor, can act as a pharmacologic "enhancer" when administered with other PIs metabolized by this enzyme, resulting in elevated plasma concentrations of the second drug at a lower dosage and with longer elimination kinetics than if the drug was administered alone. In infected adults, low dose ritonavir in combination with lopinavir, fosamprenavir, indinavir, saquinavir, either as dual PI therapy alone or combined with one or two NRTIs, has been well tolerated and has shown substantial ARV activity. Most of these studies have been conducted in treatment-experienced patients; it is unclear whether dual PIs are better than single PI regimens for initial therapy. A few dual PI regimens have been studied in a small number of children [35, 38]. However, because data on the pharmacokinetics, safety and efficacy of dual PI combinations in children are limited, use of such regimens for initial therapy is not recommended, with the exception of lopinavir/ritonavir. The PI atazanavir, and the nucleotide reverse transcriptase inhibitor tenofovir have been approved for treatment of adults; however, studies to define appropriate dosage and safety in children are underway. Additional new ARV drugs and combinations are under study, and it is highly likely that other drug combinations capable of suppressing viral replication will become available in the future and will increase treatment options for children.

When should a change in antiretroviral therapy be considered? (Tables 15.7 and 15.8)

The reasons to consider changing an ARV regimen include: (a) evidence of disease progression based on virologic, immunologic, or clinical parameters indicating therapeutic failure of the current regimen; (b) toxicity or intolerance to the current regimen; and (c) consideration of new data demonstrating that a drug or regimen is superior to the current regimen.

Failure of an ARV regimen can occur for many reasons, including problems with absorption or metabolism of a drug due to inherent characteristics of the individual or pharmacokinetic interactions with concomitant medications leading to subtherapeutic drug levels; pre-existing or acquired drug resistance; and/or problems with patient adherence to the regimen. Adherence can be a special problem in pediatrics, yet rigorous adherence to the prescribed regimen is essential to achieve an effective ARV effect from therapy. Close family and medical follow-up are essential to ensure compliance with new therapeutic regimens.

Table 15.7. US Public Health Service guidelines for HIV-infected postpubertal adolescents and adults: considerations for changing antiretroviral therapy

Virologic considerations	1. Incomplete virologic response (not achieving HIV RNA <400 copies/ml by 24 weeks or <50 copies/ml by 48 weeks in a treatment naïve patient starting therapy)[a]
	2. Virologic rebound (repeated detection of viremia after achieved virologic suppression)[b]
Immunologic considerations	1. Failure to increase the CD4 cell count by 25–50 cells/mm^3 over the first year of therapy
	2. Experiencing a decrease in CD4+ cell count below the baseline CD4+ cell count on therapy
Clinical considerations	1. Occurrence or recurrence of HIV-related events (after at least 3 months on an antiretroviral regimen), excluding immune reconstitution syndromes

Modified from [2].

[a] Baseline HIV RNA may impact the time course of response, and some patients may take longer than others to suppress viremia.

[b] The degree of plasma HIV RNA increase should be considered, and the health care provider may consider short-term observation in a patient whose plasma HIV RNA increases from undetectable to low-level detectability (e.g., 500–5000 copies/ml) at 4 months. In this situation, the patient should be followed very closely.

Virologic considerations for changing therapy

Virologic response should be assessed 4 weeks after initiating or changing therapy; however, the time to maximal virologic response will vary depending on the baseline HIV RNA value when therapy started. Because HIV RNA levels in perinatal infection are extremely high compared to most infected adults, the initial response of infected infants and young children to initiation of ART may be slower than that observed in adults. If baseline HIV RNA levels are very high (e.g., >1 000 000 copies/ml), virologic response may not be observed until after 8 to 12 weeks or more of therapy.

Suppression of plasma HIV RNA to undetectable levels may be achieved less often in children despite potent combination therapy due to the high viral loads in children, but significant clinical benefit may be seen with decrements in HIV RNA that do not result in undetectable levels. Therefore, the initial HIV RNA level of the child at the start of therapy as well as the nadir achieved on therapy should be taken into consideration when contemplating potential drug changes. Given the observation that HIV-infected infants often have much higher viral loads than adults, it may be difficult to decrease the viral loads of many infants to below detectable limits. Rapid modifications of ART might not achieve this goal and could unnecessarily and prematurely exhaust the patient's therapeutic options. However, it should be recognized that failure to maximally suppress viral replication might be associated with increased risk for viral

Table 15.8. US Public Health Service guidelines for HIV-infected infants, children and young adolescents: considerations for changing antiretroviral therapy

Virologic considerations[a]	1. Less than a minimally acceptable virologic response after 8–12 weeks of therapy. For children receiving aggressive antiretroviral therapy, such a response is defined as a less than tenfold ($1.0 \log_{10}$) decrease from baseline HIV RNA levels
	2. HIV RNA not suppressed to undetectable levels after 4–6 months of antiretroviral therapy[c]
	3. Repeated detection of HIV RNA in children who initially had undetectable levels in response to antiretroviral therapy[c]
	4. Substantial reproducible increase[c] in plasma viremia from the nadir of suppression, defined as: • For children <2 years old, an increase of >fivefold (>$0.7 \log_{10}$) copies/ml • For children ≥2 years old, an increase of >threefold (>$0.5 \log_{10}$) copies/ml
Immunologic considerations[a]	1. Change in pediatric CDC Immune Category[d]
	2. For children with CD4+ percentage <15% (pediatric CDC Immune Category 3), a persistent decline of 5% or more in CD4+ cell percentage (e.g., from 15% to 10%)
	3. A rapid and substantial decrease in absolute CD4+ lymphocyte count (e.g., >30% decline <6 months)
Clinical considerations	1. Progressive neurodevelopmental deterioration
	2. Growth failure defined as persistent decline in weight-growth velocity despite adequate nutritional support and without other explanation
	3. Disease progression, as defined by advancement from one pediatric CDC Clinical Category to another[e]

Reference [1].

[a] At least two measurements (at least one week apart) should be performed before considering a change.

[b] The initial HIV RNA level of the child at the start of therapy as well as the level achieved with therapy should be considered when contemplating potential drug changes.

[c] Continued observation with more frequent evaluation of HIV RNA levels should be considered if the HIV RNA increase is limited (i.e., less than 5000 copies/ml). The presence of repeatedly detectable or increasing RNA levels suggests the development of resistance mutations.

[d] Minimal changes in CD4+ percentile that may result in CDC Immune Category change (e.g., from 26% to 24%, or 16% to 14%) may not be as concerning as a major rapid substantial change in CD4+ percentile within the same Immune Category (e.g., a drop from 35% to 25% in a short period of time).

[e] In patients with stable immunologic and virologic parameters, progression from one clinical category to another may not in itself represent an indication to change therapy.

mutations and selection for drug-resistant viral variants. Resistance testing is recommended in children, as in adults, in the setting of persistent or increasing HIV RNA levels [1].

Following achievement of a maximal virologic response, HIV RNA levels should be measured at least every 3 months to monitor continued response to therapy. At least two measurements taken at least a week apart should be performed before considering a change. Intrapatient biologic variation in HIV RNA levels may be greater in young children than adults, making it somewhat more difficult to define a significant change in HIV RNA copy number in children, and HIV RNA declines even without therapy in children with perinatal HIV infection during the first few years of life, with the most rapid decline in the first 15–24 months of life [39–41]. Therefore, the definition of a significant plasma HIV RNA change for pediatric patients differs by age (see Chapter 1). For children <2 years old, a significant change is defined as >fivefold (0.7 $\log_{10}$) on repeated testing, whereas for children ≥2 years old, a change >threefold (0.5 $\log_{10}$) is significant.

Immunologic considerations for changing therapy

In HIV-infected adults, disease progression risk has been shown to increase directly with baseline plasma HIV RNA concentration and inversely with baseline CD4+ lymphocyte number; at any given HIV RNA level, patients with lower CD4+ counts have poorer prognosis. CD4+ lymphocyte count and plasma HIV RNA concentration also predict disease progression and mortality in children [39, 42, 43].

Interpretation of CD4+ lymphocyte changes in pediatric patients is complicated by the normal age-related changes in absolute number; CD4+ lymphocyte percentage is more stable and less affected by age (see Chapter 1). ART should not be changed due to an apparent decline in CD4+ lymphocyte values unless the change is validated by at least two repeated measurements obtained at least a week apart.

Clinical considerations for changing therapy

In infected adults and adolescents, clinical deterioration, defined as a new AIDS-defining diagnosis acquired after treatment is initiated, is an indication for a change in therapy. However, if the patient has had a good virologic response to therapy, the appearance of a new opportunistic infection may not reflect a failure of therapy, but persistence of severe immunocompromise. In children with stable immunologic and virologic parameters, development of HIV-related infectious complications may not in itself represent an indication to change therapy.

Central nervous system dysfunction and growth failure are common manifestations of HIV infection in children and have been shown to improve with therapy [31, 32, 16]. Thus, deterioration in these latter parameters may be more useful than development of opportunistic infections in determining therapeutic failure in children. Persistent or progressive neurologic deterioration is defined as the presence of two or more of the following: impairment in brain growth (e.g., assessed by serial head circumference measurements or neuroimaging); decline of cognitive function documented by psychometric testing; or clinical motor dysfunction.

Choosing a new antiretroviral regimen

When a change is due to toxicity or intolerance

The nature and severity of the toxicity or intolerance are important considerations in decisions about alterations in therapy. Alternative explanations for clinical or laboratory abnormalities, such as intercurrent infections or toxicity secondary to concomitant medications, must be considered. Severe and potentially fatal toxicities such as pancreatitis, hepatic failure, lactic acidosis, or severe skin rash or Stevens–Johnson syndrome require discontinuation of therapy. ABC should never be restarted following a hypersensitivity reaction, since hypotension, renal and respiratory insufficiency, and death has occurred within hours of rechallenge. Similarly, nevirapine should not be restarted in children who experience a severe skin rash; who develop cutaneous bullae or target lesions, mucosal involvement, or symptoms consistent with hypersensitivity; or who have had nevirapine-associated hepatitis. When therapy requires discontinuation, all drugs should be stopped temporarily to avoid development of drug resistance; following resolution of the toxicity, restarting the drug regimen with change of a single drug is permissible. The substituted drug should ideally be in a similar class (e.g., substitute one NRTI for another NRTI) but have different toxicity or tolerance characteristics. In some cases, substitution within a class may not be advisable (for example, most clinicians would not use another drug in the NNRTI class in a patient receiving nevirapine who develops Stevens–Johnson syndrome).

For non-life-threatening toxicities in patients with adequate virologic, immunologic and clinical responses, all efforts should be made to continue the current therapeutic regimen. This should include adjunctive therapies directed at the observed toxicity, such as erythropoietin and/or transfusions for treatment of anemia, or granulocyte colony stimulating factor for neutropenia. Some toxicities may be transient in nature, and therapy may be safely continued with close monitoring (e.g., nausea secondary to therapy with certain PIs), while other toxicities may require a temporary or permanent reduction in dose. Due to concerns about the development of resistance with subtherapeutic drug levels, ARV drugs should only be reduced to the lower end of their therapeutic range, and adequacy of continued ARV activity should be confirmed by monitoring HIV RNA levels or drug levels, if available.

The toxicities of ARV drugs can occur at different frequencies in children and adults and/or have different implications for children. Chapters 11 and 13 detail toxicities observed in pediatric patients with the currently available ARV drugs.

When a change is due to virologic, immunologic, or clinical disease progression

An assessment of adherence problems is important in choosing a new therapeutic regimen. When changing therapy, all medications taken by the patient should be reviewed for possible drug interactions with the new regimen. Alterations in drug absorption, distribution, metabolism or elimination induced by one drug can result in altered pharmacokinetics of one or more other drugs; pharmacodynamic synergy or antagonism between ARV agents could affect toxicity or effectiveness. Drugs metabolized by cytochrome P450, such as NNRTIs and PIs, have particularly significant interactions with many drugs (see Chapter 12).

ARV history and the impact of change on future treatment are important when choosing a new regimen. Replacement with a regimen containing drugs the child has not previously received would be ideal. However, the number of available drug options may be restricted due to prior ARV drug experience and limited data on pharmacokinetics and safety of some combination regimens in children, and it may not be possible to provide a completely new regimen. In that case, the failing regimen should be changed to incorporate at least two new drugs. Change in, or addition of, a single drug to a failing regimen is suboptimal and not recommended, as it promotes development of resistance to the new agent. For children failing initial therapy, change in dual NRTI backbone and of the drug class of the third drug (e.g., change of PI to NNRTI, or vice versa) should be feasible. However, there is no consensus about the best approach to salvage therapy for children with more ARV experience. Interchange of NNRTI drugs should be avoided due to cross-resistance. The mutation patterns associated with PI resistance overlap; resistance to one may result in reduced susceptibility to some or all of the other currently available PIs. High-level cross-resistance exists between ritonavir and indinavir.

Data from some, but not all, studies in adults experiencing virologic failure have demonstrated a modest short-term virologic benefit with use of genotypic or phenotypic resistance testing to guide choice of a new therapeutic regimen compared to clinical judgment alone [44, 45]. Resistance testing should be considered in children when changing a failing regimen [1]. However, interpretation of the results can be difficult because the mutations that lead to resistance are not fully understood and there is a potential for cross-resistance to other drugs to be conferred by certain mutations. Additionally, while the presence of viral resistance to a particular drug suggests that the drug is unlikely to successfully suppress viral replication, the absence of resistance to a drug does not ensure that its use will be successful. Consultation with an HIV specialist is advised for interpretation of test results. Resistance assays should be performed while the patient is receiving the drug regimen, because in the absence of drug pressure wild type virus is likely to replace resistant strains and mask the presence of resistant virus (see Chapter 14).

For children with extensive prior treatment with all three ARV drug classes, approaches have included the following: continuing the current regimen if partial virologic suppression was achieved and the patient is immunologically and clinically stable; use of "mega-HAART" (treatment with four to six ARV drugs in an attempt to overcome resistance and suppress viral replication, often including two NRTIs, an NNRTI and two to three PIs); use of "drug holidays" to see if wild-type virus will again predominate (although, since all prior species are archived and can rapidly re-emerge, many would argue that this approach should not be considered); recycling previously tolerated medications; or discontinuing therapy. Data suggest that HIV with multidrug resistance mutations has reduced replication capacity and pathogenicity compared to wild-type virus. Some patients who have failed multiple ARV drug regimens and have actively replicating, drug-resistant virus have had low rates of clinical progression and stabilization of CD4+ cell numbers if viral load is sustained 0.5 log below the patient's pretreatment value [46].

Conclusions

Although the pathogenesis of HIV infection and the general virologic and immunologic principles underlying the use of ART are similar for all HIV-infected individuals, there are unique considerations for HIV-infected infants, children, and adolescents. Most children acquire HIV infection through perinatal exposure, which raises the possibility of initiating therapy during the period of primary infection if sensitive diagnostic tests are used to determine infection status early in life. Because perinatal infection occurs during the development of the infant immune system, both the clinical manifestations and course of immunologic and virologic markers of infection differ from those in adults. These differences must be taken into consideration when using immunologic and virologic markers for therapeutic decision making in children. Additionally, changes in drug pharmacokinetics during the transition from the newborn period to adulthood require specific evaluation of drug dosing and toxicities in infants and children. Finally, unique issues related to adherence exist for pediatric patients that need to be addressed to achieve optimal response to therapy.

REFERENCES

1. Centers for Disease Control and Prevention. Guidelines for the use of antiretroviral agents in pediatric HIV infection. *Morb. Mortal. Wkly Rep*, 1998; **47** (No. RR-4):1–42 (updates available at http://AIDSInfo.nih.gov).

2. Centers for Disease Control and Prevention. Guidelines for using antiretroviral agents among HIV-infected adults and adolescents. Recommendations of the Panel on Clinical Practices for Treatment of HIV. *Morb. Mortal. Wkly Rep*, 2002;**51** (No. RR-7):1–55 (updates available at http://AIDSInfo.nih.gov).

3. Sharland, M., Castelli, G., Ramos, J. T., Blanche, S., Gibb, D. M. PENTA guidelines for the use of antiretroviral therapy in paediatric HIV infection – 2004. Available on line: http://www.ctu.mrc.ac.uk/PENTA.

4. Melvin, A. J., Lennon, S., Mohan, K. M., Purnell, J. Q. Metabolic abnormalities in HIV type 1-infected children treated and not treated with protease inhibitors. *AIDS Res Hum. Retroviruses* 2001;**17**:1117–1123.

5. Arpadi, S. M., Cuff, P. A., Horlick, M., Wang, J., Kotler, D. P. Lipodystrophy in HIV-infected children is associated with high viral load and low CD4+-lymphocyte count and CD4+-lymphocyte percentage at baseline and use of protease inhibitors and stavudine. *J. Acquir. Immune Defic. Syndr. Hum. Retrovirol.* 2001;**27**:30–34.

6. Mora, S., Sala, N., Bricalli, D., Zuin, G., Chiumello, G., Vigano, A. Bone mineral loss through increased bone turnover in HIV-infected children treated with highly active antiretroviral therapy. *AIDS* 2001;**15**:1823–1829.

7. Cossarizza, A., Pinti, M., Moretti, L. *et al.* Mitochondrial functionality and mitochondrial DNA content in lymphocytes of vertically infected human immunodeficiency virus-positive children with highly active antiretroviral therapy-related lipodystrophy. *J. Infect. Dis.* 2002;**185**:299–305.

8. Brambilla, P., Bricalli, D., Sala, N. *et al.* Highly active antiretroviral-treated HIV-infected children show fat distribution changes even in absence of lipodystrophy. *AIDS* 2001;**15**:2415–2422.

9. Parker, M. M., Wade, N., Lloyd, R. M., Jr. *et al.* Prevalence of genotypic drug resistance among a cohort of HIV-infected newborns. *J. AIDS*, 2003; **32**(3):292–297.

10. Paediatric European Network for Treatment of AIDS (PENTA). Comparison of dual nucleoside-analogue reverse-transcriptase inhibitor regimens with and without nelfinavir in children with HIV-1 who have not previously been treated: the PENTA 5 randomised trial. *Lancet*, 2002; **359**(9308):733–70.

11. Nachman, S. A., Stanley, K., Yogev, R. *et al.* Nucleoside analogs plus ritonavir in stable antiretroviral-experienced HIV-infected children – a randomized controlled trial. *J. Am. Med. Assoc.* 2000;**283**:492–498.

12. Saez-Llorens, X., Violari, A., Deetz, C. O. *et al.* Forty-eight-week evaluation of lopinavir/ritonavir, a new protease inhibitor, in human immunodeficiency virus-infected children. *Pediatr. Infect. Dis. J.*, 2003; **22**(3):216–224.

13. Krogstad, P., Lee, S., Johnson, G. *et al.* Nucleoside-analogue reverse transcriptase inhibitors plus nevirapine, nelfinavir, or ritonavir for pretreated children infected with human immunodeficiency virus type 1. *Clin. Infect. Dis.* 2002;**34**:991–1001.

14. Wiznia, A., Stanley, K., Krogstad, P. *et al.* Combination nucleoside-analogue reverse transcriptase inhibitor(s) plus nevirapine, nelfinavir, or ritonavir in stable, antiretroviral-experienced HIV-infected children: week 24 results of a randomized controlled trial – PACTG 377. *AIDS Res. Hum. Retroviruses* 2000;**16**:1113–1121.

15. Floren, L. C., Wiznia, A., Hayashi, S. *et al.* Nelfinavir pharmacokinetics in stable human immunodeficiency virus-positive children: pediatric AIDS Clinical Trials Group protocol 377. *Pediatrics* 2003;**112**:e220–227: http://www.pediatrics.org/cgi/content/full/112/3/e220.

16. Verweel, G., van Rossum, A. M. C., Hartwig, N. *et al.* Treatment with highly active antiretroviral therapy in human immunodeficiency virus type 1-infected children is associated with a sustained effect on growth. *Pediatrics* 2002;**109** (2). URL: http://www.pediatrics.org/cgi/content/full/109/2/e25.

17. Miller, T. L., Mawn, B. E., Orav, E. J. *et al.* The effect of protease inhibitor therapy on growth and body composition in human immunodeficiency virus type 1-infected

children. *Pediatrics* 2001;**107**(5). URL: http://www.pediatrics.org/cgi/content/full/107/5/e77.

18. Jankelevich, S., Mueller, B. U., Mackall, C. L. *et al.* Long-term virologic and immunologic responses in human immunodeficiency virus type 1-infected children treated with indinavir, zidovudine and lamivudine. *J. Infect. Dis.* 2001;**183**:1116–1120.

19. Starr, S. E., Fletcher, C. V., Spector, S. A. *et al.* Combination therapy with efavirenz, nelfinavir, and nucleoside reverse transcriptase inhibitors in children infected with human immunodeficiency virus type 1. *N. Engl. J. Med.* 1999;**341**:1874–1881.

20. Friedl, A. C., Ledergerber, B., Flepp, M. *et al.* Response to first protease inhibitor- and efavirenz-containing antiretroviral combination therapy – the Swiss HIV Cohort Study. *AIDS* 2001;**15**:1793–1800.

21. Starr, S. E., Spector, S. A. *et al.* Efavirenz liquid formulation in human immunodeficiency virus-infected children. *Pediatr. Infect. Dis. J.*, 2002;**21**(7):659–663.

22. Verweel, G., Sharland, M., Lyall, H. *et al.* Nevirapine use in HIV-1-infected children. *AIDS* 2003;**17**:1639–1647.

23. Saez-Llorens, X., Nelson, R. P., Emmanuel, P. *et al.* A randomized, double-blind study of triple nucleoside therapy of abacavir, lamivudine, and zidovudine versus lamivudine and zidovudine in previously treated human immunodeficiency virus type 1-infected children. *Pediatrics* 2001;**107**:e4. URL: http://www.pediatric.org/cgi/content/full/107/1/e4.

24. van Rossum, A. M., Dieleman, J. P., Fraaij, P. L. *et al.* Persistent sterile leukocyturia is associated with impaired renal function in human immunodeficiency virus type 1-infected children treated with indinavir. *Pediatrics*, 2002;**110** (2 pt 1):e19.

25. Van Leth, F., Phanuphak, P., Ruxrungthan, K. *et al.* Comparison of first-line antiretroviral therapy with regimens including nevirapine, efavirenz, or both drugs, plus stavudine and lamivudine: a randomised open-label trial, the 2NN Study. *Lancet.* 2004; **363** (9417): 1253–1263.

26. Sulkowski, M. S., Thomas, D. L., Mehta, S. H. *et al.* Hepatotoxicity associated with nevirapine or efavirenz-containing antiretroviral therapy: role of hepatitis C and B infections. *Hepatology*, 2002;**35**(1):182–189.

27. Saavedra, J., McCoig, C., Mallory, M. *et al.* Clinical experience with triple nucleoside (NRTI) combination ZDV/3TC/abacavir (ABC) as initial therapy in HIV-infected children. *41st Interscience Conference on Antimicrobial Agents and Chemotherapy.* Chicago, IL, September 22–25, 2001 (Abstract 1941).

28. Wells, C. J., Sharland, M., Smith, C. J. *et al.* Triple nucleoside analogue therapy with zidovudine (AZT), lamivudine (3TC), and abacavir (ABC) in the paediatric HIV London South Network (PHILS-NET) cohort. *XIV International AIDS Conference.* Barcelona, Spain, July 7–12, 2002 (Abstract TuPeB4625).

29. Paediatric European Network for Treatment of AIDS (PENTA). Comparison of dual nucleoside analogue reverse transcriptase inhibitor regimens with and without nelfinavir in children with HIV-1 who have not previously been treated: the PENTA 5 randomised trial. *Lancet* 2002;**359**:733–740.

30. National Institute of Allergy and Infectious Diseases. Physician letter, AACTG protocol 5095, March 13, 2003. Available at: http://www.nlm.nih.gov/databases/alerts/hiv.html.

31. McKinney, R. E., Johnson, G. M., Stanley, K. *et al.* A randomized study of combined zidovudine-lamivudine versus didanosine monotherapy in children with symptomatic therapy-naïve HIV-1 infection. *J. Pediatr.* 1998;**133**:500–508.

32. Englund, J., Baker, C., Raskino, C. *et al.* Zidovudine, didanosine or both as initial treatment for symptomatic HIV-infected children. *N. Engl. J. Med.* 1997;**336**:1704–1712.

33. Kline, M. W., Brundage, R. C., Fletcher, C. V. *et al.* Combination therapy with saquinavir soft gelatin capsules in children with human immunodeficiency virus infection. *Pediatr. Infect. Dis. J.* 2001;**20**:666–671.

34. Grub, S., DeLora, P., Ludin, E. *et al.* Pharmacokinetics and pharmacodynamics of saquinavir in pediatric patients with human immunodeficiency virus infection. *Clin. Pharmacol. Ther.* 2002;**71**:122–130.

35. Hoffmann, F., Notheis, G., Wintergerst, U. *et al.* Comparison of ritonavir plus saquinavir- and nelfinavir plus saquinavir-containing regimens as salvage therapy in children with human immunodeficiency virus type 1 infection. *Pediatr. Infect. Dis. J.* 2000;**19**:47–51.

36. Moyle, G., Use of HIV protease inhibitors as pharmacoenhancers. *AIDS Reader* 2001;February:87–98.

37. Church, J. A., Cunningham, C., Hughes, M. *et al.* Safety and antiretroviral activity of chronic subcutaneous administration of T-20 in human immunodeficiency virus 1-infected children. *Pediatr. Infect. Dis. J.* 2002;**21**:653–659.

38. van Rossum, A. M. C, de Groot, R., Hartwig, N. G. *et al.* Pharmacokinetics of indinavir and low-dose ritonavir in children with HIV-1 infection. *AIDS* 2000;**14**:2209–2219.

39. Mofenson, L. M., Korelitz, J., Meyer, W. A. *et al.* The relationship between serum human immunodeficiency virus type 1 (HIV-1) RNA level, CD4 lymphocyte percent, and long-term mortality risk in HIV-1-infected children. *J. Infect. Dis.* 1997;**175**:1029–1038.

40. Shearer, W. T., Quinn, T. C., LaRussa, P. *et al.* Viral load and disease progression in infants infected with human immunodeficiency virus type 1. *N. Engl. J. Med.* 1997;**336**:1337–1342.

41. McIntosh, K., Shevitz, A., Zaknun, D. *et al.* Age- and time-related changes in extracellular viral load in children vertically infected by human immunodeficiency virus. *Pediatr. Infect. Dis. J.* 1996;**15**:1087–1091.

42. Palumbo, P. E., Raskino, C., Fiscus, S. *et al.* Predictive value of quantitative plasma HIV RNA and CD4+ lymphocyte count in HIV-infected infants and children. *J. Am. Med. Assoc.* 1998;**279**:756–761.

43. HIV Paediatric Prognostic Markers Collaborative Study Group. Short-term risk of disease progression in HIV-1-infected children receiving no antiretroviral therapy or zidovudine monotherapy: estimates according to CD4 percent, viral load, and age. *Lancet* 2003; **362**: 1605–1600.

44. Durant, J., Clevenbergh, P., Halfon, P. *et al.* Drug-resistance genotyping in HIV-1 therapy: the VIRADAPT randomised controlled trial. *Lancet* 1999;**353**:2195–2199.

45. Cohen, C. J., Hunt, S., Sension, M. *et al.* A randomized trial assessing the impact of phenotypic resistance testing on antiretroviral therapy. *AIDS* 2002;**16**:579–588.

46. Yeni, P. G., Hammer, S. M., Carpenter, C. C. J. *et al.* Antiretroviral treatment for adult HIV infection in 2002: updated recommendations of the International AIDS Society-USA Panel. *J. Am. Med. Assoc.* 2002;**288**:222–235.

16 Therapeutic drug monitoring

Stephen C. Piscitelli, Pharm.D.

Discovery Medicine – Antivirals, GlaxoSmithKline, Research Triangle Park, NC

Therapeutic drug monitoring (TDM) refers to the adjustment of drug doses based on measured plasma concentrations to attain values within a "therapeutic window." Clinicians have used these principles for years to adjust doses of many drugs, however, TDM has not generally been used for monitoring the treatment of chronic infectious diseases. There is growing evidence that TDM may be useful in some circumstances to ensure HIV-infected patients have adequate blood concentrations for efficacy without producing toxicity. This may be especially true for children where there is wide variability in plasma concentrations. A number of critical questions remain to be addressed before TDM is used routinely in HIV infection.

Retrospective studies have demonstrated plasma concentrations of antiretroviral drugs correlate with antiviral activity [1–4]. It is clear that drug concentrations are an important predictor of response to HIV treatment. However, these findings are quite different than assessing the value of using TDM in the clinic to guide antiretroviral therapy for an individual.

Drugs as TDM candidates

Some antiretrovirals share many of the characteristics of drugs that require monitoring of plasma levels, including variable inter-subject pharmacokinetics, serious consequences if there is a lack of effect or drug toxicity, documented relationships between drug concentration and effect or toxicity, identification of a therapeutic range, and the availability of rapid and accurate assays.

Plasma concentrations of protease inhibitors (PIs) may vary by more than ten-fold between individuals receiving the same dose [5]. This is especially true for children who have been shown to have wide interpatient variability in pharmacokinetic parameters of protease inhibitors [6]. There is also a common misconception that boosting with ritonavir (RTV) decreases the interpatient variability. While the mean concentration has

Handbook of Pediatric HIV Care, ed. Steven L. Zeichner and Jennifer S. Read.
Published by Cambridge University Press. © Cambridge University Press 2006.

been shown to increase with RTV added, the overall variability remains high [7]. Thus, even with RTV boosting, there will likely be some patients with suboptimal plasma concentrations.

There are obvious serious consequences for patients if plasma concentrations are above or below the optimal range. Sustained low plasma concentrations will invariably lead to the development of resistance and high concentrations may result in toxicity.

The identification of a therapeutic range remains problematic. Treatment-experienced patients, infected with virus that has high, but not insurmountable levels of resistance to antiretrovirals, are likely to need much higher concentrations for an antiviral response compared to treatment-naïve patients. In addition, target concentrations may be different between patients due to demographic factors such as weight and gender.

Which antiretrovirals are candidates for TDM?

PIs and non-nucleoside reverse transcriptase inhibitors (NNRTIs) meet many of the conditions for TDM and could be monitored during therapy. There are many retrospective studies demonstrating that PI concentrations [1–4] and, more recently, NNRTI concentrations, correlate with antiviral effect [8]. The long half-life of NNRTIs combined with their generally high concentrations ensure that most patients with wild-type virus will have therapeutic concentrations even if their adherence is less than perfect. However, TDM for NNRTIs is important because the small percentage of patients with suboptimal levels are at clear risk for the rapid development of resistance and treatment failure, since a single amino acid substitution in reverse transcriptase is sufficient to render the virus highly resistant to currently available NNRTIs. This raises the dilemma of whether all patients should receive TDM to identify the small percentage who will benefit the most.

Nucleoside reverse transcriptase inhibitors (NRTIs) are actually pro-drugs that must be converted intracellularly to their active forms. Thus, the concentration in the plasma does not accurately reflect the concentration of the active moiety at the site of action. Monitoring of NRTIs is not recommended [9, 10]. However there may be certain instances such as evaluation of toxicity or adherence when assessment of plasma concentrations would be helpful.

Unique TDM issues for children

The rapid development and maturation of liver enzyme activity and renal function, combined with changes in body fat and protein, complicate the dosing of HIV-infected children and make plasma concentrations difficult to predict. There may also be differences in drug absorption between children and adults due to changes in gastric pH, gastric emptying time, or other factors. Attempts to dose children by applying pharmacokinetic data from adults have consistently shown poor results. Similarly, dosages based on pharmacokinetic data from older children may not apply to young children and infants. Clinical trials with nelfinavir and efavirenz using mg/kg doses based on adults have shown that adequate concentrations are often not achieved [11, 12]. In some cases, dosing based on BSA may be more consistent than dosing based on weight. Indinavir has also been shown to require increased doses or shorter dosing intervals in children compared to adults to achieve similar concentrations [13]. For these reasons, a consensus panel on TDM in HIV infection agreed that children represent a population that may benefit the most from TDM [14].

Clinical trials of TDM

The beneficial role of TDM in HIV clinical practice remains to be demonstrated. Over the past 5 years, a number of studies have described relationships between antiretroviral drug concentrations and antiviral effect. Results from four prospective, randomized trials of TDM in HIV-infected patients have been reported. In the ATHENA trial, data have been reported in treatment-naïve patients who were randomized to TDM or no TDM and were receiving indinavir or nelfinavir [15, 16]. Indinavir and nelfinavir doses were adjusted based on the "concentration ratio" (see "Target concentrations and plasma sampling" below). At 12 months, subjects in the TDM arms had significantly better viral load responses than the standard of care arms. Improved outcome with TDM for indinavir was primarily driven by reduced toxicity where for nelfinavir, results were primarily due to fewer virological failures in the TDM group.

Conversely, PHARMADAPT, which used trough plasma PI concentrations to modify salvage therapy, did not show a significant improvement in virologic outcomes at 12 weeks [17]. The lack of a difference may have occurred because only 22% of patients receiving TDM had a therapy modification, dosage modifications did not occur until 8 weeks into therapy, and a target concentration for wild-type virus was used.

A prospective trial in HIV-infected patients evaluated TDM of all drugs in a three-drug regimen [18]. Forty treatment-naïve patients were randomized to receive indinavir, zidovudine, and lamivudine by concentration-guided therapy or per standard fixed doses. Of 33 evaluable patients, 15 of 16 in the TDM arm and 9 of 17 in the standard dose arm had HIV RNA levels < 50 copies/ml at week 52 ($P = 0.017$).

The GENOPHAR study randomized patients failing therapy with viral load >1000 RNA copies/ml to either treatment based on genotyping or treatment based on genotyping and TDM [19]. At week 24, the genotype alone group had 34/59 (58%) patients with viral load <200 copies/ml while 40/61 (66%) of the genotype with TDM patients were undetectable ($P = $ NS).

These clinical trials demonstrate that TDM may be useful in some settings and not others. It is understandable that TDM alone could be useful in treatment-naïve patients where standard doses can achieve high enough concentrations to block replication of wild-type virus. However, in treatment-experienced patients, it is likely that some measurement of the sensitivity of the virus must be used in conjunction with drug levels for optimal treatment. The concept of a monitoring tool that incorporates both plasma concentrations and resistance testing is described below.

The IQ ratio

Recent studies have evaluated the phenotype or "virtual" phenotype used along with the plasma concentration as a potential tool to optimize drug therapy. The ratio of the Cmin (trough level) to the protein binding-adjusted IC_{50} is often called the inhibitory quotient or IQ. A number of variations in calculating the IQ have been described including the "virtual IQ" and the "normalized IQ" [20]. Both of these variations use the fold-change in the sensitivity of the virus compared to wild-type from the Virtual Phenotype[TM] (Virco) test in their equations and attempt to correct for protein binding.

Regardless of the specific equation, a number of small trials have demonstrated relationships between IQ and clinical outcome for lopinavir, amprenavir, and indinavir [21–25]. In these studies, resistance testing or drug level measurement alone was not associated with improved outcome, while IQ was predictive. These trials suggest that integration of the drug level and virus susceptibility to the drug may provide more complete information than either measurement used alone. Two large multicenter IQ trials initiated by the AIDS Clinical Trials Group (ACTG) will further evaluate the clinical utility of the IQ ratio in HIV-infected patients.

Plasma levels and toxicity

In contrast to relationships between plasma concentrations and antiviral activity, there is limited information linking drug levels with toxicity. Higher indinavir concentrations have been associated with urological complaints compared to patients with no urological adverse events [26]. A study in subjects receiving a regimen of stavudine, lamivudine, saquinavir and nelfinavir reported that abdominal pain was associated with higher plasma levels of saquinavir and nelfinavir [27]. Increased concentrations of ritonavir have also been reported to be associated with gastrointestinal complaints [28]. While these data may be intriguing, it remains difficult to use plasma concentrations to predict, avoid, or reduce toxicity. Some clinicians are willing to increase doses based on low drug levels but may be reluctant to decrease the dose if levels are high, for fear of compromising efficacy. It is also important to note that some toxicities, such as hyperlipidemia and fat redistribution, are unlikely to have a definitive dose–response relationship with plasma levels.

Table 16.1. Proposed target trough concentrations in treatment-naive patients

Drug	Concentration (ng/ml)
Protease inhibitors	
Amprenavir	150–400
Indinavir	80–120
Lopinavir/ritonavir	1000–2000
Nelfinavir	700–1000
Ritonavir	1500–2100 (full dose)
Saquinavir	100–250
Non-nucleoside reverse transcriptase inhibitors	
Efavirenz	1000–1100
Nevirapine	3400

Source: Reference [29].

Target concentrations and plasma sampling

Retrospective studies have provided some target concentrations for treatment-naïve patients [29]. Table 16.1 shows general therapeutic ranges that the clinician can use for TDM in treatment-naïve patients. For treatment-experienced patients, these concentrations are likely too low. In the experienced population, plasma concentrations should be used along with resistance testing. A simple method of using drug levels with phenotyping to guide therapy has been previously described [29].

The specific parameter to monitor, whether it be peak, trough, or area under the curve (AUC), has not been adequately defined. There appears to be general agreement that trough concentrations correlate best with antiviral effect. This seems reasonable from a biologic rationale in keeping concentrations of the antiretroviral above a threshold level throughout the dosage interval to avoid any breakthrough replication. The trough is also the easiest to collect from a practicality and feasibility standpoint. However, collection of a trough sample relies upon the patient to accurately recall the time of their last dose. Without directly observed dosing, the use of patient-recorded dosing times may lead to a trough concentration that was drawn several hours away from the true trough. Such errors clearly complicate interpretation of drug levels. A definitive study to address this question has not been performed. Data to support the use of the trough concentration for modeling also include in vivo modeling of protease inhibitors and a clinical trial of BID vs. TID indinavir [30, 31]. In this study, the BID regimen was inferior in antiviral activity and had lower trough values although the AUCs were similar between the regimens.

Another approach to TDM sampling is the concentration ratio [14]. This method compares the plasma concentration of an individual patient at any time during the dosing interval to a mean value that was determined in subjects who had extensive pharmacokinetic sampling after a directly observed dose. From this control group, a reference concentration–time curve is constructed that can be compared to a patient sample at any time after administration. For example, an individual's sample collected at 4 hours after their last dose would be compared to the mean four-hour value from the reference group. The patient's dose might be adjusted if the concentration was above or below some predetermined confidence interval of the reference value at four hours.

Pharmacokinetic modeling is another method for TDM sampling where one or more concentrations are collected at random times after a dose (i.e., two and four hours after dosing) [14]. Using a mathematical model and previous information on the drug's pharmacokinetics, the trough concentration can be estimated. This approach has an advantage in that other parameters (AUC, maximum concentration (C_{max}), plasma clearance) can also be estimated and used to guide therapy. This method can be very accurate if more than one sample is obtained. The model does require validation and pharmacokinetics expertise for calculation and interpretation. Collection of multiple samples may also be inconvenient for patients and medical staff in a busy clinic.

Problems, concerns, and unresolved issues

A number of practical and logistical challenges may limit the widespread use of TDM for antiretroviral therapy. A primary limitation of TDM is that it does not provide information on long-term adherence. A patient could not have taken their drugs correctly for weeks, but may do so for the 2 or 3 days immediately before their clinic appointment if they know a TDM sample will be taken. The drug concentration in such a patient would appear to be adequate although the patient may be failing therapy due to non-adherence. Another problem could be the upward adjustment of a dose in a patient who was non-adherent, based on low levels, and then develops subsequent toxicity when the patient starts to adhere to the new dose. A successful TDM program needs to be coupled with adherence monitoring so that plasma concentrations can be accurately interpreted.

Intrapatient variability for key pharmacokinetic parameters also appears to be large for some antiretrovirals, particularly in pediatric populations, suggesting that clinical decisions should be made only after two or more trough levels are collected and not after a single determination. Intrapatient variability may be large because concentrations can be affected by small changes in diet, time of administration, concomitant illnesses, or other unknown factors. However, intrapatient variability has been reported to be modest when these factors are controlled for, and most importantly, is smaller than interpatient variability [32].

Logistical issues cannot be ignored in the use of TDM. Currently, there are no rapid tests for antiretroviral drug levels that can be performed in the hospital or clinic. Samples must be shipped to a reference laboratory for measurement. Table 16.2 shows

Table 16.2. Commercial or academic laboratories that measure antiretroviral concentrations for individual patients

Consolidated Laboratories, Van Nuys, CA
Mayo Clinic, Rochester, MN
National Jewish Hospital, Denver, CO
Specialty Labs, Santa Monica, CA
TDM Service, University of Liverpool, UK

a number of commercial laboratories that measure concentrations of antiretrovirals for a fee. Several academic centers also perform these tests for research purposes. Accurate sample collection, timely processing, storage and shipping of plasma, and rapid turnaround times for assay results must be assured. A more important factor is the quality of the reference laboratory. Since there is no common assay method among laboratories, the clinician needs some assurance that the results being reported back are accurate. An international quality assurance program has been developed whereby participating laboratories received samples with spiked amounts of various PIs and NNRTIs [33]. Laboratories send their results back to a central site and are given a report of how well their method compared to the actual concentrations. A similar program exists for laboratories participating in ACTG trials. Clinicians should select a laboratory that participates in such a program and has demonstrated that it can produce accurate results.

Practical issues for the clinician

Adjustment of drug doses should only be performed in a thoughtful and methodical manner. The clinician should first identify the reason for the measurement. This could be an inadequate response, dose-limiting toxicity, potential drug interaction, starting a new regimen in a special population (children, pregnant women, patients with organ dysfunction), or others (Table 16.3). In general, TDM should not be used for adherence testing as the concentration only describes the patient's drug administration in the past 1–2 days.

If TDM is to be performed, the sample should be collected at steady-state which generally is at least two weeks into a new regimen. The time of the patient's last dose should be recorded and a trough sample should be collected. The sample should be sent to a TDM laboratory following the processing and shipping instructions of the specific facility.

When the patient's concentration is reported, clinicians should carefully consider several factors before adjusting the dose (Table 16.4). These include an understanding

Table 16.3. Clinical situations for TDM in HIV-infected patients

Experimental regimens
Confirm adequate concentrations in children
Confirm adequate concentrations in pregnant women
Document levels in patients with organ dysfunction
In conjunction with resistance testing in patients failing therapy (IQ ratio)
Provide additional information in patients experiencing drug toxicity
Evaluation for unknown drug interactions (mega-HAART, enzyme inducers, herbal remedies, etc.)

Table 16.4. Questions to ask before altering a dose based on a TDM result

Did the patient follow the drug's dietary restrictions?
Was the sample collected at the correct time (trough value)?
Has the patient been adherent with his/her therapy?
Was the dose observed or was the dose taken at the correct time?
Is the pill burden of the new regimen reasonable?

of the patient's adherence, the current pill burden, and the quality of the sample collection. The dosage change should not be dramatic and limited to a 15%–20% increase in the dose of the drug or the addition of a second drug such as low-dose ritonavir to optimize the pharmacokinetics. The drug level should be repeated in 2–4 weeks to evaluate the change. It is important to note that TDM in clinical practice is mainly focused on PIs, however concentrations of NNRTIs have also been reported to correlate with outcome [8].

Conclusions

There is increasing interest in TDM as a tool for improving therapy for HIV-infected patients. A number of trials have shown that TDM is both feasible and can improve outcomes, however, large randomized trials are ongoing and will provide more definitive answers. The treatment of HIV-infected patients is complicated. It is critical to understand that successful TDM programs cannot exist by themselves but must be used in conjunction with other interventions such as adherence counseling, management of adverse effects, resistance testing, and treatment of concomitant illnesses.

REFERENCES
1. Burger, D. M., Hoetelmans, R. M. W., Hugen, P. W. H. *et al.* Low plasma concentrations of indinavir are related to virological treatment failure in HIV-1 infected patients on indinavir-containing triple therapy. *Antiviral Ther.* 1998;**3**:315–320.

2. Durant, J., Clevenbergh, P., Garraffo, R. *et al.* Importance of protease inhibitor plasma levels in HIV-infected patients treated with genotypic-guided therapy: pharmacological data from the Viradapt study. *AIDS* 2000; **14**:1333–1339.

3. Hoetelmans, R. M. W., Reijers, M. H., Weverling, G. J. *et al.* The effect of plasma drug concentrations on HIV-1 clearance rate during quadruple drug therapy. *AIDS* 1998;**12**:F111–F115.

4. Schapiro, J. M., Winters, M. A., Stewart, F. *et al.* The effect of high-dose saquinavir on viral load and CD4+ T-cell counts in HIV-infected patients. *Ann. Intern. Med.* 1996;**124**:1039–1050.

5. Acosta, E. P., Henry, K., Weller, D. *et al.* Indinavir concentrations and antiviral effect. *Pharmacotherapy* 1999;**19**:708–712.

6. Acosta, E. P., Nachman, S., Wiznia, A. *et al.* Pharmacokinetic evaluation of nelfinavir in combination with nevirapine or ritonavir in HIV infected children. *In 40th Interscience Conference on Antimicrobial Agents and Chemotherapy*, Toronto, Canada, September 17–20, 2000 [Abstract 1642].

7. Gibbons, E. S., Reynolds, H. E., Tija, J. F. *et al.* The Liverpool therapeutic drug monitoring service – a summary of the service and examples of use in clinical practice. 5th International Congress on Drug Therapy in HIV infection. *AIDS* 2000; **14**(Suppl 4):S89.

8. Marzolini, C., Telenti, A., Decosterd, L. A. *et al.* Efavirenz plasma levels can predict treatment failure and central nervous system side effects in HIV-1-infected patients. *AIDS* 2001;**15**:71–75.

9. Drusano, G. L., Yuen, G. J., Lambert, J. S., Seidlin, M., Dolin, R., Valentine, F. T. Relationship between dideoxyinosine exposure, CD4 counts, and p24 antigen levels in human immunodeficiency virus infection. *A phase I trial. Ann. Intern. Med.*. 1992; Apr 1;**116**: 562–566.

10. Hoetelmans, R. M., Burger, D. M., Meenhorst, P. L., Beijnen, J. H. Pharmacokinetic individualisation of zidovudine therapy. Current state of pharmacokinetic-pharmacodynamic relationships. *Clin. Pharmacokinet.* 1996;**30**:314–327.

11. Brundage, R. C., Fletcher, C. V., Fenton, T. *et al.* Efavirenz and nelfinavir pharmacokinetics in HIV infected children under 2 years of age. *In 7th Conference on Retroviruses and Opportunistic Infections.* San Francisco, CA, February 2000 [Abstract 719].

12. Rongkavilit, C., Van Heeswijk, R. P. G., Risuwanna, P. *et al.* The safety and pharmacokinetics of nelfinavir in a dose escalating study in HIV-1 exposed newborn infants. HIV-NAT 007. *In 2nd International Workshop on Clinical Pharmacology of HIV Therapy*. Nordwijk, the Netherlands, April 2001 [Abstract 3.1].

13. Fletcher, C. V., Brundage, R. C., Remmel, R. P. *et al.* Pharmacological characteristics of indinavir, didanosine, and stavudine in human immunodefiency infected children receiving combination therapy. *Antimicrob. Agents Chemother*. 2000;**44**:1029–1034.

14. Back, D., Gatti, G., Fletcher, C. *et al.* Therapeutic drug monitoring in HIV infection: current status and future directions. *AIDS* 2002; **16**(Suppl. 1):S5–S37.

15. Burger, D. M., Hugen, P. W. H., Droste, J. *et al.* Therapeutic drug monitoring of indinavir in treatment naïve patients improves therapeutic outcome after 1 year: results from ATHENA. *In 2nd International Workshop on Clinical Pharmacology of HIV Therapy*, Noordwijk, the Netherlands, April 2–4, 2001 [Abstract 6.2a].

16. Burger, D. M., Hugen, P. W. H., Droste, J. *et al.* Therapeutic drug monitoring of nelfinavir 1250 bid in treatment naïve patients improves therapeutic outcome after 1 year: results

from ATHENA. *In 2nd International Workshop on Clinical Pharmacology of HIV Therapy*, Noordwijk, the Netherlands, April 2–4, 2001 [Abstract 6.2b].

17. Clevenbergh, P., Durant, J., Garraffo, R. *et al.* Usefulness of protease inhibitor therapeutic drug monitoring? PharmAdapt: A prospective multicentric randomized controlled trial: 12 week results. *In 8th Conference on Retroviruses and Opportunistic Infections*. Chicago, IL, Feb 4–8, 2001 [Abstract 260B].

18. Fletcher, C. V., Anderson, P. L., Kakuda, T. N. *et al.* Concentration-controlled compared with conventional antiretroviral therapy for HIV infection. *AIDS* 2002; **16**:551–560.

19. Bossi, P., Peytavin, G., Delaugerre, C. *et al.* GENOPHAR: a randomized study of plasmatic drug measurements associated with genotypic resistance testing in patients failing antiretroviral therapy. *In 9th Conference on Retroviruses and Opportunistic Infections*. Seattle, WA, February 24–27, 2002 [Abstract 585-T].

20. Piscitelli, S. C. The role of therapeutic drug monitoring in the management of HIV-infected patients. *Curr. Infect. Dis. Rep.* 2002;**4**:353–358.

21. Kempf, D., Hsu, A., Isaacson, J. *et al.* Evaluation of the inhibitory quotient as a pharmacodynamic predictor of the virological response to protease inhibitor therapy. *In 2nd International Workshop on Clinical Pharmacology of HIV Infection*. Noordwijk, the Netherlands, April 2–4, 2001 [Abstract 7.3].

22. Kempf, D., Hsu, A., Jiang, P. *et al.* Response to ritonavir intensification in indinavir recipients is highly correlated with inhibitory quotient. *In 8th Conference on Retroviruses and Opportunistic Infections*. Chicago, IL, February 4–8, 2001 [Abstract 523].

23. Phillips, E., Tseng, A., Walker, S. *et al.* The use of virtual inhibitory quotient in antiretroviral experienced patients taking amprenavir/lopinavir combinations. *In 9th Conference on Retroviruses and Opportunistic Infections*. Seattle, WA, February 24–28, 2002 [Aabstract 130].

24. Piscitelli, S. C., Metcalf, J. A., Hoetelmans, R. H. *et al.* Relative inhibitory quotient is a significant predictor of outcome for salvage therapy with amprenavir plus either ritonavir or nelfinavir plus amprenavir. *In 8th ECAAC*, Athens, Greece, 2002.

25. Castagna, A., Danise, A., Hasson, H. *et al.* The normalized inhibitory quotient of lopinavir is predictive of viral load response over 48 weeks in a cohort of highly experienced HIV-1 infected individuals. *In 9th Conference on Retroviruses and Opportunistic Infections*. Seattle, WA, February 24–28, 2002 [Abstract].

26. Dieleman, J. P., Gyssens, I. C., van der Ende. *et al.* Urological complaints in relation to indinavir plasma concentrations in HIV-infected patients. *AIDS* 1999; **13**:473–478.

27. Reijers, M. H., Weigel, H. M., Hart, A. A. *et al.* Toxicity and drug exposure in a quadruple drug regimen in HIV-1 infected patients participating in the ADAM study. *AIDS* 2000; **14**:59–67.

28. Gatti, G., Di Biagio A., Casazza, R. *et al.* The relationship between ritonavir plasma levels and side-effects: implications for therapeutic drug monitoring. *AIDS* 1999;**13**:2083–2089.

29. Acosta, E. P., Gerber, J. G. Position paper on therapeutic drug monitoring of antiretroviral agents. *AIDS Res. Hum. Retrovirus* 2002;**18**:825–834.

30. Drusano, G., D'Aregenio, D., Preston, S. *et al.* Use of drug effect interaction modelling with Monte Carlo Simulation to examine the impact of dosing interval on the projected antiviral activity of the combination abacavir and amprenavir. *Antimicrob. Agents Chemother.* 2000; **44**:1655–1659.

31. Haas, D. W., Arathoon, E., Thompson, M. A. *et al.* Comparative studies of two-times daily versus three times daily indinavir in combination with zidovudine and lamivudine. *AIDS* 2000; **14**: 1973–1978.

32. Acosta, E. P., Kakuda, T. N., Brundage, R. C. *et al.* Pharmacodynamics of human immunodeficiency virus type 1 protease inhibitors. *Clin. Infect. Dis.* 2000;**30** (Suppl. 2):S151–S159.

33. Aarnouste, R., Burger, D., Verweij-Van Wissen, C. *et al.* An international interlaboratory quality control program for therapeutic drug monitoring in HIV infection. *8th Conference on Retroviruses and Opportunistic Infections.* Chicago, IL, February 4–8, 2001 [Abstract 734].

17 HIV postexposure prophylaxis for pediatric patients

Peter L. Havens, M.S., M.D.

Medical College of Wisconsin and MACC Fund Research Center, Milwaukee, WI

Kenneth L. Dominguez, M.D., M.P.H.

Division of HIV/AIDS Prevention, Centers for Disease Control and Prevention, Atlanta, GA

Acknowledgment: Modified from *Pediatrics* volume 111, pages 1475–1489, Copyright 2003 with permission of the publisher.

Introduction

This chapter addresses HIV postexposure prophylaxis (PEP) in the following situations: injury from discarded needles, bite wounds, sexual exposure, and inadvertent exposure to human milk from an HIV-infected woman. In each setting, the risk of HIV transmission is directly related to the probability that the exposure source has HIV infection and that transmission of a sufficient amount of infectious virus occurred in a manner that could result in infection in the recipient. Because no studies have directly measured the effectiveness of PEP in decreasing the risk of HIV transmission in non-occupational settings or after mucosal exposure, the potential benefit of PEP in modifying transmission risk is extrapolated from data regarding HIV pathogenesis in animals, from information about PEP for needle-stick injuries in occupational settings, and from studies of mother-to-child transmission (MTCT) of HIV. Guidelines for prophylaxis after exposure to HIV in occupational and non-occupational settings have been published by the US Public Health Service (USPHS) [1–3], the American Academy of Pediatrics [4], the NY State Department of Health [5], and others [6].

Factors affecting HIV transmission risk after potential exposure

Type of source material

Not all body fluids from persons with HIV infection are equally infectious (Table 17.1). Blood and fluids contaminated with blood from persons with HIV infection are assumed to contain HIV and are associated with the highest risk of HIV transmission.

Handbook of Pediatric HIV Care, ed. Steven L. Zeichner and Jennifer S. Read.
Published by Cambridge University Press. © Cambridge University Press 2006.

Table 17.1. Materials from persons with HIV infection that could contain HIV [1]

Usually infectious materials[a]	Other potentially infectious material[b]	Usually non-infectious materials
Concentrated HIV in a laboratory specimen	Semen	Saliva
Blood[b]	Vaginal secretions	Urine
Fluid contaminated with blood	Cerebrospinal fluid	Feces
	Synovial fluid	Tears
	Pleural fluid	Sweat
	Peritoneal fluid	Vomitus
	Pericardial fluid	Nasal secretions
	Amniotic fluid	Sputum
	Human milk	
	Unfixed body tissue	

[a] Most likely to be associated with a risk of HIV transmission.

[b] May contain HIV, but less likely to be associated with risk of HIV transmission.

Exposure to other potentially infectious materials (Table 17.1) is associated with a lower risk of HIV transmission. Blood-free saliva, urine, feces (including diarrhea), and vomitus are highly unlikely to transmit HIV.

Volume of source material

Exposure to a large volume of infectious material carries a greater risk of HIV transmission than does exposure to a smaller volume. Injuries with large-gauge, hollow-bore needles are 14 times more likely to result in HIV transmission as injuries with smaller-gauge, hollow needles, solid suture needles, or solid objects such as a scalpel [7].

Concentration of virus in source material

Percutaneous exposure to blood from a person with late-stage HIV infection (presumably with high plasma virus load) increases transmission risk by more than fivefold (Table 17.2). Per heterosexual act for persons 15 to 24 years of age, the risk of HIV transmission varies from 0.01% at viral loads <1700 copies/ml to 0.3% at viral loads >38 500 copies/ml [8]. Maternal HIV viral load is important in determining the risk of MTCT [9, 10]. While treatment with antiretroviral drugs can decrease the concentration of virus in blood and body fluids, HIV transmission has occurred after exposure to blood or infectious body fluids from HIV-infected persons with plasma viral loads below the level of detection, perhaps from cell-associated virus [11]. Although there is a correlation between plasma and genital viral load, HIV may be detected in genital secretions even when undetectable in plasma [12].

Table 17.2. Percutaneous exposure to blood infected with HIV: risk factors for HIV transmission [7]

Risk factor	Adjusted odds ratio[a]	95% confidence interval
Deep injury	15	6.0–41
Visible blood on device	6.2	2.2–21
Procedure involving needle in artery or vein	4.3	1.7–12
Terminal illness in source patient	5.6	2.0–16
Postexposure use of zidovudine	0.19	0.06–0.52

[a] Based on logistic regression analysis of 33 case patients and 665 controls reported by national surveillance systems in France, Italy, the UK, and the USA.

Viability of virus in source material

Most syringes will not contain HIV even after being used to draw blood from a person with HIV infection. HIV RNA was detected in only 3.8% of 80 discarded disposable syringes that had been used by healthcare professionals for intramuscular or subcutaneous injection of patients with HIV [13]. When HIV is exposed to air, the 50% tissue culture infective dose decreases by one log every 9 hours [14]. In the laboratory setting, HIV has been shown to survive for up to 28 days in syringes containing as little as 20 µl of blood [15]. However, HIV proviral DNA could not be found in 28 syringes discarded in public places and in 10 syringes from a needle exchange program for injection drug users [16]. Two small studies have found no evidence of HIV transmission after injuries from needles of discarded syringes [17, 18]. There have been no confirmed reports of HIV acquisition from percutaneous injury by a needle found in the community [4].

Type of contact (Table 17.3)

Blood transfusion from an HIV-infected donor carries a 95% risk of HIV transmission [19]. The risk of MTCT of HIV is between 13% and 45% in the absence of interventions to prevent such transmission [20]. Needle sharing in the context of injection drug use is estimated to have a transmission probability of 0.67% per injection [21]. Sharp percutaneous exposure (needle stick, scalpel) to blood infected with HIV is associated with a transmission risk of 0.32% (95% CI: 0.20%–0.50%) [7, 22, 23]. The risk of HIV transmission from unprotected sexual exposure is highest with receptive anal intercourse (0.5%–3.2%), intermediate with receptive vaginal intercourse (0.05%–0.15%), and lowest for insertive vaginal intercourse (0.03% to 0.09%) [24–29]. The per-act risk of HIV transmission from oral sex is not known, although HIV rarely has been transmitted from orogenital sexual exposure [30–36]. The per-episode risk of HIV transmission from a single exposure of a child to human milk is estimated at approximately 0.004% to 0.006% [37]. There are no reports of HIV transmission from a single episode of exposure to HIV-infected human milk in a healthcare professional handling human milk [38].

Table 17.3. Type of exposure and risk of HIV transmission per exposure event when the source is HIV-infected [4]

Type of HIV exposure	Risk of transmission (%)
Blood transfusion [19]	95
Perinatal exposure [20]	13–45
Needle sharing (injection drug use) [21]	0.67
Needle stick (health care professional) [7, 22–23]	0.32
Unprotected receptive anal intercourse [8, 25, 27–29]	0.5–3.2
Unprotected receptive vaginal intercourse [25, 26]	0.05–0.15
Unprotected insertive vaginal intercourse [25, 26]	0.03–0.09
Ingestion of human milk [37]	0.004–0.006

Transmission of HIV by human bites has been described [39–42], although such transmission seems to be extremely rare, even when saliva is contaminated with the biter's blood [38], perhaps because saliva inhibits HIV infectivity [43].

Risk of HIV transmission after mucous membrane exposure is low, probably near 0.1% or less [44–46]. Transmission has occurred after contact between blood and non-intact skin (eczema, abrasions, etc.), but infectious blood in contact with intact skin has not been reported to result in HIV transmission and is not considered an exposure with risk of transmission [1].

Rationale for PEP to prevent HIV transmission

During acute HIV infection, the viral doubling time is approximately 10 hours, and approximately 19 newly infected cells will develop from each HIV-infected cell [47], so within 48 hours of infection, there will be $>1.3 \times 10^6$ HIV-infected cells. Therefore, it follows that early administration of potent antiretroviral drugs would be important for successful PEP [48].

Animal models of PEP

In animals, antiretroviral therapy initiated after virus inoculation can prevent or ameliorate infection when drugs of adequate potency are administered immediately [49] or within a few hours of exposure [50–52] and continued for a few days [53] to weeks [54, 55]. PEP was most effective if begun immediately or within 24 to 36 hours of HIV exposure [56, 57], and had less or no benefit if begun after 72 hours [57, 58]. Animals developing HIV infection despite receiving PEP may have evidence of infection delayed for up to 16 weeks after virus inoculation [57]. However, even potent therapy may not be able to prevent transmission if the virus inoculum is high [55, 59, 60]. PEP in animals is most efficacious when continued for 28 days, compared with shorter durations

[56], suggesting that "prophylactic" therapy is modifying, and not preventing, primary infection [61, 62], allowing the host to eliminate HIV early in infection. The development of a cellular immune response in HIV-exposed but ultimately uninfected animals [63–65] and humans [66–68] lends further support to this concept. If these regimens for prophylaxis are truly acting to abort early HIV infection, then antiretroviral regimens chosen for prophylaxis should be similar to those that have been shown to be effective for treatment of established HIV infection.

Prevention of MTCT of HIV as a model of PEP

Single drug antiretroviral prophylaxis regimens are efficacious in preventing MTCT of HIV [69, 70]. Receipt of dual- and triple-drug regimens is associated with lower risks of transmission compared to receipt of single-drug regimens or no antiretroviral drugs [71]. Among infants born to HIV-infected women without antepartum or intrapartum receipt of zidovudine, initiation of postnatal zidovudine prophylaxis within 12 to 24 hours after birth and continued for 6 weeks has been associated with a lower rate of MTCT of HIV [72, 73].

PEP: potential for failure

Although postexposure zidovudine treatment of HIV-exposed healthcare professionals was associated with an 81% lower risk of HIV transmission [7], failures have occurred [74]. Such failures may result from large inoculum size [75], late institution of therapy or failure to take prescribed therapy [76], transmission of zidovudine-resistant virus [77], or other as yet unidentified factors [2].

Although the feasibility of prophylaxis after non-occupational exposure to HIV has been demonstrated [78], there are no data regarding the efficacy or effectiveness of PEP in the non-occupational setting, even though this therapy is being offered in various communities [79]. Failures of such prophylaxis have been reported [80], as have apparent successes [48]. The theoretic concern that offering PEP to sexually active persons would increase risk-taking behavior has not been observed in practice [81]. However, the cost of prophylaxis after non-occupational exposures is high [82], and adverse effects are relatively common [83] and can, rarely, be fatal [2, 84].

Recommendation for prophylaxis after non-occupational exposure to HIV in pediatric patients

The risk of HIV transmission after an exposure varies by the type and severity of exposure (Tables 17.1–17.3) and by the likelihood that the source is infected with HIV (Table 17.4). Evaluation of the type of exposure and the exposure fluid (Table 17.1) allows for estimation of the risk of HIV transmission after a potential exposure (Table 17.5). PEP should not be used for persons with HIV exposures that have a low risk of HIV transmission, or for persons who seek care too late for the anticipated interruption of transmission (>72 hours after reported exposure; Table 17.6). While PEP can be considered for exposures to material from persons with unknown HIV infection status,

Table 17.4. Characteristics of the exposure source and risk of HIV transmission [4]

HIV infection status of exposure source	Risk of HIV transmission
Not HIV-infected Known not to be infected with HIV[a]	No risk
HIV status unknown/unknown source HIV infection status unknown, HIV risk status unknown	Not quantified

HIV status unknown: low risk
    HIV infection status unknown, but known not to have risk
        factors[b]
	Low

HIV status unknown: high risk
    HIV infection status unknown but known to have one or
        more risk factors[b]
	Intermediate

HIV-infected Known to be infected with HIV[c]	High

[a] HIV infection is documented by presence of specific antibody to HIV in persons older than 18 months and by positive plasma HIV RNA polymerase chain reaction (PCR) assay results, positive cell-associated HIV DNA PCR assay results, or detection of plasma HIV p24 antigen in persons of any age.

[b] Risk factors for HIV infection include male homosexual activity, injection drug use, blood transfusion or blood product infusion before 1985, or sexual activity with a member of a high-risk group. Some persons who have sex with members of a high-risk group do not identify themselves as at risk, because they are unaware of the risk history of their sexual partner. Their risk of HIV infection is related to the prevalence of HIV infection in their immediate community.

[c] Absence of HIV infection is identified by laboratory documentation of negative HIV antibody or negative HIV DNA PCR assay results from a specimen collected close to the time of the exposure and in the absence of interval high-risk behavior or symptoms compatible with acute retroviral infection syndrome.

PEP is only recommended for exposures to material from persons with HIV infection (Table 17.7), so efforts should be made to learn the infection status of the exposure source. Benefits of PEP likely are restricted to situations in which the risk of transmission is high, the intervention can be initiated promptly, and adherence to the regimen is likely. In individual cases of potential exposure, the perceived risks of HIV acquisition may be great enough to justify the burden and potential toxicity of PEP. The final decision to undertake PEP in a specific patient depends on the clinician's recommendation and the exposed person's and/or parent's evaluation of the risk of transmission versus the toxicity and burden of therapy. A careful discussion of the risks and benefits of therapy guides the decision making regarding PEP and allows appropriate postexposure care (Table 17.8). If PEP is begun, it should be started as soon as possible after the exposure (within hours, and definitely within 72 hours), and therapy should be continued

Table 17.5. Exposure type and exposure risk category for HIV [4]

Exposure type	Exposure risk category
Cutaneous exposure	
Fluid on intact skin	No risk identified
Bite without break in skin	
Skin with compromised integrity (eczema, chapped skin, dermatitis, abrasion, laceration, open wound)	Low to intermediate
Traumatic skin wound with bleeding in donor and recipient[a]	High
Mucous membrane exposure	
Kissing	No risk identified
Oral sex	
Human milk: single ingestion	Low
Splash to eye or mouth	
Receptive vaginal sex without trauma	Intermediate
Receptive anal intercourse	
Traumatic sex with blood (sexual assault)	High
Percutaneous exposure[b]	
Superficial scratch with sharp object, including a needle found in the community	No risk identified
Puncture wound with solid needle	
Puncture wound with hollow needle without visible blood	Low
Body piercing	
Bite with break in skin	
Puncture wound with hollow needle with visible blood	Intermediate
Puncture wound with large-bore hollow needle with visible blood on needle, or needle recently used in source patient artery or vein	High

[a] For example, in a fight, a blow to the mouth might break a tooth that bleeds and lacerate the fist that also bleeds. If there was mixing of blood, both persons may be at risk.

[b] See text for considerations used in assigning the appropriate risk category for a percutaneous exposure.

for 28 days. If consultation with a clinician experienced in the care of children and adolescents with HIV is not immediately possible, a supply of medications sufficient to last until consultation occurs could be dispensed to the patient.

Sexual exposure

HIV infection is sexually transmitted, and sexual abuse is a recognized mode of transmission of HIV to children [85]. Sexual abuse may be more likely to result in HIV transmission in girls than in women because of thin vaginal epithelium in children and cervical ectopy in adolescents, and because children may be repeatedly abused by the same person over a long period [38]. In proven cases of sexual assault by a person

Table 17.6. Suggested approach to HIV postexposure prophylaxis (PEP) on the basis of characteristics of the exposed patient [4][a]

Characteristics of exposed patient	Suggested approach
Exposure >72 hours ago; or	No PEP
Exposed person refuses PEP; or	
Exposed person unwilling or unable to commit to 28 days of therapy and appropriate follow-up.	
Exposure ≤72 hours ago; and	Consider PEP in appropriate exposure setting (Tables 17.5 and 17.7)
Exposed person voluntarily accepts PEP; and	
Exposed person commits to 28 days of therapy and appropriate follow-up.	

[a] Animal data suggest PEP started later than 72 hours after exposure is less effective in preventing infection [56–58].

Table 17.7. Suggested approach[a] to postexposure prophylaxis (PEP) on the basis of exposure risk category and HIV infection status of the source [4]

Exposure risk category[b]	HIV infection status of source[c]	Suggested approach
No risk identified	Any	No PEP
Any	Not HIV-infected	No PEP
Low, intermediate, or high	Unknown	Consider PEP
Low or intermediate risk	HIV-infected	Consider PEP
High risk	HIV-infected	Recommend PEP

[a] PEP is not recommended if the exposure occurred >72 hours ago, the exposed person refuses PEP, or if the exposed person is unwilling or unable to commit to 28 days of therapy and appropriate follow-up (Table 17.6). When considering PEP, the approach is suggested on the basis of type and severity of exposure, fluid involved, and HIV infection status of the exposure source, as outlined in Tables 17.1–17.4. Characteristics of the exposed patient are also considered, as described here and in the text. Given the absence of compelling data on effectiveness of PEP, clinicians may make different, reasonable, decisions in similar clinical circumstances.
[b] See Table 17.5.
[c] See Table 17.4.

known or suspected to have HIV infection, PEP may be considered up to 72 hours after the exposure but is likely to be most effective if given sooner, preferably within a few hours after exposure [86, 87]. If the exposure source has genital ulcer disease or another sexually transmitted infection or if the exposure included tissue damage, the risk of HIV transmission is greater [36], increasing the potential benefit of PEP relative to the

Table 17.8. Management of patients with possible exposure to HIV [4]

Exposure management issue	Implementation comment
Treat exposure site	Wash wounds with soap and water; flush mucous membranes with water. Give tetanus booster if appropriate.
Evaluate exposure source if possible	Determine the HIV infection status of the exposure source. If unknown, testing with appropriate consent should be offered if possible.
Evaluate exposed person	– Perform HIV serologic testing to identify current HIV infection – Provide or refer for counseling to address stress and anxiety – Discuss prevention of potential secondary HIV transmission – Discuss prevention of repeat exposure, if appropriate – Report incident to legal or administrative authorities as appropriate to the setting of the exposure and the severity of the incident
Consider postexposure prophylaxis	– Explain potential benefits and risks – Discuss issues of drug toxicity and medication compliance – Measure complete blood cell count, creatinine, and alanine transaminase (ALT) concentration as baseline for possible drug toxicity – Begin prophylaxis as soon as possible after exposure, preferably within 1 to 4 hours; prophylaxis begun more than 72 hours after exposure is unlikely to be effective – Arrange for follow-up with HIV specialist and psychologist, if appropriate – Educate about prevention of secondary transmission (sexually active adolescent should avoid sex, or use condoms, until all follow-up test results are negative) – Report to PEP registry at Centers for Disease Control and Prevention
Choose therapy	– Consider drug potency and toxicity, regimen complexity and effects on compliance, and possibility of drug resistance in the exposure source. Supply 3–5 days of medication immediately, instructing patients to obtain remainder of medication at follow-up visit

Table 17.8. (*cont.*)

Follow-up	– Perform initial follow-up within 2–3 days to review drug regimen and adherence, evaluate for symptoms of drug toxicity, assess psychosocial status, and arrange appropriate referrals, if needed
	– Continue therapy for 28 days
	– Monitor for drug adverse effects at 4 weeks with complete blood cell count and alanine transaminase concentration
	– Evaluate for psychological stress and medication compliance with weekly office visits or telephone calls
	– Consider referral for counseling if needed
	Repeat HIV serologic testing at 6 weeks, 12 weeks, and 6 months after exposure [103, 104]

burden of therapy and risks of drug toxicity. Such modifying factors might strengthen the force of the recommendation in a given clinical setting.

For adolescents with a history of a single sexual exposure, PEP can be considered, and, if given, should be started as soon as possible after the exposure but certainly within 72 hours [88, 89]. Such exposure might occur from sexual abuse or by accidental exposure in a consensual relationship (e.g., a broken condom). For persons with ongoing consensual sexual exposure to HIV, PEP is not indicated, and behavioral interventions to decrease repeated exposure probably are more appropriate [90].

Percutaneous exposures

The risk of HIV transmission from a puncture wound from a needle found in the community is significantly lower than the estimated 0.32% HIV transmission risk after needle stick injury in a healthcare professional from a person with HIV infection (Table 17.3). Although it is unlikely that a true estimate of risk can be established, transmission will be related to the factors previously outlined in the text and in Tables 17.2 and 17.4.

In evaluating a puncture wound, the following factors are considered in assessing the potential for HIV transmission (less risk, greater risk): the depth of the wound (superficial scratch, deep puncture); the presence of blood on the needle (no visible blood, visible blood); the characteristics of the blood on the needle (dried, fresh); the type of needle (solid bore, hollow bore); and the location in which the needle was used in the source patient's body (not in artery or vein, in artery or vein). The risk of HIV transmission from a discarded needle in public places (often referred to as a "found" needle) seems to be low, and such transmission has not been reported to CDC. Therefore, PEP is not routinely recommended in this situation [4]. However, if the needle and/or syringe are found to have visible blood and the source is known to be HIV-infected, PEP might be considered. Testing the syringe for HIV is not practical or reliable and is not recommended [4].

Bite wounds are another percutaneous body fluid exposure that may occur in children, but the risk of HIV transmission after exposure to saliva is very low. In the absence of blood in saliva and blood in the bite wound, PEP is not indicated. However, if there is blood exchange from a bite, both the person bitten and the person biting should be considered at risk of transmission of HIV and considered for PEP [4]. Use in this setting would be extremely unusual and is potentially indicated only when there is significant exposure to deep, bloody wounds in persons with HIV infection.

Adolescents may be percutaneously exposed to potentially infectious fluids by needle sharing for injection drug use (including anabolic steroids) or for body piercing. The per-contact probabilities of HIV transmission in Table 17.3 apply in this setting, and for a single percutaneous exposure to blood of a person at risk for or known to have HIV infection, PEP can be considered. For adolescents with ongoing needle sharing and potential exposure to HIV, PEP is not routinely recommended, and behavioral interventions to decrease repeated exposures are more appropriate than is postexposure drug therapy after a single episode [90].

Human milk exposures

Because HIV can be transmitted via human milk, even a single exposure to human milk should be considered to confer a potential (albeit very low) risk of HIV transmission (Table 17.3). Such exposure is possible in a hospital if stored, unpasteurized human milk is given to the wrong infant or if an infant is accidentally breastfed by a woman with HIV infection who is not the child's mother. Exposure also could occur if a mother developed HIV infection while breastfeeding or if a breastfeeding mother with established HIV infection breastfed her child (e.g., if she was unaware of her HIV infection status). However, in most areas of the USA, the prevalence of HIV infection in pregnant women is less than 2 per 1000 [91]. Most breastfeeding women will have been tested for HIV during pregnancy [92], and women known to be HIV-infected will have been counseled not to breastfeed [93]. Therefore, the actual likelihood that exposure to HIV would occur by this route is extremely low in the USA.

For women with known HIV infection, the best approach to preventing transmission is to avoid breastfeeding. For a woman who continues to breastfeed, potent antiretroviral therapy for herself could decrease viral load and therefore decrease the risk of MTCT. Prolonged therapy in an infant so exposed is of unknown benefit, but is being evaluated in several clinical trials (see Chapter 4). For an infant with a single exposure to human milk from a woman with HIV infection, the magnitude of risk is estimated to be approximately 100 times lower than that for other mucous membrane exposures (Table 17.3), and PEP is likely not warranted (Tables 17.5–17.7) [4].

Choice of antiretroviral medications for PEP

No clinical studies are available to determine the best antiretroviral regimen for PEP. The most extensive data in terms of potential efficacy and safety are for zidovudine monotherapy [7, 72]. However, if the efficacy of PEP is in aborting early mucosal, submucosal, subcutaneous, or lymphatic HIV infection, then potent three-drug suppressive therapies, such as two nucleoside analogue reverse transcriptase inhibitors

(NRTIs) with a protease inhibitor (PI), should be used, because such regimens have been shown to be more likely to suppress HIV replication than have monotherapy or dual therapy. The effectiveness of a drug regimen in practice will be related to the efficacy of the drugs and the probability of completion of the course of therapy, and the improved ease of use and potentially lower toxicity of a two-drug regimen may balance out the theoretically higher efficacy of three-drug PEP, favoring the use of two drugs instead of three in select circumstances.

The US PHS recommends two (zidovudine and lamivudine) or three (zidovudine, lamivudine, and either nelfinavir mesylate or indinavir sulfate) drugs for PEP in the occupational setting, with the choice of regimen based on the assessment of risk of HIV transmission [1–3]. The American Academy of Pediatrics [4] generally recommends a three-drug regimen (zidovudine, lamivudine, and nelfinavir mesylate) for PEP, but is permissive of PEP with two drugs in select circumstances. The New York State AIDS Institute guidelines [5] recommend a three-drug regimen for PEP in pediatric patients (zidovudine, lamivudine, and nelfinavir mesylate). (See Formulary Appendix 1 for doses – of antiretroviral drugs.) If current and/or previous therapy used by the source patient is known and drug resistance is a concern, alternatives to the standard regimen could be considered in consultation with a specialist in the care of HIV-infected pediatric patients.

Prophylaxis with zidovudine alone or in combination with other drugs was associated with at least one adverse effect in 49% of 674 healthcare professionals treated after occupational exposure to HIV, and 20% stopped prophylaxis prematurely because of adverse effects [94]. Adverse effects can be severe, including potentially fatal lactic acidosis and hepatitis from mitochondrial toxicity of NRTIs [95] and fatal hypersensitivity reactions from nevirapine [84]. Concern about adverse effects may contribute to low initiation rates for PEP [96], and premature cessation of prophylaxis may occur because of difficulty in adhering to complex drug regimens [97] (see Chapter 7), problems with drug toxicity (see Chapters 11 and 13), or other factors [87, 98–100].

If alternative antiretroviral drugs must be considered, ease of administration and potential toxicity should be considered.

NRTIs

Stavudine or didanosine are reasonable alternative NRTIs for use if resistance to zidovudine or lamivudine is suspected. Zidovudine and stavudine should never be used in combination with one another because of intracellular antagonism. Because of the potential for a severe hypersensitivity reaction, abacavir sulfate should be avoided in PEP regimens.

PIs

Indinavir is associated with crystalluria and nephrolithiasis, and requires extra hydration and for these reasons is usually avoided for PEP in children and adolescents. Gastrointestinal intolerance may be a problem with ritonavir and lopinavir/ritonavir.

The liquid formulation of amprenavir has high levels of vitamin E, contains propylene glycol in a concentration that exceeds World Health Organization standards for use in infants, and should not be used in children under four years of age; therefore, it is not recommended for routine use in PEP regimens. PIs have multiple potential interactions with other drugs (see Chapter 12).

NNRTIs

Nevirapine has been associated with severe life-threatening cases of hepatotoxicity, including liver failure and death in patients receiving nevirapine as part of a PEP regimen or as treatment of HIV infection, and nevirapine should not be used as part of a PEP regimen [84, 101].

Implementation and follow-up [4]

Key components of the initial management of a pediatric PEP patient include rapid assessment of the patient and rapid PEP administration, ascertainment of the HIV infection status of the exposure source, and wound care. Because of the need to begin HIV PEP as quickly as possible after an exposure, office or clinic staff should be instructed to act immediately on telephone calls concerning possible HIV exposure, and the clinician should not wait until the end of the clinic day to return a call. Such staff education might be incorporated into OSHA-mandated bloodborne pathogen training. Emergency departments should have protocols concerning possible need for HIV PEP, and a "starter kit" of three days of antiretroviral medicines should be available at all times to ensure immediate institution of PEP. A discussion of risks and benefits of PEP with the family of an exposed toddler will differ from the discussion with a potentially exposed adolescent, whose family may be specifically excluded from knowledge of the whole event. Treating adolescents in this setting should follow state and local laws regarding confidentiality of medical care. The HIV infection status of the exposure source should be sought. If the source person is known but their HIV status unknown, then HIV testing with appropriate counseling and consent should be requested. Testing for hepatitis B and hepatitis C should be performed as appropriate, following standard guidelines [102]. Wounds should be washed completely with soap and water. Mucous membranes should be flushed with water or saline solution. Administration of a tetanus booster and other wound care should be provided as needed (Table 17.8).

After PEP is initiated, careful follow-up is crucial to ensure that the rest of the medications can be obtained easily and that consultation with a specialist in pediatric and adolescent HIV care occurs, to monitor toxicity, and to provide support for medication adherence and psychological stress. Initial follow-up is recommended within two to three days to assess adherence, to evaluate for drug toxicity, to assess the psychosocial status of the pediatric patient and his/her and family, and to arrange appropriate referrals if needed. To support patient adherence to medications, visits to the clinician's office/clinic or patient–clinician telephone calls should occur at weekly intervals. If local experts in the use of antiretroviral agents in children are unavailable for consultation, the University of California–San Francisco has a hot line (1-888-HIV-4911), supported by the CDC and the Health Resources and Services Administration, and that is staffed 24 hours a day to help clinicians through the decision pathways and to provide information on choice of therapy.

Laboratory testing for drug toxicity should be performed at baseline and two weeks (optional) and four weeks after starting therapy, and at a minimum should include complete blood cell count and an alanine transaminase concentration. Persons treated with indinavir should be monitored for hematuria because of the risk of nephrolithiasis. Careful attention needs to be paid to complaints of abdominal pain, which might prompt evaluation for pancreatitis. Monitoring for seroconversion to HIV includes testing for HIV by enzyme immunoassay, indicated at baseline and at six weeks, at 12 weeks, and at six months after exposure. Such diagnostic testing will identify most persons who develop HIV infection after an exposure, although a small fraction of infected persons may not develop detectable antibody until more than six months after exposure [103, 104], and testing also could be performed 12 months after the potential exposure.

In a significant exposure, the person at risk of HIV acquisition also becomes a potential source of HIV transmission to others. This needs to be discussed, and methods of preventing possible secondary transmission of HIV should be outlined, including abstinence or use of condoms for sexually active adolescents. The potential for acquisition of HIV infection can lead to psychological stress, which may require intensive counseling during the immediate postexposure period and until follow-up testing is negative six months after the exposure. In selected instances of possible HIV exposure, legal or administrative issues may be raised, and careful documentation is important. For exposures in the hospital setting, hospital administrative policies should be consulted. For adolescents, support from family or friends might be encouraged, but the adolescent's right to privacy should be respected.

Summary

The risk of HIV transmission from non-occupational, non-perinatal exposure is generally low. Transmission risk is modified by factors related to the exposure source and extent. Determination of the HIV infection status of the exposure source may not be possible, and data on transmission risk by exposure type may not exist. Except in the setting of MTCT of HIV, no studies have demonstrated the safety and efficacy of postexposure use of antiretroviral drugs for the prevention of HIV transmission in the non-occupational setting. Antiretroviral drugs have significant toxicity. The decision to initiate prophylaxis needs to be made in consultation with the patient, family, and a clinician with experience in the management of HIV-exposed and -infected pediatric patients. If instituted, prophylaxis should be started as soon as possible after an exposure – no later than 72 hours – and continued for 28 days. Most recommendations suggest use of three-drug PEP regimens, although two-drug regimens may be considered in certain circumstances. Recommendations regarding prevention of secondary transmission should be provided. Careful follow-up is needed for psychological support, encouragement of drug adherence, toxicity monitoring, and serial HIV antibody testing.

REFERENCES

1. Centers for Disease Control and Prevention. Public Health Service guidelines for the management of health-care worker exposures to HIV and recommendations for post-exposure prophylaxis. *Morb. Mortal. Wkly Rep.* 1998;**47**(RR-7):1–33.

2. Centers for Disease Control and Prevention. Updated US Public Health Service guidelines for the management of occupational exposures to HBV, HCV, and HIV and recommendations for postexposure prophylaxis. *Marb. Mortal. Wkly.* Rep. 2001;**50**(RR-11): 1–52.

3. Centers for Disease Control and Prevention. Antiretroviral postexposure prophylaxis after sexual, injection-drug use, or other non-occupational exposure to HIV in the United States: recommendations from the U.S. Department of Health and Human Services. 2005;**54** (RR-2): 1–20.

4. Havens, P. L. and the Committee on Pediatric AIDS, American Academy of Pediatrics. Postexposure prophylaxis in children and adolescents for nonoccupational exposure to human immunodeficiency virus. *Pediatrics* 2003, **111**:1475–1489.

5. New York State Department of Health AIDS Institute. HIV Postexposure prophylaxis for children beyond the neonatal period: Tables and recommendations. 2002. accessed 5-7-03. http://hivguidelines.org/public_html/center/clinical-guidelines/ped_adolescent_hiv_guidelines/html/peds_pep/pdf/peds_pep_tables.pdf.

6. Merchant, R. C., Keshavarz, R. Human immunodeficiency virus postexposure prophylaxis for adolescents and children. *Pediatrics* 2001;**108**:e38. http://www.pediatrics.org/cgi/content/full/108/2/e38.

7. Cardo, D. M., Culver, D. H., Ciesielski, C. A. *et al.* A case-control study of HIV seroconversion in health care workers after percutaneous exposure. CDC Needle stick Surveillance Group. *N. Engl. J. Med.* 1997;**337**:1485–1490.

8. Gray, R. H., Wawer, M. J., Brookmeyer, R. *et al.* Probability of HIV-1 transmission per coital act in monogamous, heterosexual, HIV-1-discordant couples in Rakai, Uganda. *Lancet.* 2001;**357**:1149–1153.

9. Mofenson, L. M., Lambert, J. S., Stiehm, E. R. *et al.* Risk factors for perinatal transmission of human immunodeficiency virus type 1 in women treated with zidovudine. Pediatric AIDS Clinical Trials Group Study 185 Team. *N. Engl. J. Med.* 1999;**341**:385–393.

10. Garcia, P. M., Kalish, L. A., Pitt, J. *et al.* Maternal levels of plasma human immunodeficiency virus type 1 RNA and the risk of perinatal transmission. Women and Infants Transmission Study Group. *N. Engl. J. Med.* 1999;**341**:394–402.

11. Ioannidis, J. P. A., Abrams, E. J., Ammann, A. *et al.* Perinatal transmission of human immunodeficiency virus type 1 by pregnant women with RNA virus loads <1000 copies/ml. *J. Infect. Dis.* 2001;**183**(4): 539–545.

12. Hart, C. E., Lennox, J. L., Pratt-Palmore, M. *et al.* Correlation of human immunodeficiency virus type 1 RNA levels in blood and the female genital tract. *J. Infect. Dis.* 1999;**179**:871–882.

13. Rich, J. D., Dickinson, B. P., Carney, J. M., Fisher, A., Heimer, R. Detection of HIV-1 nucleic acid and HIV-1 antibodies in needles and syringes used for non-intravenous injection. *AIDS* 1998;**12**:2345–2350.

14. Resnick, L., Veren, K., Salahuddin, S. Z., Tondreau, S., Markham, P. D. Stability and inactivation of HTLV-III/LAV under clinical and laboratory environments. *J. Am. Med. Assoc.* 1986;**255**:1887–1891.

15. Abdala, N., Stephens, P. C., Griffith, B. P., Heimer, R. Survival of HIV-1 in syringes. *J. Acquir. Immune Defic. Syndr. Hum. Retrovirol.* 1999;**20**:73–80.

16. Zamora, A. B., Rivera, M. O., Garcia-Algar, O., Cayla Buqueras, J., Vall Combelles, O., Garcia-Saiz, A. Detection of infectious human immunodeficiency type 1 virus in discarded syringes of intravenous drug users. *Pediatr. Infect. Dis. J.* 1998;**17**:655–657.

17. Walsh, S. S., Pierce, A. M., Hart, C. A. Drug abuse: a new problem. *Br. Med. J. (Clin. Res. Ed.).* 1987;**295**:526–527.

18. Montella, F., DiSora, F., Recchia, O. Can HIV-1 infection be transmitted by a "discarded" syringe? *J. Acquir. Immune Defic. Syndr.* 1992;**5**:1274–1275.

19. Donegan, E., Stuart, M., Niland, J. C. *et al.* Infection with human immunodeficiency virus type 1 (HIV-1) among recipients of antibody-positive blood donations. *Ann. Intern. Med.* 1990;**113**:733–739.

20. The Working Group on Mother-to-Child Transmission of HIV. Rates of mother-to-child transmission of HIV-1 in Africa, America, and Europe: results from 13 perinatal studies. The Working Group on Mother-to-Child Transmission of HIV. *J. Acquir. Immune Defic. Syndr. Hum. Retrovirol.* 1995;**8**:506–510.

21. Kaplan, E. H., Heimer, R. A model-based estimate of HIV infectivity via needle sharing. *J. Acquir. Immune Defic. Syndr.* 1992;**5**:1116–1118.

22. Tokars, J. I., Marcus, R., Culver, D. H. *et al.* Surveillance of HIV infection and zidovudine use among health care workers after occupational exposure to HIV-infected blood. The CDC Needle stick Surveillance Group. *Ann. Intern. Med.* 1993;**118**:913–919.

23. Bell, D. M. Occupational risk of human immunodeficiency virus infection in healthcare workers: an overview. *Am. J. Med.* 1997;**102**:9–15.

24. Katz, M. H., Gerberding, J. L. The care of persons with recent sexual exposure to HIV. *Ann. Intern. Med.* 1998;**128**:306–312.

25. Mastro, T. D., de Vincenzi, I. Probabilities of sexual HIV-1 transmission. *AIDS* 1996;**10**:S75-S82.

26. DeGruttola, V., Seage, G. R., III, Mayer, K. H., Horsburgh, C. R., Jr. Infectiousness of HIV between male homosexual partners. *J. Clin. Epidemiol.* 1989;**42**:849–856.

27. Wiley, J. A., Herschkorn, S. J., Padian, N. S. Heterogeneity in the probability of HIV transmission per sexual contact: the case of male-to-female transmission in penile–vaginal intercourse. *Stat. Med.* 1989;**8**:93–102.

28. Peterman, T. A., Stoneburner, R. L., Allen, J. R., Jaffe, H. W., Curran, J. W. Risk of human immunodeficiency virus transmission from heterosexual adults with transfusion-associated infections. *J. Am. Med. Assoc.* 1988;**259**:55–58.

29. Downs, A. M., DeVincenzi, I. Probability of heterosexual transmission of HIV: relationship to the number of unprotected sexual contacts. *J. Acquir. Immune Defic. Syndr. Hum. Retrovirol.* 1996;**11**:388–395.

30. Lane, H. C., Holmberg, S. D., Jaffe, H. W. HIV seroconversion and oral intercourse. *Am. J. Publ. Hlth.* 1991;**81**:658.

31. Keet, I. P., Albrecht van Lent, N., Sandfort, T. G., Coutinho, R. A., van Griensven, G. J. Orogenital sex and the transmission of HIV among homosexual men. *AIDS* 1992;**6**:223–226.

32. Goldberg, D. J., Green, S. T., Kennedy, D. H., Emslie, J. A., Black, J. D. HIV and orogenital transmission [lett]. *Lancet* 1988;**2**:1363.

33. Berrey, M. M., Shea, T. Oral sex and HIV transmission [lett]. *J. Acquir. Immune Defic. Syndr. Hum. Retrovirol.* 1997;**14**:475.

34. Lifson, A. R., O'Malley, P. M., Hessol, N. A., Buchbinder, S. P., Cannon, L., Rutherford, G. W. HIV seroconversion in two homosexual men after receptive oral intercourse with ejaculation: implications for counseling concerning safe sexual practices. *Am. J. Publ. Hlth.* 1990;**80**:1509–1511.

35. DeGruttola, V., Mayer, K. H. Human immunodeficiency virus and oral intercourse [lett]. *Ann. Intern. Med.* 1987;**107**:428–429.

36. Royce, R. A., Sena, A., Cates, W. Jr, Cohen, M. S. Sexual transmission of HIV. *N. Engl. J. Med.* 1997;**336**:1072–1078.

37. Richardson, B. A., John-Stewart, G., Hughes, J. P. *et al.* Breast-milk infectivity in human immunodeficiency virus type 1-infected mothers. *J. Infect. Dis.* 2003;**187**:736–740.

38. Dominguez, K. L. Management of HIV-infected children in the home and institutional settings. Care of children and infections control in schools, day care, hospital settings, home, foster care, and adoption. *Pediatr. Clin. North. Am.* 2000; **47**:203–239.

39. Anonymous. Transmission of HIV by human bite. *Lancet* 1987;**2**:522.

40. Vidmar, L., Poljak, M., Tomazic, J., Seme, K., Klavs, I. Transmission of HIV-1 by human bite [lett]. *Lancet.* 1996;**347**:1762.

41. Richman, K. M., Rickman, L. S. The potential for transmission of human immunodeficiency virus through human bites. *J. Acquir. Immune Defic. Syndr.* 1993;**6**:402–406.

42. Abel, S., Cesaire, R., Cales-Quist, D., Bera, O., Sobesky, G., Cabie, A. Occupational transmission of human immunodeficiency virus and hepatitis C virus after a punch. *Clin. Infect. Dis.* 2000;**31**:1494–1495.

43. Yeh, C. K., Handelman, B., Fox, P. C., Baum, B. J. Further studies of salivary inhibition of HIV-1 infectivity. *J. Acquir. Immune Defic. Syndr.* 1992;**5**:898–903.

44. Centers for Disease Control and Prevention. Transmission of HIV possibly associated with exposure of mucous membrane to contaminated blood. *Morb. Mortal. Wkly Rep.* 1997;**46**:620–623.

45. Henderson, D. K., Fahey, B. J., Willy, M. *et al.* Risk for occupational transmission of human immunodeficiency virus type 1 (HIV-1) associated with clinical exposures. A prospective evaluation. *Ann. Intern. Med.* 1990;**113**:740–746.

46. Ippolito, G., Puro, V., De Carli, G. The risk of occupational human immunodeficiency virus infection in health care workers. The Italian Study Group on Occupational Risk of HIV Infection. *Arch. Intern. Med.* 1993;**153**:1451–1458.

47. Little, S. J., McLean, A. R., Spina, C. A., Richman, D. D., Havlir, D. V. Viral dynamics of acute HIV-1 infection. *J. Exp. Med.* 1999;**190**:841–850.

48. Katzenstein, T. L., Dickmeiss, E., Aladdin, H. *et al.* Failure to develop HIV infection after receipt of HIV-contaminated blood and postexposure prophylaxis. *Ann. Int. Med.* 2000;**133**:31–34.

49. Van Rompay, K. K., Marthas, M. L., Lifson, J. D. *et al.* Administration of 9-[2-(phosphonomethoxy)propyl]adenine (PMPA) for prevention of perinatal simian immunodeficiency virus infection in rhesus macaques. *AIDS Res. Hum. Retrovirus.* 1998;**14**:761–773.

50. Tavares, L., Roneker, C., Johnston, K., Lehrman, S. N., de Noronha, F. 3′-Azido-3′deoxythymidine in feline leukemia virus-infected cats: a model for therapy and prophylaxis of AIDS. *Cancer Res.* 1987;**47**:3190–3194.

51. Shih, C. C., Kaneshima, H., Rabin, L. *et al.* Postexposure prophylaxis with zidovudine suppresses human immunodeficiency virus type 1 infection in SCID-hu mice in a time-dependent manner. *J. Infect. Dis.* 1991;**163**:625–627.

52. Van Rompay, K. K., Otsyula, M. G., Marthas, M. L., Miller, C. J., McChesney, M. B., Pedersen, N. C. Immediate zidovudine treatment protects simian immunodeficiency virus-infected newborn macaques against rapid onset of AIDS. *Antimicrob. Agents Chemother.* 1995;**39**:125–131.

53. Bottiger, D., Johansson, N. G., Samuelsson, B. *et al.* Prevention of simian immunodeficiency virus, SIV$_{sm}$, or HIV-2 infection in cynomolgus monkeys by pre- and postexposure administration of BEA-005. *AIDS* 1997;**11**:157–162.

54. Black, R. J. Animal studies of prophylaxis. *Am. J. Med.* 1997;**102**:39–44.

55. Sinet, M., Desforges, B., Launay, O., Colin, J. N., Pocidalo, J. J. Factors influencing zidovudine efficacy when administered at early stages of Friend virus infection in mice. *Antiviral Res.* 1991;**16**:163–171.

56. Tsai, C. C., Emau, P., Follis, K. E. *et al.* Effectiveness of postinoculation (R)-9-(2-phosphonylmethoxypropyl) adenine treatment for prevention of persistent simian immunodeficiency virus SIV$_{mne}$ infection depends critically on timing of initiation and duration of treatment. *J. Virol.* 1998;**72**:4265–4273.

57. Otten, R. A., Smith, D. K., Adams, D. R. *et al.* Efficacy of postexposure prophylaxis after intravaginal exposure of pig-tailed macaques to a human-derived retrovirus (human immunodeficiency virus type 2). *J. Virol.* 2000;**74**:9771–9775.

58. Martin, L. N., Murphey-Corb, M., Soike, K. F., Davison-Fairburn, B., Baskin, G. B. Effects of initiation of 3′-azido, 3′-deoxythymidine (zidovudine) treatment at different times after infection of rhesus monkeys with simian immunodeficiency virus. *J. Infect. Dis.* 1993;**168**:825–835.

59. Fazely, F., Haseltine, W. A., Rodger, R. F., Ruprecht, R. M., Postexposure chemoprophylaxis with ZDV or ZDV combined with interferon-alpha: failure after inoculating rhesus monkeys with a high dose of SIV. *J. Acquir. Immune Defic. Syndr.* 1991;**4**:1093–1097.

60. Ruprecht, R. M., Bronson, R. Chemoprevention of retroviral infection: success is determined by virus inoculum strength and cellular immunity. *DNA Cell Biol.* 1994;**13**:59–66.

61. Niu, M. T., Stein, D. S., Schnittman, S. M. Primary human immunodeficiency virus type 1 infection: review of pathogenesis and early treatment intervention in humans and animal retrovirus infections. *J. Infect. Dis.* 1993;**168**:1490–1501.

62. Schacker, T., Collier, A. C., Hughes, J., Shea, T., Corey, L. Clinical and epidemiologic features of primary HIV infection. *Ann Intern Med.* 1996;**125**:257–264.

63. Ruprecht, R. M., Chou, T. C., Chipty, F. *et al.* Interferon-alpha and 3'-azido-3'-deoxythymidine are highly synergistic in mice and prevent viremia after acute retrovirus exposure. *J. Acquir. Immune Defic. Syndr.* 1990;**3**:591–600.

64. Mathes, L. E., Polas, P. J., Hayes, K. A., Swenson, C. L., Johnson, S., Kociba, G. J. Pre- and postexposure chemoprophylaxis: evidence that 3'-azido-3'-dideoxythymidine inhibits feline leukemia virus disease by a drug-induced vaccine response. *Antimicrob. Agents Chemother.* 1992;**36**:2715–2721.

65. Grob, P. M., Cao, Y., Muchmore, E. *et al.* Prophylaxis against HIV-1 infection in chimpanzees by nevirapine, a nonnucleoside inhibitor of reverse transcriptase. *Nature Med.* 1997;**3**:665–670.

66. Clerici, M., Giorgi, J. V., Chou, C. C. *et al.* Cell-mediated immune response to human immunodeficiency virus (HIV) type 1 in seronegative homosexual men with recent sexual exposure to HIV-1. *J. Infect. Dis.* 1992;**165**:1012–1019.

67. Pinto, L. A., Sullivan, J., Berzofsky, J. A. *et al.* ENV-specific cytotoxic T lymphocyte response in HIV seronegative health care workers occupationally exposed to HIV-contaminated body fluids. *J. Clin. Invest.* 1995;**96**:867–876.

68. D'Amico, R., Pinto, L. A., Meyer, P. *et al.* Effect of zidovudine postexposure prophylaxis on the development of HIV-specific cytotoxic T-lymphocyte responses in HIV-exposed healthcare workers. *Infect. Control Hosp. Epidemiol.* 1999;**20**:428–430.

69. Connor, E. M., Sperling, R. S., Gelber, R. *et al.* Reduction of maternal-infant transmission of human immunodeficiency virus type 1 with zidovudine treatment. Pediatric AIDS Clinical Trials Group Protocol 076 Study Group. *N. Engl. J. Med.* 1994;**331**:1173–1180.

70. Guay, L. A., Musoke, P., Fleming, T. *et al.* Intrapartum and neonatal single-dose nevirapine compared with zidovudine for prevention of mother-to-child transmission of HIV-1 in Kampala, Uganda: HIVNET 012 randomised trial. *Lancet* 1999;**354**:795–802.

71. Cooper, E. R., Charurat, M., Mofenson, L. *et al.* Combination antiretroviral strategies for the treatment of pregnant HIV-1-infected women and prevention of perinatal HIV-1 transmission. *J. Acquir. Immune Defic. Syndr.* 2002;**29**:484–494.

72. Wade, N. A., Birkhead, G. S., Warren, B. L. *et al.* Abbreviated regimens of zidovudine prophylaxis and perinatal transmission of the human immunodeficiency virus. *N. Engl. J. Med.* 1998;**339**:1409–1414.

73. Wade, N. A., Birkhead, G. S., French P. T. Short courses of zidovudine and perinatal transmission of HIV [response to letters]. *N. Engl. J. Med.* 1999;**340**:1043–1043.

74. Ippolito, G., Puro, V., Heptonstall, J., Jagger, J., De Carli, G., Petrosillo, N. Occupational human immunodeficiency virus infection in health care workers: worldwide cases through September 1997. *Clin. Infect. Dis.* 1999;**28**:365–383.

75. Lange, J. M., Boucher, C. A., Hollak, C. E. *et al.* Failure of zidovudine prophylaxis after accidental exposure to HIV-1. *N. Engl. J. Med.* 1990;**322**:1375–1377.

76. Jochimsen, E. M., Luo, C. C., Beltrami, J. F., Respess, R. A., Schable, C. A., Cardo, D. M. Investigations of possible failures of postexposure prophylaxis following occupational exposures to human immunodeficiency virus. *Arch. Intern. Med.* 1999;**159**:2361–2363.

77. Erice, A., Mayers, D. L., Strike, D. G. *et al.* Brief report: primary infection with zidovudine-resistant human immunodeficiency virus type 1. *N. Engl. J. Med.* 1993;**328**:1163–1165.

78. Kahn, J. O., Martin, J. N., Roland, M. E. *et al.* Feasibility of postexposure prophylaxis (PEP) against human immunodeficiency virus infection after sexual or injection drug use exposure: the San Francisco PEP Study. *J. Infect. Dis.* 2001;**183**:707–714.

79. Kunches, L. M., Meehan, T. M., Boutwell, R. C., McGuire, J. F. Survey of nonoccupational HIV postexposure prophylaxis in hospital emergency departments. *J. Acquir. Immune Defic. Syndr.* 2001;**26**:263–265.

80. Fournier, S., Maillard, A., Molina, J. M. Failure of postexposure prophylaxis after sexual exposure to HIV. *AIDS* 2001;**15**:430.

81. Waldo, C. R., Stall, R. D., Coates, T. J. Is offering post-exposure prevention for sexual exposures to HIV related to sexual risk behavior in gay men? *AIDS* 2000;**14**:1035–1039.

82. Braitstein, P., Chan, K., Beardsell, A. *et al.* How much is it worth? Actual versus expected costs of a population-based post-exposure prophylaxis program [Abstr 270P]. *Can. J. Infect. Dis.* 2001;**12**(Suppl B):45B–46B.

83. Braitstein, P., Chan, K., Beardsell, A. *et al.* Side effects associated with post-exposure prophylaxis in a population-based setting [Abstr 271P]. *Can. J. Infect. Dis.* 2001;**12**(Suppl B):46B.

84. Centers for Disease Control and Prevention. Serious adverse events attributed to nevirapine regimens for postexposure prophylaxis after HIV exposures – worldwide, 1997–2000. *Morb. Mortal. Wkly Rep.* 2001;**49**:1153–1156.

85. Lindegren, M. L., Hanson, I. C., Hammett, T. A., Beil, J., Fleming, P. L., Ward, J. W. Sexual abuse of children: intersection with the HIV epidemic. *Pediatrics.* 1998;102(4). Available at: http://www.pediatrics.org/cgi/content/full/102/4/e46

86. Gostin, L. O., Lazzarini, Z., Alexander, D., Brandt, A. M., Mayer, K. H., Silverman, D. C. HIV testing, counseling, and prophylaxis after sexual assault. *J. Am. Med. Assoc.* 1994;**271**:1436–1444.

87. Bamberger, J. D., Waldo, C. R., Gerberding, J. L., Katz, M. H. Postexposure prophylaxis for human immunodeficiency virus (HIV) infection following sexual assault. *Am. J. Med.* 1999;**106**:323–326.

88. Katz, M. H., Gerberding, J. L. Postexposure treatment of people exposed to the human immunodeficiency virus through sexual contact or injection-drug use. *N. Engl. J. Med.* 1997;**336**:1097–1100.

89. Evans, B., Darbyshire, J., Cartledge, J. Should preventive antiretroviral treatment be offered following sexual exposure to HIV? Not yet! *Sex Transm. Infect.* 1998;**74**:146–148.

90. Lurie, P., Miller, S., Hecht, F., Chesney, M., Lo, B. Postexposure prophylaxis after nonoccupational HIV exposure: clinical, ethical, and policy considerations. *J. Am. Med. Assoc.* 1998;**280**:1769–1773.

91. Gwinn, M., Wortley, P. M. Epidemiology of HIV infection in women and newborns. *Clin. Obstet. Gynecol.* 1996;**39**:292–304.

92. Centers for Disease Control and Prevention. Revised recommendations for HIV screening of pregnant women. *Morb. Mortal. Wkly Rep.* 2001;**50**(RR-19):63–85.

93. Centers for Disease Control and Prevention. Recommendations of the US Public Health Service Task Force on the use of zidovudine to reduce perinatal transmission of human immunodeficiency virus. *Morb. Mortal. Wkly Rep.* 1994;**43**(RR-11):1–20.

94. Ippolito, G., Puro, V. Zidovudine toxicity in uninfected healthcare workers. Italian Registry of Antiretroviral Prophylaxis. *Am. J. Med.* 1997;**102**:58–62.

95. Henry, K., Acosta, E. P., Jochimsen, E. Hepatotoxicity and rash associated with zidovudine and zalcitabine chemoprophylaxis [lett]. *Ann. Intern. Med.* 1996;**124**:855.

96. Forseter, G., Joline, C., Wormser, G. P. Tolerability, safety, and acceptability of zidovudine prophylaxis in health care workers. *Arch. Intern. Med.* 1994;**154**:2745–2749.

97. Sepkowitz, K. A., Rivera, P., Louther, J., Lim, S., Pryor, B. Postexposure prophylaxis for human immunodeficiency virus: frequency of initiation and completion of newly recommended regimen. *Infect. Control Hosp. Epidemiol.* 1998;**19**:506–508.

98. Babl, F. E., Cooper, E. R., Damon, B., Louie, T., Kharasch, S., Harris, J. A. HIV postexposure prophylaxis for children and adolescents. *Am. J. Emerg. Med.* 2000;**18**:282–287.

99. Wiebe, E. R., Comay, S. E., McGregor, M., Ducceschi, S. Offering HIV prophylaxis to people who have been sexually assaulted: 16 months' experience in a sexual assault service. *CMAJ* 2000;**162**:641–645.

100. Myles, J. E., Hirozawa, A., Katz, M. H., Kimmerling, R., Bamberger, J. D. Postexposure prophylaxis for HIV after sexual assault. *J. Am. Med. Assoc.* 2000;**284**:1516–1518.

101. Benn, P. D., Mercey, D. E., Brink, N., Scott, G., Williams, I. G. Prophylaxis with a nevirapine-containing triple regimen after exposure to HIV-1. *Lancet* 2001;**357**:687–688.

102. American Academy of Pediatrics. *Red Book 2003: Report of the Committee on Infectious Diseases.* Elk Grove Village, IL.: American Academy of Pediatrics; 2003.

103. Busch, M. P., Satten, G. A. Time course of viremia and antibody seroconversion following human immunodeficiency virus exposure. *Am. J. Med.* 1997;**102**:117–126.

104. Ciesielski, C. A., Metler, R. P. Duration of time between exposure and seroconversion in healthcare workers with occupationally acquired infection with human immunodeficiency virus. *Am. J. Med.* 1997;**102**:115–116.

Part IV
Clinical manifestations of HIV infection in children

18 Cutaneous diseases

Andrew Blauvelt

Department of Dermatology, Oregon Health and Science University, Portland, Oregon

The skin of HIV-infected individuals, both young and old, is a major target organ for numerous infectious, inflammatory, and neoplastic processes. Thus, dermatologists and other clinicians who are adept at diagnosing and treating skin diseases play an extremely important role in the overall care of these patients. For example, many HIV-infected individuals are unaware of their serologic status and present initially with a dermatologic complaint (e.g., the rash of primary HIV infection, herpes zoster). It is thus the responsibility of the astute clinician to inquire about underlying HIV infection. For children, a pediatrician or dermatologist may be the first to suggest HIV disease when evaluating a baby with a particularly recalcitrant case of diaper dermatitis. A second important role for those evaluating the skin of HIV-infected patients is in the recognition of cutaneous clues that are signs of severe systemic infection or cancer (e.g., cutaneous lesions of cryptococcosis or disseminated candidiasis). Prompt and accurate diagnosis through biopsy and microscopic examination of the skin may be life-saving in these types of cases. Lastly, clinicians caring for patients with skin diseases associated with HIV disease may provide tremendous symptomatic relief to their patients by correctly diagnosing and treating particularly severe conditions, such as generalized pruritus, widespread genital warts, or numerous disfiguring lesions of molluscum contagiosum on the face.

As with adults, the majority of the cutaneous manifestations of HIV disease are observed in children with greater degrees of immunosuppression [1–4]. In children with AIDS, more than 90% are likely to develop a problem that involves the skin. However, while no single dermatologic condition is pathognomonic for HIV disease, cutaneous infections predominate. Following a brief section on general principles in the dermatologic care of HIV-infected children, specific features of many of the common dermatoses that affect these patients will be outlined.

Handbook of Pediatric HIV Care, ed. Steven L. Zeichner and Jennifer S. Read.
Published by Cambridge University Press. © Cambridge University Press 2006.

Table 18.1. General guidelines for the proper evaluation of dermatologic diseases in HIV-infected children

Always have a parent or guardian in the exam room to assist.

Examine the patient in a well-lit room. The oral cavity and many skin lesions are only seen with good lighting.

It is not absolutely necessary to wear gloves while doing a skin exam on an HIV-infected child, however, gloves should always be worn if there is a potential for transmission of blood or body fluids, or when a potentially infectious agent, such as scabies or varicella-zoster virus, is suspected.

Completely examine all skin and mucous membrane surfaces. A complete skin exam should be done regardless of whether the lesions are localized or generalized. In particular, don't forget the nails, scalp, oral mucosa, genital area, and feet.

So that a particularly focused examination can be done to search for a suspected lesion or pathogen, know the history well.

Always refer the patient for a consultation with a dermatologist if there is significant doubt as to proper diagnosis and/or treatment.

General principles

The approach to evaluating the skin of a child with HIV infection should be standardized. Important general principles for examination of the skin are listed in Table 18.1. Primary care clinicians should maintain a low threshold for formally consulting a dermatologist to assist in the diagnosis and care of HIV-infected children with skin diseases. When performing the physical examination, an important goal is to determine and accurately describe the type and nature of the primary skin lesion. Primary and secondary skin lesions are listed in Table 18.2, along with examples of diseases that manifest with each particular lesion. In addition to identifying primary and secondary lesions, other important aspects of the lesions should be noted, including the shape of the individual lesions (e.g., annular, linear, arciform), the distribution of the lesions (e.g., localized, generalized, grouped, zosteriform, photodistributed), and the color of the lesions (erythematous, violaceous, brown). The correct characterization of the disease leads to a useful list of differential diagnoses, and allows the clinician to communicate information accurately to other doctors. Although physical examination remains the most important "tool" in assessing the skin of patients, a few basic carefully performed bedside procedures can greatly aid in obtaining correct diagnoses. An outline of the materials used in these procedures and basic guidelines for performing them are provided in Tables 18.3 and 18.4, respectively.

Table 18.2. Primary and secondary skin lesions

Type of primary or secondary lesion	Representative diseases	Typical distinguishing features
Papule (raised lesion <1 cm in diameter)	Verruca vulgaris	Verrucous surface
	Molluscum contagiosum	Smooth surface with central umbilication
	Scabies	Pruritic, excoriated, with burrows
	Insect bites	Pruritic, grouped, on extremities
	Drug eruption	Small, erythematous, on trunk
	Psoriasis	Erythematous, with thick gray scale
	Viral exanthem	Small, erythematous
	Cryptococcosis	Smooth with necrotic centers
	Histoplasmosis	Acneiform
	Kaposi's sarcoma	Smooth, violaceous
Nodule (raised lesion 1–2.5 cm in diameter)	Kaposi's sarcoma	Smooth, violaceous
	Prurigo nodularis	Pruritic, on extremities
Tumor (raised lesion >2.5 cm in diameter)	Kaposi's sarcoma	Violaceous, associated edema
Macule (flat lesion <1 cm in diameter)	Drug eruption	Erythematous, on trunk
	Kaposi's sarcoma	Violaceous
	Viral exanthem	Erythematous, on trunk
Patch (flat lesion >1 cm in diameter)	Kaposi's sarcoma	
Plaque (raised planar lesion)	Psoriasis	Erythematous, with thick gray scale
	Dermatophytosis	Annular, with peripheral scale
	Kaposi's sarcoma	Violaceous
	Cellulitis	Erythematous, edematous, painful
Vesicle (clear fluid-filled lesion <1 cm in diameter)	Herpes simplex	Grouped, painful
	Varicella	Disseminated, erythematous base
	Herpes zoster	Dermatomal, painful
	Impetigo	Golden crust
Bulla (clear fluid-filled lesion >1 cm in diameter)	Impetigo	Golden crust

(*cont.*)

Table 18.2. (*cont.*)

Type of primary or secondary lesion	Representative diseases	Typical distinguishing features
Pustule (white fluid-filled lesion)	Candidiasis	Satellite lesions near inflammation
	Bacterial folliculitis	Centered around hair follicles
	Psoriasis	With typical scaly papules and plaques
Wheal (hive)	Idiopathic urticaria	Erythematous, edematous, transient
Burrow (linear array of papules)	Scabies	Pruritic, linear
Scale (superficial layers of epidermis)	Seborrheic dermatitis	Greasy, in scalp and eyebrows
	Psoriasis	Thick, gray
	Dermatophytosis	On periphery of lesion
	Xerosis	Fine, diffuse
Crust (dried exudate)	Impetigo	Golden
	Herpes simplex	Grouped
Erosion (loss of epidermis)	Herpes simplex	Painful
Ulcer (loss of epidermis extending into dermis)	Herpes simplex	Painful, chronic coarse
Scar (collagen deposition in dermis)	Herpes zoster	Dermatomal
Excoriations (scratch marks)	Scabies	Associated burrows
	Insect bites	Grouped, on extremities
	Atopic dermatitis	Associated xerosis, systemic signs of atopy
Lichenification (accentuation of skin lines)	Atopic dermatitis	Associated xerosis, systemic signs of atopy

Infectious diseases that predominantly involve the skin and oral mucosa

Fungal infections

Candidiasis

Mucocutaneous candidiasis is the most common dermatologic manifestation in HIV-infected children [5–7]. *Candida albicans* is the most frequently isolated organism. Oral candidiasis typically presents as friable white plaques on the oral mucosa, which is termed the pseudomembranous form of the disease (Fig. 18.1). Less commonly, oral candidiasis presents as erythematous atrophic plaques, papillary hyperplasia, chronic hyperplastic plaques, median rhomboid glossitis, or angular cheilitis. On the skin surface, lesions appear as ill-defined erythematous plaques with surrounding

Table 18.3. Basic materials that are extremely useful as diagnostic aids when evaluating dermatologic diseases in HIV-infected children

Microscope and glass slides
10% potassium hydroxide (KOH) to examine skin and mucous membrane scrapings for
    fungal infection
Gram stain kit to examine bacterial contents of pustules and to examine suspected
    herpesvirus lesions for multinucleated giant cells (Tzanck preps)
Mineral oil to examine skin scrapings for scabies or Demodex infestation
Materials for tissue culture
    Sterile cups for fungal culture
    Bacterial culture swabs
    Viral culture medium for herpes simplex/varicella-zoster virus
Materials for skin biopsy
    2% lidocaine with epinephrine
    30-gauge needles
    3–4-mm punch biopsy devices
    Suture kit
    Cup with 10% formaldehyde
Dermatology textbook for reference

"satellite" pustules; the diaper area and other intertriginous areas are typically affected. In children from ages 2 to 6, chronic candidal paronychia (i.e., nail fold infection) with secondary nail dystrophy may occur. In all clinical types of disease, observing spores and non-septated non-branching pseudohyphae on potassium hydroxide (KOH) examination of superficial scale or roofs of pustules confirms the diagnosis. Importantly, mucocutaneous candidiasis in HIV-infected children, when persistent or recurrent, is a sign of relatively severe immunodeficiency. Hoarseness or trouble swallowing should prompt a search for disease involving the larynx or esophagus. Depending on the extent and severity of infection, treatment of candidiasis consists of topical (e.g., 2% ketoconazole cream twice daily) or systemic antifungal agents.

Dermatophytosis

Dermatophyte infections occur frequently in HIV-infected children, most often after the age of 2 years [1, 2]. *Trichophyton rubrum* is the most common organism isolated. The scalp (tinea capitis), feet (tinea pedis), and nails (onychomycosis) are often affected. In the scalp, lesions usually appear as non-inflammatory scaly plaques with secondary alopecia (Fig. 18.2). Typical kerion formation, as observed in HIV-uninfected children, is not common in children with AIDS. Lesions on the feet and other skin surfaces commonly appear as annular plaques with scales on the advancing borders of the lesions. In the nails, infection may occur beneath the nail plate (subungual onychomycosis) or within the superficial nail plate (white superficial onychomycosis) (Fig. 18.3). This

Table 18.4. Basic guidelines for performing bedside dermatologic procedures

Preparation	Candidate diseases	Ideal procedure
KOH	Dermatophytosis, candidiasis	1. Choose peripheral scale or roofs of intact pustules. 2. Scrape scales or roofs with No. 15 scalpel blade and place contents onto glass slide containing 10% KOH. 3. Place cover slip on slide and gently heat with match. 4. Examine at low power for hyphae (dermatophytosis) or pseudohyphae and spores (candidiasis) and confirm at high power if necessary.
Gram stain	Bacterial infections	1. Choose intact pustule or abscess. 2. Express pus/exudate and smear onto glass. 3. Fix and stain slide using Gram stain kit. 4. Examine at high power with oil for bacteria.
Tzanck	Herpesviral infections	1. Choose newest lesions, preferably intact vesicles. 2. Remove roofs and scrape bases of blisters with No. 15 scalpel blade and smear cellular material onto glass slide. 3. Fix and stain slide using Gram stain kit. 4. Scan at low power for multinucleated giant cells and confirm at high power.
Mineral oil	Scabies	1. Choose intact papules or papulovesicles, preferably at the ends of burrows. 2. Superficially shave tops of these lesions with No. 15 scalpel blade and place contents onto glass slide containing mineral oil. 3. Examine at low power for mites, eggs, and feces.
	Demodex	1. Scrape superficial scales from affected areas onto glass slide containing mineral oil. 2. Examine at low power for mites.

latter disease, in particular, is not a specific marker for HIV infection, although it often indicates severe underlying immunodeficiency. Diagnosis can be confirmed by the observation of septated branching hyphae on KOH examination of superficial scale obtained from the advancing borders of lesions (Fig. 18.4), or by fungal culture of scales. Therapy consists of topical (e.g., 2% ketoconazole cream twice daily) or oral antifungal agents.

A. Blauvelt

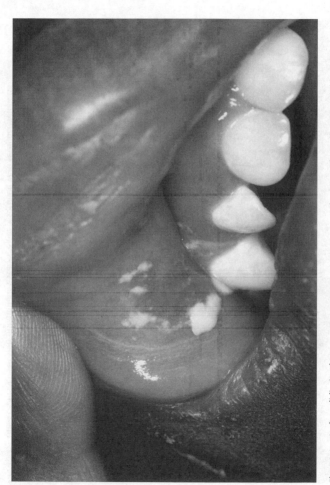

Fig. 18.1. Oral candidiasis. The most common mucocutaneous manifestation of HIV disease in children, mucosal candidiasis typically appears as white friable plaques that are easily removed with scraping.

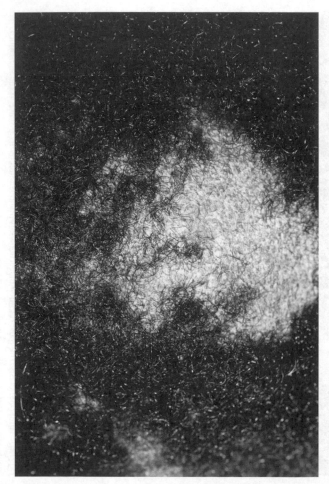

Fig. 18.2. Tinea capitis. Classic non-inflammatory scaly plaque associated with secondary alopecia.

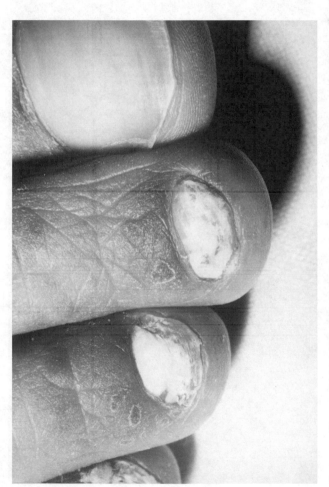

Fig. 18.3. White superficial onychomycosis. Tinea infection involves the superficial nail plate in this type of fungal nail infection, and is a harbinger for severe underlying immunodeficiency

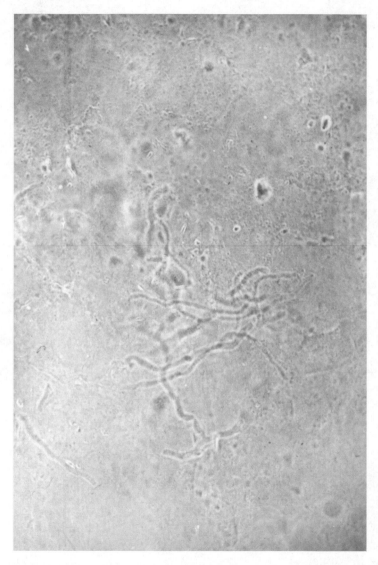

Fig. 18.4. KOH preparation – dermatophyte. Typical hyphae isolated from scales of a superficial dermatophyte infection.

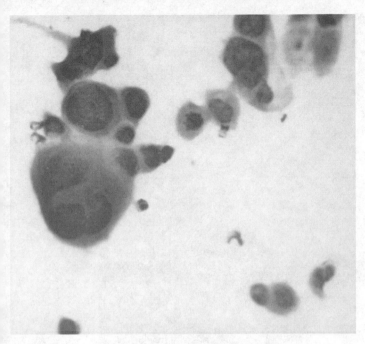

Fig. 18.5. Tzanck preparation – herpes simplex infection. Multinucleated giant cells scraped from the floor of an erosion caused by herpes simplex virus. Similar cells are observed from lesions caused by varicella-zoster virus.

Penicillium marneffei

Penicillium marneffei is a dimorphic fungus endemic in southeast Asia. Disseminated infections in children with AIDS in this region are not uncommon, with skin lesions appearing in 67% of cases [8]. Lesions appear as papules with central umbilication (i.e., molluscum-like) on the face and extremities, and are a major clue to the diagnosis. Diagnosis can be confirmed by skin biopsy in conjunction with special stains to identify organisms, or by fungal culture of affected skin.

Viral infections

Herpes simplex virus

Primary herpetic gingivostomatitis is fairly common and may be particularly severe in HIV-infected children [5–7]. Children present with painful ulceration of the lips, tongue, palate, and buccal mucosa. Secondary dehydration may occur when patients avoid eating and drinking because of pain. Diagnosis can be confirmed by observing multinucleated giant cells (scraped from the base of ulcerations) on Tzanck preps (Fig. 18.5),

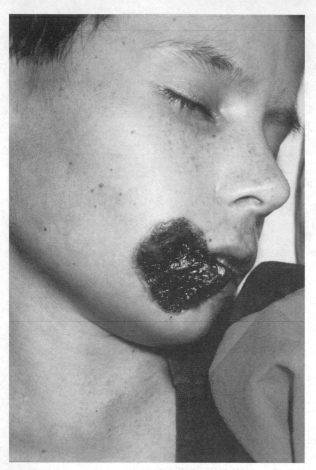

Fig. 18.6. Chronic herpes simplex virus infection. Chronic ulcerative lesion in a child with AIDS.

or by viral culture. Recurrent herpes simplex virus infection may involve any cutaneous site, regardless of whether disease is caused by herpes simplex 1 or herpes simplex 2. Acute lesions typically present as painful grouped vesicles. As individual lesions age, they become pustular and erosive. Chronic herpes simplex virus infection may not have the classic grouped distribution, and thus may present diagnostic difficulties for the physician. In these cases, lesions often present as chronic painful ulcers and crusted painful erosions (Fig. 18.6). It is important to always consider herpes simplex virus infection in any HIV-infected child with these types of lesions. Treatment of herpes simplex infection is outlined in Chapter 34.

Varicella-zoster virus

Varicella (chicken pox) is primary infection with varicella zoster virus and may be more prolonged and more severe in HIV-infected children compared to disease in HIV-uninfected children [1, 2]. Patients should be closely monitored for systemic disease, including pneumonia, hepatitis, central nervous system involvement, pancreatitis, and secondary bacterial infection. Primary lesions of varicella are vesicles with surrounding erythema, usually disseminated, and have been figuratively described as "dew drops on rose petals" (Fig. 18.7). Recurrent varicella-zoster virus infection (which is rare in healthy children) may present as herpes zoster or chronic disseminated infection. The former occurs as painful vesicles and deep crusted erosions in a dermatomal distribution and often leads to scarring in HIV-infected children. The latter presents as crusted erosions and/or verrucous papules and plaques (Fig. 18.8, see color insert) [9], and is not observed in immunocompetent individuals. As with herpes simplex virus infection, diagnosis of varicella-zoster virus infection can be confirmed by observing multinucleated giant cells on Tzanck preps (see Fig. 18.5), or by viral culture. Treatment of varicella-zoster virus infections is outlined in Chapter 34.

Kaposi's sarcoma-associated herpesvirus

Kaposi's sarcoma-associated herpesvirus (KSHV), also known as human herpesvirus 8 (HHV-8), is a newly described γ-herpesvirus that has been linked to all clinical types of KS [10]. Infection with KSHV is uncommon in HIV-infected children from the United States and western Europe and KS is rare. In sub-Saharan Africa (especially in Uganda, Zimbabwe, and Zambia), however, KSHV infection and KS are endemic and relatively common [11, 12]. In these regions, because of the HIV epidemic, KS has become one of the most common pediatric neoplasms. As in HIV-infected gay men, KS in children presents as violaceous patches, plaques, papules, nodules, and tumors (Fig. 18.9). Of note, disease in both HIV-infected and HIV-uninfected African children can be aggressive and often involves the lymph nodes, the so-called lymphadenopathic variant of KS.

Human papillomavirus

Warts are caused by human papillomavirus infection within keratinocytes, and are relatively common in HIV-infected children [1, 2]. Lesions appear as multiple verrucous papules (Fig. 18.10). At times, lesions are smooth, flat (Fig. 18.11), or pedunculated. The hands, feet, face, and genitalia are commonly involved, although warts my occur on any part of the body. Genital warts (also known as condyloma acuminata) in children may or may not be a sign of sexual abuse, and thus this possibility should be considered in a straightforward, but not accusatory, manner. Topical therapy for warts in HIV-infected children is often ineffective, yet individual lesions can be destroyed using cryotherapy (i.e., application of liquid nitrogen) or electrodesiccation.

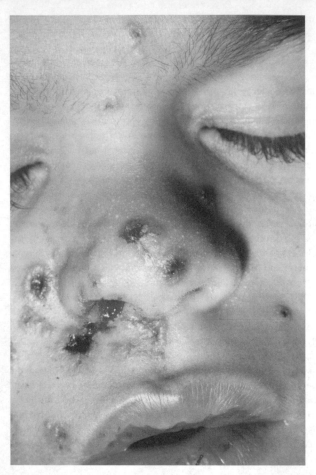

Fig. 18.7. Varicella (chicken pox). Varicella may be particularly severe and prolonged in children infected with HIV.

Molluscum contagiosum virus

Molluscum contagiosum is a DNA poxvirus that also infects keratinocytes, and like human papillomavirus, is relatively common in children with HIV disease [1,2]. Lesions classically appear as numerous dome-shaped umbilicated papules (Fig. 18.12), most commonly on the face. If doubt exists as to the correct diagnosis, white material can be expressed from individual lesions, placed onto a slide, and examined for typical molluscum bodies under a microscope (Fig. 18.13). Like human papillomavirus, no

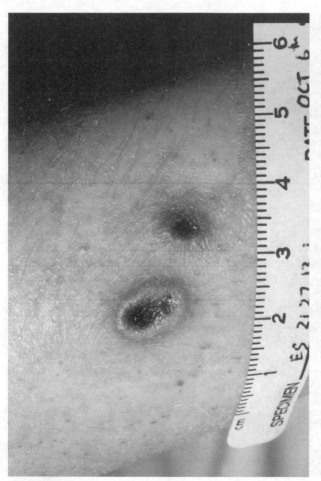

Fig. 18.8. Chronic varicella zoster virus infection. Recurrent varicella-zoster virus infection commonly occurs as scattered crusted erosions and ulcers in children with AIDS.

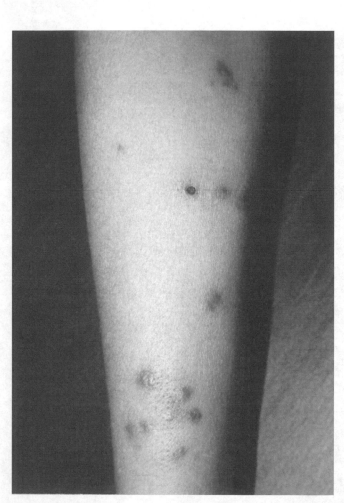

Fig. 18.9. Kaposi's sarcoma. Although uncommon in US children with AIDS, Kaposi's sarcoma can occur in children and lesions appear as violaceous patches, plaques, papules, or nodules.

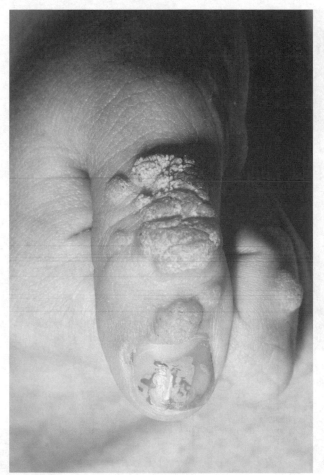

Fig. 18.10. Verruca vulgaris. Warts in HIV-infected children are common and are often resistant to treatment.

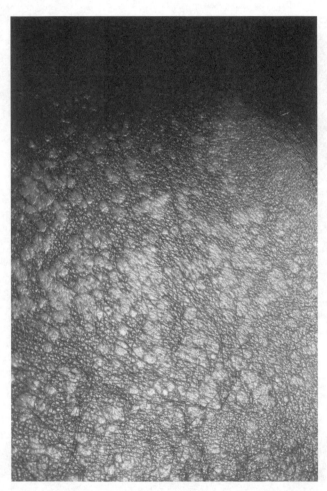

Fig. 18.11. Verruca plana (flat warts). Flat warts are relatively common on the face of HIV-infected children and appear as non-inflammatory, smooth, flat-topped papules.

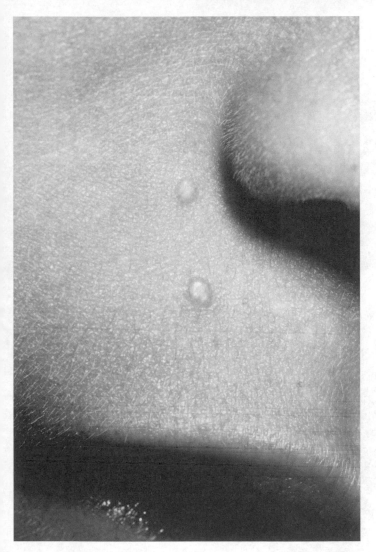

Fig. 18.12. Molluscum contagiosum. Smooth dome-shaped papules with central umbilication are classic for molluscum, and are very common in children with HIV disease.

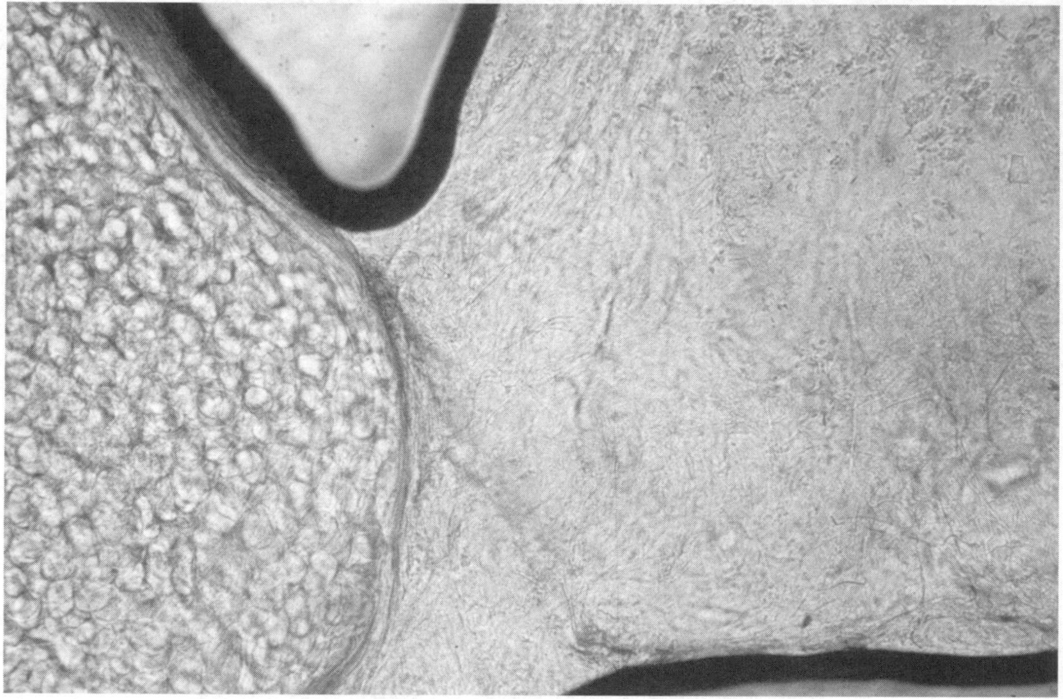

Fig. 18.13. Molluscum preparation White material can be expressed from the center of molluscum lesions, placed onto a slide with KOH, and examined for molluscum bodies, which are oval keratinocytes (left side of the picture) infected with molluscum contagiosum virus.

universally effective topical therapy exists for molluscum; however, individual lesions can be destroyed by cryosurgery or electrodesiccation.

Measles

In developing countries, measles is often more severe in HIV-infected children compared to those without infection [13]. Children may or may not present with a typical morbilliform rash. Mortality, which can be as high as 70% in these cases, is most often secondary to measles giant cell pneumonia.

Bacterial infections

The clinical manifestations of cutaneous bacterial infections are most often similar in HIV-infected and -uninfected children. *Staphylococcus aureus* and *Streptococcus pneumoniae* infection cause impetigo (Fig. 18.14), folliculitis, abscesses, wound infection, and cellulitis. Bacterial infection should be suspected when cutaneous erythema, edema, and tenderness are present, and confirmation can be made by bacterial culture if lesions exhibit frank pus or exudate. Treatment consists of oral antibiotics with good activity against *S. aureus*, e.g., dicloxacillin for 10–14 days.

Diseases caused by arthropods

Scabies

Scabies is common in HIV-infected children and is caused by the mite *Scabies sarcoptei* [1, 2]. Transmission occurs by contact with an infected individual. Cutaneous manifestations may be relatively mild (e.g., localized pruritus, scattered excoriations, excoriated papules, or areas of dermatitis). Mild infestations may be easily misdiagnosed, since usually fewer than ten mites are present on a given individual in a mild infestation. Lesions typically occur on the wrists, axillae, areolae, genitalia, and waist. By contrast, Norwegian, or crusted, scabies often manifests with widespread superficial friable scales (Fig. 18.15), less pronounced pruritus, lesions on the scalp, and thousands of mites within lesions. Norwegian scabies is a marker for severe underlying immunodeficiency. Ideally, diagnosis of scabies should be confirmed with a scabies preparation. Preparations are considered positive if any one following are observed under the microscope: mite (Fig. 18.16), mite eggs (Fig. 18.17), or mite feces. The patient and all household contacts should be treated with 5% permethrin cream or lindane, and all bedding should be washed the morning following treatment. One total body application, followed by an additional application one week later, is curative. Single doses of oral ivermectin are also effective.

Insect bite reactions

Exaggerated responses to bites by mosquitoes and other insects are commonly observed in HIV-infected children. Diagnosis should be suspected when observing grouped erythematous papules (often with prominent excoriations) on the distal extremities (Fig. 18.18). The lesions are also commonly secondarily infected with

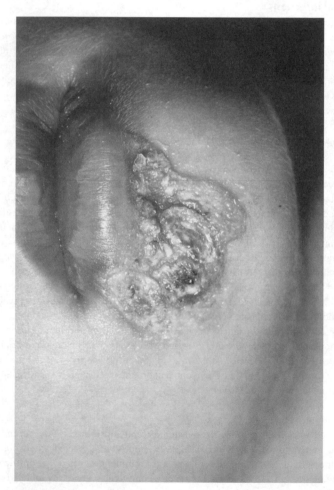

Fig. 18.14. Impetigo. Classic presentation of impetigo secondary to *S. aureus* infection in a child with HIV disease.

Fig. 18.15. Norwegian scabies. Unlike typical scabies, children with Norwegian scabies have prominent scaly non-pruritic lesions, lesions on the scalp, and numerous mites within lesions. Norwegian scabies is a sign of severe underlying immunodeficiency.

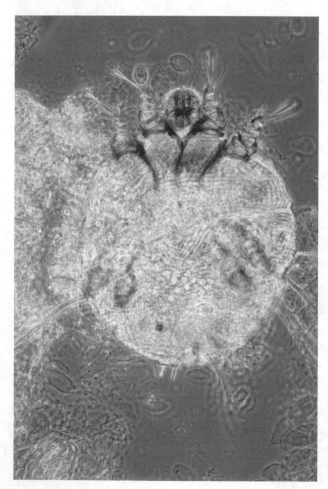

Fig. 18.16. Scabies preparation – mite. Typical appearance of a scabies mite.

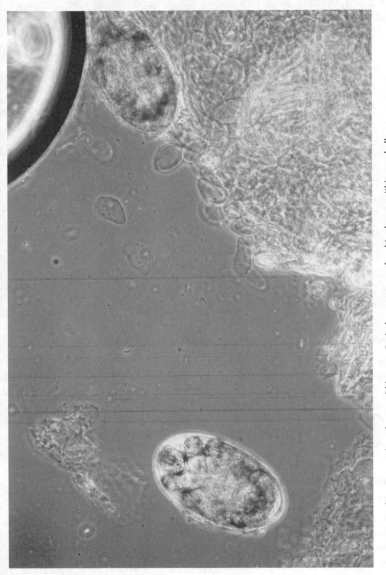

Fig. 18.17. Scabies preparation – larvae within eggs. Typical appearance of scabies larvae within eggshells.

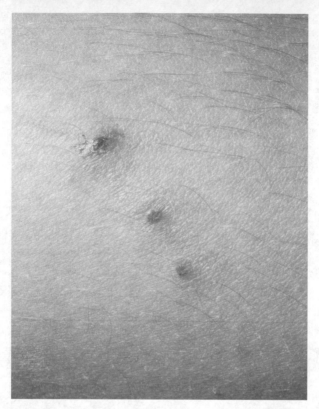

Fig. 18.18. Insect bites. To avoid unnecessary treatment, it is important to distinguish insect bites from cutaneous bacterial or viral infection. Lesions are often pruritic, grouped, and located on the distal extremities.

S. aureus. Chronic scratching of these lesions may lead to the development of prurigo nodularis. These types of reactions appear to be more prevalent in children who reside in southern US states (particular Florida and Texas) and in Africa.

Non-infectious diseases that predominantly involve the skin and oral mucosa

Drug eruptions

Drug eruptions occur commonly in HIV-infected individuals [1, 2]. Trimethoprim–sulfamethoxazole is particularly notorious, although nearly every medication is capable of causing a widespread erythematous maculopapular eruption (Fig. 18.19).

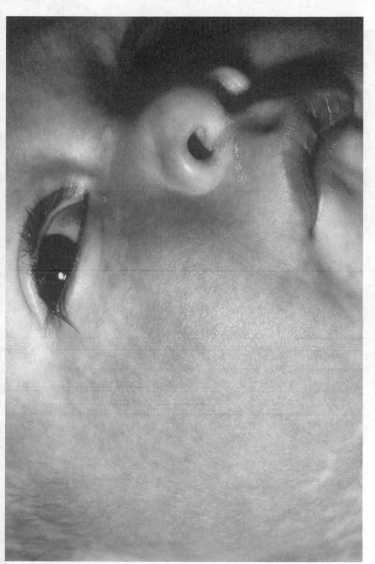

Fig. 18.19. Drug eruption secondary to trimethoprim-sulfamethoxazole. Drug eruptions are extremely common in HIV-infected children and often occur 7–14 days following the onset of initial treatment.

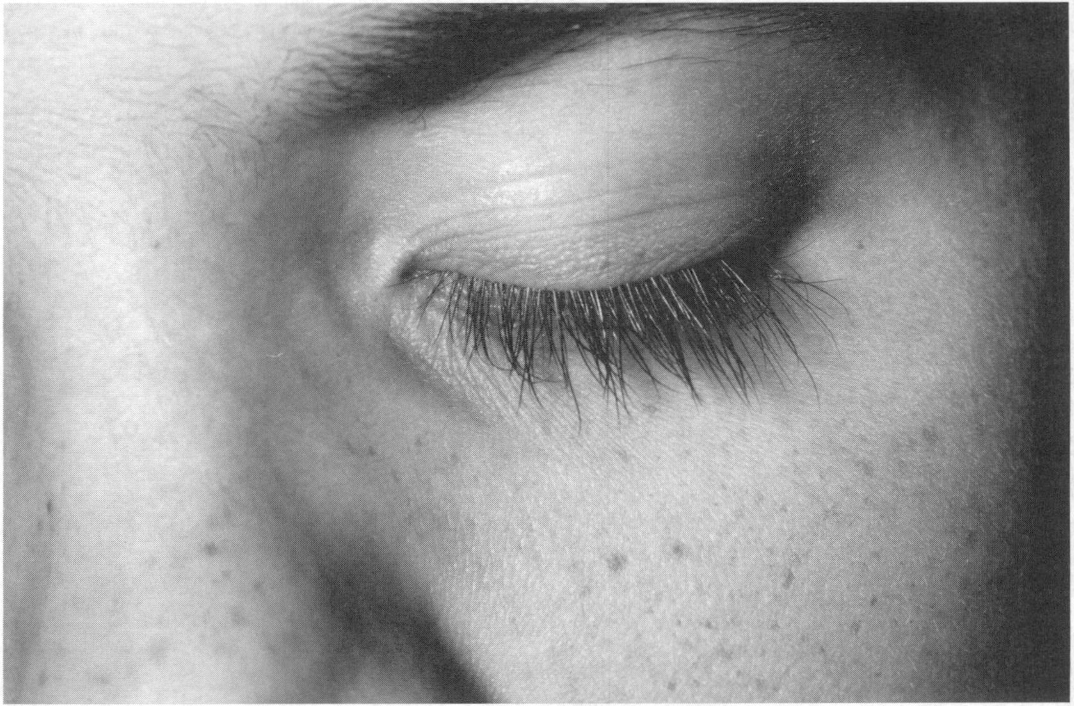

Fig. 18.20. Trichomegaly of the eyelashes. A peculiar condition observed in children with AIDS, as well as children with other severe underlying immunodeficiencies.

Typically, the onset of the rash occurs 7–14 days following initiation of the medication and 1–2 days following re-introducing the medication. Of note, in patients previously sensitized to trimethoprim-sulfamethoxazole, many clinicians are able to successfully re-initiate therapy by systematically administering drug in incremental doses, beginning with extremely low doses.

Important clinical variants of drug reactions include photosensitive eruptions (which appear to be increasingly common), fixed drug eruptions, erythema multiforme (with classic "targetoid" lesions), Stevens–Johnson syndrome (with mucosal involvement), and toxic epidermal necrolysis. The latter is an extremely severe and dangerous drug reaction that manifests with widespread blistering (and subsequent loss) of skin and mucous membranes, often complicated by fluid and electrolyte imbalance, as well as secondary infection. In particular, non-nucleoside reverse transcriptase inhibitors (e.g., nevirapine) have been implicated in many cases of Stevens–Johnson syndrome. Drug should be stopped at the first sign of mucosal symptoms, which may include itching or burning sensations prior to the development of visible lesions.

Lipodystrophy associated with protease inhibitor therapy has recently been reported in HIV-infected children [14, 15]. This complication is discussed more fully in Chapter 13.

Miscellaneous disorders

Many other dermatologic diseases have been reported in children infected with HIV. Some of these include seborrheic dermatitis, psoriasis, xerosis, generalized pruritus, urticaria, vasculitis, vitiligo, dysplastic nevi, aphthous ulcers, oral hairy leukoplakia, alopecia, and trichomegaly of the eyelashes. The latter condition is a peculiar lengthening of the eyelashes (Fig. 18.20), with no known cause, associated with severe underlying immunodeficiency. HIV-infected children are also often the target of child abuse, and therefore physicians should be aware of cutaneous signs of trauma when examining these individuals. Lastly, in developing countries, nutritional deficiency often exacerbates existing skin conditions or leads to specific cutaneous signs. For examples, protein deficiency (kwashiorkor) is associated with dry scaling skin and thinning of the hair, vitamin C deficiency (scurvy) causes a follicular petechial eruption and bleeding gums, and zinc deficiency (acrodermatitis enteropathica) causes a genital and acral rash with diarrhea.

Acknowledgments

Special thanks to Dr. Maria Turner for many of the photographs, lively discussions on this topic, and careful reading of the manuscript.

REFERENCES

1. Prose, N. S. Mucocutaneous disease in pediatric human immunodeficiency virus infection. *Pediatr. Clin. North Am.* 1991;**38**(4):977–990.

2. Prose, N. S. Cutaneous manifestations of HIV infection in children. *Dermatol. Clin.* 1991;**9**(3):543–550.

3. Wananukul, S., Thisyakorn, U. Mucocutaneous manifestations of HIV infection in 91 children born to HIV-seropositive women. *Pediatr. Dermatol.* 1999;**16**(5):359–363.

4. Stefanaki, C., Stratigos, A. J., Stratigos, J. D. Skin manifestations of HIV-1 infection in children. *Clin. Dermatol.* 2002;**20**(1):74–86.

5. Greenspan, D., Greenspan, J. S. HIV-related oral disease. *Lancet* 1996;**348**(9029):729–733.

6. Ramos-Gomez, F. J., Petru, A., Hilton, J. F., Canchola, A. J., Wara, D., Greenspan, J. S. Oral manifestations and dental status in paediatric HIV infection. *Int. J. Paediatr. Dent.* 2000;**10**(1):3–11.

7. Shiboski, C. H., Wilson, C. M., Greenspan, D., Hilton, J., Greenspan, J. S., Moscicki, A. B. HIV-related oral manifestations among adolescents in a multicenter cohort study. *J. Adolesc. Hlth.* 2001;**29**(3 Suppl):109–114.

8. Sirisanthana, V., Sirisanthana, T. Disseminated *Penicillium marneffei* infection in human immunodeficiency virus-infected children. *Pediatr. Infect. Dis. J.* 1995;**14**(11):935–940.

9. Grossman, M. C., Grossman, M. E. Chronic hyperkeratotic herpes zoster and human immunodeficiency virus infection. *J. Am. Acad. Dermatol.* 1993;**28**(2 Pt 2):306–308.

10. Moore, P. S., Chang, Y. Detection of herpesvirus-like DNA sequences in Kaposi's sarcoma in patients with and without HIV infection. *N. Engl. J. Med.* 1995;**332**(18):1181–1185.

11. Ziegler, J. L., Katongole-Mbidde, E. Kaposi's sarcoma in childhood: an analysis of 100 cases from Uganda and relationship to HIV infection. *Int. J. Cancer.* 1996;**65**(2):200–203.

12. He, J., Bhat, G., Kankasa, C. *et al.* Seroprevalence of human herpesvirus 8 among Zambian women of childbearing age without Kaposi's sarcoma (KS) and mother-child pairs with KS. *J. Infect. Dis.* 1998;**178**(6):1787–1790.

13. Dray-Spira, R., Lepage, P., Dabis, F. Prevention of infectious complications of paediatric HIV infection in Africa. *AIDS,* 2000;**14**(9):1091–1099.

14. Jaquet, D., Levine, M., Ortega-Rodriguez, E. *et al.* Clinical and metabolic presentation of the lipodystrophic syndrome in HIV-infected children. *AIDS* 2000;**14**(14):2123–2128.

15. Arpadi, S. M., Cuff, P. A., Horlick, M., Wang, J., Kotler, D. P. Lipodystrophy in HIV-infected children is associated with high viral load and low CD4+ -lymphocyte count and CD4+ -lymphocyte percentage at baseline and use of protease inhibitors and stavudine. *J. Acquir. Immune Defic. Syndr.* 2001;**27**(1):30–34.

19 Neurologic problems

Lucy Civitello, M.D.

Department of Neurology, Children's National Medical Center, Washington, DC
and National Institutes of Health, Bethesda, MD

Introduction

Neurodevelopmental abnormalities have been a well-known and frequent complication of pediatric HIV infection, causing significant morbidity and mortality [1]. However, significant progress has been made in the treatment of pediatric HIV disease, changing the prevalence and natural history of neurological complications.

Central nervous system (CNS) manifestations of HIV disease can be subdivided into two main groups: (a) those indirectly related to the effects of HIV on the brain, such as CNS opportunistic infections (OIs), malignancies, and cerebrovascular disease, and (b) those directly related to HIV brain infection.

Peripheral nervous system (PNS) abnormalities occur relatively frequently in adult HIV-infected patients and are usually related to antiretroviral therapy, HIV disease, or OIs [2]. Although much less common in infants and children, neuropathies and myopathies occur, with similar etiologies [3].

Secondary CNS disorders

Opportunistic infections of the CNS

Children with HIV disease have fewer problems with CNS OIs compared with adults, probably because OIs represent reactivation of previous, relatively asymptomatic infections. CNS OIs can present significant problems in children; their incidence may increase because children with HIV disease are living longer. Generally, OIs are seen in patients with severe immunocompromise (age-corrected CD4+ lymphocyte counts less than 200 cells/μl), and in infants and younger children due to congenital infection.

The most common CNS OI in chlidren is cytomegalovirus (CMV) infection, which may present as a subacute or chronic encephalitis/ventriculitis, an acute ascending radiculomyelitis, or as an acute or subacute neuritis [4, 5] (see also Chapter 34). Other

Handbook of Pediatric HIV Care, ed. Steven L. Zeichner and Jennifer S. Read.
Published by Cambridge University Press. © Cambridge University Press 2006.

viruses (herpes simplex virus (HSV), varicella-zoster virus (VZV), may also cause an acute or subacute encephalitis [6]. Progressive multifocal leukoencephalopathy (PML), caused by a papova virus (the JC virus) has been reported only rarely in the pediatric AIDS population [7].

The next most common CNS OIs in children are fungal infections (*Candida* and *Aspergillus* meningitis and abscess) [4]. Cryptococcal meningitis, although seen in 5% to 10% of adult AIDS patients, appears to be less common in pediatric AIDS patients (see also Chapter 33).

Toxoplasma encephalitis, a protozoan CNS infection, is the most common cause of intracranial mass lesions in adults with AIDS, occurring in ten to fifty percent of patients. This infection has only been reported in about one percent of HIV-infected children [8].

Bacterial CNS infections are also relatively uncommon in children with HIV disease. Unusual bacterial pathogens need to be considered in these immunocompromised hosts, such as *Mycobacterium tuberculosis,* atypical *Mycobacteria,* syphilis, *Bartonella, Listeria monocytogenes* and *Nocardia asteroides* [9].

Neoplasms

Primary CNS lymphoma is the most common cause of CNS mass lesions in pediatric AIDS patients and is the second most common cause of focal neurologic deficits, after stroke [10] (see also Chapter 29). These are usually high grade, multifocal B-cell tumors, which present with the subacute onset of change in mental status or behavior, headache, seizures, and new focal neurologic signs. The tumors have a predilection for the deep gray matter (basal ganglia and thalamus). On neuroimaging studies, they enhance with contrast and are associated with edema and mass effect. The prognosis is poor [11]. Treatment options include steroids, radiation therapy and chemotherapy. Metastatic lymphomas tend to cause more peripheral meningeal involvement and are rare in children with HIV disease.

Cerebrovascular disease

Strokes are the most common cause of clinical focal neurologic deficits in children with HIV infection [10, 12]. Strokes may be secondary to hemorrhage or ischemia. Ischemic strokes may be embolic, or may be secondary to an infectious vasculitis (for example, VZV). AIDS patients may also develop a hypercoagulable state secondary to acquired protein C, and/or protein S deficiencies. In addition, there is a characterisitic vasculopathy seen in HIV-infected children resulting in aneurysmal dilatation of vessels of the circle of Willis, with or without ischemic infarction or hemorrhage [13]. The etiology of this vasculopathy is unclear but it may be due to direct viral invasion of vessel walls (Fig. 19.1).

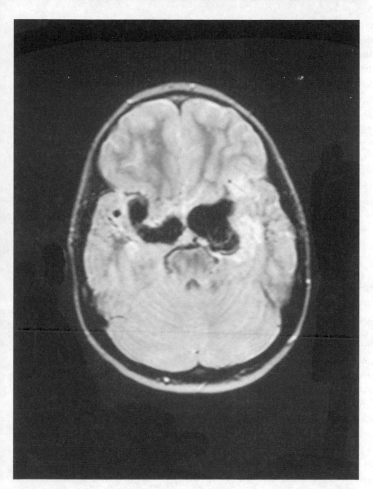

Fig. 19.1. Magnetic resonance imaging scan of large aneurysmal dilatations of multiple vessels of the Circle of Willis in an adolescent boy with transfusion-acquired HIV infection. (Image courtesy of Department of Radiology, National Institutes of Health.)

Primary HIV-related CNS disease

HIV-related CNS disease has been a prominent feature in pediatric patients with HIV infection. Even early on in the epidemic, it was recognized that the frequent neurodevelopmental abnormalities seen in these children were due to the direct effects of HIV infection on the brain and not due to OIs or malignancies.

Epidemiology

The prevalence of HIV-related CNS disease in children was estimated at 50%–90% in early studies [14]. By the mid 1990s, the prevalence was estimated to be between 20% and 50% in the USA [15, 16]. Since the advent of highly active antiretroviral therapy (HAART), the incidence of encephalopathy is lower [17]. In general, children less than 3 years of age have higher rates of CNS disease than older children and adolescents [15–17]. Patients with more advanced degrees of immune suppression have higher rates of encephalopathy [18]. It is important to note that HIV-related CNS disease may be the presenting manifestation of HIV infection. Early onset of HIV infection (i.e., infection occurring in utero) increases a child's risk for poor neurodevelopmental outcome within the first thirty months of life [19].

Early onset of neurologic signs and symptoms in HIV-infected infants less than 1 year of age seems to have a different significance and pathophysiology than those occurring later on in children and adults [20]. CNS disease in older children and adolescents seems to be more similar to the dementia and motor cognitive dysfunction seen in adults, both clincally and pathophysiologically.

Clinical manifestations

The classic triad of pediatric HIV-related encephalopathy includes developmental delays (particularly motor and expressive language), acquired microcephaly, and pyramidal tract motor deficits [1]. There is a broad spectrum of clinical manifestations and severity of CNS disease in infants and children addressed by a new classification system for pediatric HIV-related CNS disease developed at the HIV and AIDS Malignancy Branch (HAMB) of the National Cancer Institute (NCI) to assess CNS status. Patients are classified as having encephalopathy (static or progressive), CNS compromise, or as not being apparently affected (for details see Chapter 10, Table 19.1).

The subacute progressive type of encephalopathy is often seen in infants and young children naïve to antiretroviral therapy [1, 14, 21]. The hallmarks of this disorder include loss of previously acquired milestones, particularly motor and expressive language, with progressive non-focal motor dysfunction (spastic quadriplegia or hypotonia in young infants and spastic diplegia or hypotonia in older infants and children). The course of this disorder is usually slower, developing over weeks to months, and more insidious than the course observed with OIs, tumors, or strokes.

Children with HIV-related encephalopathy may have prominent oromotor dysfunction, facial diparesis, and abnormal eye movements, including nystagmus and impaired upgaze [14]. Impaired brain growth leads to acquired microcephaly. Progressive cognitive deterioration occurs, along with social regression and apathy. Extrapyramidal movement disorders, such as bradykinesia (which may be responsive to L-dopa), cerebellar signs and symptoms, and seizures, occur less frequently [22]. Seizures may occur in about sixteen percent of children with HIV-related CNS disease. About half of these are provoked by febrile illnesses. Recurrent, unprovoked seizures are rarely due to HIV

Table 19.1. Clinical manifestations of HIV-related encephalopathy

---

Progressive encephalopathies

Subacute progressive
Loss of milestones
Progressive motor dysfunction
Oromotor dysfunction
Acquired microcephaly
Cognitive deterioration
Apathy
Progressive long tract signs
Movement disorders (uncommon)
Cerebellar signs (uncommon)
Seizures (uncommon)
More rapid course (weeks to months)

Plateau
No loss of skills
No or slower acquisition of skills
Decline in rate of cognitive development
Motor dysfunction (non-progressive)
Acquired microcephaly
More indolent course

Static encephalopathy
Fixed deficits
No loss of skills
Skills acquired at a stable but slow rate
Deficient, but stable IQ
Motor dysfunction (non-progressive)
Static course
Many potential etiologies

CNS disease; more often they are due to other factors, such as complications of prematurity, CNS OIs, etc. [14]. Rarely, infants and young children exhibit generalized subcortical myoclonus, which clincially resembles infantile spasms. EEGs are typically normal and myoclonus resolves with antiretroviral treatment alone. In the school-aged child, the first complaints may be a decline in academic achievement, change in behavior, and/or psychomotor slowing. Eventually, progressive cognitive impairment and new pyramidal tract signs (hyperreflexia and gait disturbances) occur.

The course of the plateau type of progressive encephalopathy is more indolent with either the absence of acquisition of new developmental skills or a slower rate of acquisition of skills than previously. The rate of cognitive development declines, as does the rate of brain growth. Motor involvement is common, particularly spastic diplegia

Children with static encephalopathy tend to have fixed neurodevelopmental deficits with no loss of skills. Development continues at a stable but slow rate. IQs are stable but low. Motor dysfunction is common, but not progressive. Whereas the etiology of progressive encephalopathy is related to the direct effects of HIV brain infection, the etiology of static encephalopathy can be varied and can include in utero exposure to drugs, alcohol, and/or infections, prematurity and perinatal difficulties. Other factors to consider include genetics, nutrititional, endocrinologic, and metabolic factors. Environmental and psychosocial factors may also affect development.

Children with HIV-related CNS compromise typically have normal overall cognitive functioning, but they may have had a significant decline in one or more psychological tests, or they may have significant impairments in selective neurodevelopmental functions. The specific domains of impairment seen in children with HIV disease include expressive (greater than receptive) language, attention, adaptive functioning (socialization, behavior, quality of life) and memory [23].

Patients with CNS compromise may have abnormal findings on neurologic examination (such as pathologic deep tendon reflexes with extensor plantar responses) that do not affect their day-to-day functioning. Patients who were functioning in the average cognitive range at baseline, but who improve after beginning or changing antiretroviral therapy are also classified in this category.

Children are classified as apparently not affected when their cognitive function is at least within normal limits, they have had no decline in function, have a normal neurologic examination and have had no therapy-related improvements in function.

Psychiatric disturbances (depression, bipolar disorder, anxiety, and adjustment disorders) occur in pediatric AIDS patients, but may be under-reported, particularly in adolescents [21]. Acute psychosis can be due to varying etiologies (CNS OIs, tumors, medication side effects, nutritional deficiencies, or active HIV CNS infection).

Neuroradiologic findings

Neuroradiologic studies provide essential information concerning HIV-related CNS disease. The most common abnormalites seen on CT scans in symptomatic, treatment-naïve children are ventricular enlargement, cortical atrophy, white matter attenuation, and basal ganglia calcifications [24]. Calcifications are seen primarily in vertically infected children or premature babies who were infected via transfusion in the neonatal period. They are not seen in adults [25] (Fig. 19.2).

In general, greater degrees of CT brain scan abnormalities are seen with more advanced stages of HIV disease [26]. In addition, the severity of CT abnormalities has been correlated with lower levels of general cognitive abilities and language functioning in children with symptomatic HIV infection [18, 23, 27].

Cortical atrophy, but not calcification, is correlated with CSF RNA viral concentration [28], suggesting that active HIV CNS replication is at least partly responsible for the development of cortical atrophy. Calcifications may not be related to active HIV

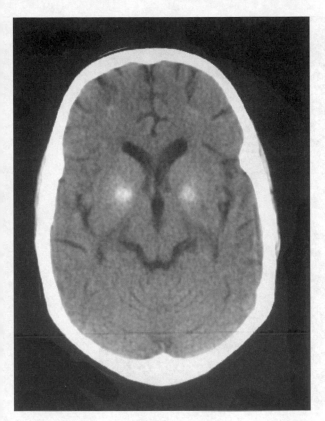

Fig. 19.2. Computerized axial tomographic scan depicting cortical atrophy and basal ganglia calcifications in a preschool child with vertically-acquired HIV infection. (Image courtesy of Gilbert Vezina, M.D., Children's National Medical Center.)

replication, but rather may indicate past infection of the immature brain, perhaps indicating a special vulnerability of the infant basal ganglia to HIV infection.

A decreased prevalence of CT scan abnormalities has been found in children treated with combination nucleoside analogue antiretroviral therapy, even prior to the availability of HAART including protease inhibitors (PIs) [29]. Similar abnormalities are seen on magnetic resonance imaging (MRI) scans, although calcifications are not as well seen as on CT scans. White matter abnormalities are more readily seen on MRIs. Mild white matter changes in children are not necessarily correlated with cognitive dysfunction, although extensive white matter changes may be associated with cognitive impairments [30] (Fig. 19.3).

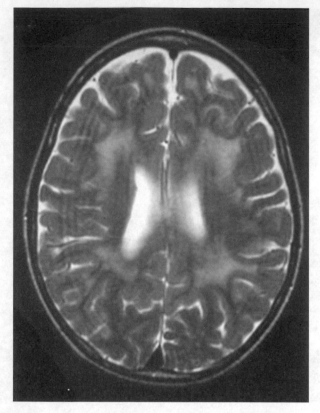

Fig. 19.3. Magnetic resonance imaging scan of a school-aged child with vertically-acquired HIV infection depicting bright signal in the periventricular white matter. (Image courtesy of Gilbert Vezina, M.D., Children's National Medical Center.)

CSF studies

Routine CSF studies may show nonspecific abnormalities, including a mild pleocytosis or elevated protein level, but are usually normal. In adults, an aseptic meningitis can be seen at the time of seroconversion, but this is rarely seen in children.

Children and adults with abnormal brain function have increased levels of HIV RNA in the CSF compared to those patients with normal brain function [31]. Therefore, CSF viral load may be predictive of CNS status. In adults elevated baseline CSF HIV RNA levels predict progression to neuropsychological impairment one year later [32]. In addition, markers of immune activation in the CSF (and serum) such as tumor necrosis factor, beta-2-microglobulin, neopterin, quinolinic acid and certain chemokines have been correlated with CNS disease in both adults and children.

Diagnosis of HIV-related CNS disease

The diagnosis of HIV-related CNS disease remains a clinical diagnosis, based on history, physical, and neurological examinations, and age-appropriate neuropsychologic testing. Other causes of CNS disease should be ruled out, such as CNS OIs, malignancies, cerebrovascular disease, and non-HIV-related conditions (static encephalopathies due to effects of prematurity, maternal drug use, other congenital infections, genetic, nutritional, and endocrinologic factors). Neuroimaging is indicated to rule out OIs, tumors, and stroke, and to identify the characteristic features of HIV-related CNS disease. CSF studies should be done to rule out OIs.

Neuropathology

HIV "encephalitis" consists of perivascular inflammatory cell infiltrates composed of microglia, macrophages, and multinucleated giant cells (micoglial nodules) [33]. These infiltrates occur in the subcortical white matter, the deep gray nuclei (putamen, globus pallidus), and pons. The characteristic finding in pediatric CNS disease is a calcific basal ganglia vasculopathy, consisting of vascular and perivascular mineralization, sometimes extending into the white matter. This corresponds to the basal ganglia calcifications seen on brain CT scans and is not seen in adults.

HIV leukoencephalopathy consists of myelin loss and reactive astrocytosis. In adults, neuronal loss is seen in the hippocampi and the orbitofrontal cortex, along with loss of dendritic arborizations. These features are difficult to appreciate in pediatric patients because there are few standards for neuronal cell counts.

Neuropathogenesis

HIV enters the brain early during the course of HIV infection in adults, either as free viral particles or within infected monocytes, which then set up residence in the brain as macrophages. Only two brain cell types, the microglia/macrophage and the astrocyte have clearly been shown to be infected by HIV [34]. In microglia, a productive and cytopathic infection results, but in astrocytes a latent or restricted infection exists. However, despite the prominent neuronal cell loss and evidence of neuronal apoptosis, neurons are not thought to be directly infected by HIV. There are a large number of glial cells in the CNS, so there are potentially a large number of HIV-infected cells in the CNS. The brain may act as an important viral reservoir.

Products released from HIV-infected glial cells may be responsible for causing neurotoxicity and ultimately neuronal cell death [34]. These products may be derived from the virus or the host and can set up a chain of events leading to potentially reversible neuronal dysfunction at sites distant from infected cells.

Infected, activated glial cells release viral proteins (gp120, Tat), as well as several host-derived neurotoxic factors [35]. These factors include the proinflammatory cytokines

(TNF-alpha, IL-1, IL-6, IFN-gamma and alpha), arachidonic acid and its metabolites, quinolinic acid (an agonist of excitatory amino acid receptors), nitric oxide, and chemokines [36]. The chemokines, monocyte chemoattractant protein-1 (MCP-1), macrophage inflammatory protein-1 alpha (MIP-1-alpha), and MIP-1-beta may be important in CNS disease [31]. Host genetic factors may predispose to the development of, or protect the host from, developing CNS disease.

HIV CNS infection is worsened by cell-to-cell interactions between HIV-infected macrophages and astrocytes, which initiate a self-perpetuating cascade of neurotoxic events in the brain. These events ultimately lead to an increase in the extracellular concentration of the excitatory amino acid glutamate which, through activation of the N-methyl-D-aspartate (NMDA) receptor and non-NMDA excitatory amino acid receptors, leads to increases in intracellular calcium concentrations and eventually disruption of mitochondrial function, generation of nitric oxide and other free radicals, and eventual activation of apoptotic and other cellular pathways [34–37].

Treatment of HIV-related CNS disease

There are three main types of therapy for HIV CNS disease: (a) antiretroviral, (b) neuroprotective, and (c) symptomatic.

Antiretroviral therapy

HIV encephalopathy is at least, in part, related to active viral replication in the brain. The CNS behaves as a separate compartment from the rest of the body in HIV disease [38]. Plasma viral loads may not reflect the degree of viral replication in the brain. The brain may act as a viral reservoir and may theoretically reseed the plasma, potentially with species of pathophysiologic significance, for example virus-bearing drug resistance mutations. At times of high plasma viral load, virus may traffick into the CNS through a disrupted blood–brain barrier (BBB). If HIV CNS disease is a concern, patients should be treated with drugs able to cross the BBB and reach effective concentrations in the CSF and brain. Some evidence suggests that HIV CNS disease may be worse when the peripheral viral load is high, perhaps due to continued seeding of the CNS from the periphery. Aggressive and effective efforts to decrease peripheral viral load may have beneficial effects upon CNS HIV disease.

The nucleoside analogue reverse transcriptase inhibitors (NRTIs) zidovudine (AZT, ZDV, Retrovir) and stavudine (d4T, Zerit) have relatively good CSF penetration [39, 40]. ZDV has been beneficial in pediatric patients with HIV-related encephalopathy [39]. Early epidemiologic studies in Europe demonstrated decreased prevalence of dementia in adult AIDS patients after ZDV was introduced [41]. Limited studies document the clinical efficacy of d4T in CNS disease in pediatric patients. Other NRTIs, didanosine (ddI, Videx), zalcitabine (ddC, Hivid), lamivudine (3TC, Epivir) have less CSF penetration, but may have some beneficial effects in HIV-associated dementia. A more recently

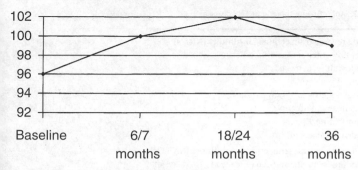

Fig. 19.4. Effect of indinavir treatment on full-scale IQ from baseline to 6/7 months, to 18/24 months and to 36 months ($n=20$). There was a significant improvement in Full Scale IQ over time (P less than 0.02). (See reference [29].)

developed NRTI, abacavir (ABC, Ziagen) crosses the BBB and offers potential for CNS coverage [42].

Of the non-nucleoside reverse transcriptase inhibitors (NNRTIs), nevirapine (NVP, Viramune) has the best potential for treatment of CNS disease. Efavirenz (EFV, Sustiva, Stocrin) and delavirdine (DLV, Resriptor) have less CNS penetration.

Protease inhibitors (PIs) have poor CSF penetration; indinavir (Crixivan) has the best penetration among PIs [42]. Ritonavir (Norvir) and indinavir were the first two PIs used in pediatric clinical trials. Full-scale IQs significantly improved with either drug (used in combination with two NRTIs) but then appeared to plateau, possibly due to the development of drug resistance [29] (Fig. 19.4).

Highly active antiretroviral therapy (HAART) has been found to be beneficial in the treatment of HIV CNS disease in many studies in adults [43]. In a large retrospective study, the prevalence of AIDS dementia and neuropathy, and toxoplasma encephalitis have decreased since the introduction of HAART. There have been few reported studies of the effect of HAART on cognitive functioning in HIV-infected children.

HAART including an NRTI or NNRTI with good CSF penetration is indicated in the treatment of children with HIV-related CNS disease (Table 19.2). ZDV, d4T, abacavir and nevirapine have the best CSF penetration among NRTIs and NNRTIs. The choice of individual drug depends on the history of prior antiretroviral use and on drug resistance patterns. There is no clear-cut evidence to suggest that regimens containing multiple CSF-penetrating drugs are superior to those with single CSF-penetrating drugs [40].

Neuroprophylaxis

Once CNS disease is present, antiretroviral regimens may improve neurocognitive dysfunction. However, since there is an improved survival rate for patients with HIV disease

Table 19.2. Antiretroviral therapy of CNS disease

Nucleoside reverse transcriptase inhibitors (NRTIs)
(In descending order of potential efficacy in CNS disease)
    AZT (zidovudine, Retrovir)
    d4T (stavudine, Zerit)
    Abacavir (Ziagen)
    ddI (didanosine, Videx)
    3TC (lamivudine, Epivir)
    ddC (zalcitabine, Hivid)

Non-nucleoside reverse transciptase inhibitors (NNRTIs)
(In descending order of potential efficacy in CNS disease)
    Nevirapine (Viramune)
    Efavirenz (Sustiva, Stocrin)
    Delavirdine (Rescriptor)

Protease inhibitors
(In descending order of potential efficacy in CNS disease)
    Indinavir (Crixivan)
    Ritonavir (Norvir)
    Saquinavir (Fortovase, Invirase)
    Nelfinavir (Viracept)
    Amprenavir (Agenerase)

---

who are treated with HAART, it is possible that CNS disease is being delayed but not prevented. Therefore, the prophylactic value of antiretroviral therapy on the CNS is becoming a more important issue. Zidovudine appears to have some beneficial prophylactic effects for HIV CNS disease [41, 44].

The prophylactic value of HAART for HIV CNS disease appears to occur in a subgroup of patients with subclinical psychomotor slowing and with clinical motor signs. However, this prophylactic effect may be time-limited, which could be related to the development of drug resistance. HAART may not have a prophylactic effect for patients with more sustained subclinical psychomotor slowing [45].

Neuroprotection

Neuroprotective strategies (adjunctive therapies) are directed toward the effects of viral proteins and other cellular "toxins," such as cytokines, on neuronal function. These strategies are largely investigational at this time and are not recommended for general use. These agents include steroids, pentoxifylline and thalidomide (TNF-alpha antagonists), the calcium channel blocker nimodipine, memantine (an NMDA receptor antagonist), antioxidants, and antipoptotic agents. Additional potential agents include other cytokine anatagonists, antichemokine agents, other NMDA receptor antagonists, nitric oxide synthase inhibitors, and inhibitors of arachidonic acid metabolites.

Symptomatic treatment

Symptomatic treatment includes treatment of pain, movement disorders, seizures, spasticity, attention deficit/hyperactivity disorder (ADHD), and psychiatric/behavioral disorders. In general, the same agents can be used in the HIV-infected child as in the general population. However, one should always keep in mind the potential for bone marrow suppression, liver and pancreatic toxicities, as well as their effect on metabolism of antiretrovirals, particularly PIs. One should also keep in mind that patients with CNS involvement may be very sensitive to psychotropic medications.

Children with severe neurodevelopmental deficits may benefit from physical, occupational, and speech therapy. Educational remediation is indicated for children with ADHD and/or learning disabilities. Optimal nutrition is extremely important. Other causes of neurodevelopmental disorders, such as endocrinologic and metabolic disturbances, (hypothyroidism, vitamin and cofactor deficiencies) should be carefully sought out and treated. Psychostimulants, such as methylphenidate, have been used in HIV-infected adults with lethargy and progressive slowing.

Other nervous system abnormalities

Myelopathies

Vacuolar myelopathy, seen in up to 30% of adult AIDS patients at autopsy in the past, is rarely seen in children [46]. Spinal corticospinal tract degeneration is one of the characteristic features seen in pediatric AIDS patients at autopsy but this is not usually a clinical diagnosis [47]. Myelopathies can also be due to OIs (HSV, CMV, VZV) or tumors.

Peripheral neuropathies

Peripheral neuropathies are less common in children than adults with HIV infection. Several patterns of neuropathy can be seen in pediatric patients [3]. The most common pattern is a distal sensory or axonal neuropathy, possibly related to antiretroviral use and/or HIV infection itself. Carpal tunnel syndrome is less common. A subacute demyelinating neuropathy due to HIV infection is rare. Paresthesias and pain are the most common presenting complaints, followed by weakness or loss of motor milestones.

Antiretrovirals implicated in peripheral neuropathy include, but are not limited to, the NRTIs ddI, ddC, and d4T. Peripheral neuropathies due to these agents can be severe and may require discontinuation of the drug.

Myopathies

Numerous muscle disorders have been described in adults with HIV infection, including HIV myopathy, ZDV and d4T-induced mitochondrial myopathy, and secondary myopathies (due to OIs or lymphoma) [48, 49]. Typically, these patients present with progressive muscle weakness, and sometimes with pain and elevated CPK. These muscle disorders can occur in children, but are less common.

Summary

The incidence of HIV-related CNS disease has declined since the advent of HAART. However, CNS disease may become more prevalent as life-expectancy increases and as drug resistance occurs. HAART improves neurocognitive function in at least a subset of patients with CNS disease. Nervous system involvement, when it does occur, can have a profound impact on quality of life as well as on survival. Accurate diagnosis and management of neurologic disease in pediatric patients remains a challenge. The development of new therapies for HIV CNS disease remains an important priority.

REFERENCES

1. Epstein, L. G., Sharer, L. R., Oleske, J. M. *et al.* Neurological manifestations of HIV infection in children. *Pediatrics* 1986;**78**:678–687.

2. Simpson, S. M., Olney, R. K. Peripheral neuropathies associated with HIV infection. *Neurol. Clin.* 1992;**10**:685–711.

3. Floeter, M. K., Civitello, L. A., Everett, C. R. *et al.* Peripheral neuropathy in children with HIV infection. *Neurology* 1997;**49**:207–212.

4. Kozlowski, P. B., Sher, J. H., Dickson, D. W. *et al.* CNS infections in pediatric HIV infection: a multicenter study. In Kozlowski, P. B., Snider, D. A., Vietze, P. M., Wisniewski, H. M., eds, *Brain in Pediatric AIDS*. Basel: Karger, 1990:132–146.

5. Holland, N. R., Power, C., Matthews, V. P. *et al.* CMV encephalitis in AIDS. *Neurology* 1994;**44**:507–514.

6. Annunziato, P. W., Gershon, A. A. Herpesvirus infections in children infected with HIV. In Wilfert, C. M., Pizzo, P. A., eds. *Pediatric AIDS: The Challenge of HIV Infection in Infants, Children and Adolescents*. Baltimore: Williams and Wilkins, 1998;205–225.

7. Berger, J. R. F., Scott, G., Albrecht, J. *et al.* PML in HIV-1 infected children. *AIDS* 1992;**6**:837–842.

8. Simonds, R. J., Gonzalo, O. *Pneumocystis carinii* pneumonia and Toxoplasmosis. In Wilfert, C. M., Pizzo, P. A., eds. *Pediatric AIDS: The Challenge of HIV Infection in Infants, Children and Adolescents*. Baltimore: Williams and Wilkins, 1998;251–265.

9. Cohen, B. A., Berger, J. R. Neruologic opportunistic infections in AIDS. In Gendelman, H. E., Lipton, S. A., Epstein, L., Swindells, S., eds. *The Neurology of AIDS*. New York: Chapman and Hall, 1988:303–332.

10. Dickson, D. W., Llen, A. J. F., Werdenheim, K. M. *et al.* CNS pathology in children with AIDS and focal neurologic signs: stroke and lymphoma. In Kozlowski, P. B., Snider,

D. A., Vietze, P. M., Wisniewski, H. M., eds. *Brain in Pediatric AIDS*. Basel:Karger, 1990: 147–157.

11. Epstein, L. G., DiCarlo, F. J., Joshi, V. V. *et al*. Primary lymphoma of the central nervous system in children with AIDS. *Pediatrics* 1988; 355–363.

12. Park, Y. D., Belman, A. L., Kim, T. S. *et al*. Stroke in pediatric AIDS. *Ann. Neurol.* 1990;**28**:303–311.

13. Husson, R. N., Saini, R., Lewis, L. L. Cerebral artery aneurysms in children infected with HIV. *J. Pediatr.* 1992;**121**:927–930.

14. Civitello, L. A., Brouwers, P., Pizzo, P. A. Neurologic and neuropsychologic manifestations in 120 children with symptomatic HIV infection. *Ann. Neurol.* 1993;**34**:481.

15. England, J. A., Baker, C. J., Raskino, C. *et al*. Clinical and laboratory characteristics of a large cohort of symptomatic HIV-infected infants and children. *Pediatr. Infect. Dis. J.* 1996;**15**:1025–1036.

16. Blanche, S., Newell, M., Mayaux, M. *et al*. Morbidity and mortality in European children vertically infected by HIV-1. *Acquir. Immune Defic. Syndr. Hum. Retrovirol.* 1997;**14**:442–450.

17. Sacktor, N., Lyles, R. H., Skolasky, R. *et al*. HIV-associated neurologic disease incidence changes: multicenter AIDS cohort study, 1990–1998. *Neurology* 2001;**56**:257–260.

18. Brouwers, P., Tudor-Williams, G., DiCarli, C. *et al*. Relation between stage of disease and neurobehavioral measures in children with symptomatic HIV disease. *AIDS* 1995;**9**:713–720.

19. Smith, R., Malee, K., Charurat, M. *et al*. Timing of perinatal HIV-1 infection and rate of neurodevelopment. *Pediatr. Infect. Dis. J.* 2000;**19**:862–871.

20. Tardieu, M., Le Chenadec, J., Persoz, A. *et al*. HIV-1-related encephalopathy in infants compared with children and adults. *Neurology* 2000;**54**:1089–1095.

21. Mintz, M., Clinical features and treatment interventions for HIV-associated neurologic disease in children. *Semin. Neurol.* 1999;**19**:165–176.

22. Mintz, M., Tardieu, M., Hoyt, L. *et al*. Levodopa therapy improves motor function in HIV-infected children. *Neurology* 1996;**47**:1583–1585.

23. Wolters, P., Brouwers, P., Moss, H., Pizzo, P. Differential receptive and expressive language functioning of children with symptomatic HIV disease and relation to CT scan brain abnormalities. *Pediatrics* 1995;**95**:112–119.

24. DeCarli, C., Civitello, L. A., Brouwers, P., Pizzo, P. A. The prevalence of computed axial tomographic abnormalities in 100 consecutive children symptomatic with the human immunodeficiency virus. *Ann. Neurol.* 1993;**34**:198–205.

25. Civitello, L., Brouwers, P., DeCarli, C., Pizzo, P. Calcification of the basal ganglia in children with HIV infection. *Ann. Neurol.* 1994;**36**:506.

26. Brouwers, P., Tudor-Williams, G., DeCarli, C. *et al*. Interrelations among patterns of change in neurocognitive, CT brain imaging, and CD4 measures associated with antiretroviral therapy in children with symptomatic HIV infection. *Adv. Neur. Immunol.* 1994;**4**:223–231.

27. Brouwers, P., De Carli, C., Civitello, L. *et al*. Correlation between computed tomographic brain scan abnormalities and neuropsychological function in children with symptomatic HIV disease. *Arch. Neurol.* 1995;**52**:39–44.

28. Brouwers, P., Civitello, L., DeCarli, C. *et al.* Cerebrospinal fluid viral load is related to cortical atrophy and not to intracerebral calcifications in children with symptomatic HIV disease. *J. Neurovirol.* 2000; **6**:390–397.

29. Civitello, L. A., Wolters, P., Serchuck, L. *et al.* Long-term effect of protease inhibitors on neuropsychological function and neuroimaging in pediatric HIV disease. *Ann. Neurol.* 2000;**48**:513.

30. Brouwers, P., van der Vlugt, H., Moss, H. *et al.* White matter changes on CT brain scans are associated with neurobehavioral dysfunction in children with symptomatic HIV disease. *Child Neuropsychol.* 1995; **1**:93–105.

31. DeLuca, A., Ciancio, B. C., Larussa, D. *et al.* Correlates of independent HIV-1 replication in the CNS and of its controls by antiretrovirals. *Neurology* 2002;**59**:342–347.

32. Ellis, R. J., Moore, D. J., Childers, M. E. *et al.* Progression to neuropsychologic impairment in HIV infection predicted by elevated CSF levels of HIV RNA. *Arch. Neurol.* 2002;**59**:923–928.

33. Sharer, L. R. Neuropathologic aspects of HIV-1 infection in children. In Gendelman, H. E., Lipton, S. A., Epstein, L., Swindells, S., eds. *The Neurology of AIDS*. New York:Chapman and Hall, 1998.

34. Nath, A. Pathobiology of HIV dementia. *Semin. Neurol.* 1999;**19**:113–127.

35. Nath, A., Haughey, N. J., Jones, M. *et al.* Synergistic neurotoxicity by HIV proteins Tat and gp 120: protection by memantine. *Ann. Neurol.* 2000;**47**:186–194.

36. Genis, P., Jett, M., Bernton, E. W. *et al.* Cytokines and arachidonic metabolites produced during HIV-infected macrophage–astroglia interactions: implications for the neuropathogenesis of HIV disease. *J. Exp. Med.* 1992;**176**:1703–1718.

37. Bukrinsky, M. I., Notte, H. S., Schmidtmayerova, H. *et al.* Regulation of nitric oxide synthase activity in HIV-1 infected monocytes: implications for HIV-associated neurologic disease. *J. Exp. Med.* 1995;**181**:735–745.

38. Stingele, K., Haas, J., Zimmerman, T. *et al.* Independent HIV replication in paired CSF and blood viral isolates during antiretroviral therapy. *Neurology* 2001;**56**:355–361.

39. McKinney, R. E., Maha, M. A., Connor, E. M. *et al.* A multicenter trial of oral zidovudine in children with HIV infection. *N. Engl. J. Med.* 1991;**324**:1018–1925.

40. Sacktor, N., Tarwater, P. M., Skolasky, M. A. *et al.* CSF antiretroviral drug penetrance and the treatment of HIV-associated psychomotor slowing. *Neurology* 2001;**57**:542–544.

41. McArthur, J. C., Sacktor, N., Selnes, O. HIV-associated dementia. *Semin. Neurol.* 1999;**19**:129–150.

42. Enting, R. H., Hoetelmans, M. W., Lange, J. M. A. *et al.* Antiretroviral drugs and the CNS. *AIDS* 1998;**12**:1941–1955

43. Suarez, S., Baril, L., Stankoff, B. *et al.* Outcome of patients with HIV-1-related cognitive impairment on HAART. *AIDS* 2001;**15**:195–200.

44. Simpson, D. M., HIV-associated dementia: review of pathogenesis, prophylaxis and treatment studies of zidovudine therapy. *Clin. Infect. Dis.* 1999;**29**:19–34.

45. Geisen, H. J., Hefter, H., Jablonski, H., Arendt, G. HAART is neuroprophylactic in HIV-1 infection. *J. AIDS* 2000 **23**:380–385.

46. Petito, C. K., Navia, B. A., Cho, E. S. *et al.* Vacuolar myelopathy pathologically resembling subacute combined degeneration in patients with AIDS. *N. Engl. J. Med.* 1985;**312**:874–879.

47. Dickson, D. W., Belman, A. L., Tin, T. S. *et al.* Spinal cord pathology in pediatric AIDS. *Neurology* 1989;**39**:227–235.
48. Dalakas, M. C., Illa, I., Pezeshkpour, G. H. *et al.* Mitochondrial myopathy caused by long-term zidovudine therapy. *N. Engl. J. Med.* 1990;**322**:1098–1105.
49. Walter, E. B., Drucker, R. P., McKinney, R. E. *et al.* Myopathy in HIV-infected children receiving long-term zidovudine therapy. *J. Pediatr.* 1991;**119**:152–155.

20 Ophthalmic problems

Howard F. Fine, M.D. M.H.S.

Ophthalmology, Wilmer Eye Institute, Johns Hopkins, Baltimore, M.D.

Susan S. Lee, BS, and Michael R. Robinson, M.D.

National Eye Institute, NIH, Bethesda, M.D.

Introduction

Ophthalmic disease is common in patients with HIV infection, occurring in up to 75% of patients over the course of their illness [1]. As in other organ systems, a hallmark of the ocular sequelae of HIV infection is the presence of opportunistic infections by bacteria, viruses, fungi, and parasites, which may occur in up to 30% of HIV-positive individuals [2, 3]. HIV-positive children may acquire infections that are also common in immunocompetent patients, although the severity is often greatly increased.

Because children rarely complain of ocular symptoms, eye disease such as cytomegalovirus (CMV) retinitis, is often diagnosed at a more advanced stage. This chapter gives an overview of the ocular manifestations of HIV in children.

Epidemiology

Ophthalmologic disease in HIV-infected children can involve any part of the eye. The ocular manifestations of HIV infection in children are listed in Table 20.1; few of the disorders occur in more than 5% of children. The most common ophthalmologic diseases in HIV-infected children affect the posterior segment (vitreous, retina, and choroid).

Clinical examination

Routine screening eye examinations are suggested because sight-threatening complications like CMV retinitis can be asymptomatic, and early diagnosis and treatment can prevent loss of sight. Sight-threatening diseases occur most frequently in children with advanced HIV infection and low CD4+ lymphocyte counts. Regular screening examinations should be performed by an experienced ophthalmologist according to Table 20.2 [4].

Handbook of Pediatric HIV Care, ed. Steven L. Zeichner and Jennifer S. Read.
Published by Cambridge University Press. © Cambridge University Press 2006.

Table 20.1. Ocular manifestations of pediatric HIV infection

Lids / Conjunctiva
    Molluscum contagiosum
    Hypertrichosis
    Kapos's sarcoma
Cornea / sclera
    Keratoconjunctivits sicca[a]
    Herpes keratitis
    Herpes zoster ophthalmicus
    Corneal microsporidiosis
Vitreous / retina / choroid
    CMV retinitis[a]
    Immune recovery uveitis
    Toxoplasmosis
    Progressive outer retinal necrosis (PORN)
    HIV microangiopathy[a]
    Frosted branch angiitis
Orbit
    Fungi (aspergillosis, mucormycosis)
    Bacteria (*P. aeruginosa, T. pallidum, S. aureus*)
    Parasites (*Toxoplasma gondii*)
    Protozoa (*Pneumocystis carinii*)
Neoplasms
    Burkitt's / Burkitt's-like lymphoma
    Kaposi's sarcoma
Neuro-ophthalmology
    Papilledema
    Optic neuropathy
    Motor neuropathies
    Field defects
    Nystagmus
    Gaze paresis
    Horner's syndrome
Developmental
    AIDS-associated embryopathy
Drug ocular toxicity
    Rifabutin
    Cidofovir
    Didanosine
    Atovaquone

[a] Occurs in more than 5% of patients.

Table 20.2. Screening examination frequency

Age <6 years	CD4% < 21 q2–3 months	CD4% ≥ 21 q6 months
Age ≥6 years	CD4+ cells < 50 cells/μl q2–3 months	CD4+ cells ≥ 50 cells/μl q6 months

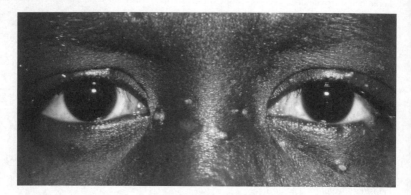

Fig. 20.1. External photograph of molluscum contagiosum involving the eyelids. A chronic keratoconjunctivitis can occur with lesions on the eyelid margin.

The complete ophthalmic examination consists of a slit lamp examination for anterior segment disease and a dilated retinal examination primarily to rule out asymptomatic CMV retinitis.

External diseases

Ocular sequelae of HIV in the lids and conjunctiva of children are not common.

Molluscum contagiosum, a growth of cutaneous papules and nodules with central umbilication, is caused by a pox virus (Fig. 20.1). It can occur near the lid margin and be associated with a chronic follicular conjunctivitis [5]. Lesions may be treated with excision or cryotherapy.

HIV can damage lacrimal glands, leading to keratoconjunctivitis sicca (dry eye), which is often relieved with lubrication [6]. This must be distinguished from epithelial keratitis, caused by the herpes viruses including herpes simplex virus (HSV), CMV, and varicella-zoster virus (VZV), which can be associated with significant pain, reduced corneal sensation, dendritic corneal lesions, and secondary glaucoma. Treatment may include topical trifluorothymidine and oral acyclovir or valacyclovir [7]. VZV keratitis is commonly observed with herpes zoster ophthalmicus, a painful, vesicular dermatitis in the distribution of the ophthalmic division of the trigeminal nerve.

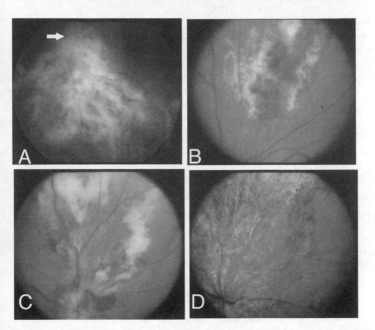

Fig. 20.2. CMV retinitis. (a) Retinal photograph of a patient with CMV retinitis involving the optic disc (arrow) with counting fingers vision. The patient was treated with intravenous ganciclovir and the vision improved to 20/40 with residual optic disc pallor. (b) Retinal photograph showing an area of CMV retinitis in the midperiphery. This patient was asymptomatic and was diagnosed during a routine screening examination. (c) Retinal photograph showing CMV retinitis extending from the optic disc to the superior quadrants. (d) Retinal photograph of the patient shown in Fig. 20.2(c) after treatment with intravenous ganciclovir. Note the retinal hemorrhages and necrosis are replaced by an atrophic chorioretinal scar.

CMV retinitis

CMV retinitis in children with HIV is less common than in adults, yet is still the most common HIV-related ocular infection. The prevalence of CMV retinitis in HIV-positive children in the pre-HAART era was approximately 3% to 5%. After the introduction of HAART in 1996, the occurrence of CMV retinopathy has been dramatically reduced [2]. The disease is usually associated with low CD4 counts, <50 cells/μl. While older children may complain of floaters and decreased peripheral or central vision, young children often present without subjective visual complaints despite advanced retinitis [8].

CMV retinitis may progress in several ways. Indolent or smoldering CMV is usually peripheral with a granular appearance and progresses slowly, at a rate of 1–3 mm/month

Table 20.3. Treatment of CMV retinitis

Systemic therapy:		
Systemic agent	*Dose*	*Toxicity*
Ganciclovir	Intravenous: 5 mg/kg body weight bid for 14–21 days, then 5 mg/kg maintenance	Neutropenia, thrombocytopenia
	Oral: FDA approved in adults only at 3–6 g/day. Consult pediatric ID specialist	
Foscarnet	Intravenous: 60 or 90 mg/kg body weight bid for 14–21 days, then 90–120 mg/kg maintenance	Nephrotoxicity, electrolyte imbalance (hypocalcemia, hypokalemia, hypomagnesemia)
Cidofovir	Intravenous: 5 mg/kg weekly for 2 weeks, then 5 mg/kg every 2 weeks maintenance	Intravenous: nephrotoxicity, uveitis
Local therapy		
Intraocular agent	*Dose*	*Toxicity*
Ganciclovir	Injection: 400–800 µg/0.1 ml 2–3 times/week for 2–3 weeks, then 400–800 µg/0.1 ml 1–2 times/week maintenance	Local: vitreous hemorrhage, retinal detachment, endophthalmitis
	Implant: releases 1.4 µg/h over 5–8 months, 1–3 week course of intravenous ganciclovir may be used in the perioperative period	
Foscarnet	Injection: 2.4 mg/0.1 ml 2–3 times/week, then 1.2–2.4 mg/0.05–0.10 ml 1–2 times/week for maintenance	
Cidofovir	Injection: 10–20 µg/0.1 ml every 3–6 weeks	

without therapy. Fulminant retinitis is marked by a confluent, yellow-white, geographic opacification which follows vascular arcades and may be associated with mild vitritis (Fig. 20.2) [9]. Serious sequelae of CMV retinitis include vitreous hemorrhages, often at the edge of advancing retinitis, and retinal detachments, which occurred in almost 40% of adult patients without HAART at 1 year. Risk factors for detachment include the area of retinitis involvement and lower CD4+ T-cell counts [10]. Fortunately, with HAART therapy the risk of retinal detachment has decreased by about 60% [11].

Treatment of CMV retinitis is outlined in Table 20.3. Systemic therapy is generally given as an initial induction for 2–3 weeks, followed by maintenance therapy at a lower dosage. Note that maintenance therapy can be safely stopped in those patients with stable retinitis who have recovered CD4 counts on HAART [12]. Local anti-viral therapy

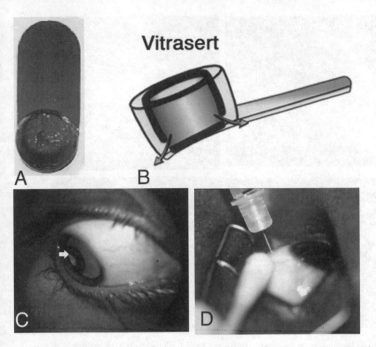

Fig. 20.3. Local antiviral therapy. (a) Vitrasert implant (Bausch and Lomb, Rochester NY)– delivers ganciclovir for the treatment of CMV retinitis for up to 8 months. (b) The release of ganciclovir occurs at the base of the implant and clinical trials have shown the implant to be superior in efficacy to systemic therapy for the treatment of CMV retinitis. (c) External photograph showing the implant through a dilated pupil (arrow). The implant is sutured to the scleral and projects into the vitreous cavity releasing ganciclovir. (d) External photograph showing an intravitreal injection of ganciclovir into the eye in a patient with refractory CMV retinitis. The injections are performed at least weekly under local anesthesia and are not suitable for children under the age of ~15 years without general anesthesia.

is effective and can avoid the serious adverse effects of systemic administration (Fig. 20.3). Orally administered valganciclovir has been shown to be as effective as intravenous ganciclovir in adult patients [13], however clinical trials in a pediatric population have not been reported.

Immune recovery uveitis

Patients with CMV retinitis and depressed CD4 counts who subsequently regain immune function on HAART therapy can develop inflammation in the eye (uveitis) comprised of vitreous inflammatory cells (vitritis) and edema of the optic disk and macula [14, 15]. This condition, termed immune recovery uveitis, can be sight-threatening,

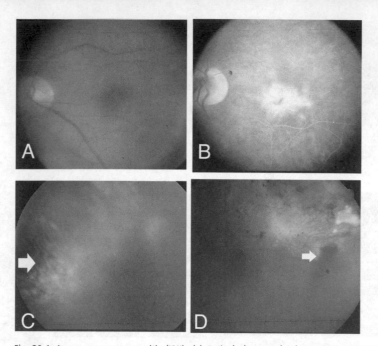

Fig. 20.4. Immune recovery uveitis (IRU). (a) Retinal photograph of a patient with IRU. This patient had inactive CMV retinitis in the periphery, a mild vitritis, reduced visual acuity to 20/60 from cystoid macular edema and an epiretinal membrane; all features commonly seen with IRU. (b) A fluorescein angiogram retinal photograph of a patient with IRU and reduced visual acuity. Leakage of fluorescein in the central macula is consistent with cystoid macular edema, a consistent finding in IRU patients with reduced vision. (c) A retinal photograph of a patient with IRU with inactive CMV retinitis (arrow). The remarkable finding in this patient was a moderate vitritis obscuring retinal details. (d) A retinal photograph of a patient with IRU that developed recurrent vitreous hemorrhages. A small area of neovascularization is present at the edge of the healed CMV scar (arrow), a less common finding in patients with IRU. Retinal details inferiorly obscured by overlying vitreous hemorrhage.

but may be treated with topical, periocular, and or systemic corticosteroids (Fig. 20.4) [15].

Other diseases of the posterior segment

HIV microangiopathy, a microvascular retinal ischemia evidenced by cotton wool spots (nerve fiber layer infarcts) and hemorrhages, is seen much less commonly in HIV-positive children than adults. Retinal venous occlusive disease has also been reported with HIV infection (Fig. 20.5).

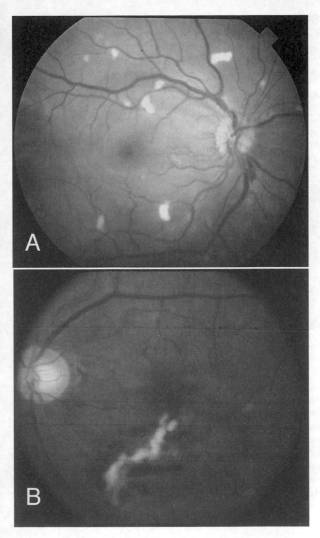

Fig. 20.5. HIV microangiopathy. (a) Retinal photograph showing cotton wool spots and a retinal hemorrhage, common findings in patients with CD4 lymphocyte counts < 100 cells/μl. (b) Retinal photograph showing a branch retinal vein occlusion, an uncommon manifestation of HIV microangiopathy.

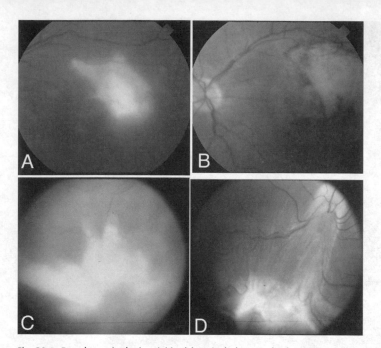

Fig. 20.6. Toxoplasmosis chorioretinitis. (a) Retinal photograph of a patient with a presumptive diagnosis of CMV retinitis responding poorly to specific anti-CMV medications. Patient was referred and workup revealed a positive toxoplasmosis titer. (b) Retinal photograph of patient discussed in Fig. 20.6(a) With a presumptive diagnosis of toxoplasmosis chorioretinitis, following 3 months of treatment with anti-toxoplasmosis medications, the lesion showed resolution with a chorioretinal scar remaining in the posterior pole. Unfortunately, the lesion had extended into the central macula and the vision was reduced to counting fingers. (c) Retinal photograph of a patient who presented to the ER following a seizure. Brain imaging showed a large solitary abscess. Ophthalmologic consultation was requested for complaints of reduced acuity in one eye. Examination showed an exudative subretinal lesion in the macula not typical of CMV retinitis. Further workup revealed a positive toxoplasmosis titer and a brain biopsy confirmed toxoplasmosis. (d) Retinal photograph of patient discussed in Fig. 20.6(c) Six months following treatment with anti-toxoplasmosis medications, the chorioretinitis resolved with traction of the macula inferiorly.

HIV-infected children are at significant risk for ocular infection with the protozoan *Toxoplasma gondii* [16]. Toxoplasma causes necrotizing retinochoroiditis, which may be unilateral or bilateral; unifocal, multifocal, or diffuse; and is often associated with retinal detachments and marked anterior chamber and vitreal inflammation (Fig. 20.6).

Children with HIV are at risk for acquiring progressive outer retinal necrosis (PORN) [17], a rapidly progressive necrotizing retinopathy. The infection is with either

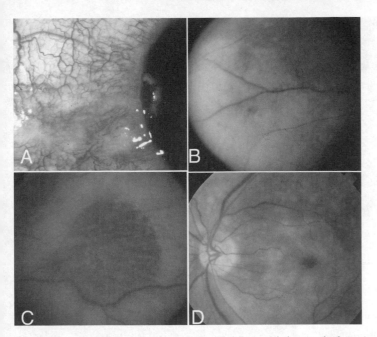

Fig. 20.7. Progressive outer retinal necrosis (PORN). (a) External photograph of a patient with zoster ophthalmicus who developed scleral and corneal involvement during the healing phase of the skin disease. (b) Retinal photograph of the patient discussed in Fig. 20.7(a). He complained of floaters in one eye 3 months after the onset of the zoster ophthalmicus and examination showed a unilateral retinitis involving the deep retinal structures consistent with PORN. Note the relative sparing of the retinal vessels and lack of hemorrhage, typical of this disease. (c) Retinal photograph of a patient with a history of varicella-zoster in the T10 dermatome. The patient subsequently developed an outer retinal necrosis in both eyes consistent with PORN. (d) Retinal photograph of the patient discussed in Fig. 20.7(c) The retinitis progressed rapidly towards the macula and within 2 months, this eye had no light perception despite aggressive use of a combination of anti- HSV, HZV, and CMV medications.

varicella-zoster or herpes simplex, and clinically appears as ill-defined, posterior retinal lesions that rapidly progress to full-thickness retinal necrosis (Fig. 20.7). The visual prognosis is extremely poor, despite aggressive treatment with antivirals (acyclovir, foscarnet) to halt progression and photocoagulation to prevent retinal detachment.

Orbit

Orbital infections in HIV-positive patients include: fungi (aspergillosis, mucormycosis) often invading from the sinuses/orbits to the brain; bacteria (*Pseudomonas*

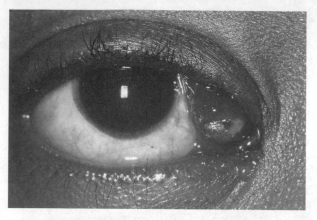

Fig. 20.8. External photograph of a Kaposi's sarcoma lesion in the medial orbit extending anteriorly. These lesions can be treated with systemic chemotherapy or radiation.

aeruginosa, Rhizopus arrhizus, Treponema pallidum, Staphylococcus aureus) causing orbital cellulitis; parasites (*Toxoplasma gondii*) engendering cysts, panophthalmitis, and orbital cellulitis; and protozoa (*Pneumocystis carinii*) inducing granulomatous orbital inflammation [3].

Although orbital infections are relatively rare, the most common and life threatening are due to invasive fungi. In the setting of irreversible immunosuppresion, the mortality rate is high despite aggressive surgical debridement, including orbital exenteration, and antifungal therapies [18].

Neoplasms

Some ocular neoplasms in children with HIV are life threatening. Diagnosis can be difficult and delayed when neoplasms masquerade as more common ophthalmic conditions.

Burkitt's/Burkitt's-like lymphoma in children with AIDS has been reported to masquerade as acute bacterial sinusitis and orbital cellulitis. [19].

Kaposi's sarcoma (KS), a common neoplasm in AIDS, may be mistaken for other ocular conditions. On the eyelid, KS may resemble a chalazion. On the conjunctiva, KS can mimic a foreign body granuloma, subconjunctival hemorrhage, or cavernous hemangioma (Fig. 20.8). Conjunctival lesions are usually located in the inferior fornix. Since ophthalmic KS is slowly progressive, treatment usually consists of observation alone or focal irradiation for entropion prevention or cosmesis [20].

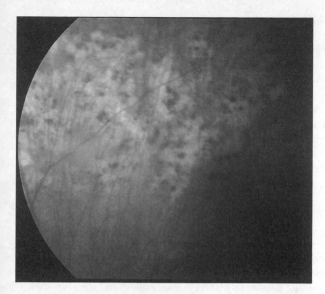

Fig. 20.9. Retinal photograph of DDI toxicity associated with didanosine (DDI) therapy. The well-circumscribed depigmented lesions with some hyperpigmented borders are typically observed.

Neuro-ophthalmology

Neuro-ophthalmic signs are present in 2%–12% of patients with AIDS [4, 21, 22]. Findings include: meningeal involvement (papilledema, optic neuropathy, motor neuropathies); thalamic-midbrain masses (cranial nerve III involvement); pontine tegmental lesions (pontine gaze paresis, internuclear ophthalmoplegia, nystagmus); cerebellar masses (abnormal spontaneous eye movements); cerebral masses (homonymous hemianopia, papilledema); and pupillary abnormalities (Horner's syndrome). Etiologies include lymphoma, cryptococcus, toxoplasmosis, neurosyphilis, progressive multifocal leukoencephalopathy (PML), CMV, herpes viruses, and HIV infection itself [21, 23]. Cryptococcal meningitis is prevalent in adult HIV patients and can be associated with an optic neuropathy that can lead to blindness [24].

Drug ocular toxicity

Several of the commonly used antimicrobials in HIV-positive patients are associated with ocular toxicity.

In children, rifabutin can induce bilateral corneal endothelial deposits, which are initially peripheral and stellate in nature [25]. Rifabutin can also cause a mild to severe uveitis that may be associated with hypopyon, vitritis, and/or retinal vasculitis [26].

Didanosine (DDI) has been shown to induce retinal lesions and decrease retinal function in approximately 7% of children. The medication adversely affects the retinal pigment epithelium (RPE), causing initial peripheral atrophy and secondary RPE hypertrophy and neurosensory retinal loss (Fig. 20.9).

Cidofovir, both intravenously and intravitreally administered, has been associated with intraocular inflammation in adults, causing iritis, vitritis, and/or hypotony. Concurrent treatment with probenecid may reduce the incidence of toxicity. Treatment of the inflammation with topical corticosteroids is often effective [27].

Summary

Understanding the diseases of the eye that occur with HIV infection is crucial to properly diagnose and promptly treat potentially blinding disorders. Diseases such as CMV retinitis can be especially difficult to diagnose in the pediatric population because they are largely asymptomatic. Routine screening eye examinations and aggressive therapy are mandatory to save vision.

REFERENCES

1. Mines, J. A., Kaplan, H. J. Acquired immunodeficiency syndrome (AIDS): the disease and its ocular manifestations. *Int. Ophthalmol. Clin.* 1986;**26**(2):73–115.

2. Robinson, M. R., Ross, M. L., Whitcup, S. M. Ocular manifestations of HIV infection. *Curr. Opin. Ophthalmol* 1999;**10**(6):431–437.

3. Kronish, J. W., Johnson, T. E., Gilberg, S. M., Corrent, G. F., McLeish, W. M., Scott, K. R. Orbital infections in patients with human immunodeficiency virus infection. *Ophthalmology* 1996;**103**(9):1483–1492.

4. Pizzo, P. A., Wilfert, C. A., ed. *Ocular Manifestations of HIV in the Pediatric Population.* 3rd edn. Baltimore: Williams & Wilkins, 1998.

5. Robinson, M. R., Udell, I. J., Garber, P. F., Perry, H. D., Streeten, B. W. Molluscum contagiosum of the eyelids in patients with acquired immune deficiency syndrome. *Ophthalmology* 1992;**99**(11):1745–1747.

6. Cunningham, E. T., Jr., Margolis, T. P. Ocular manifestations of HIV infection. *N. Engl. J. Med.* 1998;**339**(4):236–244.

7. Chern, K. C., Conrad, D., Holland, G. N., Holsclaw, D. S., Schwartz, L. K., Margolis, T. P. Chronic varicella-zoster virus epithelial keratitis in patients with acquired immunodeficiency syndrome. *Arch. Ophthalmol.* 1998;**116**(8):1011–1017.

8. Du, L. T., Coats, D. K., Kline, M. W. *et al.* Incidence of presumed cytomegalovirus retinitis in HIV-infected pediatric patients. *J. Aapos.* 1999;**3**(4):245–249.

9. Kanski, J. J., *Clinical Ophthalmology: A Systemic Approach.* 4th edn. Boston: Butterworth Heinemann publishers, 1999.

10. The Studies of Ocular Complications of AIDS (SOCA) Research Group in Collaboration with the AIDS Clinical Trials Group (ACTG). Rhegmatogenous retinal detachment in patients with cytomegalovirus retinitis: the Foscarnet-Ganciclovir Cytomegalovirus Retinitis Trial. *Am. J. Ophthalmol.* 1997;**124**(1):61–70.

11. Kempen, J. H., Jabs, D. A., Dunn, J. P., West, S. K., Tonascia, J. Retinal detachment risk in cytomegalovirus retinitis related to the acquired immunodeficiency syndrome. *Arch. Ophthalmol.* 2001;**119**(1):33–40.

12. Whitcup, S. M., Fortin, E., Lindblad, A. S. *et al.* Discontinuation of anticytomegalovirus therapy in patients with HIV infection and cytomegalovirus retinitis. *J. Am. Med. Assoc.* 1999;**282**(17):1633–1637.

13. Martin, D. F., Sierra-Madero, J., Walmsley, S. *et al.* A controlled trial of valganciclovir as induction therapy for cytomegalovirus retinitis. *N. Engl. J. Med.* 2002;**346**(15):1119–1126.

14. Jabs, D. A., Van Natta, M. L., Kempen, J. H. *et al.* Characteristics of patients with cytomegalovirus retinitis in the era of highly active antiretroviral therapy. *Am. J. Ophthalmol.* 2002;**133**(1):48–61.

15. Robinson, M. R., Reed, G., Csaky, K. G., Polis, M. A., Whitcup, S. M. Immune-recovery uveitis in patients with cytomegalovirus retinitis taking highly active antiretroviral therapy. *Am. J. Ophthalmol.* 2000;**130**(1):49–56.

16. Girard, B., Prevost-Moravia, G., Courpotin, C., Lasfargues, G. [Ophthalmologic manifestations observed in a pediatric HIV-seropositive population]. *J. Fr. Ophtalmol.* 1997;**20**(1):49–60.

17. Hammond, C. J., Evans, J. A., Shah, S. M., Acheson, J. F., Walters, M. D. The spectrum of eye disease in children with AIDS due to vertically transmitted HIV disease: clinical findings, virology and recommendations for surveillance. *Graefes Arch. Clin. Exp. Ophthalmol.* 1997;**235**(3):125–129.

18. Robinson, M. R., Fine, H. F., Ross, M. L. *et al.* Sino-orbital-cerebral aspergillosis in immunocompromised pediatric patients. *Pediatr. Infect. Dis. J.* 2000;**19**(12):1197–1203.

19. Robinson, M. R., Salit, R. B., Bryant-Greenwood, P. K. *et al.* Burkitt's/Burkitt's-like lymphoma presenting as bacterial sinusitis in two HIV-infected children. *AIDS Patient Care STDS* 2001;**15**(9):453–458.

20. Shuler, J. D., Holland, G. N., Miles, S. A., Miller, B. J., Grossman, I. Kaposi sarcoma of the conjunctiva and eyelids associated with the acquired immunodeficiency syndrome. *Arch. Ophthalmol.* 1989;**107**(6):858–862.

21. Keane, J. R. Neuro-ophthalmologic signs of AIDS: 50 patients. *Neurology* 1991;**41**(6):841–845.

22. Kestelyn, P., Lepage, P., Karita, E., Van de Perre, P. Ocular manifestations of infection with the human immunodeficiency virus in an African pediatric population. *Ocul. Immunol. Inflamm.* 2000;**8**(4):263–273.

23. Smith, D. D., Robinson, M. R., Scheibel, S. F., Valenti, W. M., Eskin, T. A. Progressive multifocal leukoencephalopathy (PML) in two cases of cortical blindness. *AIDS Patient Care* 1994;**8**(3):110–113.

24. Kestelyn, P., Taelman, H., Bogaerts, J. *et al.* Ophthalmic manifestations of infections with *Cryptococcus neoformans* in patients with the acquired immunodeficiency syndrome. *Am. J. Ophthalmol.* 1993;**116**(6):721–727.

25. Smith, J. A., Mueller, B. U., Nussenblatt, R. B., Whitcup, S. M. Corneal endothelial deposits in children positive for human immunodeficiency virus receiving rifabutin prophylaxis for *Mycobacterium avium* complex bacteremia. *Am. J. Ophthalmol.* 1999;**127**(2):164–169.

26. Arevalo, J. F., Russack, V., Freeman, W. R. New ophthalmic manifestations of presumed rifabutin-related uveitis. *Ophthalmic Surg. Lasers.* 1997;**28**(4):321–324.

27. Davis, J. L., Taskintuna, I., Freeman, W. R., Weinberg, D. V., Feuer, W. J., Leonard, R. E. Iritis and hypotony after treatment with intravenous cidofovir for cytomegalovirus retinitis. *Arch. Ophthalmol.* 1997;**115**(6):733–737.

21 Oral health and dental problems

Jane C. Atkinson, D.D.S.

National Institute of Dental and Craniofacial Research, National Institutes of Health, Bethesda, MD

Anne O'Connell, B.D.S., M.S.

Department of Public and Child Dental Health; Lincoln Place, Dublin, Ireland

Many children with HIV have oral manifestations of the infection (Table 21.1), including some that are part of the 1994 CDC classification system [1]. Since the introduction of antiretroviral therapy and highly active antiretroviral therapy (ART and HAART), the prevalence of these oral manifestations has decreased. However, in many countries where therapy is less than ideal, such as Romania, Brazil, and Mexico, HIV-associated oral lesions are more common, with prevolenic ranging from 55%–61% [2–4]. Their presence can still be used as markers for progression of disease. Referral to a dentist before 1 year of age is recommended for all children, but this is especially important for the HIV-infected child. Careful examination of the soft tissues and teeth is essential.

Oral mucosal lesions

Fungal infections

Oral candidiasis (thrush) is by far the most common oral opportunistic infection in HIV-infected children [5–8]. Prevalence estimates in this group range from 28%–67% (Table 21.1), and its presence is associated with low or declining CD4 counts [7, 8]. The diagnosis and treatment of *Candida* infections are discussed in detail in Chapter 33.

Oral candidal infections can appear as a red patch (erythematous, Fig. 21.1), a white patch that rubs off (pseudomembranous) or as red patches at the corners of the mouth (angular chelitis). Often, patients are asymptomatic, but they may experience oral burning or soreness. The diagnosis of oral candidiasis is based on clinical appearance and the presence of hyphae on a smear prepared with potassium hydroxide. *Candida* species are isolated most commonly; however, many other species are recovered from the oral cavity [7]. All laboratory results must be correlated with the clinical presentation

Handbook of Pediatric HIV Care, ed. Steven L. Zeichner and Jennifer S. Read.
Published by Cambridge University Press. © Cambridge University Press 2006.

Table 21.1. Oral manifestations of HIV-infected children

Diagnosis	Prevalence	Features
Oral mucosal changes		
• Candidiasis	28%–67%	White patches that rub off, red patches intraorally or redness at corners of mouth.
• Herpetic stomatitis	3%–5%	Both primary and recurrent forms may be more dramatic in HIV-infected children.
• Aphthous ulcers	Up to 15%	Ulcers of unknown etiology that can be more severe in HIV-infected children
• Hairy leukoplakia	0%–2%	White plaques on the lateral border of the tongue that do not rub off
• Other viral infections	Very rare	CMV, VZV can cause oral changes
• Tumors	Very rare	Kaposi's sarcoma and non-Hodgkin's lymphoma are very rare in this population
Gingival changes		
• Gingivitis	>80%	Erythematous gingival changes from plaque on teeth
• Linear gingival erythema	Up to 25%	Specific to HIV infection
• HIV-associated periodontitis	Rare	Rapidly advancing periodontal disease
Tooth changes		
• Decay	Common	Tooth breakdown can be obvious. Pain is not normally a presenting complaint
• Abscesses	Fairly common	Can cause fever and pain
• Delayed exfoliation and eruption	Fairly common	Primary teeth may be retained well into teenage years
Parotid gland enlargement	2%–11%	
• Lymphocytic-mediated		Painless enlargements; Clear saliva can be expressed from glands. MRI can be used to confirm presence of cysts.
• Bacterial infection		Pain on palpation; often, pus can be expressed from glands. May or may not be accompanied by fever

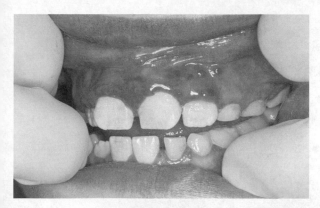

Fig. 21.1. Erythematous candidiasis on the gingiva and buccal mucosa of a child with HIV infection.

since HIV-positive patients have greater numbers of *Candida* species in the oral cavity, even in the absence of clinical infection [9]. Treatment can be with systemic or topical antifungal agents, but treatment is complicated with the emergence of resistant strains (see Chapter 33).

Viral infections

Oral viral infections are not found as frequently as fungal infections [5–9]. Herpes simplex infection is the most common, with a similar presentation in children with or without HIV. However, the disease can be more severe and debilitating for patients with HIV infection. Primary herpetic stomatitis is characterized by fever, lymphadenopathy, and gingival fluid-filled vesicles, which quickly rupture and ulcerate. The vesicular fluid is the best source of virus for culture. After primary infection, the virus establishes a latent infection in the trigeminal ganglion until reactivation. Typically, intraoral recurrent HSV lesions are found on keratinized tissues of the mouth, but lesions may be more severe and involve any oral mucosal surfaces of children with HIV. Extraoral lesions are found on the lips, and heal in 7–14 days without scarring (Fig. 21.2). Burning and tingling may precede vesicle formation. While coating agents such as Benadryl and Kaopectate (mixed 1:1) can be used as a rinse to decrease discomfort of small intraoral lesions, viscous xylocaine should be discouraged in young children. Intraoral herpes zoster occurs rarely in children, but was reported recently in a study of Romanian children [4]. It may present as small, crusted, painful ulcerated areas of keratinized intraoral tissues in a unilateral pattern that follows the distribution of the trigeminal nerve. The systemic therapy of herpesvirus infections is discussed in detail in Chapter 34.

Epstein–Barr virus (EBV) is the causative agent of oral hairy leukoplakia (OHL) [10, 13]. It is very rare in children with HIV infection. Clinically, the lesion is a white patch along the lateral borders of the tongue that does not wipe off. Diagnosis requires

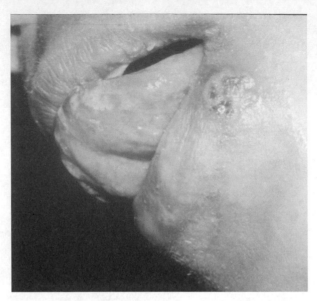

Fig. 21.2. A 10-year-old child displays oral features typical of HIV infection: oral candidiasis on the lateral border of the tongue and at the corners of mouth, and a large, recurrent herpetic lesion extraorally.

identification of EBV genome in a biopsy specimen or cytologic smear, and lesions are not treated typically.

Sometimes, the cause of intraoral ulcerations in both children and adults with HIV infection is not established, despite repeated diagnostic procedures. Rare infectious processes that should be considered include tuberculosis, systemic mycotic infections such as histoplasmosis, and cytomegalovirus infection. Treatment of these lesions with topical anesthetics, antimicrobial rinses or topical corticosteroids may be necessary if they are persistent and symptomatic, and no etiology is established.

Neoplasms

In contrast to adults, neoplasms associated with HIV infection are rarely found in the oral cavity of pediatric patients. However, intraoral Kaposi's sarcoma and non-Hodgkin's lymphoma have been reported [11, 12].

Salivary gland pathology

Saliva is essential for the maintenance of oral health, having lubricating, physical cleansing, and antibacterial and antiviral properties. Salivary flow may be reduced by the medications used in the treatment of HIV. Medications with potent anticholinergic effects such as diphenhydramine can reduce salivary flow by 50%, which can enhance the development of dental caries or candidal infections.

Although many children with HIV infection may have decreased salivary gland function as a consequence of medication usage, a subset develop enlargement of the salivary glands. Prevalence estimates in controlled studies are 2% to 14% of children with HIV infection [5–8]. Some enlargements are secondary to a lymphocytic infiltration of the salivary glands; others are the result of bacterial infection. Enlargements from infiltrates can be persistent, uni- or bilateral, and accompanied by xerostomia or pain. The lymphocytic infiltrations may develop cysts containing lymphoid aggregates that can be visualized by magnetic resonance imaging. Clear saliva can be milked from the glands. In contrast, glands infected with bacteria may demonstrate a purulent discharge at the duct openings when massaged (Fig. 21.2). Mumps could be considered in child who has not received the measles–mumps–rubella (MMR) vaccine. Finally, salivary gland tumors do occur in children, regardless of their HIV status. If glands continue to enlarge or a mass is detected on imaging, a fine-needle aspiration or biopsy of the gland must be performed.

The etiology of a salivary gland enlargement will dictate its treatment. Bacterial parotitis usually occurs because of a retrograde infection with oral flora, which typically is sensitive to the penicillins, clindamycin or second-generation cephalosporins. Treatment of lymphocyte-mediated enlargements is rarely indicated. Frequent intake of fluids (preferably water) throughout the day is recommended.

Periodontal tissues

The severity of periodontal (gum) diseases depends on the presence of certain periodontal pathogens and the immune status of the host. Gingivitis, the most common form of periodontal disease in the general pediatric population, is caused by an accumulation of oral bacteria and food particles at the gum line. Usually, good oral hygiene can reverse the inflammation and return the gingiva to health. Up to 25% [13] of HIV-infected pediatric patients present linear gingival erythema (LGE), a form of gum disease that is unique to HIV infection. LGE is characterized by a distinct red band of gingiva that bleeds easily. The inflammation is disproportional to the amount of plaque present, and resolution may not occur with conventional therapy. A more rare form of gingivitis, necrotizing ulcerative gingivitis (NUG), presents with destruction of one or more interdental papilla, tissue sloughing, halitosis and often pain. Treatment of both conditions includes meticulous oral hygiene, antibacterial mouth rinses (chlorhexidine), antibiotic therapy and frequent dental cleanings. Very rarely, necrotizing ulcerative periodontitis (NUP), a severe periodontal disease with rapid destruction of periodontal tissues and supporting bone, is found in children with HIV infection [13]. Frequent monitoring by a dentist is essential to prevent progression and ultimate tooth

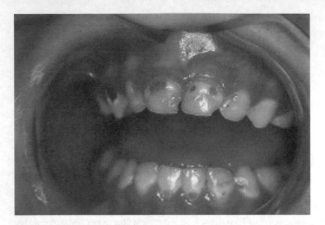

Fig. 21.3. Caries of the primary dentition of an HIV-infected child. Caries is evident on the anterior teeth, indicating a very high rate of caries development. These lesions may have been prevented by proper feeding practices and good oral hygiene.

loss. Neutropenia, which sometimes occurs in HIV-infected children, can predispose children to severe pediatric periodontal disease.

Dental development

Delays in the eruption and exfoliation of primary teeth and eruption of permanent teeth, particularly in symptomatic children, have been noted in HIV-infected teeth [14–17]. Prevention of dental disease in the primary dentition, therefore, is critical since these teeth will be retained in the mouth for longer than normal.

Teeth

Dental decay is frequently present in children with HIV infection and at levels higher than the general population in the primary dentition [14, 18]. It may present as early childhood caries, in which decay occurs on smooth surfaces normally not prone to caries (Fig. 21.3). Many factors have been suggested to explain the unusually high caries incidence in the HIV-infected population, including nutritional supplementation, sweetened pediatric medications, lack of saliva and declining immune system, frequency of fermentable carbohydrates intake, prolonged bottle feeding, and poor oral hygiene [16–18]. It may present as nursing caries, in which decay occurs on smooth surfaces normally not prone to caries (Fig. 21.3). Caries rates of HIV-infected children and their siblings have been compared. While one study reported that HIV-infected children had increases in caries compared to their non-infected siblings [17], others have noted high rates in both groups [16]. Caries are more prevalent in children with advanced HIV disease [18].

Prevention

All HIV-infected children should have an oral evaluation within the first year to ensure proper treatment. Primary caregivers should be encouraged to:

1. Enrol children in a prevention program that teaches good oral hygiene practices, along with control of dietary sugars. The use of fluorides and the placement of sealants on teeth will minimize the risk of dental caries and the possible dental pain. Prevention is easier than provision of restorative care for the pediatric HIV-infected patient, who often needs intravenous sedation for dental treatments and may have other complications such as neutropenia and thrombocytopenia.

2. Limit the frequency of ingestion of viscous sugar sweetened liquids or those with low pH (such as sodas, pediatric syrups). Topical treatment of oral candidiasis requires that the antifungal pastilles be retained in the mouth for long periods of time to be effective. These preparations are highly sweetened to disguise the taste and encourage compliance with therapy. Unsweetened vaginal troches can be used in older children. However, this is not always acceptable to young patients.

3. Limit the use of the bottle to daytime hours. Children should never be put to bed with the bottle. Remind caregivers of the risks of nursing caries when bottles containing juice or high calorie nutritional supplements are given to children. Administer highly sweetened pediatric medications by syringe to bypass the teeth and minimize the time in the oral cavity.

4. Encourage frequent intake of water to facilitate clearance of food, medicines and other substances that can initiate tooth decay.

Conclusions

Children with HIV infection may have inadequate oral health. Soft tissue lesions, especially oral candidiasis, occur frequently in this patient group, and should be treated appropriately. Untreated dental caries is found more often in children from poor families, primarily because they do not have dental insurance or access to a dentist [19]. The HIV-infected child is additionally at risk for periodontal problems. Serious oral sequela can be averted by preventive dental services and regular dental visits.

REFERENCES

1. Centers for Disease Control and Prevention. Revised classification system for HIV in children. *Morb. Mortal. Wkly Rep.* 1994;**43** (RR-12):1–10.
2. Bretz, W. A., Flaitz, C., Moretti, A., Corby, P., Schneider, L. G., Nichols, C. M. Medication usage and dental caries outcome-related variables in HIV/AIDS patients. *AIDS Patient Care STDS* 2000;**44**:549–554.

3. Costa, L. R., Villena R. S., Sucasas, P. S., Birman, E. G. Oral findings in pediatric AIDS: a case control study in Brazilian children. *ASDC J. Dent. Child.* 1998;**65**:186–190.

4. Flaitz, C., Wullbrandt, B., Sexton, J., Bourdon, T., Hicks, J. Prevalence of orodental findings in HIV-infected Romanian children. *Pediatr. Dent.* 2001;**23**:44–50.

5. European Collaborative Study. Children born to women with HIV-1 infection: natural history and risk of transmission. *Lancet* 1991;**337**:253–260.

6. Ramos-Gomez, F. J., Hilton, J. F., Canchola, A. J., Greenspan, D., Greenspan, J. S., Maldonado, Y. A. Risk factors for HIV-related orofacial soft-tissue manifestations in children. *Pediatr. Dent.* 1996;**18**:121–126.

7. Moniaci, D., Cavallari, M., Greco, D. *et al.* Oral lesions in children born to HIV-1 positive women. *J. Oral Pathol. Med.* 1993;**22**:8–11.

8. Barasch, A., Safford, M. M., Catalanotto, F. A., Fine, D. H., Katz, R. V. Oral soft tissue manifestations in HIV-positive vs. HIV-negative children from an inner city population: a two-year observational study. *Pediatr. Dent.* 2000;**22**:215–220.

9. Eversole, L. R., Viral infections of the head and neck among HIV-seropositive patients. *Oral Surg. Oral Med. Oral Pathol.* 1992;**73**:155–163.

10. Greenspan, J. S., Greenspan, D., Lennette, E. T. *et al.* Replication of Epstein–Barr virus within the epithelial cells of oral hairy leukoplakia, an AIDS-associated lesion. *N. Engl. J. Med.* 1985;**313**:1564–1571.

11. Italian Multicentre Study. Epidemiology, clinical features and prognostic factors of paediatric HIV infection. *Lancet* 1988;**ii**:1043–1045.

12. Atkinson, J.C., Valdez, I.H., Childers, E. Oral cavity and associated structures. In Moran, C., Mullick, F., eds. *Systemic Pathology of HIV Infection and AIDS in Children.* Washington, DC: Armed Forces Institute of Pathology, 1997:55–71.

13. Schoen, D. H., Murray, P. A., Nelson, E., Catalanotto, F., Katz, R. V., Fine, D. H. A comparison of periodontal disease in HIV-infected children and household peers: a two-year report. *Pediatr. Dent.* 2000;**22**:365–369.

14. Valdez, I. H., Pizzo, P. A., Atkinson, J. C. Oral health of pediatric AIDS patients: a hospital-based study. *ASDC J. Dent. Child.* 1994;**61**:114–118.

15. Hauk, M. J., Moss, M. E., Weinberg, G. A., Berkowitz, R. J. Delayed tooth eruption: association with severity of HIV infection. *Pediatr. Dent.* 2001;**23**:260–262.

16. Tofsky, N., Nelson, E. M., Lopez, R. N., Catalanotto, F., Fine, D. H., Katz, R. V. Dental caries in HIV-infected children versus household peers: two-year findings. *Pediatr. Dent.* 2000;**22**:207–214.

17. Madigan, A., Murray, P. A., Houpt, M. I., Catalanotto, F., Fuerman, M. Caries experience and cariogenic markers in HIV-positive children and their siblings. *Pediatr. Dent.* 1996;**18**:129–136.

18. Hicks, M. J., Flaitz, C. M., Carter, A. B. *et al.* Dental caries in HIV-infected children: a longitudinal study. *Pediatr. Dent.* 2000;**22**:359–364.

19. US Department of Health and Human Services. *Oral Health in America: A Report of the Surgeon General.* Rockville MD: US Department of Health and Human Services; 2000. National Institutes of Health publication 00–4713.

22 Otitis media and sinusitis

Ellen R. Wald, M.D.

Division Allergy, Immunology and Infectious Diseases, Children's Hospital of Pittsburgh,
Pittsburgh, PA

Barry Dashefsky, M.D.

Division of Pulmonology, Allergy, Immunology and Infectious Diseases, UMDNJ – New Jersey
Medical School, Newark, NJ, USA

Introduction and background

Otitis media and sinusitis are among the most common minor bacterial infections affecting children with normal immune function. To date, there has been a paucity of systematic study of these infections in immunocompromised hosts in general. However, substantial experience and a limited literature suggest that, in their acute, chronic, and recurrent forms, they also occur commonly in children who are infected with HIV.

Epidemiology of acute otitis media and sinusitis

Acute otitis media (AOM) is a very common occurrence in immunocompetent children, with peak frequency during the first 2 years of life. In addition to young age, risk factors for AOM include male gender, a history of severe or recurrent AOM in siblings, early age of first AOM, absence of breast feeding, winter season, race (with high rates among Eskimos and other Native Americans, as well as Australian aborigines), daycare attendance, lower socioeconomic status, and craniofacial anomalies [1].

There are three controlled studies that describe the relative frequency of AOM among HIV-infected children [2–4]. All clearly indicate that, although this common childhood condition does not affect a greater proportion of children infected with HIV than normal children, it does recur significantly more often among children with symptomatic HIV infection.

Acute sinusitis is an extremely common problem among young children with normal immunity. It has been estimated that 5%–10% of viral upper respiratory infections (URIs) in young children (which occur six to eight times annually) are complicated by bacterial sinusitis [5]. There is some evidence that episodes of sinusitis occur more

Handbook of Pediatric HIV Care, ed. Steven L. Zeichner and Jennifer S. Read.
Published by Cambridge University Press. © Cambridge University Press 2006.

frequently among HIV-infected children than among immunologically uncompromised children [4]. In a trial of intravenous immunoglobulin (IVIG) prophylaxis for serious bacterial infections in HIV-infected children, clinically diagnosed acute sinusitis represented 39% of the episodes of "serious" infection and occurred irrespective of CD4 count, HIV disease severity classification, and receipt of IVIG [6, 7].

Pathogenesis and natural history of AOM and sinusitis

In the immunocompetent host, AOM is attributable to dysfunction of the eustachian tube, which is responsible for: (a) ventilation; (b) clearance of secretions produced locally; and (c) protection of the middle ear from nasopharyngeal contents [8]. Viral infection of the upper respiratory tract is the major pathogenetic factor which produces both physiologic and anatomic obstruction of the eustachian tube and effusion within the middle ear. Aspiration of heavily colonized nasopharyngeal contents into the middle ear leads to a suppurative process manifested as AOM. A similar pathogenesis probably occurs in the immunocompromised host.

In the usual case of sinusitis, either a viral URI or allergy leads to mucositis, resulting in obstruction of the sinus ostia. Colonizing nasopharyngeal flora, which have gained access to the formerly sterile sinuses, proliferate, producing a local inflammatory reaction which damages the mucosa and thereby further impairs ciliary function and local phagocytic activity [5, 9].

Clinical presentation

Otitis media

In both immunocompetent and immunocompromised hosts, AOM often presents with the abrupt onset of otalgia, fever, or irritability in association with typical otoscopic findings described below. Suppurative complications of AOM include tympanic membrane perforation, cholesteatoma, mastoiditis, and intracranial suppuration including meningitis, brain, subdural or extradural abscess, sinus thrombosis, and phlebitis [10].

Sinusitis

There are two patterns of illness with which acute sinusitis presents in immunocompetent children – either persistent or severe symptoms. Persistent symptoms represent the more common presentation, which is characterized by the presence of unimproving cough and/or rhinorrhea for 10 to 30 days. Breath may be malodorous. If present, fever is usually low grade. Facial pain and headache are unusual complaints. Less commonly, acute sinusitis may present with features of a more severe nature – high fever (>39 °C) and purulent nasal discharge concurrently for 3–4 consecutive days. Intense headache (supra- or retroorbital), toxicity, or periorbital edema may be features of this presentation.

In immunocompromised hosts, including children with HIV infection, the clinical presentation of sinusitis is most often indistinguishable from that in immunocompetent patients. Unfortunately, the physical examination is usually not helpful in differentiating acute sinusitis from a viral URI. Fungal sinusitis is suggested by the presence of nasal mucosa that are focally pale, gray or black; have decreased or absent pain sensation; and do not bleed following trauma.

Sinusitis in either the immunocompetent or immunocompromised host may be complicated by extension of infection to adjacent bone, the orbit, or the central nervous system (CNS) (in the form of an epidural abscess, brain abscess, meningitis, cavernous sinus thrombosis, optic neuritis, or carotid aneurysm). Orbital involvement is signaled by the onset of proptosis, ophthalmoplegia, ocular tenderness or decreased visual acuity.

Diagnostic considerations in AOM and sinusitis

Otitis media

The diagnosis of otitis media is based on otoscopic findings. The tympanic membrane is assessed with respect to its contour, color, transparency, architecture, and, most importantly, mobility. Decreased mobility implies the presence of middle ear effusion, which is almost always present in both acute and chronic otitis media. Marked fullness or bulging of a white or yellow, sometimes hyperemic, tympanic membrane are typical findings in AOM.

Tympanocentesis should be performed selectively in both immunocompetent and immunocompromised hosts for diagnostic and therapeutic purposes. The major indications for tympanocentesis are: (a) failure to respond to medical therapy, (b) suppurative complications such as mastoiditis or CNS abscess, (c) suspicion of an unusual pathogen, (d) otitis media in patients who are seriously ill, or (e) for relief of severe pain [8]. Aspirated fluid should be used for culture and Gram stain. Radiographs or computerized tomography (CT) scanning may be required occasionally to confirm the presence of mastoiditis or intracranial complications.

Sinusitis

The diagnosis of acute bacterial sinusitis is most often made solely on the basis of a clinical presentation with the characterized persistent symptoms described previously. Physical examination seldom helps distinguish acute bacterial sinusitis from viral rhinosinusitis (a "cold"). In acute sinusitis, radiographic findings include diffuse opacification, mucosal thickening of at least 4–5 mm, or, rarely in children, an air–fluid level. The presence of these abnormalities in a child with either persistent or severe symptoms is associated with a bacterial infection of the maxillary sinuses in 70% of cases [5]. Often, the diagnosis of sinusitis is inferred on the basis of clinical criteria alone. This practice is justified by the strong correlation (88% agreement) between abnormal sinus radiographs and features of persistent sinusitis described above in children less than six years of age [5].

Sinus radiographs should not routinely be used to confirm the diagnosis of clinically suspected sinusitis in children less than 6 years of age with persistent symptoms; some authorities advocate their selective use in all children older than six years suspected of having sinusitis on the basis of presentation with persistent symptoms, and in all children of any age who present with severe symptoms [11]. These recommendations apply to both immunocompetent and immunocompromised hosts.

CT scans with contrast enhancement should be reserved for evaluation of persistent or recurrent sinusitis not responsive to medical management or associated with suspected complications of the orbit or brain (situations in which surgical intervention is being considered) [11].

Although not routinely used for diagnostic purposes, maxillary sinus aspiration can be safely and effectively performed by a pediatric otolaryngologist as an outpatient procedure using a transnasal approach after careful decontamination and adequate local anesthesia of the area below the inferior turbinate, which the trocar traverses. Aspirated material should be processed promptly for aerobic and anaerobic bacterial cultures as well as for Gram stain. Recovery of organisms in a density of at least 10^4 cfu/ml is considered indicative of infection [5].

Indications for sinus aspiration and perhaps biopsy are similar to those for tympanocentesis (see above). These indications are similar to those for immunocompetent patients. In such cases, aspirated and biopsied material should be processed to facilitate the identification of bacteria, fungi, viruses, mycobacteria, *Legionella* sp., parasites, protozoa, and possibly *P. jiroveci* and should be submitted for histologic examination. When fungal infection is suspected a biopsy of nasal mucosa should be similarly evaluated [12].

Microbiologic considerations

In immunocompetent children, *Streptococcus pneumoniae*, *Haemophilus influenzae* and *Moraxella catarrhalis* predominate at all ages and in both acute and chronic otitis media [12, 13] (see Table 22.1). Respiratory viruses have been isolated from middle ear or nasopharyngeal specimens from approximately 20% of cases of AOM. Recurrent episodes of AOM, as well as 20%–66% of cases of chronic otitis media are caused by the same array of bacterial species as is found in AOM [10]. Chronic suppurative otitis media (CSOM), characterized by persistent otorrhea through a perforated tympanic membrane, is usually attributable to *Pseudomonas aeruginosa*, staphylococci, or *Proteus* spp.; anaerobic organisms have been documented in up to 50% of cases [12]. Occasionally, *Aspergillus* and *Candida* species and, rarely, blastomycosis have been

Table 22.1. Oral antimicrobial therapy for acute otitis media and acute sinusitis in children

Antimicrobial	Daily dosage (mg/kg/day)	Maximum daily dose (mg)	Number daily doses
Amoxicillin (many brands)	45–90	1750	2
Amoxicillin/clavulanate potassium (Augmentin®)	45/6.5–90/6.5	4000	2
Cefdinir (Omnicef®)	14	600	1
Cefpodoxime proxetil (Vantin®)	10	800	2
Cefuroxime axetil (Ceftin®)	30	1000	2
Clarithromycin (Biaxin®)	15	1000	2
Azithromycin (Zithromax®)	10 mg/kg × 1 day[a] 5 mg/kg × 4 days	500/250	1

[a] Azithromycin is prescribed at 10 mg/kg as a single daily dose on day 1; the four subsequent daily doses are prescribed at 5 mg/kg per day. The maximum dose for day 1 is 500 mg; the maximum dose for day 2–5 is 250 mg.

implicated in CSOM, either alone or in combination with bacterial pathogens [12]. In children with HIV who have AOM, the prevalence of the three most common pathogens is similar to that observed in uninfected children [2, 14]. (Table 22.1) One study suggests that *S. aureus* is significantly more often associated with AOM in HIV-infected children who are severely immunosuppressed [14].

The microbiology of acute sinusitis is very similar to that of AOM. There have been no systematic studies documenting the microbiology of sinusitis in HIV-infected adults or children. It is likely that they become infected with the same organisms that usually infect immunocompetent hosts, as well as uncommon and opportunistic pathogens that have been implicated in a variety of compromised hosts [12].

Treatment of middle ear and sinus infections

Most episodes of AOM or acute sinusitis in non-toxic children infected with HIV are managed without specific microbiologic data with an orally administered antimicrobial agent that is predictably active against the most likely pathogens. *H. influenzae* and *M. catarrhalis* are resistant to amoxicillin on the basis of beta-lactamase production approximately 35%–50% and 90%–100% of the time, respectively [11, 15]. *S. pneumoniae* are not susceptible to penicillin between 8% and 38% (average 25%) of the time because of alteration of penicillin binding proteins. Fifty percent of resistant strains are intermediate in resistance and 50% are highly resistant. Risk factors for infection with penicillin-resistant pathogens include attendance at day care, treatment with antimicrobials within the previous 90 days, and age less than 2 years

[11]. Candidate antimicrobial agents and dosage recommendations are presented in Table 22.1 [11, 15, 16].

In general, amoxicillin, administered at either a standard dose of 45 mg/kg per day or at a high dose of 90 mg/kg per day, both in two divided doses for 10 to 14 days, is the agent of choice for empiric treatment of the first episode of AOM or acute sinusitis in a child with uncomplicated, mildly-to-moderately severe infection who does not attend daycare. A permissive dosage range allows the practitioner to individualize therapy. Early in the respiratory season, lower doses of amoxicillin will suffice in children who are older than 2 years, have not recently received antibiotics and do not attend daycare. For patients with penicillin allergy (provided it is not type 1 hypersensitivity), alternatives to amoxicillin include cefdinir (14 mg/kg per d in a single or two divided doses), cefuroxime (30 mg/kg per d in two divided doses), or cefpodoxime (10 mg/kg per d in two divided doses). For patients with histories of serious allergic reactions to penicillins, clarithromycin (15 mg/kg per d in two divided doses) or azithromycin (10 mg/kg per d on day one and 5 mg/kg per d on days 2 through 5 as a single daily dose) can be used (notwithstanding the fact that the US Food and Drug Administration has not approved azithromycin for use in sinusitis). Patients known to be infected with penicillin-resistant *S. pneumoniae* can be treated with clindamycin (30–40 mg/kg per day in three divided doses).

For episodes of AOM or acute sinusitis that fail to improve within 48 to 72 hours of initiation of standard dose amoxicillin, that recur within 90 days of a previous episode treated with antimicrobials, that are moderate or more severe, or that occur in daycare attendees, a broader-spectrum, orally administered antimicrobial should be prescribed. High-dose amoxicillin-clavulanate (90 mg/kg per d of amoxicillin in combination with 6.5 mg/kg per d of clavulanate in divided doses) is an ideal choice. It is important to note that amoxicillin-clavulanate comes in several liquid and tablet formulations that differ in their fixed ratios of amoxicillin to clavulanate (varying from 2:1 to 12.9:1). Only the new Augmentin ES-600® oral suspension formulation (containing 600 mg of amoxicillin and 42.9 mg of clavulanate per 5 ml) affords an easy means of prescribing amoxicillin at the recommended high dose while avoiding diarrhea associated with the doses of clavulanate that exceed 10 mg/kg per day. Alternatives include cefdinir, cefuroxime or cefpodoxime. For patients intolerant of oral therapy, treatment may begin with ceftriaxone (50 mg/kg per day) intravenously or intramuscularly until orally administered antimicrobials can be reliably instituted. Neither trimethoprim-sulfamethoxazole nor erythromycin-sulfisoxazole, are appropriate antimicrobial choices for treatment of AOM and sinusitis when illness is severe or there has been failure to respond to amoxicillin.

Decisions about the duration of antimicrobial therapy for AOM and acute sinusitis need to be individualized. Recognizing the demonstrated efficacy of relatively short courses of treatment for uncomplicated AOM in children older than 5 years of age, recent guidelines have endorsed courses of treatment as brief as five to seven days for clinically responsive episodes of AOM in immunocompetent children of that age [16]. However, children with symptomatic HIV are at significantly increased risk for recurrences of AOM and bacterial sinusitis, as well as for the development of complications and treatment failures, with amoxicillin. In general, we recommend treating recurrent episodes of AOM or acute sinusitis in this population according to the general clinical practice guideline advocated for managing sinusitis in normal hosts [11], i.e., with a broader-spectrum antimicrobial for a duration of 10 to 21 days (or for at least 1 week beyond the complete resolution of symptoms). In the case of an HIV-infected child who appears systemically ill or toxic at presentation or during treatment of AOM or acute sinusitis, tympanocentesis or sinus aspiration should be performed, aspirated fluid should be cultured, and a parenterally administered broad-spectrum antimicrobial (e.g., cefotaxime, ceftazidime, ceftriaxone or high-dose ampicillin-sulbactam) should be initiated empirically. (If the tympanic membrane has perforated spontaneously, the canal should be suctioned, cleaned, and a sample of middle ear fluid obtained for culture.) Specific treatment is given as directed by results of cultures and susceptibility testing.

In immunocompetent children, persistence of middle-ear effusion following treatment of AOM despite resolution of signs and symptoms of suppuration is present in up to 50% of cases immediately upon completion of therapy, and gradually resolves in all but 10% over 3 months [17, 18]. Antimicrobials are not indicated for middle effusion in the absence of signs and symptoms of recurrent AOM [16]. If the effusion persists for more than 3 months and is associated with a significant hearing loss, a second course of treatment with a broader-spectrum antimicrobial may be given. When middle ear effusion persists for more than 3 months despite treatment with antimicrobials, especially when bilateral, occurring in a young child, or associated with hearing loss, myringotomy (usually with tympanostomy tube placement) should be considered. These same recommendations apply to children infected with HIV.

To date, *P. jiroveci* has not been reported to cause ear infections in children infected with HIV. The few such adults who have been described appear to have responded to oral trimethoprim-sulfamethoxazole with or without dapsone, or to intravenously administered pentamidine.

CSOM should be managed in conjunction with an otolaryngologist who will obtain a specimen for culture, perform daily aural toilet, and undertake serial examinations. Topical therapy with ofloxacin is advised [15]. If the otorrhea does not begin to resolve in 48–72 hours, parenteral antibiotics, initially selected empirically for activity against *P. aeruginosa* and *S. aureus* (e.g., ticarcillin disodium/clavulanate potassium or piperacillin/tazobactam or cefepime), and subsequently chosen according to culture and antimicrobial susceptibility results, may be necessary to effect a cure. Antimicrobial therapy is usually continued for 7 days beyond resolution of the otorrhea. Tympanomastoidectomy is sometimes required if otorrhea persists or recurs despite parenteral therapy.

Sinus infections

Routine use of inhaled decongestants is not recommended for patients with sinusitis; however, in selected cases (severe nasal congestion or periorbital swelling) their use for a few days may be helpful. Systemic and local antihistamines, intranasal corticosteroids, and sodium cromolyn are not recommended for acute sinusitis.

Rarely, when patients with acute sinusitis do not respond to parenteral therapy, surgical drainage may be necessary to restore physiologic function to a paranasal sinus. Currently, functional endonasal sinus surgery may be helpful in carefully selected children with chronic sinusitis [5, 19].

When fungal sinusitis is highly suspected or documented, treatment with amphotericin B should be instituted in an accelerated fashion to quickly achieve a daily dose of 1 mg/kg. 5-Fluorocytosine may provide additional benefit as adjunctive therapy. Liposomal amphotericin should be used when use of conventional amphotericin B is either contraindicated or complicated by abnormal renal function. Fluconazole and intraconazole should be reserved for occasions when susceptibility has been demonstrated or can be reliably predicted. Extensive surgical debridement is usually required. Hyperbaric oxygen may be helpful in cases of rhinocerebral mucormycosis [12].

Prevention of otitis media and sinusitis

The use of chemoprophylaxis is recommended in immunocompetent hosts for highly selected cases that meet stringent criteria of three or more well documented episodes of AOM or acute sinusitis within six months or four episodes within 12 months [16, 20]. We recommend similarly rigorous criteria for initiating chemoprophylaxis in immunocompromised hosts, including children with HIV infection. Agents for which efficacy had been demonstrated (albeit, prior to the current era of substantial antibiotic resistance) include amoxicillin (at a dose of 20 mg/kg once daily) and sulfisoxazole (at a dose of 50–75 mg/kg per d in two divided doses). At least one publication has reported a failure of prophylaxis with amoxicillin compared to placebo presumably because of the prevalence of resistant middle ear isolates (both beta-lactamase producing *H. influenzae* and *M. catarrhalis* and penicillin-resistant *S. pneumoniae*) [21]. Although concern for its toxicity has led some authorities to caution against the use of trimethoprim-sulfamethoxazole, or sulfisoxazole alone, for preventing recurrences of otitis media, it has demonstrated efficacy for this purpose when given daily (admittedly, documented at a time of less prevalent antimicrobial resistance). Although its ability to prevent otitis media when administered less frequently (as in thrice-weekly schedules often used in HIV-infected patients for prophylaxis against *P. carinii* pneumonia) is unknown, daily administration, if tolerated, is recommended and would provide satisfactory protection for both concerns. In those highly selected instances when prophylaxis is initiated, it should generally be given throughout the respiratory infection season (winter) for those who experience the usual seasonal pattern of otitis media and sinusitis. It should be given for at least 1 year for those whose disease occurs year-round.

Myringotomy and tube placement is recommended for patients whose frequency of recurrent AOM is not substantially reduced by chemoprophylaxis and for selected patients with chronic effusion (e.g., those with significant hearing loss).

Heptavalent pneumococcal conjugate vaccine (PCV7) is recommended for universal use in children less than 24 months of age and selectively for others at high risk of invasive pneumococcal disease, including all individuals of any age with HIV infection [22]. A history of frequent otitis media or sinusitis is not currently a formally recommended indication for its administration to children older than 2 years who do not satisfy other "high risk" criteria. However, the impact of immunizing infants with PCV7 on reducing the frequency and morbidity associated with AOM has been well documented in two large studies in the United States [23] and Finland [24]. Routine administration of PCV7 as well as 23-valent pneumococcal polysaccharide vaccine to all HIV-infected children according to published guidelines [22] is strongly recommended.

Summary

The clinical presentation, diagnosis, microbiology, and management of episodes of AOM and bacterial sinusitis in immunocompetent children and those who are infected with HIV is very similar. In an era of increasing resistance to antimicrobial agents, it is appropriate to obtain samples of middle ear fluid or maxillary sinus aspirates in patients who do not respond to the first or second antibiotic empirically selected for treatment. These data will help inform the selection of specific antimicrobial agents.

REFERENCES

1. Teele, D. W., Klein, J. O., Rosner, B., and the Greater Boston Otitis Media Study Group. Epidemiology of otitis media during the first seven years of life in children in Greater Boston: a prospective cohort study. *J. Infect. Dis.* 1989;**160**:83–94.
2. Principi, N., Marchisio, P., Tornaghi, R., Onorato, J., Massironi, E., Picco, P. Acute otitis media in human immunodeficiency virus-infected children. *Pediatrics* 1991;**88**:566–571.
3. Barnett, E. D., Klein, J. O., Pelton, S. I., Luginbuhl, L. M. Otitis media in children born to human immunodeficiency virus-infected mothers. *Pediatr. Infect. Dis. J.* 1992;**11**:360–364.
4. Chen, A. Y., Ohlms, L. A., Stewart, M. G., Kline, M. W. Otolaryngologic disease progression in children with human immunodeficiency virus infection. *Arch. Otolaryngol. Head Neck Surg.* 1996;**122**:1360–1363.
5. Wald, E. R., Sinusitis in children. *N. Engl. J. Med.* 1992;**326**:319–323.

6. The National Institute of Child Health and Human Development Intravenous Immunoglobulin Study Group. Intravenous immune globulin for the prevention of bacterial infections in children with symptomatic human immunodeficiency virus infection. *N. Engl. J. Med.* 1991;**325**:73–80.

7. Mofenson, L. M., Korelitz, J., Pelton, S., Moye, J., Jr, Nugent, R., Bethel, J. Sinusitis in children infected with human immunodeficiency virus: clinical characteristics, risk factors, and prophylaxis. *Clin. Infect. Dis.* 1995;**21**:1175–1181.

8. Bluestone, C. D., *Otitis Media in Infants and Children*, ed. Bluestone, C., Klein, J. 2nd edn. W.B. Saunders Co., 1995.

9. Wald, E. R., Diagnosis and management of sinusitis in children. *Adv. Pediatr. Infect. Dis.* 1996;**12**:1–20.

10. Parsons, D. S., Wald, E. R. Otitis media and sinusitis: similar diseases. *Otolaryngol. Clin. N. Am.* 1996;**29**:11–25.

11. American Academy of Pediatrics Subcommittee on Management of Sinusitis and Committee on Quality Improvement. Clinical Practice Guideline: Management of Sinusitis. *Pediatrics* 2001;**108**:798–808.

12. Wald, E.R. Infections of the sinuses, ears, and hypopharynx. In Shelhamer, J., Pizzo, P. A., Parrillo, J. E., Masur, H., eds. *Respiratory Disease in the Immunosuppressed Host*. Philadelphia: J. B. Lippincott Co. 1991;450–468.

13. Wald, E. R., *Haemophilus influenzae* as a cause of acute otitis media. *Pediatr. Infect. Dis. J.* 1989;**8**:S28–S30.

14. Marchisio, P., Principi, N., Sorella, S., Sala, E., Tornaghi, R. Etiology of acute otitis media in human immunodeficiency virus-infected children. *Pediatr. Infect. Dis. J.* 1996;**15**: 58–61.

15. Dowell, S. F., Butler, J. C., Giebink, G. S. *et al.* Acute otitis media: management and surveillance in an era of pneumococcal resistance – a report from the drug-resistant *Streptococcus pneumoniae* Therapeutic Working Group. *Pediatr. Infect. Dis. J.* 1999; **18**:1–9.

16. Dowell, S. F., Marcy, S. M., Phillips, W. R. *et al.* Otitis media – principles of judicious use of antimicrobial agents. *Pediatrics* 1998;**101**:165–171.

17. Klein, J. O., Bluestone, C. D. Management of otitis media in the era of managed care. *Adv. Pediatr. Infect. Dis.* 1996;**12**:351–386.

18. Barlow, D., Duckert, L., Kreig, C., Gates, G. Ototoxicity of topical otomicrobial agents. *Acta Otolaryngol* 1995;**115**:231–235.

19. Lusk, R. P., The surgical management of chronic sinusitis in children. *Pediatr. Ann.* 1998;**27**:820–827.

20. Paradise, J. L., Antimicrobial drugs and surgical procedures in the prevention of otitis media. *Pediatr. Infect. Dis. J.* 1989;**8**:S35–S37.

21. Roark, R., Berman, S. Continuous twice daily or once daily amoxicillin prophylaxis compared with placebo for children with recurrent acute otitis media. *Pediatr. Infect. Dis. J.* 1997;**16**:376–381.

22. American Academy of Pediatrics. Policy statement: Recommendations for the prevention of pneumococcal infections, including the use of pneumococcal conjugate vaccine (Prevnar), pneumococcal polysaccharide vaccine, and antibiotic prophylaxis. *Pediatrics* 2000;**106**:362–366.

23. Black, S., Shinefield, H., Ray, P. *et al.* Efficacy, safety and immunogenicity of heptavalent pneumococcal conjugate vaccine in children: Northern California Kaiser Permanente Vaccine Study Group. *Pediatr. Infect. Dis. J.* 2000;**19**:187–195.
24. Eskola, J., Kilpi, T., Palmu, A. *et al.* Efficacy of a pneumococcal conjugate vaccine against acute otitis media. *N. Engl. J. Med.* 2001; **344**:403–409.

23 Cardiac problems

Gul H. Dadlani, M.D.

Congenital Heart Institute of Florida, All Children's Hospital and University of South Florida,
St. Petersburg, FL, USA

Steven E. Lipshultz, M.D.

Sylvester Comprehensive Cancer Center University of Miami and Miller School of Medicine, Holtz
Children's Hospital, University of Miami-Jackson Memorial Medical Center, FL, USA

Introduction

As the survival of HIV-infected patients improves, the cardiovascular complications of
HIV infection are becoming an increasingly common cause of morbidity and mortality.
The prevalence of cardiovascular disease is estimated to be more than 90% in pediatric
HIV patients [1–3]. The spectrum of cardiovascular disorders includes abnormalities
in left ventricular performance, wall thickness, contractility, dilated cardiomyopathy,
myocarditis, pericarditis, and rhythm disturbances. Cardiac complications have surpassed pulmonary disease as the leading cause of death in HIV-infected patients [4].
The recognition of cardiovascular complications can be very difficult because many
patients are asymptomatic until late in the disease course. In addition, the cardiac
symptoms can be inadvertently attributed to other causes such as pulmonary or infectious etiologies. Early detection of these symptoms is only possible if clinicians have a
fundamental understanding of the wide array of cardiovascular complications associated with HIV infection. The initiation of routine screening and monitoring will allow
clinicians the ability to intervene and hopefully prevent or delay the onset of these
complications in the future.

Risk factors

Several risk factors for cardiovascular disease among HIV-infected children have been
described. The triad of encephalopathy, wasting, and low CD4 counts in children with
HIV have been shown to be associated with an increased the risk of cardiovascular
complications and decreased survival [5]. Encephalopathy can lead to an autonomic
neuropathy, which may precipitate arrhythmias or even sudden death [5]. Children with
a prior history of a serious cardiac event or who have rapid progression of their disease
(an AIDS defining condition, other than lymphoid interstitial pneumonia/pulmonary

Handbook of Pediatric HIV Care, ed. Steven L. Zeichner and Jennifer S. Read.
Published by Cambridge University Press. © Cambridge University Press 2006.

hyperplasia or severe immunosuppression, in the first year of life) are at increased risk of severe cardiac complications from their HIV infection [6]. Co-infection with other viruses is associated with increased cardiac morbidity and mortality in HIV patients [7]. The highest risk of cardiac or non-cardiac mortality following a viral co-infection is associated with Epstein–Barr virus (EBV) [5]. Cytomegalovirus (CMV) is a significant predictor of cardiac events when associated with wasting and a prior history of cardiac abnormality [7]. Left ventricular dysfunction and increased left ventricular wall thickness as detected by echocardiography (ECHO) are also independent risk factors for all-cause mortality in pediatric HIV patients [8]. Cardiotoxic medications used to treat HIV or associated diseases (malignancies) may be another risk factor for the development of cardiovascular complications.

Types of cardiovascular disease

One common cardiac manifestation of HIV infection in children is left ventricular (LV) dysfunction [8]. This is defined as decreased systolic or diastolic function of the ventricle as identified by echocardiography. LV dysfunction is usually asymptomatic and can occur at any stage of the HIV infection. Increased LV wall thickness can occur with or without LV dysfunction. Both of these echocardiographic findings are useful long-term predictors of mortality in HIV-infected children [8]. The relationship of these changes in LV structure and function remain unknown, but may include any of the risk factors discussed above. Progression of LV dysfunction results in alterations in heart rate, LV preload, LV afterload, and in decreased LV contractility [8, 9].

As LV dysfunction advances, patients can develop a cardiomyopathy. A cardiomyopathy is a disease process that affects the structure or function of the myocardium. It may be idiopathic or caused by a secondary process such as a systemic disease, infection, toxin, metabolic process or ischemia. A dilated cardiomyopathy, which occurs with HIV infection, is enlargement of the left or both ventricles with decreased contractility. This can present with symptoms of congestive heart failure (CHF), which include tachypnea, diaphoresis, pallor, organomegaly, edema, and failure to thrive or wasting.

Myocarditis (inflammation of the myocardium), is another common complication associated with HIV infection. The inflammation can be transient or can lead to a cardiomyopathy. Myocarditis can be caused by a variety of agents including: direct HIV infection of the myocyte; viral co-infection with adenovirus, CMV, EBV, coxsackievirus, herpesvirus or parvovirus; opportunistic infections with *Toxoplasma gondii, Cryptococcus neoformans, Mycobacterium tuberculosis,* and *Mycobacterium avium intracellulare*; drug-related toxicities; nutritional deficiencies; or autoimmune reactions [10–12]. The presentation of myocarditis can range from completely asymptomatic echocardiographic findings, severe congestive heart failure or even sudden death.

Arrhythmias represent a life-threatening complication of HIV infection. HIV encephalopathy can produce an autonomic neuropathy, which has been associated with sinus arrhythmias, bradycardia, hypotension and cardiac arrest [5]. Many medications used by HIV patients have the potential to provoke arrhythmias. Pentamidine, amphotericin B, ganciclovir, and trimethoprim-sulfamethoxazole have been shown to cause atrial and ventricular arrhythmias [10, 11]. Pentamidine, especially when given intravenously, can prolong the QT_c interval and induce torsades de pointes, a polymorphic form of ventricular tachycardia [13]. Cardiomyopathies may induce premature ventricular beats and ventricular tachycardia. A history of chest pain, palpitations, syncope, near-syncope, dyspnea, or dizzy spells can indicate an underlying arrhythmia.

Pericarditis, inflammation of the pericardium, and pericardial effusions, fluid collections within the pericardial space, also occur in HIV patients. The etiologies are similar to those for myocarditis and include: HIV, viral or bacterial co-infections, opportunistic infections, malignancy, malnutrition, hypothyroidism, and autoimmune reactions [14]. Children can present with symptoms of chest pain radiating to the neck or shoulder, a pericardial friction rub upon auscultation, pulsus paradoxicus, dyspnea, cough and tachypnea.

Endocarditis is commonly seen in adult HIV patients with a history of intravenous drug abuse, but can be encountered in the pediatric population, especially if there is a pre-existing history of congenital heart disease. The most common agents causing endocarditis are *Staphylococcus aureus, Streptococcus* species, *Haemophilus influenzae*, fastidious organisms of the HACEK group (*Haemophilus parainfluenzae, Haemophilus aphrophilus, Haemophilus paraphrophilus, Actinobacillus actinomycemcomitans, Cardiobacterium hominis, Eikenella* species, *Kingella kingae*) and opportunistic infections such as *Cryptococcus* and *Candida* [14]. Patients usually present with persistent fever, fatigue, heart murmur, splenomegaly, signs of systemic micro-emboli (petechiae, Osler nodes, Janeway lesions, and splinter hemorrhages), and a history of congenital heart disease.

Hypertension can affect many pediatric HIV patients. Hypertension is defined as a systolic and/or diastolic blood pressure that is greater than the 95th percentile for age on at least three different occasions. Hypertension can be caused by medications, vasculitis, early or accelerated atherosclerosis, renal disease, autonomic nervous system disturbances, or protease inhibitor-induced insulin resistance with increased sympathetic activity and sodium retention [14]. Affected patients are usually asymptomatic and are found on routine screening.

Cardiac malignancies (Kaposi's sarcoma and lymphoma), primary pulmonary hypertension with right ventricular dysfunction, premature coronary artery disease or atherosclerosis, and lipid abnormalities are all cardiac complications that are frequently encountered in adults but less so in the pediatric HIV population. Lipid abnormalities and other metabolic complications of antiretroviral therapy are discussed in Chapter 13. The clinician must keep these other complications in mind as the survival of the pediatric HIV population continues to improve and these patients enter adulthood.

Table 23.1. Findings on history suggestive of cardiovascular disease: differential diagnosis

Symptoms	Potential cardiovascular etiology	Other etiologies
Fatigue, dyspnea with exertion	Congestive heart failure	Malnutrition, chronic illness, anemia, depression
Pallor	Congestive heart failure	Malnutrition, chronic illness, anemia
Cyanosis	Structural heart disease	Lung disease, methemoglobulinemia
Persistent respiratory symptoms: cough, wheezes, tachypnea, dyspnea.	Congestive heart failure	Lung disease
Diaphoresis with feedings	Congestive heart failure	Chronic illness, lung disease
Nausea/vomiting	Organomegaly from congestive heart failure	Gastrointestinal disease
Syncope/presyncope	Arrhythmia, low cardiac output.	Neurologic disease, anemia, hypoglycemia
Failure to thrive	Any form of heart disease	Chronic illness, endocrine, renal, or gastrointestinal disease
Chest pain	Pericarditis, myocarditis, arrhythmia, ischemia	Gastrointestinal or lung disease, costochondritis

Evaluation of the pediatric HIV patient for cardiovascular problems

Detecting cardiovascular complications of HIV can be difficult because subclinical disease may be present many years before symptoms arise. Symptoms may be masked by the involvement of other organ systems (see Tables 23.1 and 23.2). All evaluations should include a comprehensive cardiovascular history and physical examination. The diagnosis and management of HIV-related cardiovascular disorders are summarized in Table 23.3. Routinely scheduled echocardiograms should also be included for all HIV patients. The addition of laboratory, non-invasive, and invasive cardiac studies should be determined by the risk factors identified with the history and physical examination (see Table 23.3). A thorough review of the patient's medications should also be completed as many of the medications used in the treatment of HIV infection can have potential cardiovascular side effects. Table 23.4 summarizes some of the more commonly used classes of drugs in HIV patients and their associated cardiac side effects.

Echocardiography (ECHO) is the most important screening tool for cardiovascular complications of HIV. It is capable of identifying LV systolic dysfunction and increased

Table 23.2. Physical examination findings suggestive of cardiovascular disease: differential diagnosis

Sign	Cardiovascular etiology	Other etiologies
Tachycardia	All forms of heart disease	Anemia, sepsis, fever, dehydration, medications
Bradycardia	All forms of heart disease	Neurologic or pulmonary diseases, medications
Hypertension	Cardiomyopathy	Neurologic or renal diseases, medications
Hypotension	All forms of heart disease	Dehydration, sepsis, or neurologic disease
Jugular venous distention	Congestive heart failure pericardial tamponade	Liver disease, malnutrition with ascites
Rales, wheezes, rhonchi	Congestive heart failure	Lung disease
Abnormal or displaced precordial impulse	Pericarditis, myocarditis, cardiomyopathy	Sepsis, pneumothorax
Abnormal S2	Structural heart disease, cardiomyopathy	Increased pulmonary pressures
S3/S4	Congestive heart failure	Sepsis, fever, anemia, dehydration
Murmur	Structural heart disease endocarditis, cardiomyopathy	Lung disease, anemia, normal physiology
Organomegaly	Congestive heart failure	Sepsis, liver disease
Poor perfusion	Low cardiac output due to heart disease	Low cardiac output due to sepsis or anemia
Disorientation	Low cardiac output due to heart disease	Low cardiac output due to sepsis, or neurological disease (encephalopathy)
Edema, ascites, decreased urine output	Congestive heart failure	Renal or liver disease, malnutrition, anasarca

LV wall thickness. These echocardiographic findings are typically asymptomatic, but have been reported to be present more than a year before the patient's death [8, 9]. Early identification of these findings may allow time for prevention or therapeutic interventions. ECHO can identify the following conditions: pericardial effusions, valvular heart disease, endocarditis, right ventricular dysfunction, endocardial masses or thrombus formation, and LV diastolic dysfunction. Our recommended schedule for echocardiograms is as follows: a baseline echocardiogram at the time of HIV diagnosis, with asymptomatic HIV-infected children having a follow-up echocardiogram every

1 to 2 years until they become symptomatic [15]. Once they have been diagnosed with symptoms related to their HIV infection, annual echocardiograms are recommended [11]. Any patient found to have a cardiovascular abnormality should be followed by a pediatric cardiologist.

Electrocardiography and Holter monitoring are used to detect abnormalities in the cardiac conduction system or rhythm disturbances. An electrocardiogram (ECG) may be useful as a baseline study at the time of HIV diagnosis and prior to the introduction of new medications if the potential of prolongation of the QT_c interval exists. Holter monitors provide a 24-hour or other long-term electrocardiographic recording of a patient's rhythm. Holter monitors are useful if a patient provides a history of symptoms that are consistent with an arrhythmia.

Exercise stress testing can assess the degree of cardiac reserve, determine the exercise potential of patients with LV dysfunction and screen for ischemic changes that may be a marker of premature atherosclerosis [15]. Metabolic stress tests in adults have revealed that individuals with a maximal oxygen uptake (VO_2 max) of less than 14 ml/kg per m^2 have significantly reduced survival [15]. The use of exercise or metabolic studies should be considered in any HIV-infected patient with arrhythmias or LV dysfunction under the guidance of a pediatric cardiologist.

Cardiac catheterization with endomyocardial biopsy can be a useful invasive diagnostic procedure if HIV-infected patients have had congestive heart failure of an unclear etiology for more than 2 weeks [7]. The biopsy results can lead to a diagnosis of myocarditis from a specific or non-specific cause. This information may allow the clinician to initiate or redirect the current therapeutic regimen.

Pericardiocentesis can be both a diagnostic and therapeutic invasive procedure for HIV patients with pericardial effusions. Emergent pericardiocentesis may be needed if signs of pericardial tamponade are present.

Non-invasive screening for premature atherosclerosis may be considered in older children as they begin to enter adolescence. New non-invasive technologies are available to image the coronary arteries and to initially assess for premature atherosclerosis without the need for angiography. For example, electron beam computed tomography is an ultrafast computed tomography scanning method with limited availability in the USA, which is capable of detecting calcium deposits within the walls of the coronary arteries. The calcium deposits can be quantitated as a calcium score, which can be predictive of future coronary artery events. Other technologies such as contrast enhanced computed tomography and magnetic resonance angiography can produce non-invasive images of the coronary artery anatomy and identify areas of obstruction.

Serum laboratory tests also can be useful for detecting micronutrient deficiencies, electrolyte abnormalities, myocardial injury, lipid abnormalities, ongoing inflammation, and potential thrombotic markers. Selenium and carnitine are two micronutrients that can be screened for as potential causes of a cardiomyopathy. Patients with

Table 23.3. Diagnosis and management of cardiovascular disease

Types of cardiovascular disease	Signs and symptoms	Diagnostic tests	Possible etiologies	Clinical management
Abnormalities of left ventricular structure and function	May progress to CHF	ECHO will show decreased left ventricular function and increased wall thickness. Blood measurements of cardiac troponin T (or I) and pro-brain natriuretic peptide.	Unknown; see text (risk factors)	Possibly ACE inhibitor or beta antagonist therapy
Cardiomyopathy	May progress to CHF	CXR may show cardiomegaly, increased pulmonary blood flow. ECHO will show decreased left ventricular function. Blood measurements of cardiac troponin T (or I) and pro-brain natriuretic peptide.	Unknown; see text (risk factors)	Supportive therapy
Myocarditis	Intercurrent viral-type illness, murmur, CHF, arrhythmia. May present *in extremis* or as sudden death.	Same as cardiomyopathy. Laboratory: elevated WBC and other indications of sepsis. Blood measurements of cardiac troponin T (or I) and pro-brain natriuretic peptide.	Mostly viral etiologies, such as CMV, adenovirus, EBV, parvovirus, herpes-virus, coxsackievirus	Treat underlying cause, if possible. IVIG in monthly doses. Steroid therapy unclear.

Condition	Symptoms	Diagnostic tests	Etiology	Treatment
Pericarditis and pericardial effusions	Chest pain, shoulder pain, hacking cough, diaphoresis, pericardial rub, fever, CHF, hemodynamic instability	CXR: enlarged cardiac silhouette without increased intravascular markings. ECHO: pericardial effusion. Blood measurements of cardiac troponin T (or I) and pro-brain natriuretic peptide.	May be secondary to inflammatory, infectious, malignant, immune, or thyroid abnormalities	Treat the underlying agent if possible. Careful use of diuretics, antiinflammatory and steroids. Pericardiocentesis for diagnostic or if hemo-dynamically compromising
Endocarditis	+/- fever, new murmur, petechiae, CHF	ECHO: valvular abnormalities LABS: blood cultures may be positive.	Usually *S. aureus*, but also subtypes of *Streptococcus*	Antimicrobial therapy. Surgery if severely hemodynamically compromised.
Premature atherosclerosis	Asymptomatic	EBCT will detect calcium deposits in coronary arteries	Unknown	Modify traditional risk factors: smoking, diabetes, hypertension, cholesterol/LDL, physical inactivity, obesity.
Hypertension	Asymptomatic	Routine blood pressure monitoring in the office	Medications; vasculitis	Lifestyle modification, reduced salt intake, antihypertensive medications
Arrhythmias or conduction disturbances	Syncope, pre-syncope, palpitations, chest pain	ECG and Holter monitoring	Autonomic neuropathy, medication side effects, infections irritating the sinus node, AV node or myocardium.	Early referral to a pediatric cardiologist or electrophysiologist and a thorough review of all medication side effects.
Lipid abnormalities	Asymptomatic	Routine screening of serum lipid panels	Medication side effects, especially protease inhibitors	Lifestyle modification, initiation of lipid lowering agents to reduce risk of atherosclerosis.

Table 23.3. Cardiovascular interactions of commonly used drugs in HIV-infected patients

Medications	Cardiac side effects
Nucleoside reverse transcriptase inhibitors	Zidovudine – skeletal muscle myopathy, myocarditis, and dilated cardiomyopathy. Zalcitabine – short-term free radical cardiotoxicity
Non-nucleoside reverse transcriptase inhibitors	Delavirdine and vasoconstrictors can cause ischemia
Protease inhibitors	Implicated in premature atherosclerosis, dyslipidemia, insulin resistance, diabetes mellitus, fat wasting, and fat redistribution.
Antibiotics	Erythromycin: orthostatic hypertension, ventricular tachycardia, bradycardia, torsades(with drug interactions). Rifampin: reduces digoxin therapeutic effect. Clarithromycin: QT prolongation and torsades. Trimethoprim/sulfamethoxazole: orthostatic hypertension, anaphylaxis, QT prolongation, torsades, hypokalemia. Sparfloxacin (fluoroquinolones): QT prolongation
Antifungal agents	Amphotericin B: digoxin toxicity(interaction), hypertension, arrhythmia, renal failure, hypokalemia, thrombophlebitis, bradycardia, angioedema, and dilated cardiomyopathy. Ketoconazole, fluconazole, itraconazole: QT prolongation and torsades de pointes.
Antiviral agents	Foscarnet: reversible cardiac failure, electrolyte imbalances. Ganciclovir: ventricular tachycardia, hypotension.
Antiparasitic agents	Pentamidine: hypotension, QT prolongation, arrhythmias, torsades, ventricular tachycardia, hyperglycemia, hypoglycemia, sudden death. Effects are enhanced by hypomagnesemia and hypokalemia.
Chemotherapeutic agents	Vincristine: arrhythmia, myocardial infarction, cardiomyopathy, and cardiac autonomic neuropathy. Anthracyclines: myocarditis, cardiomyopathy, and cardiac failure.
Systemic corticosteroids	Steroids: ventricular hypertrophy, cardiomyopathy, and hyperglycemia.

LV dysfunction should have a cardiac troponin T level drawn to evaluate for active myocardial injury secondary to myocarditis [16]. A cardiac troponin T level of greater than 0.01 ng/ml in children is elevated. General markers of inflammation, such as highly sensitive C-reactive protien [hsCRP], also are elevated in patients with active myocarditis (11). Lipid panels should be done routinely on all patients who are receiving protease inhibitors. Pro-brain natriuretic peptide is useful in the assessment of cardiomyopathy.

Management of the pediatric HIV patient with cardiac problems

Prevention of cardiovascular complications is at the cornerstone of the management of HIV-infected children. At the present time, no uniform HIV-specific preventive or therapeutic guidelines have been published. Our recommendations are based on clinical experience and evidence-based results from the general pediatric population. The reduction of traditional coronary artery risk factors for adults may benefit children with HIV since they are at risk for premature atherosclerosis. These risk factor include smoking, hypertension, elevated total and LDL cholesterol, low HDL cholesterol, diabetes, and advancing age [17]. Exercise and a healthy diet can decrease cardiovascular risk and also can stimulate the immune system. Routine screening of the blood pressure, lipid panels and a regular schedule for echocardiograms as other ways of early identification of cardiac problems in HIV-infected patients were discussed previously in this chapter.

Abnormalities of LV structure and function, cardiomyopathies, and myocarditis

Immunomodulatory therapy with intravenous immunoglobulin (IVIG) has shown significant promise for two specific sub-groups of pediatric HIV patients with cardiac problems [15]. Pediatric HIV patients without congestive heart failure showed less frequent echocardiographic abnormalities of left ventricular structure and function with monthly administration of IVIG (2 grams/kilogram per dose) [15, 18]. HIV-infected children with myocarditis and congestive heart failure symptoms that are refractory to traditional anticongestive therapy can achieve resolution of the myocarditis with IVIG therapy [15, 18]. We would consider IVIG use in these situations, although future research is needed to better define more exact guidelines. In addition, clinicians should initiate focused anti-infective therapy directed against any identified co-infecting pathogens and should medically manage any congestive heart failure symptoms [19].

Pericardial effusions

Pericardial effusions in HIV-infected patients are usually asymptomatic and well-tolerated from a cardiovascular standpoint. The treatment of underlying infections or malignancies that could be causing the pericarditis should be the first priority for the clinician. HAART for HIV infection also may need to be initiated. Effusions may resolve in as many as 42% of HIV-infected patients, often spontaneously [14]. Traditional therapies such as diuretics and steroids should be used cautiously in this patient population. The steroids may cause further immunosuppression and diuretics may rapidly reduce the patient's intravascular volume. The indications for pericardiocentesis include pericardial tamponade, diagnostic evaluation of the pericardial fluid, or persistent, poorly tolerated large effusions [14].

Endocarditis

HIV-infected patients with endocarditis can be very difficult to treat. The causative agent should be identified and treated aggressively (usually with a minimum of 6 weeks of IV antibiotics). The initiation of HAART may improve the patient's immunological status. Patients should be followed with serial echocardiograms. In larger children or young adults, transesophageal echocardiography may need to be utilized to effectively view the heart valves. Early referral to both an infectious disease specialist and a pediatric cardiologist will help direct therapeutic management. Cardiothoracic surgical intervention is only indicated for severe valve dysfunction leading to intractable heart failure that is resistant to medical therapy.

Arrhythmias

Early referral to a pediatric cardiologist or electrophysiologist is crucial because of the vast array of different arrhythmias an HIV patient can develop. A baseline ECG always should be obtained by the primary provider in any patient with symptoms of arrhythmias or conduction disturbances. A thorough review of the patient's medications and their cardiac side effects should be completed (see Table 23.4). Assessment of electrolytes, drug toxicology screen, and use of complementary and alternative therapiers should be performed. Any patient with a history of syncope should receive urgent attention.

Hypertension and lipid abnormalities and premature atherosclerosis

The clinician caring for HIV-infected pediatric patients must remember that hypertension, lipid abnormalities, and premature atherosclerosis can occur in this pediatric population. As antiretroviral therapy improves, children will continue to increase their survival and therefore will be susceptible to these traditional adult diseases. Routine office screening of blood pressure should occur at every office visit. Serum lipid panels should be drawn at diagnosis and then followed routinely, especially if the patient is on a protease inhibitor. Electron beam computed tomography has been able to detect coronary artery calcifications in pediatric patients with coronary artery injuries from Kawasaki disease and could be a useful screening tool for pediatric patients with advanced HIV disease [20]. However, future research will need to determine the clinical utility of this technology in HIV patients. Detection of the abnormalities can lead to early initiation of antihypertensive medications or lipid-lowering agents, which may improve overall morbidity in the future.

Referral to a pediatric cardiologist

Referral to a pediatric cardiologist should be considered based upon any of the following:

1. Findings on history:
   - Any previous cardiac disease
   - Encephalopathy
   - Severe wasting and malnutrition
   - Vague chest pain, malaise, fatigue, lethargy, weakness.
2. Findings on physical examination:
   - Respiratory symptoms for more than 7 days that are not attributable to a pulmonary or infectious process
   - Signs and symptoms of congestive heart failure
   - Evidence of structural or congenital heart disease
   - Frequent arrhythmias or inappropriate tachycardias
   - Episodes of cyanosis, syncope, seizure
   - Pulmonary hypertension with recurrent bronchopulmonary infections
   - Friction rub, hacking cough, pulsus paradoxicus, poor peripheral perfusion (consistent with pericardial effusion).
3. Findings on echocardiography:
   - Left ventricular systolic dysfunction
   - Left ventricular hypertrophy
   - Other echocardiographic abnormalities including: pericardial effusions, valvular heart disease, congenital heart disease, regional wall motion abnormalities, and intracardiac thrombi or masses.
4. Laboratory findings:
   - Elevated cardiac troponin T
   - Elevated pro-brain natriuretic peptide

Summary

Cardiovascular complications are common in pediatric HIV patients. Clinicians need to be aware of subclinical cardiac abnormalities such as LV dysfunction, LV hypertrophy, hypertension and lipid abnormalities, which may be present many years prior to the presentation of overt clinical symptoms. Routine screening with blood pressure monitoring, lipid panels, blood markers of myocardial injury and cardiomyopathy, and echocardiograms may provide early detection of many cardiac problems. In addition, clinicians must be aware of the cardiovascular signs and symptoms that can be obscured by other organ system failures in HIV-infected patients. In the future, early detection and treatment of cardiac disease may prevent much of the associated morbidity and mortality.

REFERENCES

1. Lipshultz, S. E., Chanock, S., Sanders, S. P. *et al.* Cardiovascular manifestations of human immunodeficiency virus in infants and children. *Am. J. Cardiol.* 1989;**63**:1489–1497.

2. Starc, T. J., Lipshultz, S. E., Kaplan, S. *et al.* Cardiac complications in children with human immunodeficiency virus infection. *Pediatrics* 1999;**104**(2): e14.

3. Starc, T. J., Lipshultz, S. E., Easley, K. A. *et al.* Incidence of cardiac abnormalities in children with human immunodeficiency virus infection: the prospective P2C2 HIV study. *J. Pediatr.* 2002;**141**(3): 327–334.

4. Langston, C., Cooper, E. R., Goldfarb, J. *et al.* Human immunodeficiency virus-related mortality in infants and children: data from the pediatric pulmonary and cardiovascular complications of vertically transmitted HIV P2C2 study. *Pediatrics* 2001;**107**(2): 328–338.

5. Luginbuhl, L. M., Orav E. J., McIntosh, K., Lipshultz, S. E. Cardiac morbidity and related mortality in children with HIV infection. *J. Am. Med. Assoc.* 1993;**269**:1869–1875.

6. Keesler, M. J., Fisher, S. D., Lipshultz, S. E. Cardiac manifestations of HIV infection in infants and children. *Ann. NY Acad. Sci.* 2001;**946**:169–178.

7. Moorthy, L. N., Lipshultz, S. E. Cardiovascular monitoring of HIV-infected patients. In Lipshultz, S. E., ed. *Cardiology in AIDS.* New York: Chapman and Hall, 1998:345–384.

8. Lipshultz, S. E., Easley, K. A., Orav, E. J. *et al.* Cardiac dysfunction and mortality in HIV-infected children. The prospective P^2C^2 HIV multicenter study. *Circulation* 2000;**102**:1542–1548.

9. Fisher, S. D., Easley, K. A., Orav, E. J., *et al.*, Pediatric pulmonary and cardiovascular complications of vertically transmitted HIV infection (P2C2 HIV) study group. *Am. Heart J.* 2005;**150**(3):439–447.

10. Lipshultz, S. E., Easley, K. A., Orav, E. J., *et al.*, Pediatric pulmonary and cardiovascular complications of vertically transmitted HIV infection (P2C2 HIV) study group. *Lancet* 2002; **360**(9330): 368–373.

11. Al-Attar, I., Orav, E. J., Exil, V., Vlach, S. A., Lipshultz, S. E. Predictors of cardiac morbidity and related mortality in children with acquired immunodeficiency syndromes. *J. Am. Coll. Cardiol.* 2003;**41**(9):1598–1605.

12. Aretz, H. T., Myocarditis: the Dallas criteria. *Hum. Pathol.* 1987;**18**:619–624.

13. Kasten-Sportes, C., Weinstein C. Molecular mechanisms of HIV cardiovascular disease. In Lipshultz, S.E., ed. *Cardiology in AIDS.* New York: Chapman & Hall, 1998: 265–282.

14. Barbaro, G., Fisher, S. D., Lipshultz, S. E. Pathogenesis of HIV-associated cardiovascular complications. *Lancet Infect. Dis.* 2001;**1**;115–124.

15. Lipshultz, S. E., Fisher, S. D., Lai, W. W., Miller, T. L. Cardiovascular risk factors, monitoring, and therapy for HIV-infected patients. *AIDS* 2003;**17** (Suppl. 1): S96–S122.

16. Lipshultz, S. E., Rifai, N., Sallan, S.E. *et al.* Predictive value of cardiac troponin T in pediatric patients at risk for myocardial injury. *Circulation* 1997;**96**;2641–2648.

17. Pearson, T., New tools for coronary risk assessment. *Circulation* 2002;**105**:886–892.

18. Lipshultz, S. E., Orav, E. J., Sanders, S. P. *et al.* Immunoglobulins and left ventricular structure and function in pediatric HIV infection. *Circulation* 1995;**92**:2220–2225.

19. Rosenthal, D., Chrisant, M. R., Edens, E., *et al.* International Society for Heart and Lung Transplantation: practice guidelines for management of heart failure in children. *J. Heart Lung Transpl.* 2004;**23**(12):1313–1333.

20. Dadlani, G. H., Gingell, R. L., Orie, J. D. *et al.* Coronary artery calcifications in the long-term follow-up of Kawasaki disease. *Am. Heart J.* 2005: in press.

24 Pulmonary problems

Lauren V. Wood, M.D.

National Cancer Institute, Belhesda, MD

Introduction

Despite advances in the treatment of HIV disease and the implementation of highly active antiretroviral therapy as the standard of care in resource-rich countries, pulmonary diseases continue to cause significant morbidity and mortality in HIV-infected pediatric patients [1]. Common pulmonary diseases seen in pediatric HIV patients include: (a) lymphoproliferative processes (lymphoid interstitial pneumonitis (LIP), pulmonary lymphoid hyperplasia (PLH)); (b) conventional infectious processes; (c) viral, bacterial, and fungal opportunistic infections pathogens; (d) disorders such as asthma/ reactive airway disease worsened by the immune dysregulation accompanying HIV infection.

Pneumocystis carinii pneumonia (PCP) remains the most common pulmonary complication of pediatric HIV infection in the United States [2]. Pulmonary tuberculosis exceeds recurrent bacterial infections or PCP as the primary clinical manifestation of pediatric HIV disease in tuberculosis-endemic countries [3]. Improvements in prophylaxis and in HIV clinical management have led to a substantial decrease in the incidence of PCP [4]. LIP is the second most common pulmonary complication of pediatric HIV infection [2] and historically has been associated with improved survival in affected patients, including those in developing countries [5].

Recent studies suggest that LIP is a cytokine-mediated process mediated by immune responses against HIV antigens and/or other pathogens (e.g. EBV) [6].

Pediatric HIV patients may develop a variety of immune-related pulmonary disorders. These include T-cell alveolitis due to HIV-specific cytotoxic and NK-like CD8+ CTLs, activated alveolar macrophage accumulation, hyperproduction of macrophage-derived cytokines, pulmonary neutrophilia, and the loss of NK and HIV-specific CTL activities [6]. These conditions impair host responses to pulmonary pathogens, lead to the release of proinflammatory cytokines, and worsen gas exchange, producing pulmonary function declines.

Handbook of Pediatric HIV Care, ed. Steven L. Zeichner and Jennifer S. Read.
Published by Cambridge University Press. © Cambridge University Press 2006.

Common respiratory problems

Pediatric HIV patients may present with a variety of non-specific respiratory symptoms, including cough, dyspnea, sputum production, and/or wheezing. These symptoms may result from both pulmonary and non-pulmonary causes. Respiratory symptoms in an HIV-infected child may result from unusual opportunistic infections, lympho-proliferative disorders, immune-mediated conditions, or from processes seen in HIV-unifected children. Common causes of respiratory symptoms may include upper respiratory infections, reactive airway disease, bronchitis, sinusitis, and bacterial pneumonias [7]. Practitioners should consider both the unusual processes associated with HIV infection and the more common disorders.

Other primary disease processes may produce respiratory symptoms. Cardiac disease can cause respiratory signs and symptoms (tachypnea, dyspnea, wheezing, rales) and increased interstitial markings and small pleural or lingular effusions on chest radiographs. Pulmonary malignancies may produce respiratory complaints. They include non-Hodgkin's lymphomas, tumors of smooth muscle origin, or mucosa-associated lymphoid tissue (MALT) lesions, and Kaposi's sarcoma, a rare problem in children. Malignancies can present as hilar adenopathy, isolated parenchymal nodules, mediastinal masses or, less commonly, diffuse interstitial disease. Foreign body aspiration is a classic cause of respiratory distress in children. Metabolic derangements (systemic acidosis) can produce hyperventilation characterized by deep, rapid respirations (Kussmaul breathing).

Lymphoid interstitial pneumonitis (LIP)

Lymphoid (or lymphocytic) interstitial pneumonitis is the most common lymphopro-liferative, non-infectious pulmonary disorder seen in HIV infection and its description pre-dated the AIDS era [8]. It occurs in the absence of a detectable opportunistic infection or neoplasm and is characterized histologically by diffuse infiltration with mature, predominately CD8+ T-lymphocytes, plasma cells and histiocytes in alveolar septa and along lymphatic vessels [9]. LIP is very common in pediatric HIV infection and has been found in up to 30%–40% of HIV-infected infants and children with pulmonary disease [5]. LIP describes a spectrum of disorders involving pulmonary lymphocytic infiltrates of interstitial lung parenchyma and hyperplasia of bronchus-associated lymphoid tissue and the surrounding alveolar spaces or stroma, termed pulmonary lymphoid hyperplasia (PLH) [10]. While the distinction between LIP and PLH is clear histologically, the disorders are indistinguishable clinically, and most clinicians refer to the disorders interchangeably. In the 1994 Revised Classification System LIP is classified as a Category B symptom indicative of an HIV-related immunologic deficit [11].

The clinical manifestations of LIP can range from asymptomatic disease with isolated radiographic abnormalities to severe bullous lung disease with pulmonary

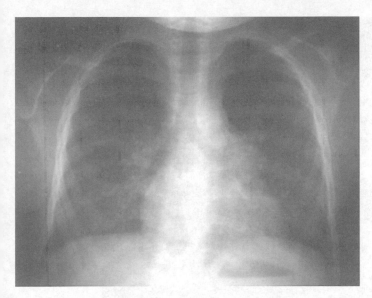

Fig. 24.1. PA Chest radiograph of LIP: bilateral, diffuse reticulonodular interstitial infiltrates associated with severe LIP.

insufficiency. Children with symptomatic LIP often present during the second or third year of life with insidious onset of mild cough, fatigue, dyspnea and tachypnea. These respiratory symptoms are associated with generalized lymphadenopathy, hepatosplenomegaly, parotid gland enlargement (parotitis) and lymphocytosis [12]. The chest physical examination is usually normal. Wheezing, oxygen desaturation with cyanosis, and digital clubbing may also be present in more advanced stages of disease. Chest radiographs show fine, bilateral reticulonodular or alveolar infiltrates that are more prominent in the lower lobes (Fig. 24.1), but may have no abnormalities other than hyperinflation. When present, these reticulonodular infiltrates are often difficult to differentiate from other infectious pneumonias due to *Pneumocystis carinii*, *Candida* spp., CMV and *Mycobacterium* spp. Chest CT confirms the interstitial pattern observed on X-ray and is useful for monitoring disease severity and extent (Fig. 24.2). Patients with LIP can have significant pulmonary dysfunction with decreased oxygen saturation at rest, a decrease in diffusing capacity, and increased alveolar–arterial oxygen gradient. Currently, biopsy is rarely used to confirm the diagnosis. The diagnosis is usually a presumptive one based on clinical criteria supported by radiographic lung findings.

The clinical course of LIP in children is highly variable, but generally benign. LIP can resolve spontaneously, worsen episodically, or worsen slowly and progressively

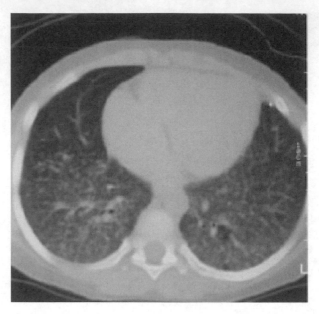

Fig. 24.2. Chest CT of LIP: chest CT correlation of radiographic findings in Fig. 24.1.

with intercurrent pulmonary infections and bronchiectasis, resulting in intermittent pulmonary decompensation or hypoxic respiratory failure [13]. LIP-related clinical and radiological manifestations can improve over time independent of LIP disease severity or HIV disease status.

Broad anecdotal clinical experience indicates that LIP-PLH responds to systemic corticosteroids [14], but no controlled studies have been performed. Bronchodilators and intermittent corticosteroid bursts are used for mild to moderately symptomatic LIP (e.g., intermittent cough or wheezing). Prolonged treatment with steroids is usually reserved for patients with significant hypoxemia and symptoms of pulmonary insufficiency, including tachypnea, dyspnea on exertion, or exercise intolerance. A typical regimen uses 2 mg/kg per day of prednisone administered for 2 to 4 weeks with subsequent tapering to 1 mg/kg per day, titrated to the lowest possible dose that results in control of clinical symptoms and resolution of hypoxemia [15]. Once an adequate response has been obtained, steroids should be weaned. Most children respond promptly within the first few weeks of treatment, although some with severe, advanced lung disease may be refractory to therapy. Steroids should be discontinued if no response is seen after 4 to 6 months [4]. Successful clinical treatment is often associated with an improvement in radiographic abnormalities.

Infectious pneumonias

Recurrent invasive bacterial infections

Serious bacterial infections are common in HIV-infected children and are responsible for a substantial degree of HIV-associated morbidity. Recurrent bacterial pneumonias are a Category C severe manifestation of HIV disease in the CDC classification system [11]. The bacterial pathogens that cause invasive disease in HIV-infected children are often identical to those seen in immunocompetent pediatric patients (see Chapter 30). Vaccination against *H. influenzae* type b has dramatically reduced the incidence of this disease. During evaluation for a pulmonary disorder, an induced sputum should be examined for PCP as well as cultured for routine bacterial, fungal and mycobacterial pathogens. Broad-spectrum antibiotics such as ticarcillin-clavulanic acid effective against β-lactamase-producing pathogens should be the initial choice. The addition of aminoglycosides should be considered in patients with severe immunocompromise, a history of neutropenia or those infected with resistant gram-negative bacteria. Bronchoscopic evaluation may be necessary to obtain adequate culture material, especially with severe or rapidly progressive disease.

Mycobacterial pneumonias

Other pathogens must be considered in the differential diagnosis of any HIV-infected child suspected of having bacterial pneumonia. *M. tuberculosis* infection is discussed in more detail in Chapter 31. Since tuberculosis may be the initial manifestation of HIV-associated illness, HIV-infected children with pulmonary illness should be tested for TB, and all children with TB should be tested for HIV.

Infection with non-tuberculous mycobacteria, commonly referred to as mycobacterium avium complex (MAC) which includes *M. avium*, *M. intracellulare*, *M. paratuberculosis*, *M. lepremurium*, and *M. scrofulaceum*, results in systemic infection associated with severe immunosuppression and late stage disease. Disease due to MAC is discussed in more detail in Chapter 32.

Viral and fungal pneumonias

The same viruses that cause lower respiratory tract infection in immunocompetent children also infect children with HIV infection. They include respiratory syncytial virus (RSV), parainfluenza viruses, influenza A and B, and adenovirus. These viruses may cause a primary pneumonia or worsen pulmonary pathology in the setting of a concurrent opportunistic infection or bacterial pneumonia. Infection is characterized by severe disease, potential systemic involvement and prolonged viral excretion [13]. Culture of nasopharyngeal, sputum or BAL specimens for respiratory viruses should be performed in children with persistent or significant symptoms of upper or lower respiratory tract infection, particularly during known seasonal peaks of viral disease. All patients should receive inactivated split trivalent influenza vaccine annually before the influenza season starts. Pulmonary mycoses are increasingly encountered in children

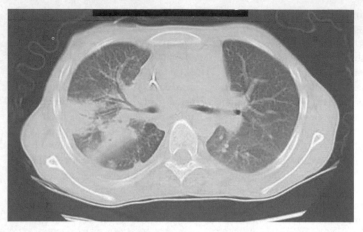

Fig. 24.3. Chest CT: lobar consolidation and bullous lung disease associated with recurrent bacterial pneumonia due to *Pseudomonas aeruginosa* and *Serratia marcesens*. Extensive infiltrates and cavitary lesions with air fluid levels and cystic bronchiectasis.

with HIV infection as a consequence of severe immunodeficiency, although the exact incidence of fungal pneumonia is unknown [2]. Histoplasmosis, cryptococcosis and coccidioidomycosis may all present with pulmonary involvement and are frequently characterized by progressive pneumonia and disseminated infection. In contrast, some fungal pathogens such as aspergillus, typically present with locally invasive pulmonary and sinus disease (Fig. 24.4) and present extremely challenging management problems [16] (see Chapter 33 for a more extensive discussion of fungal pneumonias).

Diagnostic approach to evaluation of pneumonias

HIV-infected pediatric patients presenting with suspected pneumonia represent a diagnostic challenge. Adequate diagnostic specimens must be rapidly procured and blood cultures should always be obtained. The choice of antimicrobial agent should be based on the sputum Gram stains and stains for acid-fast bacilli, and the clinical presentation. The treatment of bacterial pneumonia is discussed more extensively in Chapter 30. If the clinician suspects that fungal or viral pathogens may be the etiologic agent for the pneumonia, the evaluation may require broncheoalveolar lavage or an open thorascopic lung biopsy to differentiate simple colonization from invasive disease. This procedure should be considered promptly if disease is severe, progression is rapid, and the response to antibacterial therapy is not good.

Chronic cough

Many abnormalities of large and small airways, and pulmonary parenchymal disease can produce chronic cough [17]. Common etiologies in patients without evidence of a

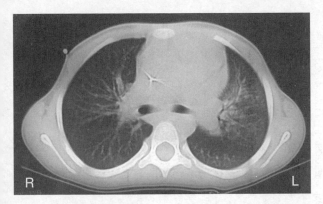

Fig. 24.4. Chest CT: invasive pulmonary aspergillosis due to *A. fumigatus*. Prominent left perihilar interstitial infiltrate with early parenchymal consolidation.

specific pulmonary disease include asthma, allergic rhinitis, chronic sinusitis, chronic bronchitis, and gastroesophageal reflux. Cough that occurs at night, after crying spells, intense play, or during exercise is suggestive of asthma [17]. Children with chronic cough who are older than 6 years should have pulmonary function testing, including an assessment of reversibility with bronchodilators, if the history is suggestive of reactive airways disease.

Chronic sinusitis is a source of significant morbidity in HIV disease and aggressive, empiric antibiotic therapy for this condition often results in a dramatic reduction in or complete resolution of cough. CT examination of the sinuses should be performed to determine the extent of disease and response to therapy, particularly in individuals with recurrent episodes.

In younger infants with chronic cough or children with radiographic patterns suggestive of recurrent aspiration pneumonia, significant gastroesophageal reflux (GER) can often be diagnosed using barium swallow or more definitively by pH probe testing. Many drugs used to treat GER are contraindicated in patients receiving certain antiretroviral agents, particularly protease inhibitors. Rare causes of wheezing include tracheomalacia or a vascular ring. Young children can also wheeze due to foreign body aspiration.

Asthma/reactive airways disease

Asthma or reactive airway disease (RAD) is a pattern of intermittent recurrent wheezing, dyspnea, dry cough or chest tightness, precipitated by triggers such as allergens, exercise, or infection [18]. It is often associated with other atopic disorders, such as allergic rhinitis, atopic dermatitis and food allergy. There are two distinct reactivity patterns: intermittent and persistent asthma. Many of the basic mechanisms underlying the

Table 24.1. Prophylaxis for pulmonary infections in HIV-infected children

Pathogen/indication	First choice	Alternatives
Pneumocystis carinii	TMP-SMX 150/750 mg/m^2 per day po BID 3 days/wk on consecutive days.	Dapsone (children ≥ 1 mos of age): 2 mg/kg (max 100 mg) po qd 4 mg/kg (max 200 mg) po q wk
Primary prophylaxis All infants aged 1–12 mos, irrespective of HIV status; 1–5 yrs CD4+ count <500 µl or 15%; 6–12 yrs CD4+ count <200 µl or 15%.	Acceptable alternative dosage schedules: Single dose po 3 days/wk on consecutive days.	Aerosolized Pentamidine (≥ 5 yrs of age) 300 mg q mos via Respirgard Nebulizer
Secondary prophylaxis After prior episode PCP	BID dosing qd or 3 days/wk on alternate days.	Atovaquone: Age 1–3 mos, >24 mo: 30 mg/kg po qd Age 4–24 mos: 45 mg/kg po qd
Mycobacterium tuberculosis _Isoniazid-sensitive_ PPD reaction ≥ 5 mm or prior positive result without treatment; **or contact** with any case of active TB **regardless of PPD result.**	Isoniazid 10–15 mg/kg (max 300 mg) po qd x 9 mos or 20–30 mg/kg (max 900 mg) po 2 days/wk × 9 mos.	Rifampin 10–20 mg/kg (max 600 mg) po qd 4–6 mos.
Isoniazid-resistant Same as above; high probability of exposure to isoniazid-resistant TB.	Rifampin 10–20 mg/kg (max 600 mg) po qd 4–6 mos.	Uncertain
Multidrug- (isoniazid/rifampin) resistant Same as above; high probability of exposure to multi-drug resistant TB.	Choice of drugs requires consultation with public health authorities and susceptibility of isolate from patient.	

Mycobacterium avium complex [4, 13, 26, 27]

Primary prophylaxis

< 1 yr CD4+ count <750 µl; 1–2 yrs CD4+ count <500 µl; 2–6 yrs CD4+ count <75 µl; ≥ 6 yrs CD4+ count <50 µl

Clarithromycin 7.5 mg/kg (max 500 mg) po BID or azithromycin 20 mg/kg (max 1200 mg) po q wk.

Azithromycin 5 mg/kg (max 250 mg) po qd; children ≥ 6 yrs, rifabutin, 300 mg po qd.

Secondary prophylaxis

After prior disseminated MAC disease

Clarithromycin 7.5 mg/kg (max 500 mg) po BID *plus* ethambutol 15 mg/kg (max 900 mg) po qd; with or without rifabutin 5 mg/kg (max 300 mg) po qd.

Azithromycin 5 mg/kg (max 250 mg) po qd *plus* ethambutol 15 mg/kg (max 900 mg) po qd; with or without rifabutin 5 mg/kg (max 300 mg) po qd.

Recurrent invasive bacterial infections

> 2 serious infections in 1-yr period

TMP-SMX 150/750 mg/m² per day po BID qd. IVIG 400 mg/kg iv q 2–4 wks.

Antibiotic chemoprophylaxis with another active agent.

Adapted from USPHS/IDSA Guidelines for the Prevention of Opportunistic Infections, November 2001.

development of the disease remain unknown. While children commonly wheeze during upper respiratory tract infections, many do not subsequently develop asthma [19].

Asthma can share a similar presentation with other problems seen in HIV patients such as LIP, PCP, chronic bronchitis, and bacterial pneumonia. Wheezing associated with a dry, non-productive cough, without fever suggests asthma as opposed to a respiratory infection. Infections can exacerbate pre-existing asthma and may be associated with acute wheezing and postinfectious bronchial hyperresponsiveness [20]. Aerosolized pentamidine for PCP prophylaxis is frequently associated with bronchospasm. Pretreatment with bronchodilators is usually successful in minimizing symptoms; discontinuation of therapy is rarely necessary.

Therapy for wheezing should be tailored to the severity of the episode and frequency of recurrences [21, 22]. Medication delivery devices such as spacers and holding chambers should be selected according to the child's ability to use them. The goals of asthma therapy are: to minimize chronic symptoms, exacerbations, the use of short-acting inhaled beta$_2$-agonists and adverse effects from medications; to eliminate limitations on activities of daily living (e.g., missed school), and to maintain normal pulmonary function [22]. Treatment guidelines for mild intermittent and mild, moderate and severe persistent asthma are outlined in Table 24.2. A stepwise approach is taken to managing asthma, with inhaled corticosteroids as the cornerstone of therapy. Pediatric doses of commonly used medications are summarized in Tables 24.3 and 24.4. Infrequent episodic asthma associated only with cough and audible wheezing, may be treated alone with intermittent, short-acting, β_2-agonist bronchodilators such as albuterol, using a metered dose inhaler or a nebulizer. Administration of oral β_2-agonists (albuterol 0.1 mg/kg per dose given tid–qid) can be considered in younger infants and children for whom aerosol therapy is difficult. Low-dose inhaled corticosteroids are the preferred treatment for mild persistent asthma, although inhaled cromolyn, or a leukotriene receptor antagonist such as monteleukast, are acceptable alternatives and may be preferable in patients predisposed to oral thrush. Moderate persistent exacerbations associated with tachypnea, use of accessory muscles or significant dyspnea in addition to wheezing should be treated with low-dose inhaled corticosteroids and long-acting inhaled beta$_2$-agonists or medium-dose inhaled corticosteroids. Alternative treatment can include low-dose inhaled corticosteroids in combination with either a leukotriene receptor antagonist or theophylline. Monitoring of serum drug levels is critical to the safe and successful use of theophylline in asthma management. Severe persistent symptoms require high dose inhaled corticosteroids, long acting inhaled beta$_2$-agonists and, if needed, oral corticosteroids. Repeated attempts should be made to reduce systemic corticosteroids and maintain control of symptoms with high-dosed inhaled corticosteroids whenever possible. Serial monitoring of response to therapy should be done using peak flow meters and pulmonary function testing. The approach to management of wheezing and reactive airway disease is the same for all children regardless of HIV infection status. However, because wheezing may often be precipitated or exacerbated by inflammation associated with acute and chronic infection, concurrent pulmonary infection should be ruled out.

Other pulmonary problems

Bronchiectasis

Bronchiectasis is a permanent abnormal dilatation of the bronchi, typically resulting from previous infection that damaged the pulmonary mucosa and the bronchial wall, irreversibly altering its shape and function. These alterations predispose to recurrent infection. Although chest radiographs often reveal evidence of bronchial wall thickening, the hallmark bronchial dilatation characteristic of bronchiectasis requires confirmation by high-resolution, thin-section CT examination. Once a diagnosis of bronchiectasis is established, patients should receive aggressive chest pulmonary toilet, prompt antimicrobial therapy for exacerbations, and antiinflammatory therapy, if indicated, for LIP or recurrent asthma. Patients with bronchiectasis should undergo routine monitoring every 6 months with high-resolution chest CTs and PFTs. Those with bronchiectasis due to recurrent bacterial pneumonias should receive monthly IVIG prophylaxis.

Spontaneous pneumothorax

Spontaneous pneumothorax (PTX) is a well-recognized complication of AIDS and may occur with *Pneumocystis carinii* infection and pulmonary cryptococcosis, or with no clear predisposing conditions [23]. This diagnosis should always be suspected and immediately confirmed in patients with cystic or bullous lung disease associated with LIP or bronchiectasis who experience an acute respiratory decompensation.

Lymphoproliferative thymic cysts

Multilocular thymic cysts (MTCs) are believed to result from an unusual response of the normal thymus gland to infection, inflammation or neoplasm [24]. MTCs are usually found in the mediastinum, are multilocular by definition and demonstrate significant inflammation and fibrosis on histopathologic examination [24]. Characteristically they are associated with Sjogren's disease and neoplasms, such as Hodgkin's disease and germinoma. MTCs appear to be a rare condition in pediatric HIV disease. It should be considered in the differential diagnosis in HIV-infected children who present with an anterior mediastinal mass.

Approach to evaluation and management of pulmonary disease

Clinicians evaluating HIV-infected children with respiratory symptoms must first determine whether those symptoms result from a common bacterial infection or an opportunistic infection. A chest X-ray should always be obtained in patients with any

Table 24.2. Management of asthma in infants and children

Asthma severity	Symptoms day / Symptoms night	Medications required to maintain long-term control	
		5 years of age and younger	Older than 5 years of age
Quick relief All Patients		Short-acting inhaled beta$_2$-agonists by nebulizer or face mask and space/holding chamber OR oral beta$_2$-agonist.	2–4 puffs short-acting inhaled beta$_2$-agonists as needed for symptoms.
Mild intermittent	≤ 2 days/week ---- ≤ 2 nights/month	No daily medication needed.	• No daily medication needed. • Severe exacerbations may occur, separated by periods of normal lung function and no symptoms. A course of systemic steroids is recommended.
Mild persistent	> 2/week but < 1/day ---- > 2 nights/month	**Preferred treatment** Low-dose inhaled corticosteroids (with nebulizer or MDI with holding chamber with or without face mask). **Alternative treatment** Cromolyn (nebulizer preferred or MDI with holding chamber) or leukotriene receptor antagonist.	**Preferred treatment** Low-dose inhaled corticosteroids. **Alternative Treatment** Cromolyn, leukotriene modifier, nedocromil, OR sustained release theophylline to serum concentrations of 5–15 mcg/ml.

		Preferred treatment
Moderate persistent	Daily ------------- > 1 night/week	Low-dose inhaled corticosteroids and long-acting beta$_2$-agonists *or* Medium-dose inhaled corticosteroids. **Alternative treatment** Low-dose inhaled corticosteroids and either leukotriene receptor antagonist or theophylline.	Low-to-medium dose inhaled corticosteroids and long-acting inhaled beta$_2$-agonists. **Alternative treatment** Increase inhaled corticosteroids within medium-dosage range *or* low-to-medium dose inhaled corticosteroids and either leukotriene modifer or theophylline.
Severe persistent	Continual ------------- Frequent	**Preferred treatment** High-dose inhaled corticosteroids *and* long-acting inhaled beta$_2$-agonists *and* if needed, corticosteroid tablets or syrup long term.	**Preferred treatment:** High-dose inhaled corticosteroids *and* long-acting inhaled beta$_2$-agonists *and* if needed, corticosteroid tablets or syrup long term.

Adapted from NAEPP Expert Panel Report July 2002 (NIH Publication No. 02-5075). Table Abbreviations: MDI (Metered Dose Inhaler).

Table 24.3. Pediatric dosages for long-term asthma control medications

Medication	Dosage form	Dose in children ($\leq$ 12 years of age)
Long-acting inhaled beta₂-agonists		
Salmeterol		1 – 2 puffs q 12hrs
	DPI 50 mcg/blister	1 blister q 12 hrs
Formoterol	DPI 12 mcg/single-use capsule	1 capsule q 12 hrs
Combined medication		
Flucatisone/salmeterol	DPI 100, 250, or 500 mcg/50mcg	1 inhalation bid; dose depends on severity of asthma
Cromolyn and nedcromil		
Cromolyn	MDI 1 mg/puff	1–2 puffs tid – qid
	Nebulizer 20 mg/ampule	1 ampule tid – qid
Nedocromil	MDI 1.75 mg/puff	1–2 puffs bid – qid
Leukotriene modifiers		
Monteleukast	4 or 5-mg chewable tablet	4 mg qhs (2–5 yrs)
	10-mg tablet	5 mg qhs (6–14 yrs)
	10 or 20-mg tablet	10 mg qhs (> 14 years)
Zafirlukast		20 mg daily (7–11 yrs) (10-mg tablet bid)
Methylxanthines		
Theophylline*	Liquids, sustained-release tablets, and capsules	Starting dose 10 mg/kg per day; usual max:
*Serum monitoring is critical; target concentration of 5–15 mcg/mL at steady state.		• < 1 yr: 0.2 (age in weeks) + 5 = mg/kg per day • $\geq$ 1 yr: 16 mg/kg per day
Systemic corticosteroids		Applies to all three corticosteroids:
Methylprednisolone	2, 4, 8,16, 32-mg tablets	• 0.25 – 2 mg/kg daily in a single dose in a.m. or qod as needed for control.
Prednisolone	5-mg tablets, 5 mg/5 ml, 15 mg/5ml	• Short-course "burst": 1–2 mg/kg per day, maximum 60 mg/day for 3–10 days.
Prednisone	1, 2.5, 5, 10, 20, 50-mg tablets; 5 mg/5 ml	

Adapted from NAEPP Expert Panel Report July 2002 (NIH Publication No. 02-5075).

Table 24.4. Comparative daily pediatric dosages for inhaled corticosteroids

Drug	Low daily dose	Medium daily dose	High daily dose
Beclomethasone CFC			
42 or 84 mcg/puff	84–336 mcg	336–672 mcg	> 672 mcg
Beclomethasone HFA			
40 or 80 mcg/puff	80–160 mcg	400–800 mcg	> 800 mcg
Budesonide DPI			
200 mcg/inhalation	200–400 mcg	400–800 mcg	> 800 mcg
Inhalation suspension for nebulization (child dose)	0.5 mg	1.0 mg	2.0 mg
Flunisolide			
250 mcg/puff	500–750 mcg	1000–1250 mcg	> 1250 mcg
Flucatisone			
MDI: 44, 110, or 220 mcg/puff	88–176 mcg	176–440 mcg	> 440 mcg
DPI: 50, 100, or 200 mcg/inhalation	100–200 mcg	200–400 mcg	> 400 mcg
Triamcinolone acetonide			
100 mcg/puff	400–800 mcg	800–1200 mcg	> 1200 mcg

Adapted from NAEPP Expert Panel Report July 2002 (NIH Publication No. 02-5075).

pulmonary complaints even if infection is not suspected. An assessment of the acuity, type and severity of symptoms should guide the practitioner's approach to management (Table 24.5). Clinically stable children with mild to moderate or chronic symptoms can often be treated empirically, assessed for response to therapy, and if unimproved, undergo more conclusive diagnostic studies. The suspected clinical condition should also determine the tests performed (Table 24.6). Clinicians should not hesitate to employ additional, more intensive studies to establish a definitive diagnosis, particularly in severely immunosuppressed patients. These studies include induced sputum examination, bronchoscopy with broncheoalveolar lavage (BAL), pulmonary function testing, arterial blood gas analysis or pulse oximetry monitoring, and open lung biopsy.

Pulmonary function tests (PFTs) provide a rapid, albeit non-specific, non-invasive method to evaluate HIV-infected children with cough or dyspnea. Children must be cooperative and generally at least 6 years of age. PFTs can be used to confirm the presence of pulmonary disease in symptomatic patients with normal chest radiographs or to detect evidence of diffuse disease in patients with localized infiltrates.

Careful measurements of the respiratory rate are useful in evaluating children with ILD. Tachypnea may reflect underlying hypoxemia. Arterial blood gas analysis or pulse oximetry, especially after exercise, can be used to measure the severity of impairment

Table 24.5. Approach to the pediatric patient with pulmonary disease

Respiratory symptoms

- Determine if acute or chronic
- Determine severity: mild, moderate, severe
- Identify symptoms: cough, chest tightness, wheezing, tachypnea, dyspnea, sputum production, digital clubbing, fever
- Identify physical examination findings: consolidation, crepitant rales, rhonchi, wheezing, pleural friction rubs, tachycardia, murmurs, gallops
- Identify precipitants and exacerbators of respiratory symptoms

Relevant clinical history

- CDC classification (Clinical and Immunologic Category)
- CD4+ T-lymphocyte count and HIV-1 RNA level
- Current antiretroviral treatment and prophylaxis for opportunistic infections
- Prior episodes of recurrent serious bacterial or opportunistic infections
- Exposure history

Fever absent
Suspect non-infectious complications

⇒

Chest radiograph

Normal or hyperinflated	Focal or diffuse infiltrates, Parenchymal nodules	Normal

Normal or hyperinflated

- Allergic rhinitis
- Acute/chronic sinusitis
- Foreign body
- Asthma/RAD
- Bronchiectasis
- Gastroesophageal reflux
- Vocal cord dysfunction
- Vascular ring
- Tracheomalacia

⇒

Focal or diffuse infiltrates, Parenchymal nodules

- LIP / PLH
- Atypical mycobacterial disease
- Cardiac disease
- Bronchiectasis
- Bronchiolitis obliterans
- Malignancy

⇒

Diagnostic studies

- CT sinuses
- PFTs
- CT chest
- ABG or pulse oximetry
- Barium swallow

- Induced sputum
- Chest CT
- PFTs
- ABG or pulse oximetry
- Echocardiogram
- Consider open lung biopsy

Fever present
Suspect infectious complications

⇒

Chest radiograph

Normal

- Acute/chronic bronchitis
- Acute/chronic sinusitis
- Viral URI
- OIs: PCP; TB, fungal infection

⇒ ⇒ ⇒ ⇒ ⇒

Focal or diffuse infiltrates

- Bacterial, fungal, viral, mycobacterial pneumonia.
- Atypical pneumonia
- Consider common *vs.* opportunistic pathogens

⇒ ⇒ ⇒ ⇒

Diagnostic studies

- Expectorated sputum, n/p wash
- Pathogen identified: treat
- No pathogen identified: treat empirically
- If no improvement consider: induced sputum ⇒ BAL

- Blood culture
- Induced sputum
- ABG or pulse oximetry
- Pathogen identified: treat
- No pathogen identified: BAL ⇒ open lung biopsy

Table 24.6. Diagnostic evaluation of HIV-associated pulmonary problems

Condition	Incidence	Diagnostic and radiographic studies
LIP-PLH	Common	• Chest radiograph, high resolution chest CT • Pulmonary function studies in older children • Assessment of arterial oxygen saturation at rest and with exercise. • Consider BAL to rule out infectious pathogens. • Open lung biopsy for definitive diagnosis.
Recurrent pneumonias	Common	• Chest radiograph • Blood cultures • Induced sputum or BAL with panmicrobial culture to assess for infectious pathogens; early am gastric aspirates to rule out M. TB. *In severe recurrent disease:* • High resolution chest CT to assess for bronchiectasis. • Pulmonary function studies to assess for restrictive lung disease and alterations in diffusion capacity and oxygen saturation.
Chronic cough	Common	• Assess and treat for acute/chronic bronchitis, allergic rhinitis. • Consider CT of sinuses to asses for acute/chronic sinusitis • Pulmonary function studies to assess for reversible, subacute bronchospasm. • Barium swallow or pH probe to rule out gastroesophageal reflux.
Asthma/wheezing	Common	• Chest radiograph to rule out acute infiltrates, foreign bodies, anatomic abnormalities. • Pulmonary function studies with assessment of response to bronchodilators. Peak flow meters should be used for ongoing monitoring in patients with chronic symptoms. • Induced sputum or BAL if indicated by radiographic studies to rule out infectious pathogens. • Consider comprehensive allergy assessment including skin testing in patients with significant clinical or family history of atopic disease.
Bronchiectasis	Uncommon	• High resolution chest CT. • Aggressive microbial screening with induced sputum or BAL with exacerbations of recurrent pneumonia to rule out unusual opportunistic pathogens.

Table 24.6. (*cont.*)

Condition	Incidence	Diagnostic and radiographic studies
Spontaneous pneumothorax	Uncommon	• Chest radiograph. • Induced sputum or BAL to rule out infectious pathogens, especially PCP.
Lymphoproliferative thymic cysts	Uncommon	• High resolution chest CT: assess for intrathoracic adenopathy and other parenchymal lung lesions.
Malignancy	Uncommon	• Etiologies to consider: non-Hodgkin's lymphoma, leiomyoma, leiomyosarcoma, mucosa-associated lymphoid tumor. *Tissue histopathology is definitive*: • CT-guided needle biopsy. • Open lung biopsy.

in gas exchange, and should be obtained in children presenting with significant tachypnea, wheezing, exercise intolerance or digital clubbing.

Although bronchoscopy may present technical challenges in pediatric patients, analysis of BAL fluid may help establish a clinical diagnosis and allow refinement of antimicrobial therapy. Patients with unrevealing induced sputum results who are unresponsive to empiric antimicrobial therapy or who have rapidly progressive disease are primary candidates for BAL. Fluid should be sent for gram, acid-fast and silver stains; routine bacterial, fungal and viral cultures; cytology; and enzyme-linked immunosorbent assays or fluorescent antibody studies for *Bordetella pertussis*, *Chlamydia*, and *Legionella*. If BAL analysis is inconclusive, open lung biopsy may be used for definitive histologic diagnosis, although thorascopic or CT-guided needle biopsy can be considered for older children and adolescents. Although associated with notable surgical morbidity, lung biopsy may provide essential information [25].

Summary

Despite advances in treatment, respiratory symptoms continue to be a very common manifestation of disease in HIV-infected children. Practitioners must determine whether these symptoms are due to an opportunistic infection or to a chronic process such as asthma, chronic bronchitis, recurrent pneumonia, bronchiectasis, or LIP. New patterns of disease will continue to emerge. Clinicians must be prepared to meet this challenge by keeping abreast of the constantly changing spectrum of pulmonary HIV disease.

REFERENCES

1. Johann-Liang, R., Cervia, J. S., Noel, G. J. Characteristics of human immunodeficiency virus-infected children at the time of death: an experience in the 1990s. *Pediatr. Infect. Dis. J.* 1997;**16**:1145–1150.

2. Shenep, J. L., Flynn, P. M. Pulmonary fungal infections in immunocompromised children. *Curr. Opin. Pediatr.* 1997;**9**(3):213–218.

3. Merchant, R. H., Oswal, J. S., Bhagwat, R. V., Karkare J. Clinical profile of HIV infection. *Indian Pediatr.* 2001;**38**:239–246.

4. Mato, S. P., Van Dyke, R. B. Pulmonary infections in children with HIV infection. *Semin. Respir. Infect.* 2002;**17**(1):33–46.

5. Scott, G. B., Hutto, C., Makuch, R. W. *et al.* Survival in children with perinatally acquired human immunodeficiency type 1 infection. *N. Engl. J. Med.* 1989;**321**:1791–1796.

6. Agostini, C., Semenzato, G. Immunologic effects of HIV in the lung. *Clin. Chest Med.* 1996;**17**(4):633–645.

7. Wallace, J. M., Rao, A. V., Glassroth, J. *et al.* Respiratory illness in persons with human immunodeficiency virus infection. *Am. Rev. Respir. Dis.* 1993;**148**:1523–1529.

8. Liebow, A. A., Carrington, C. B. Diffuse pulmonary hyporeticular infiltrations associated with dysproteinemia. *Med. Clin. North Am.* 1973;**57**:809–843.

9. Fan, L. L., Langston, C. Chronic interstitial lung disease in children. *Pediatr. Pulmonol.* 1993;**16**:184–196.

10. Schneider, R. F. Lymphocytic interstitial pneumonitis and nonspecific interstitial pneumonitis. *Clin. Chest Med.* 1996;**17**(4):763–766.

11. Centers for Disease Control and Prevention. Revised classification system for human immunodeficiency virus infection in children less than 13 years of age. *Morb. Mortal. Wkly Rep.* 1994;**43**(RR-12):1–10.

12. Abuzaitoun, O. R., Hanson, I. C. Organ-specific manifestations of HIV disease in children. *Pediatr. Clin. North Am.* 2000;**47**(1):109–125.

13. Domachowske, J. B. Pediatric human immunodeficiency virus infection. *Clin. Microbiol. Rev.* 1996;**9**:448–468.

14. Rubinstein, A., Berstein, L. J., Charytan, M. *et al.* Corticosteroid treatment for pulmonary lymphoid hyperplasia in children with the acquired immune deficiency syndrome. *Pediatr. Pulmonol.* 1988;**4**:13–17.

15. Laufer, M., Scott, G. B. Medical management of HIV disease in children. *Pediatr. Clin. North Am.* 2000;**47**(1):127–153.

16. Shetty, D., Giri, N., Gonzalez, C. E., Pizzo, P. A., Walsh, T. J. Invasive aspergillosis in human immunodeficiency virus-infected children. *Pediatr. Infect. Dis. J.* 1997;16(2):216–221.

17. Callahan, C. Etiology of chronic cough in a population of children referred to a pediatric pulmonologist. *J. Am. Board Fam. Pract.* 1996;**9**(5):324–327.

18. Warner, J. O., Naspitz, C.K. Third International Pediatric Consensus statement on the management of childhood asthma. International Pediatric Asthma Consensus Group. *Pediatr. Pulmonol.* 1998;**25**(1):1–17.

19. Martinez, F. D., Wright, A. L., Taussig, L. M. *et al.* Asthma and wheezing in the first six years of life. *N. Engl. J. Med.* 1995;**332**:133–138.

20. Huang, L., Stansell, J. D. AIDS and the lung. *Med. Clin. North Am.* 1996;**80**(4):775–801.

21. Centers for Disease Control and Prevention. AIDS-indicator conditions reported in 1996, by age group, United States. HIV/AIDS Surveillance Report. 1997;**9**(2):18.

22. National Heart, Lung, and Blood Institute. Expert Panel Report: Guidelines for the Diagnosis and Management of Asthma–Update on Selected Topics 2002. National Institutes of Health 2002;NIH Publication 02–5075:3B-24.

23. Schroeder, S. A., Beneck, D., Dozor, A.J. Spontaneous pneumothorax in children with AIDS. *Chest* 1995;**108**(4):1173–1176.

24. Suster, S., Rosai, J. Multilocular thymic cyst: an acquired reactive process: study of 18 cases. *Am. J. Surg. Pathol.* 1991;**15**:388–398.

25. Izraeli, S., Mueller, B. U., Ling, A. *et al.* Role of tissue diagnosis in pulmonary involvement in pediatric human immunodeficiency virus infection. *Pediatr. Infect. Dis. J.* 1996;**15**(2):112–116.

26. Abrams, E.J. Opportunistic infections and other clinical manifestations of HIV disease in children. *Pediatr. Clin. North Am.* 2000;**47**(1):79–108.

27. Polack, F. P., Flayhart, D. C., Zahurak, M. L., Dick, J. D., Willoughby, R. E. Colonization by *Streptococcus pneumoniae* in human immunodeficiency virus-infected children. *Pediatr. Infect. Dis. J.* 2000;**19**(7):608–612.

25 Hematologic problems

William C. Owen, M.D. and Eric J. Werner, M.D.

Division of Pediatric Hematology/Oncology, Eastern Virginia Medical School, Children's Hospital of The King's Daughters, Norfolk, VA

Most HIV-infected children and adolescents have abnormalities of their peripheral blood and/or hemostatic systems. These abnormalities may be caused by direct or indirect effects of HIV on hematopoiesis, by secondary infections, by nutritional deficits, by medications or by aberrations of the immune system. While in many cases these abnormalities are asymptomatic, on occasion they may have life-threatening consequences. This chapter will review the common hematologic consequences of HIV infection and will emphasize the diagnostic and therapeutic considerations in their management.

Anemia

Anemia is common in children infected with HIV [1]. Anemia in HIV-infected children can be due to decreased red blood cell (RBC) production, defective erythroid maturation, blood loss and increased RBC destruction (hemolysis). In many cases, the anemia is multifactorial. Potential etiologies of anemia in HIV-infected children are listed in Table 25.1. Congenital RBC disorders, such as glucose-6-phosphate dehydrogenase (G-6-PD) deficiency, may be present coincidentally.

HIV infection alters the bone marrow microenvironment impairing RBC production [2]. Cytokines such as tumor necrosis factor and interleukin-1 are elevated in HIV infection and may have an inhibitory effect on erythropoiesis [3]. Patients with HIV have a relatively poor erythropoietin response to anemia [3].

Several types of infections suppress erythropoiesis. Infectious agents such as *Mycobacterium avium intracellulare* (MAC), cytomegalovirus (CMV), and Epstein–Barr virus (EBV) can inhibit RBC production. Pure red cell aplasia due to parvovirus B19 can occur in the HIV-infected individual [4]. Medications used to treat HIV or its complications may interfere with RBC production. For instance, the dose-limiting toxicity of zidovudine is anemia, and other drugs such as trimethoprim-sulfamethoxazole (TMP-SMX), ganciclovir, and acyclovir may inhibit erythropoiesis [5]. Zidovudine frequently causes macrocytosis; in fact, lack of macrocytosis is sometimes used as an indicator

Handbook of Pediatric HIV Care, ed. Steven L. Zeichner and Jennifer S. Read.
Published by Cambridge University Press. © Cambridge University Press 2006.

Table 25.1. Causes of anemia in HIV-infected children and adolescents

Decreased erythrocyte production
  Suppression of erythropoiesis by HIV
  Suppression of erythropoiesis by other infections
    Mycobacterium avium intracellulare (MAC)
    Mycobacterium tuberculosis
    Histoplasma capsulatum
    Cytomegalovirus
    Epstein–Barr virus
    Parvovirus B19
    Other
  Medications
    Zidovudine
    Other antiretroviral medication(s)
    Ganciclovir
    Acyclovir
    Trimethoprim-sulfamethoxazole
    Other
  Bone marrow infiltration by malignancy
  Anemia of chronic disease

Ineffective erythropoiesis
  Nutritional deficiencies
    Iron
    Folate
    Cobalamin
  Thalassemia

Hemolysis
  Hypersplenism
  Autoimmune hemolytic anemia (rare)
  Congenital erythrocyte disorder
    G-6-PD deficiency
    Hemoglobinopathy
    Other
  Medications
    Primaquine
    Dapsone
    Sulfonamide
  Other
  HUS/TTP

Blood loss

of poor adherence to zidovudine. Finally, infiltration of the bone marrow by malignancy, a relatively uncommon phenomenon in children with HIV, can result in decreased RBC production.

Anemia related to defective erythroid maturation in the HIV-infected child is usually caused by nutritional deficiencies. Iron deficiency can be due to poor nutritional intake, occult intestinal blood loss, or repeated phlebotomy. Vitamin B_{12} and folate deficiencies are usually caused by poor dietary intake.

An elevated reticulocyte count indicates increased RBC production. as may occur in response to hemolysis or blood loss. Hypersplenism results in increased filtration and premature destruction of normal RBCs. While auto-antibodies are frequently detected by the Coombs test in HIV-infected children, usually they do not result in clinically significant hemolysis [3]. Rarely, autoimmune hemolytic anemia may be a feature or even a presenting finding of HIV infection in infants [5a]. Glucose-6-phosphate dehydrogenase deficiency is common in many populations. Hemolysis can result in persons deficient in G-6-PD in response to infection or multiple medications including sulfonamides, dapsone, and antimalarials [6]. Hemolytic-uremic syndrome (HUS) and thrombotic thrombocytopenia purpura (TTP) appear to occur with increased frequency in patients with HIV [6, 7]. In these disorders, there is usually a marked hemolytic anemia with schistocytes on the peripheral blood smear.

The diagnostic evaluation of anemia in the HIV-infected patient begins with a thorough history and physical exam, focusing on persistent fever, weight loss, blood loss, medications, diet, and signs or symptoms of hemolysis such as jaundice or darkening of the urine. The family history should be evaluated for anemia, hemoglobinopathy, recurrent jaundice, splenectomy, early cholecystectomy or splenomegaly.

The laboratory evaluation begins with a complete blood count, reticulocyte count, and review of the peripheral blood smear. The combination of microcytosis and hypochromia should raise the differential diagnosis of iron deficiency, thalassemia, chronic disease or, less commonly, sideroblastic anemia or lead ingestion. The standard laboratory tests for iron deficiency such as the serum iron:transferrin ratio and serum ferritin concentration may be misleading. The serum iron is often low in the anemia of chronic disease leading to a low iron:transferrin ratio even in the presence of adequate iron stores, while ferritin can be falsely normal in inflammatory states. The combination of an elevated ferritin and low total iron-binding capacity is typical of the anemia of chronic inflammation [8]. When in doubt, the clinical response to a trial of ferrous sulfate supplementation, at a dose of 4–6 mg/kg per day of elemental iron, can be both diagnostic and therapeutic. A hemoglobin electrophoresis will evaluate for the presence of abnormal hemoglobins. As most states in the USA, as well as many other countries, now have neonatal hemoglobinopathy screening, this test may have been previously performed. To evaluate the possibility of β-thalassemia trait, it is necessary to perform a quantitative hemoglobin A_2 level. A lead level determination will rule out lead intoxication, and assays of erythrocyte G-6-PD activity are available. Red blood cell or serum folate and vitamin B_{12} levels will assess the adequacy of these nutrients although false normal results may occur, especially for cobalamin. As noted above, a positive Coombs test is common, but autoimmune hemolysis is uncommon. The combination of elevated serum indirect bilirubin, decreased serum haptoglobin, and microspherocytes on the peripheral smear support the diagnosis of autoimmune hemolytic anemia, but hereditary spherocytosis may also cause these findings. For the patient with refractory anemia or unexplained fever, urine and buffy coat cultures for CMV, blood cultures or nucleic acid hybridization for MAC, and serology or PCR for parvovirus, CMV, and EBV are indicated. A bone marrow evaluation may be indicated to look for malignancy, for unexplained refractory anemia or to confirm the diagnosis of MAC, parvovirus, or histoplasmosis [9]. In addition to routine morphological evaluation, the bone marrow should be stained for iron, cultured for bacteria, MAC, viruses, and fungi, and tested for parvovirus by PCR. While morphologic abnormalities of the hematopoietic precursors are commonly seen [9a], the identification of unique diagnostic abnormalities bone marrow examination is much less common and often less invasive techniques will yield the proper diagnosis [9b].

Effective treatment depends upon a correct diagnosis. Often, effective antiretroviral therapy alone will ameliorate the anemia [5]; however, sometimes these medications, especially zidovudine, may require modification because of severe anemia. Likewise, supportive care drugs that inhibit erythropoiesis may also require modification. Iron deficiency anemia should be corrected with 4–6 mg/kg per day of elemental iron. Other nutritional deficiencies (vitamin B_{12} and folate) should likewise be corrected with supplements, and opportunistic infections should be treated appropriately. Intravenous immunoglobulin can reverse parvovirus-induced pure red blood cell aplasia [4]. Erythropoietin at 150 units/kg administered 3 days per week subcutaneously often improves the quality of life [10] and allows continuation of medications that cause anemia, primarily for patients with baseline erythropoietin levels less than 500 IU/l [11]. Dosage escalation by 50 units/kg every 4 weeks (to a maximum of 300 units/kg) until the hematocrit rises by 5%–6% or reaches a level of 36% has been recommended [3]. If the hematocrit increases to >40%, the erythropoietin should be held until the hematocrit is ≤36% and then resumed at a dose that is 50 units/kg lower. Iron sufficiency must be maintained for erythropoietin to be effective.

For patients with life-threatening anemia or for those who continue to have symptomatic anemia despite appropriate interventions, transfusions of packed RBCs can be utilized. CMV-negative or leukocyte-depleted products are desirable to decrease the risk of new CMV infection. If available, irradiated products should be used to decrease the risk of graft-versus-host disease from transfused lymphocytes, although the risk of this complication appears to be very small [3].

Neutropenia

Neutropenia, defined as an absolute neutrophil count (ANC) less than 1500 cells/mm^3, is common in HIV-infected children, with reported incidence rates of 34%–65% [5].

Table 25.2. Causes of neutropenia in HIV-infected children and adolescents

---

Impaired myelopoiesis
  HIV infection of stem cells or supporting cells
  Opportunistic infection
    Mycobacterium avium intracellulare
    Mycobacterium intracellulare
    Histoplasma capsulatum
    Cytomegalovirus
    Epstein–Barr virus
    Parvovirus B19
    Other
  Nutritional deficiencies
    Folate
    Cobalamin
  Medications
    Antiretroviral drugs
    Ganciclovir
    Trimethoprim-sulfamethoxazole
    Pentamidine
    Alpha-interferon
    Antineoplastic chemotherapy
    Other
  Malignant bone marrow infiltration

Peripheral destruction
  Hypersplenism
  Infection

Severe neutropenia is usually defined as an ANC <500/µl. Neutropenia often coexists with anemia. In addition to a decreased ANC, neutrophil function defects such as decreased bactericidal activity or abnormal chemotaxis have been described [3, 5]. Quantitative and qualitative neutrophil disorders combined with other immunological abnormalities predispose these patients to severe bacterial and fungal infections.

Potential causes of neutropenia in the HIV-infected patient are listed in Table 25.2. Neutropenia can result from impaired myelopoiesis, or peripheral destruction of the circulating neutrophils. Causes of impaired myelopoiesis include direct suppression of infected marrow progenitor cells by HIV and/or indirect effects caused by release of soluble glycoproteins that inhibit myelopoiesis in HIV-infected marrow [3]. Opportunistic infections such as CMV, EBV, MAC, and parvovirus can directly suppress myelopoiesis. Deficiencies of nutrients such as vitamin B_{12} cobalamin and folate as well as malignant infiltration impair myelopoiesis.

Drugs used to treat HIV infection or its complications often cause neutropenia. Zidovudine, ganciclovir, TMP–SMX, and pentamidine, drugs commonly employed in

HIV therapeutic regimens, are potential causes of neutropenia, as are less commonly used medications such as alpha-interferon and cancer chemotherapeutic agents. Hypersplenism may shorten neutrophil survival. Although antigranulocyte antibodies are common in children with HIV infection, their presence does not correlate with the degree of neutropenia [12].

The initial diagnostic approach begins with the history, focusing on signs or symptoms of infection, nutritional factors, and the patient's current medications. The patient should be examined for evidence of active infection, adenopathy, and organomegaly. The laboratory evaluations begin with a complete blood count with review of the peripheral smear. Appropriate cultures and/or serological tests are useful for diagnosis of bacterial, viral, and fungal etiologies. Bone marrow evaluation should be performed when two or more cell lines are suppressed or when fever of unknown origin is present [9]. Antigranulocyte antibody tests are generally not helpful [12].

Treatment of the underlying HIV infection itself with antiretroviral therapy will often improve the neutropenia. However, some antiretroviral medications cause neutropenia. Stavudine has been shown to cause less neutropenia than zidovudine [13]. The cytokine increase G-CSF circulating neutrophils and improves neutrophil function [3]. In a randomized controlled clinical trial, G-CSF, dose adjusted to maintain a neutrophil count of $2–10 \times 10^9$/l significantly reduced the incidence of severe neutropenia, severe bacterial infections and bacterial infection-related hospital days [14]. Other supportive care drugs such as TMP-SMX may need to be altered if they cause significant neutropenia. Opportunistic infections should be aggressively treated, selecting drugs which are the least myelosuppressive. Nutritional deficiencies should be corrected and malignant diseases should be appropriately treated. HIV-infected children who present with fever and severe neutropenia (i.e. an absolute neutrophil count $<500/\mu l$) should receive a prompt and thorough evaluation for a source of the fever and immediate broad-spectrum antibiotics.

Thrombocytopenia

Thrombocytopenia is present in about one-third of children and adolescents infected by HIV [1, 15]. While spontaneous remissions occur, in most instances untreated thrombocytopenia is persistent or progressive [16].

Thrombocytopenia can result from decreased platelet production, accelerated platelet destruction, platelet sequestration or a combination of these factors (Table 25.3). Structural abnormalities are seen in the megakaryocytes of HIV-infected individuals [1, 17] and HIV-1 RNA has been identified in the megakaryocytes [17]. Bone marrow infiltration by malignancy or infection can inhibit platelet production. Other than myelosuppressive cancer chemotherapy, medications infrequently inhibit platelet production.

Platelet survival is shortened in patients with HIV, even those with normal platelet counts [18]. This finding combined with elevated levels of immunoglobulin on the

Table 25.3. Causes of thrombocytopenia in HIV-infected children and adolescents

---

Impaired thrombopoiesis
  HIV infection of megakaryocytes or supporting cells
  Malignant bone marrow infiltration
  Infections
    Mycobacterium avium intracellulare
    Mycobacterium intracellulare
    Histoplasma capsulatum
    Cytomegalovirus
    Epstein–Barr virus
    Other
  Medications
    Antineoplastic chemotherapy
    Other
  Nutritional deficiencies
    Folate
    Cobalamin
Peripheral destruction
  Immune thrombocytopenia
  Disseminated intravascular coagulation
  HUS/TTP
  Splenic sequestration

---

surface of the platelet [19], the identification of antibody against platelet glycoprotein IIIa in the serum [20], and a favorable response to therapies used to treat immune thrombocytopenia [16, 21] indicate an immune mechanism for the thrombocytopenia is often present. In carefully studied HIV-infected individuals, both shortened platelet lifespan and inadequate platelet production have been documented [18, 22]. Congenital HIV infection should be considered in the differential diagnosis of an infant with persistent thrombocytopenia [22a].

In addition to immune thrombocytopenia, disseminated intravascular coagulation (DIC) can occur in the HIV patient as a complication of granulocyte colony stimulating factor therapy or infection [23]. TTP and HUS also occur in this population [7]. Splenomegaly may accentuate platelet sequestration.

Mild thrombocytopenia is generally asymptomatic, but when the platelet count falls below approximately 20 000–50 000/ μl, mucosal bleeding (epistaxis, menorrhagia, mouth bleeding) and postoperative hemorrhage may ensue. Rarely, severe thrombocytopenia leads to intracranial hemorrhage, especially in hemophilia patients affected by HIV [24]. Ellaurie *et al.* [25] also described fatal central nervous system hemorrhage in three patients with platelet counts <15 000/ μl.

The development of easy bruising, petechiae or unusual bleeding should prompt a diagnostic evaluation. The physical examination should evaluate the size, distribution, and age of petechiae and/or ecchymoses. Massive adenopathy may indicate malignancy or superimposed viral infection such as EBV or CMV. The child with DIC usually has a toxic appearance. Severe headache or neurologic abnormalities raise the possibility of intracranial hemorrhage, cerebral infarction or TTP.

The laboratory evaluation begins with a complete blood count and careful review of the peripheral blood smear. Concomitant anemia or neutropenia suggest bone marrow infiltrate, failure or infection. Red cell fragmentation is a feature of DIC or TTP/HUS. Toxic granulation, vacuoles and Döhle bodies in neutrophils suggest infection. A bone marrow aspirate and biopsy should be considered early in the HIV-infected child with thrombocytopenia. In addition to routine histologic evaluation, marrow samples should be cultured for fungi and acid fast bacilli. A DIC screen (prothrombin time, activated partial thromboplastin time, fibrinogen and D-dimer or fibrin degradation products) should be performed in the toxic-appearing child. Platelet-associated-immunoglobulin is unlikely to be helpful.

Management depends largely upon the patient's clinical status, the etiology and severity of the thrombocytopenia and physician/patient preference. For DIC, treatment of the underlying cause should be instituted immediately. Platelet and/or plasma transfusion is used to treat clinical bleeding. There may also be a role for anti-thrombin concentrates [26]. TTP is a rare life-threatening disorder, for which plasmapheresis has been shown to improve survival [7, 27]. Other treatments tried but not studied by randomized clinical trial for TTP include corticosteroids, vincristine, intravenous immunoglobulins (IVIG) and splenectomy [28].

Antiretroviral therapy can raise the platelet count [18, 29, 30] and may provide durable responses. Patients with more severe thrombocytopenia, clinical bleeding or already receiving antiretroviral therapy usually need other treatments. Corticosteroids have long been used to treat immune thrombocytopenic purpura (ITP). Initial prednisone doses of 2–4 mg/kg per day have been used [31, 32]. One approach is to administer prednisone at 2 mg/kg per day for 2 weeks then taper or discontinue the medication. High dose methylprednisolone (30 mg/kg per day for three days, maximum dose 1 gram) has also been reported to be effective in children with ITP [33], although the effectiveness of this approach in HIV-infected patients is unknown. Short-term therapy with dexamethasone has been used in HIV-infected adults with immune thrombocytopenia [34]. While steroids often improve platelet counts in the HIV-infected patient, the effect is usually transient [35]. Long-term treatment is best avoided due to the toxicity of corticosteroids, especially osteopenia and fungal infection [36].

Intravenous immunoglobulin is widely used for management of ITP. The mechanism of action likely involves blockade of the splenic Fc receptor. Advantages include a rapid response and relative safety. Responses to IVIG in HIV-infected patients with thrombocytopenia are well documented [35]. A total of 2 grams/kg of IVIG is usually administered over 2–5 days. Common adverse effects include fever, headache and vomiting. A severe headache requires immediate medical attention in the thrombocytopenic individual, as the differential diagnosis includes intracranial hemorrhage.

Other problems with IVIG include its high cost, prolonged infusion time and the very small risk of transfusion-transmitted diseases.

Intravenous anti-D has also been effective in increasing platelet counts in HIV-infected children [21]. Anti-D binds to Rh positive erythrocytes and causes splenic Fc blockade. It is not effective in patients who have the Rh negative blood type or who have undergone splenectomy. An advantage is a brief infusion time and relatively few side effects. Disadvantages include expense, although it is less expensive than IVIG, a theoretical risk of transfusion-transmitted disease and hemolysis. Generally, the decrease in hemoglobin is small and well tolerated, rarely however, significant or even life-threatening hemolysis occurs [36a]. Recently, rituximab (chimeric anti CD20 monoclonal antibody) has been used for the treatment of symptomatic, refractory HIV-associated thrombocytopenia, although the efficacy and safety of this treatment needs further study [36b].

Splenectomy should be considered for patients who do not tolerate or respond to anti-D or IVIG or who require long-term corticosteroid treatment. Ideally, splenectomy should be deferred for as long as possible in young children [37]. While splenectomy does not appear to accelerate the progression of HIV, it is associated with a risk for overwhelming bacterial infection. Other long-term complications of splenectomy such as pulmonary hypertension may yet be identified [37a]. Prior to splenectomy, patients should be immunized against *Streptococcus pneumoniae*, *Haemophilus influenzae* type b and *Neisseria meningitides* [38]. However, it should be recognized that HIV-infected patients, particularly those with significant immunosuppression, may not respond optimally to immunization [38]. Partial (subtotal) splenectomy was reported to be successful in a child with HIV-related immune thrombobocytopenia [39]. While an occasional patient will have a prolonged response to splenic irradiation [40], in most patients there is a limited increase in the platelet count and a short duration of effect [40, 41].

Coagulation abnormalities

Both bleeding and thrombotic abnormalities have been described in HIV-infected children and adolescents. A list of hemostatic abnormalities in this population is provided in Table 25.4. Acquired bleeding disorders seen in HIV-infected patients include those due to medications which inhibit platelet function, to vitamin K deficiency, or to advanced liver disease, as may occur in individuals concomitantly infected with hepatitis B and/or hepatitis C.

Lupus anticoagulants are common in HIV-infected individuals [42]. While the lupus anticoagulant causes a prolonged PTT, bleeding is not usually a problem but there is paradoxically an increased risk of thrombosis. Deficiencies of the circulating anti-coagulants protein S and heparin cofactor II are also seen in the HIV-infected population [43–45]. These deficiencies also increase the risk of thrombosis. Despite the laboratory evidence for hypercoagulability, the contribution of these factors to

Table 25.4. Coagulation abnormalities in HIV-infected children and adolescents

Bleeding disorders
  Congenital disorders
    Hemophilia
    von Willebrand disease
    Other
  Acquired disorders
    Vitamin K deficiency
    Liver disease
    Medication effect
Prothrombotic disorders
  Lupus anticoagulant
  Protein S deficiency
  Heparin cofactor-II deficiency

thrombosis in HIV-infected children is less clear. A high incidence of stroke in young adults with HIV has been shown [46]. Stroke in pediatric patients has also been described, although infection or other mechanisms may contribute to this complication [47, 48]. Patsalides *et al.*[49] found radiologic abnormalities in 11 of 426 pediatric HIV-infected patients who had undergone neuroimaging (either MRI or CT). Seven patients had a total of 26 cerebral aneurysms and 8 patients had a total of 27 infarctions identified. Most of the infarctions were related to the aneurysms. Protein C deficiency was identified in one patient and protein S deficiency in two. Only one of these patients was symptomatic. In contrast, Dubrovsky *et al.*[50] reported a series of five patients in their care who had fatal cerebral aneurysms. In a retrospective review of hospitalized HIV-infected adults, DVT was identified in nearly 1% [51]. Central venous catheters are a known risk factor for thrombosis in children.

Screening coagulation studies (PT, PTT) will not detect deficiencies of circulating anticoagulants such as anti-thrombin, protein C, protein S or heparin co-factor II; therefore, these specific proteins need to be assayed if a deficiency is to be identified. In the patient with the lupus anticoagulant, the PTT is generally prolonged and does not correct when patient plasma is diluted 1:1 with normal plasma. Confirmatory studies such as the dilute Russell viper venom time are available in many specialized laboratories.

For patients with congenital bleeding disorders, the underlying hemostatic abnormality must be considered as multiple new medications are introduced for management of HIV and its complications. Reports of severe, unusual bleeding in hemophilia patients treated with protease inhibitors have begun to surface and need further evaluation [52, 53]. The use of medications that inhibit platelet function, such as aspirin or non-steroidal anti-inflammatory agents, should be avoided in these individuals.

Anticoagulation is not routinely administered to patients with lupus anticoagulants or deficiencies of circulating anticoagulants in the absence of thrombosis, but might be considered in high-risk situations such as prolonged immobilization. However, early intervention is recommended for children and adolescents with thrombosis. A review of the management of thrombosis in children has been published [54]. For the patient with severe or recurrent thrombosis, the use of long-term anticoagulation should be entertained.

Summary

HIV infection and its treatments induce a wide range of hematologic abnormalities. The advent of improved antiretroviral therapy will likely lessen the direct effect of HIV on hematopoiesis. However, additional research is yet needed to determine the impact of these treatments on the blood. Advances in hematologic supportive care options will also improve the quality of life for HIV-infected individuals.

Acknowledgments

The authors would like to acknowledge the administrative assistance of Jessica Jones, RN and Lorraine Nelson and the editorial assistance of Randall Fisher, MD and Hal Jenson, MD.

REFERENCES

1. Ellaurie, M., Burns, E. R., Rubinstein, A. Hematologic manifestations in pediatric HIV infection: severe anemia as a prognostic factor. *Am. J. Pediatr. Hematol. Oncol.* 1990; **12**:449–453.

2. Moses, A., Nelson, J., Bagby, G. C., Jr. The influence of human immunodeficiency virus-1 on hematopoiesis. *Blood* 1998;**91**:1479–1495.

3. Coyle, T. E. Hematologic complications of human immunodeficiency virus infection and the acquired immunodeficiency syndrome. *Med. Clin. North Am.* 1997;**81**:449–470.

4. Koduri, P. R., Kumapley, R., Valladares, J., Teter, C. Chronic pure red cell aplasia caused by parvovirus B19 in AIDS: use of intravenous immunoglobulin – a report of eight patients. *Am. J. Hematol.* 1999;**61**:16–20.

5. Mueller, B.U. Hematological problems and their management in children with HIV infection. In Pizzo, P. A., Wilfert, C. M., eds. *Pediatric AIDS*. Baltimore: Williams and Wilkins Publishers 1994:591–601.

5a. Rheingold, S. R., Burnham, J. M., Rutstein, R., Manno, C. S. HIV infection presenting as severe autoimmune hemolytic anemia with disseminated intravascular coagulation in an infant. *J. Pediatr. Hematol. Oncol.* 2004;**26**:9–12.

6. Luzzatto, L. Glucose-6-phosphate dehydrogenase deficiency and hemolytic anemia. In Nathan, D. G., Orkin, S. H., eds. *Hematologic Disease of Infancy and Childhood*. Vol. 1. Philadelphia: W. B. Saunders Company, 1998:704–726.

7. Thompson, C. E., Damon, L. E., Ries, C. A., Linker, C. A. Thrombotic microangiopathies in the 1980s: clinical features, response to treatment, and the impact of the human immunodeficiency virus epidemic. *Blood* 1992;**80**:1890–1895.

8. Andrews, N.C., Bridges, K.R. Disorders of iron metabolism and sideroblastic anemia. In Nathan, D. G., Stuart, H. O., eds. *Hematology of Infancy and Childhood*. Vol. 1. Philadelphia: W. B. Saunders Company, 1998:423–469.

9. Mueller, B. U., Tannenbaum, S., Pizzo, P.A. Bone marrow aspirates and biopsies in children with human immunodeficiency virus infection. *J. Pediatr. Hematol. Oncol.* 1996;**18**:266–271.

9a. Meira, D. G., Lorand-Metze, I., Toro, A. D., Silva, M. T., Vilela, M. M. Bone marrow features in children with HIV infection and peripheral blood cytopenias. *J. Trop. Pediatr.* 2005;**51**:114–119.

9b. Volberding, P. A., Baker, K. R., Levine, A. M. Human immunodeficiency virus hematology. *Hematology (Am. Soc. Hematol. Educ. Program)* 2003:294–313.

10. Moore, R.D. Anemia and human immunodeficiency virus disease in the era of highly active antiretroviral therapy. *Semin. Hematol.* 2000;**37**:18–23.

11. Fischl, M., Galpin, J. E., Levine, J. D. *et al.* Recombinant human erythropoietin for patients with AIDS treated with zidovudine. *N. Engl. J. Med.* 1990;**322**:1488–1493.

12. Weinberg, G. A., Gigliotti, F., Stroncek, D. F. *et al.* Lack of relation of granulocyte antibodies (antineutrophil antibodies) to neutropenia in children with human immunodeficiency virus infection. *Pediatr. Infect. Dis. J.* 1997;**16**:881–884.

13. Kline, M. W., Van Dyke, R. B., Lindsey, J. C. *et al.* A randomized comparative trial of stavudine (d4T) versus zidovudine (ZDV, AZT) in children with human immunodeficiency virus infection. AIDS Clinical Trials Group 240 Team. *Pediatrics* 1998;**101**:214–220.

14. Kuritzkes, D. R., Parenti, D., Ward, D. J. *et al.* Filgrastim prevents severe neutropenia and reduces infective morbidity in patients with advanced HIV infection: results of a randomized, multicenter, controlled trial. G-CSF 930101 Study Group. *AIDS* 1998;**12**:65–74.

15. Eyster, M. E., Rabkin, C. S., Hilgartner, M. W. *et al.* Human immunodeficiency virus-related conditions in children and adults with hemophilia: rates, relationship to CD4 counts, and predictive value. *Blood* 1993;**81**:828–834.

16. Glatt, A. E., Anand, A. Thrombocytopenia in patients infected with human immunodeficiency virus: treatment update. *Clin. Infect. Dis.* 1995;**21**:415–423.

17. Zucker-Franklin, D., Cao, Y. Z. Megakaryocytes of human immunodeficiency virus-infected individuals express viral RNA. *Proc. Natl Acad. Sci. USA* 1989;**86**:5595–5599.

18. Ballem, P., Belzberg, A., Devine, D. *et al.* Kinetic studies of the mechanism of thrombocytopenia in patients with human immunodeficiency virus infection. *N. Engl. J. Med.* 1992;**327**:1779–1784.

19. Karpatkin, S. Hemostatic abnormalities in AIDS. In Colman, R. W., Hirsh, J., Marder, V. J., Salzman, E. W., eds. *Hemostasis and Thrombosis: Basic Principles and Clinical Practice*. Philadelphia: J. B. Lippincott Company, 1994:969–980.

20. Nardi, M., Karpatkin, S. Antiidiotype antibody against platelet anti-GPIIIa contributes to the regulation of thrombocytopenia in HIV-1-ITP patients. *J. Exp. Med.* 2000;**191**:2093–2100.

21. Scaradavou, A., Woo, B., Woloski, B. M. *et al.* Intravenous anti-D treatment of immune thrombocytopenic purpura: experience in 272 patients. *Blood* 1997;**89**:2689–2700.

22. Cole, J. L., Marzec, U. M., Gunthel, C. J. *et al.* Ineffective platelet production in thrombocytopenic human immunodeficiency virus-infected patients. *Blood* 1998;**91**:3239–3246.

22a. Tighe, P., Rimsza, L. M., Christensen, R. D., Lew, J., Sola, M. C. Severe thrombocytopenia in a neonate with congenital HIV infection. *J. Pediatr.* 2005;**146**:408–413.

23. Mueller, B. U., Burt, R., Gulick, L., Jacobsen, F., Pizzo, P. A., Horne, M. Disseminated intravascular coagulation associated with granulocyte colony-stimulating factor therapy in a child with human immunodeficiency virus infection. *J. Pediatr.* 1995;**126**:749–752.

24. Ragni, M. V., Bontempi, F. A., Myers, D. J., Kiss, J. E., Oral, A. Hemorrhagic sequelae of immune thrombocytopenic purpura in human immunodeficiency virus-infected hemophiliacs. *Blood* 1990;**75**:1267–1272.

25. Ellaurie, M., Burns, E. R., Bernstein, L. J., Shah, K., Rubinstein, A. Thrombocytopenia and human immunodeficiency virus in children. *Pediatrics* 1988;**82**:905–908.

26. Kreuz, W. D., Schneider, W., Nowak-Gottl, U. Treatment of consumption coagulopathy with antithrombin concentrate in children with acquired antithrombin deficiency – a feasibility pilot study. *Eur. J. Pediatr.* 1999;**158** Suppl. 3:S187–S191.

27. Prasad, V. K., Kim, I. K., Farrington, K., Bussel, J.B. TTP following ITP in an HIV-positive boy. *J. Pediatr. Hematol. Oncol.* 1996;**18**:384–386.

28. Parker, R.I. Etiology and treatment of acquired coagulopathies in the critically ill adult and child. *Crit. Care Clin.* 1997;**13**:591–609.

29. Hymes, K. B., Greene, J. B., Karpatkin, S. The effect of azidothymidine on HIV-related thrombocytopenia. *N. Engl. J. Med.* 1988;**318**:516–517.

30. Arranz C. s., J. A., Sanchez Mingo, C., Garcia Tena, J. Effect of highly active antiretroviral therapy on thrombocytopenia in patients with HIV infection. *N. Engl. J. Med.* 1999;**341**:1239–1240.

31. Blanchette, V., Imbach, P., Andrew, M. *et al.* Randomised trial of intravenous immunoglobulin G, intravenous anti-D, and oral prednisone in childhood acute immune thrombocytopenic purpura. *Lancet* 1994;**344**:703–707.

32. Beardsley, D. S., Nathan, D. G., Platelet abnormalities in infancy and childhood. In. Nathan, D. G., Orkin, S. H., eds. *Hematology of Infancy and Childhood* Vol. 2. Philadelphia: W. B. Saunders Company, 1998:1585–1630.

33. van Hoff, J., Ritchey, A. K. Pulse methylprednisolone therapy for acute childhood idiopathic thrombocytopenic purpura. *J. Pediatr.* 1988;**113**:563–566.

34. Ramratnam, B., Parameswaran, J., Elliot, B. *et al.* Short course dexamethasone for thrombocytopenia in AIDS. *Am. J. Med.* 1996;**100**:117–118.

35. Bussel, J. B., Haimi, J. S. Isolated thrombocytopenia in patients infected with HIV: treatment with intravenous gammaglobulin. *Am. J. Hematol.* 1988;**28**:79–84.

36. Singh, N., Yu, V. L., Rihs, J. D. Invasive aspergillosis in AIDS. *South. Med. J.* 1991;**84**:822–827.

36a. Gaines, A. R. Disseminated intravascular coagulation associated with acute hemoglobinemia or hemoglobinuria following Rh(O)(D) immune globulin intravenous administration for immune thrombocytopenic purpura. *Blood* 2005;**106**:1532–1537.

36b. Ahmad, H. N., Ball, C., Height, S. E., Rees, D. C. Rituximab in chronic, recurrent HIV-associated immune thrombocytopenic purpura. *Br. J. Haematol.* 2004;**127**:607–608.

37. Oksenhendler, E., Bierling, P., Chevret, S. *et al.* Splenectomy is safe and effective in human immunodeficiency virus-related immune thrombocytopenia [see comments]. *Blood* 1993;**82**:29–32.

37a. Jais, X., Ioos, V., Jardim, C. *et al.* Splenectomy and chronic thromboembolic pulmonary hypertension. *Thorax* 2005;**60**:1031–1034.

38. Immunization in special clinical circumstances. In Pickering, L. K., Peter, G., Baker, C. J., Gerber, M. A., MacDonald, N. E., Orenstein, W. O., eds. *Red Book: Report of the Committee on Infectious Diseases*. Elk Grove, IL: American Academy of Pediatrics, 2000:66–67.

39. Monpoux, F., Kurzenne, J. Y., Sirvent, N., Cottalorda, J., Boutte, P. Partial splenectomy in a child with human immunodeficiency virus-related immune thrombocytopenia. *J. Pediatr. Hematol. Oncol.* 1999;**21**:441–443.

40. Blauth, J., Fisher, S., Henry, D., Nichini, F. The role of splenic irradiation in treating HIV-associated immune thrombocytopenia. *Int. J. Radiat. Oncol. Biol. Phys.* 1999;**45**:457–460.

41. Marroni, M., Sinnone, M. S., Landonio, G. *et al.* Splenic irradiation versus splenectomy for severe, refractory HIV-related thrombocytopenia: effects on platelet counts and immunological status. *AIDS* 2000;**14**:1664–1667.

42. Bloom, E. J., Abrams, D. I., Rodgers, G. Lupus anticoagulant in the acquired immunodeficiency syndrome. *J. Am. Med. Assoc.* 1986;**256**:491–493.

43. Stahl, C. P., Wideman, C. S., Spira, T. J., Haff, E. C., Hixon, G. J., Evatt, B.L. Protein S deficiency in men with long-term human immunodeficiency virus infection. *Blood* 1993;**81**:1801–1807.

44. Sugerman, R. W., Church, J. A., Goldsmith, J. C., Ens, G. E. Acquired protein S deficiency in children infected with human immunodeficiency virus. *Pediatr. Infect. Dis. J.* 1996;**15**:106–111.

45. Toulon, P., Lamine, M., Ledjev, I. *et al.* Heparin cofactor II deficiency in patients infected with the human immunodeficiency virus. *Thromb. Haemost.* 1993;**70**:730–735.

46. Qureshi, A. I., Janssen, R. S., Karon, J. M. *et al.* Human immunodeficiency virus infection and stroke in young patients. *Arch. Neurol.* 1997;**54**:1150–1153.

47. Park, Y. D., Belman, A. L., Kim, T. S. *et al.* Stroke in pediatric acquired immunodeficiency syndrome. *Ann. Neurol.* 1990;**28**:303–311.

48. Philippet, P., Blanche, S., Sebag, G., Rodesch, G., Griscelli, C., Tardieu, M. Stroke and cerebral infarcts in children infected with human immunodeficiency virus. *Arch. Pediatr. Adolesc. Med.* 1994;**148**:965–970.

49. Patsalides, A. D., Wood, L. V., Atac, G. K., Sandifer, E., Butman, J. A., Patronas, N.J. Cerebrovascular disease in HIV-infected pediatric patients: neuroimaging findings. *Am. J. Roentgenol.* 2002;**179**:999–1003.

50. Dubrovsky, T., Curless, R., Scott, G. *et al.* Cerebral aneurysmal arteriopathy in childhood AIDS. *Neurology* 1998;**51**:560–565.

51. Saber, A. A., Aboolian, A., LaRaja, R. D., Baron, H., Hanna, K. HIV/AIDS and the risk of deep vein thrombosis: a study of 45 patients with lower extremity involvement. *Am. Surg.* 2001;**67**:645–647.

52. Wilde, J. T., Lee, C. A., Collins, P., Giangrande, P. L., Winter, M., Shiach, C.R. Increased bleeding associated with protease inhibitor therapy in HIV-positive patients with bleeding disorders. *Br. J. Haematol.* 1999;**107**:556–559.

53. Racoosin, J. A., Kessler, C.M. Bleeding episodes in HIV-positive patients taking HIV protease inhibitors: a case series. *Haemophilia* 1999; **5**:266–269.

54. Monagle, P., Michelson, A. D., Bovill, E., Andrew, M. Antithrombotic therapy in children. The 7th ACCP Conference on Antithrombotic and Thrombolytic Therapy. *Chest* 2004;**126**:645S–687S.

26 Gastrointestinal disorders

Harland S. Winter, M.D.

Division of Pediatric Gastroenterology and Nutrition, VBK 107, Massachusetts General Hospital for Children, Boston, MA

Jack Moye, Jr., M.D.

Pediatric, Adolescent, and Maternal AIDS Branch, NICHID, Bethesda, MD

Introduction

Gastrointestinal (GI) dysfunction, a common occurrence in children with HIV disease, can be related to infectious agents, malnutrition, immunodeficiency or HIV infection itself, and can result in retardation of growth, increased caloric requirements, and/or diarrhea/malabsorption. The absorption and utilization of nutrients is a primary function of the GI tract, but the immune system of the gut has been shown to be the major site of CD4+ lymphocyte depletion and viral replication [1]. The mucosal immune and enteric nervous systems interact with the epithelium to regulate intestinal function. Lymphocytes and macrophages produce cytokines and vasoactive peptides that can alter brush border epithelial cell enzyme expression, secretion, motility or mucosal blood flow. These factors ultimately affect nutrient absorption. As immune function deteriorates in the HIV-infected child, intestinal function declines to a degree greater than might be expected due to opportunistic infections alone. The goal of this chapter is to present the GI aspects of HIV disease so that clinicians will begin intervention in the early stages of the disease, thereby minimizing the impact on growth and development.

GI problems of HIV-infected children

During acute infection with HIV, GI symptoms are rare. Older children can experience a "flu-like" illness, but most infants infected through MTCT are asymptomatic. One of the earliest clinical manifestations of HIV infection in children is growth retardation and slow weight gain. These changes in growth can occur as early as two months of age and do not appear to be related to concomitant, e.g., opportunistic, infection [2–4]. Older children and adults with HIV disease have decreased lean body mass and relative preservation of fat mass [5]. Alterations in body composition in infants with

Handbook of Pediatric HIV Care, ed. Steven L. Zeichner and Jennifer S. Read.
Published by Cambridge University Press. © Cambridge University Press 2006.

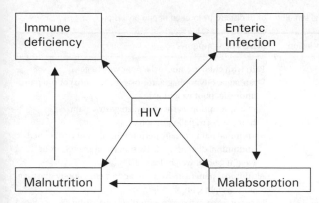

Fig. 26.1. The cycle of events leading to clinical deterioration and growth retardation in HIV-infected children.

primary HIV infection have yet to be studied directly, though progressive decrements in body mass index during the first 6 months of life have been observed in HIV-infected infants [6].

With progression of HIV infection, patients can develop enteric infections, increased caloric requirements, and malabsorption. Changes in GI function also can affect nutrient utilization and growth. Decreased acid production in the stomach (achlorhydria), by eliminating the normal gastric acid barrier, predisposes to bacterial overgrowth. Mucosal immune dysfunction can result in decreased mucosal IgA that is targeted against specific pathogens, thereby reducing one of the important mechanisms of protection against enteric pathogens. HIV-infected individuals can produce excessive amount of antibodies, but the quality or the specificity of the antibody is thought to be poor. Although not yet evaluated in the intestinal lumen of HIV-infected children, one assumes that this process pertains to the mucosal immune system as well as the systemic immune system.

The absorptive capacity of the GI tract is altered in HIV-infected children. Activity of brush border enzymes, particularly lactase, the enzyme required for metabolism of the sugar found in milk, is decreased [7]. Lactose intolerance can present challenges in selecting an appropriate diet for a child because many foods that children like contain milk or milk products. With progression of HIV, systemic immune function declines, and children develop enteric infections that exacerbate malabsorption and malnutrition. Since malnutrition further impairs immune function, particularly T-cell function, a cycle of immunodeficiency, enteric infection, malabsorption and malnutrition results in clinical deterioration and growth retardation. Other brush border enzymes responsible for absorption of proteins and other carbohydrates decrease as HIV continues to drive this cycle (Fig. 26.1).

Table 26.1. Signs and symptoms of GI disease by location of primary lesion

Location of primary lesion	Signs and symptoms
Mouth	Pain with chewing, anorexia, poor weight gain
Esophagus	Dysphagia, odynophagia, retrosternal or subxyphoid pain, anorexia, poor weight gain
Stomach	Nausea, vomiting, early satiety, epigastric pain, hematemesis, pallor, melena
Small intestine	Abdominal pain (usually periumbilical), watery diarrhea, abdominal distention, early satiety, flatulence, poor weight gain or weight loss
Colon	Abdominal pain (usually lower abdomen), bloody diarrhea, poor weight gain or weight loss
Liver	Fever of unknown origin, jaundice, dark urine, clay-colored stool, pruritis
Pancreas	Abdominal pain (usually during or after meals), anorexia, fever, weight loss, diarrhea

Careful attention to a patient's signs and symptoms should guide the approach to diagnosis and therapy. In the following section, GI tract diseases will be examined by clinical presentation. When possible, a link will be made between symptoms and pathophysiology (Table 26.1).

Evaluation and management of GI disorders (Table 26.2)

Anorexia or dysphagia

In the pediatric population, any discomfort with eating can result in anorexia. Older children can identify pain with chewing or abdominal pain, but younger children and infants can only refuse to eat. In the HIV-infected child, there are many causes of food refusal. The initial manifestation of disease in the mouth is often decreased oral intake and poor weight gain. Although HIV-infected children with parotitis can have decreased caloric intake, impaired salivary secretion of amylase rarely impacts on the digestion of starch. A careful evaluation of the mouth, gums and teeth should be included in the physical examination. Herpes simplex virus infection, linear gingival erythema, and recurrent aphthous ulcers are commonly found in the oral cavity of HIV-infected children. Culture of the lesion will help identify the pathogen. In addition, children with HIV infection frequently have poor dental hygiene and can have extensive caries, dental abscesses, and gingivitis, causing painful chewing and potential decreases in oral intake (see Chapter 21). Routine dental care is critical for proper management and should be part of the multidisciplinary team approach to caring for HIV-infected

Table 26.2. Recognition and management of GI disorders in HIV-infected children [8]

Signs and symptoms	Differential diagnosis	Evaluation	Management
Dysphagia or anorexia	Disease localized to the mouth and/or esophagus:		
	• Thrush	• Examination, scraping for KOH preparation, culture for *Candida*	• Nystatin, clotrimazole, ketoconazole, fluconazole, amphotericin B with or without flucytosine
	• Stomatitis/esophagitis	• Culture for cytomegalovirus, herpes simplex virus	• Acyclovir, ganciclovir, foscarnet
	• Hairy leukoplakia	• Examination, biopsy for Epstein–Barr virus, human papilloma virus	• May resolve without treatment
	• Periodontal disease	• Dental evaluation	• Dental hygiene, topical chlorhexidine
	• Oral ulcers	• Check CBC for neutropenia; stop zalcitabine if appropriate	• Steroids in some patients
	• Medication	• Zalcitabine (ddC), 2%–17% stomatitis	• Often self-limited
		• Zidovudine (ZDV), anorexia	• Discontinue therapy
		• Hydroxyurea, stomatitis 8%	• Discontinue therapy
		• Ritonavir (RTV), anorexia, dysgeusia 10%	• Discontinue therapy
Nausea and vomiting	Diseases localized to the stomach:		
	• *H. pylori*	• Serum antibody	• Double or triple antibiotic regimen and proton pump inhibitor
		• Upper endoscopy and biopsy	
		• Urea breath test	
		• Rapid urease test on antral biopsy	
		• Stool antigen	

(cont.)

Table 26.2. (cont.)

Signs and symptoms	Differential diagnosis	Evaluation	Management
	• Candidiasis	• Upper endoscopy and biopsy	• Clotrimazole, ketoconazole, fluconazole, amphotericin B with or without flucytosine
	• *Cryptosporidium*	• Stool analysis using concentration technique prior to staining with modified Kinyoun acid-fast stain or upper endoscopy with biopsy	• Paromomycin, azithromycin, nitazoxanide and bovine colostrum (investigational)
	Non-intestinal causes:		
	• Drug medication	• Review medications: abacavir, nausea 45%, vomiting 15%; lamivudine, zidovudine, nausea 4%–26%, vomiting 3%–8%; stavudine, 26%; adefovir and zidovudine/lamividine, mild nausea and vomiting 1–8%; nevirapine; delavirdine, nausea 7%; saquinavir; ritonavir; indinavir; amprenavir, vomiting 7%–33%; hydroxyurea, nausea 12%, vomiting; trimethoprim-sulfamethoxazole; trimethoprim-dapsone; clindamycin; primaquine; atovaquone; pentamidine isoethionate; sulfadiazine; atovaquone; azithromycin; dapsone; clarithromycin	• Discontinue therapy, substitute as appropriate
	• Central nervous system lesion	• CT scan of the head	• Dependent on cause

Diarrhea	Disease localized primarily to the small intestine:	
	• *Salmonella*	• Clinitest or fecal fat, stool cultures, ova and parasite examination, blood culture if fever present	• Pathogen specific therapy
	• *Shigella*		
	• *Campylobacter*		
	• *Giardia lamblia*		
	• *Cryptosporidium*		
	• Cytomegalovirus		
	• *Mycobacterium avium intracellulare*		
	• Lactose intolerance	• Lactose breathe hydrogen test	
	Disease localized to the colon:		
	• Cytomegalovirus	• Check for blood in the stool, fecal WBC exam, blood culture if fever present	• Acyclovir, ganciclovir, forcarnet
		• Endoscopy, culture or biopsy lesions	
	• *C. difficile*	• *C. difficile* stool toxin assay if indicated	• Metronidazole, oral vancomycin, avoid antiperistaltic agents
	• Medication	• Review medications: didanosine, 16%; stavudine (d4T), 33%; lamivudine, mild transient; abacavir, 25%; adefovir dipivoxil; and zidovidine/lamivudine; delavirdine 4%; sequinavir; ritonavir; indinavir (IDV); nelfinavir 2%–19%; amprenavir; ABT 378 lopinavir-ritonavir, 10%–20%; hydroxyurea	• Discontinue therapy if symptoms are severe or persistent

(cont.)

607

Table 26.2. (cont.)

Signs and symptoms	Differential diagnosis	Evaluation	Management
Hepatomegaly, jaundice or elevated aminotransferases	• Nutritional	• Abdominal ultrasound	• Enteral nutrition
	• Obstruction of the common bile duct: malignancy, infection	• Abdominal ultrasound	• Depends on cause and clinical status
	• Medication-related	• Review medications: zidovudine, steatosis; didanosine, 6%–20%; stavudine, 65%; abacavir, 2%–5% have hypersensitivity reaction with elevated AST/ALT; adefovir dipivoxil and zidovudine/lamivudine, 4%; nevirapine, 1%; delavirdine, <5%; ritonavir, 10%–15%; indinavir, 10%; lopinavir-ritonavir, 8%; hydroxyurea, 2%	• Discontinue medication
Abdominal pain	• Enteric pathogen	• Stool analysis	• Treatment dependent upon stool analysis
	• Medication-related	• Review medications: stavudine (d4T); lamivudine (3TC); abacavir (ABC), 15%; saquinavir (SQC); ritonavir (RTV), 20%–40%; indinavir (IDV), 4%–15%;	• With abacavir abdominal pain may decrease after weeks of therapy

Lactose intolerance	• Lactose breath test	• Lactose free diet
Pancreatitis: • idiopathic • *Cryptosporidium*	• Abdominal ultrasound • Serum lipase and amylase	• Bowel rest • Nutrition support with or without total parenteral nutrition as needed
• Cytomegalovirus	• Endoscopic retrograde cholangiopancreatography with culture and/or biopsy	
• Medication-related	• Review medications: didanosine, 4%–8%; zalcitabine, 0.5%–9%; nelfinavir; stavudine; clindamycin-primaquine; atovaquone; azithromycin; clarithromycin; pentamidine	• Discontinue implicated medication, substitute therapy as appropriate
GI bleeding		
• Hematemesis	• Upper endoscopy	• Depends on cause
• Hematochezia	• Sigmoidoscopy	• Depends on cause

From [8].

Table 26.3. Infectious agents causing esophageal injury in HIV-infected children

Bacterial agents
  Mycobacterium avium complex
  Mycobacterium tuberculosis

Viral agents
  Cytomegalovirus
  HIV
  Epstein–Barr virus
  Herpes simplex virus

Fungal agents
  Candida albicans
  Torulopsis glabrata
  Histoplasma capsulatum

Protozoal agents
  Cryptosporidium
  Pneumocystis jiroveci
  Leishmania species

children. In children in whom there is no identifiable etiology for anorexia, increased disease activity associated with circulating cytokines such as tumor necrosis factor can decrease appetite. Medications such as megestrol acetate have been prescribed in adults with AIDS wasting and appear to be effective in increasing weight. However, results are not as encouraging in the pediatric population in whom weight is increased, but linear growth is not sustained (see Chapter 9). The side effect of diabetes mellitus impacts on the use of megestrol in children and it should not be given to any child with lipodystrophy.

Pain with swallowing (odynophagia) should alert the provider to consider an invasive infectious or inflammatory process in the esophageal mucosa (e.g., *Candida* esophagitis). Although esophageal ulceration associated with gastroesophageal acid reflux can cause dysphagia, any symptoms associated with swallowing in the HIV-infected child are likely to be caused by infectious agents such as *Candida* species, cytomegalovirus, or herpes simplex virus (Table 26.3). In the oral cavity, *Candida* infection can be evident as exudative plaques on any mucosal surface, red and atrophic lesions on the palate or tongue, or erythematous fissures at the corners of the mouth, termed angular cheilitis. However, many children with candidiasis of the esophagus may not have evidence for the infection in the mouth. If lesions compatible with thrush are identified, treatment with fluconazole should be effective within 5 days. If dysphagia is not improved during this time, an upper endoscopy is recommended to identify other causes of esophagitis. A barium swallow is usually not sufficiently sensitive to identify esophageal ulcerations. If oral lesions are not identified, upper endoscopy is recommended for the child with chronic dysphagia or odynophagia. Multiple adherent white–yellow plaques can cover the lining of the esophagus and suggest a diagnosis of candidiasis. However, yeast forms on mucosal biopsy or from a mucosal scraping are essential to establish a diagnosis of invasive *Candida* species. *Candida* esophagitis often responds to oral fluconazole (3–6 mg/kg once daily, with a maximum dose of 200 mg). Intravenous amphotericin B should be reserved for those children who fail initial therapy. Improvement in immune function often results in resolution of candidiasis and should not be overlooked as an important component of treatment.

Co-infection with other pathogens is not uncommon. Discrete ulcers with well demarcated borders are suggestive of cytomegalovirus. Intranuclear inclusions with confirmatory immunohistochemical staining support a diagnosis of cytomegalovirus, but culture of mucosal biopsy is necessary for confirmation. Herpes simplex virus esophagitis can be characterized by a diffuse, hemorrhagic-appearing esophageal mucosa or by small vesicles with superficial ulcerations. As with other pathogens, mucosal biopsy and culture are confirmatory. Both herpes simplex virus and cytomegalovirus should be treated with ganciclovir, acyclovir, or foscarnet. The decision of which agent to use depends upon the degree of immunodeficiency and the presence of extraintestinal infections, such as cytomegaloviral retinitis. Rarely in children, *Histoplasma capsulatum* and *Cryptococcus neoformans* can cause painful ulcerations in the oropharynx. Zidovudine or zalcitabine can cause injury to the mouth or esophagus if not cleared rapidly into the stomach. Children should be reminded to always drink a full glass of water when taking medications. Tumors, such as Kaposi's sarcoma of the esophagus and lymphoma, are rare in HIV-infected US children, but should be considered in severely immunocompromised children with intractable progressive weight loss. In some regions of the world, such as sub-Saharan Africa, these malignancies are much more common and should occupy a more prominent consideration in the differential diagnosis of dysphagia and odynophagia.

Nausea and vomiting

Nausea and vomiting are usually caused by gastritis, enteritis, pancreatitis, dysmotility or medication. By producing acid, the stomach serves as an important barrier for the prevention of bacteria colonizing the upper GI tract. To prevent peptic injury to the esophagus from gastroesophageal reflux, clinicians can initiate acid suppression treatment with H_2 blockers or proton pump inhibitors. Prolonged and sustained hypochlorhydria, as achieved with high dose H_2 antagonists or proton pump inhibitors, can result in *Candida* overgrowth in the stomach. Other agents, such as antacids, are not as effective at neutralizing acid and rarely result in severe hypochlorhydria. *Helicobacter pylori*, a common gastric pathogen associated with chronic gastritis and duodenal ulcer, can also cause hypochlorhydria, but has been reported infrequently in the HIV-infected child [9]. Other pathogens such as cytomegalovirus, herpes simplex virus, *Candida*, or the intestinal parasite *Cryptosporidium* can present with nausea and vomiting caused by inflammation in the stomach. Upper endoscopy and mucosal biopsy is often helpful in identifying specific causes and guiding treatment. A diagnosis of *H.*

pylori infection can be established by non-invasive methods such as stool antigen or urea breath test. Serologic tests are not reliable in the pediatric population and this is most likely even more relevant for the HIV-infected child. Many of the medications used to treat children with HIV disease cause nausea and vomiting (Table 26.2). Abacavir (ABC), lamivudine (3TC), zidovudine (ZDV) and stavudine (d4T) are most commonly associated with nausea and vomiting. Although not well characterized in the pediatric population, one suspects that many of these medications injure the mucosa, resulting in gastritis and possible ulceration. When tolerated, giving medications with food can prevent some of these symptoms.

Diarrhea and GI bleeding

Diarrhea is a very common clinical manifestation of HIV disease, especially as the immune system deteriorates and viral load increases. For this reason, diarrhea has been seen throughout the pandemic as a clinical indicator of deteriorating immune function and disease progression. During this phase of the disease, the number of prescribed medications increases. Many cause diarrhea. In the early phases of HIV infection, some patients can experience an acute, self-limited diarrheal illness. With progression of HIV disease and concomitant immune dysfunction, AIDS enteropathy characterized by malabsorption can develop. The mechanism of this enteropathy is not well understood. There appears to be injury to the epithelium without identification of a specific pathogen. Perhaps the mucosal immune system plays a role in the maintenance of epithelial function, and deterioration of immune function results in epithelial dysfunction and malabsorption. In the late stages of the illness, parasitic, viral, bacterial and fungal infections contribute to diarrhea and malnutrition.

The differential diagnosis of diarrhea in the pediatric population includes infectious agents, allergic conditions (such as milk or soy intolerance in infants), lactose intolerance, inflammatory bowel disorders, antibiotic-associated colitis and malabsorption syndromes. Intestinal pathogens can be difficult to identify unless they can be found in the stool [10]. Enteric pathogens such as *Mycobacterium avium intracellulare* (MAI) and *Cryptosporidium* may not be evident in the stool in early stages of the infection but can cause profuse diarrhea. Other intestinal pathogens, such as S*almonella*, *Shigella*, *Campylobacter*, *Clostridium difficile*, and *Giardia lamblia*, are easier to identify by examinations of the stool or culture and may not cause the profound diarrhea seen in other enteric pathogens. Herpes simplex virus and cytomegalovirus can cause focal ulcerations that bleed. Patients infected with these pathogens can present with melena, hematemesis or hematochezia as well as with bloody diarrhea. Endoscopic evaluation, biopsy and culture of ulcers often establish the diagnosis. Both herpes simplex virus and cytomegalovirus can be cultured from stool of patients without mucosal ulcerations or injury. The most common enteric pathogens found in the pediatric population are listed in Table 26.2. Microsporidia, *Entamoeba histolytica*, *Isospora bella*, and malignancies such as Kaposi's sarcoma are quite rare in children and are not frequent causes of diarrhea.

In children without an identifiable enteric pathogen, testing for lactose intolerance with a non-invasive test such as the lactose breath hydrogen test can provide a clue to the cause of the symptom. HIV-infected children develop lactose intolerance earlier than expected based upon genetic predisposition. By age 5 years, many will be lactose intolerant, but many may not exhibit classical symptoms [11]. However, there does not appear to be a direct relationship between lactose intolerance, malabsorption, and delayed weight gain or growth. This observation leaves the clinician to determine if removing lactose-containing foods from the diet will result in improvement of diarrheal symptoms or eliminate an important source of calories that will eventually result in reduced caloric intake and weight loss.

The evaluation of diarrhea includes a thorough history and physical examination. Careful assessment of weight and growth provide important clues about malabsorption. Bulky, malodorous stools are found in children with pancreatic insufficiency; whereas malabsorption from injury to the small intestine usually causes watery diarrhea. Bloody diarrhea is seen in colitis. The presence of fecal leukocytes supports a diagnosis of colitis; whereas carbohydrate in the stool as demonstrated by a positive Clinitest assay for reducing substances or fecal fat detected by Sudan stain of stool supports a disorder associated with small intestinal injury. Radiographic studies have little role in the initial evaluation of diarrhea. Culture of the stool for enteric pathogens yields the best chance to identify treatable causes. For many enteric pathogens, identification may only be possible by endoscopic evaluation that permits sampling of duodenal fluid and/or mucosal tissue. Visual and biopsy findings from endoscopy can change medical management in over two-thirds of children [12].

Melena and hematemesis are usually caused by lesions in the stomach, esophagus, mouth, or nasopharynx. Neutropenic ulcers can be troublesome to manage, but rarely result in significant blood loss. Although rare in the pediatric population, tumors of the GI tract can present with GI bleeding. Kaposi's sarcoma is the most common malignancy associated with HIV disease, followed by lymphoma. The GI tract is involved about one-third of the time [13]. Blood loss can occur also with lymphoma, and the cauliflower-like masses also can cause intestinal obstruction. Smooth muscle tumors such as leiomyoma and leiomyosarcoma are rare in children, but have been described in association with GI blood loss [14].

Treatment depends on the specific cause of the diarrhea (Table 26.4). For example, several drugs are effective against giardiasis, including metronidazole (15 mg/kg per day in three doses for 5 days), which is effective in over 80% of children. Quinacrine, 2 mg/kg tid for 5 days (maximum dose 300 mg/day) and paromomycin (Humatin), 25–35 mg/kg per day in three doses for 7 days also have been used to treat *Giardia lamblia* infections.

The new anti-protozoal agent, nitazoxanide [15] has been approved by the FDA for treatment of diarrhea caused by *Cryptosporidium parvum* and *Giardia lamblia* in children 1–11 years old. This medication is available in a liquid formulation, and is well absorbed from the GI tract. Peak serum concentrations are achieved within

Table 26.4. Selected therapies for common enterocolonic pathogens in children

Pathogen	Treatment
Salmonella	ampicillin, amoxicillin, trimethoprim-sulfamethoxazole, cefotaxime, ceftriaxone
Shigella	ampicillin, trimethoprim-sulfamethoxazole, cefixime, ceftriaxone,cefotaxime, ciprofloxacin, ofloxacin
Campylobacter	erythromycin, ciprofloxacin
Giardia lamblia	metronidazole, tinidazole, furazolidone, paromomycin
Cryptosporidium	paromomycin, azithromycin, nitazoxanide (investigational), hyperimmune bovine colostrum (investigational)
Cytomegalovirus	ganciclovir, foscarnet
Mycobacterium avium intracellulare	clarithromycin or azithromycin plus ethambutol; additionally rifabutin, rifampin, clofazimine, ciprofloxacin, or amikacin

1–4 hours. The active metabolite, tizoxanide, is then glucuronidated prior to excretion in the urine (30%) and stool (60%). The mechanism of action of this nitazoxanide-salicylamide derivative is not known, but inhibition of the pyruvate:ferredoxin oxido-reductase enzyme-dependent electron transfer reactions are thought to be important. Nitazoxanide appears to be effective against other enteric pathogens such as *Isospora belli, Entamoeba histolytica, Balantidium coli*, and helminthes (*Ascaris lumbridoides, Enterobius vermicularis, Ancylostoma duodenale, Trichuris trichura, Taenia saginate, Hymenolepsis nana, Strongyloides stercoralis*, and *Fasciola hepatica)*. Yellow sclerae rarely occur, but is related to deposition of the medication and resolves upon completing treatment. Other side effects such as headache, abdominal pain, diarrhea and vomiting do not occur more frequently than placebo. The efficacy of nitazoxanide seems to differ in HIV-infected and HIV-uninfected children. In a randomized controlled trial of children less than 3 years of age with cryptosporidiosis, 100 mg nitazoxanide twice daily for 3 days resulted in improvement of 56% of the HIV-uninfected children compared to 23% of HIV-uninfected children who received placebo. However, in the HIV-infected children in the same study, there was no difference in the response rate in the groups treated with nitazoxanide or placebo. For treating giardiasis, nitazoxanide was as effective as metronidazole. The recommended dose for treating giardiasis for children 12–47 months old is 100 mg (5 ml) q12 hours for three days. For children 4–11 years old, the dose is 200 mg (10 ml) q12 hrs for 3 days. Currently nitazoxanide is not approved for use in adults [15].

Hepatomegaly and jaundice

Although hepatomegaly and mildly elevated liver function tests are common findings in HIV-infected children, chronic and progressive liver disease is unusual. Steatosis, most commonly associated with nutritional deficiencies, is one of the most common causes of an enlarged liver and elevated transaminases. Other conditions in the differential diagnosis include hepatitis B, hepatitis C, *M. avium intracellulare* infection, Epstein–Barr viral hepatitis, cytomegalovirus, and drug toxicity. Of the medications an HIV-infected child is likely to take, several are associated with elevated transaminases (e.g., rifabutin, isoniazid, fluconazole, itraconazole, ketoconazole, rifampin, trimethoprim/sulfamethoxazole, lamivudine, stavudine, zalcitabine, nevirapine, and ritonavir). Although hepatitis B can occur in HIV-infected children, the infection does not usually cause hepatocellular injury. The injury to the hepatitis B-infected hepatocyte is caused by activated lymphocytes. Because of the immunodeficiency associated with HIV infection, immune-mediated injury from hepatitis B is ameliorated. This is not the case with hepatitis C. Infants born to mothers who are co-infected with HIV and hepatitis C are at a significantly increased risk for developing hepatitis C [16]. This infection is a slow, progressive disease and problems with hepatocellular carcinoma may not be evident until adulthood. Nevertheless, all children who are infected with hepatitis C or B should be followed regularly and, based upon transaminases and their clinical course, treated with interferon or lamivudine.

Jaundice in the HIV-infected child should raise the possibility of common bile duct obstruction or cholestatic hepatitis. Gallstones, fibrosis, or inflammation of the biliary tract can result in symptoms of obstruction. Initial evaluation should include an abdominal ultrasound. Cryptosporidia can migrate into the bile duct resulting in inflammation of the epithelium and acalculous cholecystitis. Fever and right upper quadrant abdominal pain, and positive Murphy's sign should increase suspicion for this diagnosis. Cytomegalovirus can cause similar symptoms and an endoscopic retrograde cholangiopancreatography (ERCP) or biopsy of the papilla can help distinguish between these diagnostic possibilities.

Jaundice in the HIV-infected child should cause concern about an obstruction of the common bile duct or severe hepatitis. Drug-induced hepatic injury should be considered in patients with progressive liver disease. In adults, hepatitis and rarely fulminant hepatic failure with lactic acidosis have been associated with receipt of nucleoside analog reverse transcriptase inhibitors. Elevated transaminases should prompt evaluation for known causes of hepatitis, but often no cause is identified. In this setting, malnutrition or HIV itself can be causing the abnormality. If transaminases remain persistently elevated for 6 months, a liver biopsy can be beneficial in finding an etiology. Because HIV can modify the immune response, unusual opportunistic infections may be found when evaluating hepatic tissue.

Abdominal pain

Children with HIV disease can experience crampy abdominal pain in association with increased luminal secretion and enhanced peristalsis from enteric pathogens. In this setting, bowel sounds are increased in frequency, but are normal in pitch. Abdominal pain in conjunction with decreased frequency of bowel sounds or increased pitch (tinkles or rushes) should alert the clinician to the possibility of more serious causes.

Appendicitis and bowel obstruction (intussusception) can occur in the HIV-infected child, but have not been reported to occur at increased frequency. *Mycobacterium avium intracellulare* often infects the mesenteric lymph nodes before the bacteria can be identified in the mucosa. When the lymph nodes become enlarged they can cause abdominal pain; initiation of diarrhea may begin months later. The mechanism is not known, but transient intussusception led by these enlarged lymphoid aggregates can play a role. The diagnosis is difficult to establish but may be suspected by identifying enlarged mesenteric nodes on an abdominal CT scan.

Abdominal pain caused by pancreatitis can be the harbinger of clinical deterioration in an HIV-infected child. The diagnosis is established by detecting an elevated amylase and/or lipase. Since many children with HIV may have elevated salivary amylase, total serum amylase is not a reliable indicator of clinical pancreatitis in these children. Fractionation of amylase or measurement of lipase should be performed if pancreatitis is suspected. A plain radiograph of the abdomen may demonstrate a widened duodenal loop suggesting edema of the head of the pancreas. Abdominal ultrasound is better at assessing pancreatic parenchyma and size of intrapancreatic ducts. Cytomegalovirus and, less commonly, cryptosporidium can invade the biliary epithelium, resulting in inflammation and eventual obstruction of the pancreatic duct. In addition, antiretroviral drugs, especially didanosine, and medications used to treat opportunistic infections, such as pentamidine and isoniazid, have been associated with pancreatitis. Diagnosis of the infectious pathogens is dependent upon brushings or lavage of the pancreatic duct or biopsy of the papilla.

Treatment of pancreatitis is often palliative. Discontinuing medications that have been implicated in causing pancreatitis can be of some benefit, but monitoring amylase and lipase in children at risk may permit earlier intervention. Because food or using the GI tract for nutritional support exacerbates pancreatic disease, children with pancreatitis may become malnourished rapidly unless total parenteral nutrition is started early in the course of the illness. Even when an etiologic agent such as cytomegalovirus is identified, treatment with an antiviral agent is rarely effective, and management remains primarily supportive. In one series of HIV-infected children, pancreatitis was associated with a high rate of mortality within months of diagnosis [17].

Conclusions

GI disorders affect the lives of HIV-infected children by causing abdominal pain and discomfort, impairment of nutrient utilization and growth, decreasing caloric intake, and equally important, by depriving them of the simple pleasures surrounding family meal times. The goals of intervention are to recognize the subtle signs and symptoms of GI disease, and to use the multidisciplinary expertise of nutritionists, nurses, social workers, dietitians, physicians, mental health workers, and pharmacists to formulate a plan that meets the needs of the child as well as the expectations of the family.

REFERENCES

1. Veazey, R. S., DeMaria, M., Chalifous, L. V. *et al.* Gastrointestinal tract as a major site of CD4+ T-cell depletion and viral replication in SIV infection. *Science* 1998;**280**:427–431.

2. Moye, J., Rich, K. C., Kalish, L. A. Women and Infants Transmission Study Group. Natural history of somatic growth in infants born to women infected by human immunodeficiency virus. *J. Pediatr.* 1996;**128**:58–69.

3. McKinney, R. E., Robertson, J. W. R. Duke Pediatric AIDS Clinical Trials Unit. Effect of human immunodeficiency virus infection on the growth of young children, *J. Pediatr.* 1993;**123**:579–582.

4. Saavedra, J. M., Henderson, R. A., Perman, J. A., Hutton, N., Livingston, R. A., Yolken, R. H. Longitudinal assessment of growth in children born to mothers with human immunodeficiency virus. *Arch. Pediatr. Adolesc. Med.* 1995;**149**:497–502.

5. Miller, T. L., Evans, S. J., Orav, E. J., McIntosh, K., Winter, H.S. Growth and body composition in children infected with the human immunodeficiency virus-1. *Am. J. Clin. Nutr.* 1993;**57**:588–592.

6. Newell, M.-L. Mechanisms and timing of mother-to-child transmission of HIV. *AIDS* 1998;**12**:831–837.

7. Miller, T. L., Orav, E. J., Martin, S. R., McIntosh, K., Winter, H.S. Malnutrition and carbohydrate malabsorption in children with vertically transmitted human immunodeficiency virus 1 infection. *Gastroenterology* 1991;**100**:1296–1302.

8. Smith, P. D., Janoff, E. N. *Gastrointestinal infections in HIV disease*, In Blaser, M. J., Smith, P. D., Ravdin, J. I., Greenberg, H. B., Guerrant, R. L. (eds.) *Infections of the Gastrointestinal Tract*, 2nd edn. Philadelphia: Lippincott, Williams & Wilkins.

9. Marano, B. J., Jr, Smith, F., Bonanno, C. A. *Helicobacter pylori* prevalence in acquired immunodeficiency syndrome. *Am. J. Gastroenterol.* 1993;**88**:687.

10. Chang, T., Pelton, S.I., Winter, H.S. Enteric infections in HIV-infected children. In Blaser, M. J., Smith, P. D., Ravdin, J. I., Greenberg, H. B., Guerrant, R. L., eds. *Infections of the Gastrointestinal Tract*. New York: Raven Press Ltd., 1995:499–510.

11. Yolken, R. H., Hart, W., Oung, I., Schiff, C., Greenson, J., Perman, J. A. Gastrointestinal dysfunction and disaccharide intolerance in children infected with human immunodeficiency virus. *J. Pediatr.* 1991;**118**:359–363.

12. Miller, T. L., McQuinn, L. B., Orav, E. J. Endoscopy of the upper gastrointestinal tract as a diagnostic tool for children with human immunodeficiency virus infection. *J. Pediatr.* 1997;**130**:766–773.

13. Danzig, J. B., Brandt, L. J., Reinus, J. F., Klein, R. S. *et al.* Gastrointestinal malignancy in patients with AIDS. *Am. J. Gastroenterol.* 1991;**86**:715.

14. Chadwick, E. G., Connor, E. J., Hanson I.C. *et al.* Tumors of smooth-muscle origin in HIV-infected children. *J. Am. Med. Assoc.* 1990;**263**:3182.

15. Nitazoxanide (Alinia) – a new anti-protozoal agent. *Med. Lett.* 2003;**45**:29–30.

16. Mazza, C., Ravaggi, A., Rodella, A. *et al.* for the Study Group of Vertical Transmission: Prospective study of mother to infant transmission of hepatitis C virus (HCV) infection. *J. Med. Virol.* 1998;**54**:12–19.

17. Miller, T. L., Winter, H. S., Luginbuhl, L. M., Orav, E. J., McIntosh, K. Pancreatitis in pediatric human immunodeficiency virus infection. *J. Pediatr.* 1992;**120**:223–227.

27 Renal disease

Somsak Tanawattanacharoen and Jeffrey B. Kopp

Kidney Disease Section, Metabolic Diseases Branch, NIDDK, NIH, Bethesda, MD

Introduction

HIV infection is associated with a wide range of renal and metabolic disturbances [1]. Electrolyte and acid-base disorders are fairly common, particularly in hospitalized patients. These include hyponatremia, hyperkalemia, and metabolic acidosis. Acute renal failure may occur, most typically as a consequence of drug therapy. Other common syndromes include hematuria, pyuria, and proteinuria; it is important to have a plan of evaluation for each of these clinical syndromes. Glomerular disease is less common and most typically manifests as focal segmental glomerulosclerosis in African-Americans and proliferative glomerulonephritis in patients of other ethnic backgrounds.

Fluid and electrolyte disorders: water, sodium and potassium

Hyponatremia is the most common electrolyte disorder in HIV-infected patients. In a longitudinal study of pediatric HIV patients, the incidence of hyponatremia was about 25% and the major cause was the syndrome of inappropriate secretion of anti-diuretic hormone (SIADH) [2]. The other common cause is volume depletion due to gastrointestinal losses and poor fluid intake. Other causes include adrenal insufficiency and drugs, including diuretics. Evaluation of hyponatremic patients involves clinical assessment of intravascular volume status and measurement of random urine sodium and creatinine concentrations. In the setting of hyponatremia and sodium depletion (extracellular volume depletion, as manifested by orthostatic hypotension), urine sodium <10 mEq/l indicates extra-renal saline loss (e.g. diarrhea) and urine sodium >10 mEq/l suggests renal saline losses (e.g. diuretics or renal salt wasting). If a patient has SIADH, the patient will typically have hyponatremia, a normal extracellular volume status, and a urine sodium >20 meq/l. SIADH in HIV-infected patients might

Handbook of Pediatric HIV Care, ed. Steven L. Zeichner and Jennifer S. Read.
Published by Cambridge University Press. © Cambridge University Press 2006.

be due to brain or lung infection, hypothyroidism, hypocortisolism, or medication. Management includes free-water restriction and, in refractory cases, doxycycline therapy (avoid in children <8 years old).

Hyperkalemia in the setting of HIV infection can be caused by adrenal insufficiency, hyporeninemic hypoaldosteronism, or acute renal failure [3]. Hyperkalemia may also be due to medication, particularly trimethoprim [4] and pentamidine [5]. These drugs have structural similarities to potassium-sparing diuretics such as triamterene and block apical sodium channels within the collecting duct. This blockade of cellular sodium entry into the tubular cell results in reduced tubular secretion of potassium, which is linked to sodium uptake.

Acid-base disorders

Hyperchloremic, normal anion-gap, metabolic acidosis secondary to chronic diarrhea or medication is frequently seen in HIV-infected children. Some patients have associated persistent hyperkalemia suggestive of renal tubular acidosis type IV [6]. Type A lactic acidosis (associated with hypotension) is commonly due to sepsis and type B lactic acidosis (associated with normal blood pressure) has been described in association with therapy with nucleoside reverse transcriptase inhibitor therapy [7]. The diagnostic approach to a reduced serum bicarbonate includes the following: exclude hyperventilation with appropriate renal compensation; calculate serum anion gap; if there is an elevated anion gap, measure suspected anions (e.g., lactate); if anion gap is normal, then evaluate for causes of hyperchloremic metabolic acidosis (including urine pH). Therapy is indicated for acute metabolic acidosis guided by arterial blood gas pH (treat with intravenous serum bicarbonate) and for chronic metabolic acidosis with serum bicarbonate <18–20 meq/l (treat with citrate solutions). The pathogenesis of metabolic disorders associated with antiretroviral therapy is described in Chapter 13.

Acute renal failure

Acute renal failure (ARF), defined as the acute retention of nitrogenous wastes with or without oliguria, may occur in HIV-infected children, although less commonly than in adults [6–8]. The major etiologies of ARF are summarized in Table 27.1. Evaluation of these patients involves the following: clinical assessment of intravascular volume status; microscopic examination of the urine including staining for eosinophils; and measurement of random urine sodium and creatinine prior to the administration of diuretics, from which is calculated the fractional excretion of filtered sodium (FE Na = [U Na × P Cr] / [P Na × U Cr] × 100), where U Na is urine sodium, P Cr is plasma creatinine, P Na is plasma sodium, and U Cr is urine creatinine.

Prerenal ARF is associated with reduced urine output, urine sodium concentration <20 meq/l, and FE Na <1%. Intrinsic renal causes of ARF include acute tubular necrosis

Table 27.1. Acute renal failure in patients with HIV infection

Classification	Etiology
Prerenal	Intravascular volume depletion (vomiting, diarrhea, glucocorticoid deficiency)
	Capillary leak (sepsis, hypoalbuminemia, therapy with interleukin-2, interferon-α, or interferon-γ)
	Hypotension (sepsis, HIV cardiomyopathy)
	Decreased renal blood flow (non-steroidal anti-inflammatory drugs)
Renal	Acute tubular necrosis (ischemia, sepsis, antimicrobials, radiographic contrast, rhabdomyolysis)
	Interstitial nephritis (penicillins, ciprofloxacin, non-steroidal anti-inflammatory drugs, adenovirus, cytomegalovirus, polyomavirus, microsporidia, *Mycobacteria*)
	Rapidly progressive glomerulonephritis (immune complex glomerulonephritis, thrombotic thrombocytopenic purpura)
Postrenal	Tubular obstruction (sulfadiazine, acyclovir, tumor lysis)
	Extrinsic ureteral and pelvic obstruction (e.g., lymphoma or massive lymphadenopathy)
	Intrinsic reteral obstruction (e.g., stone, fungus ball due to *Candida*, blood clot, sloughed papilla, indinavir crystals)

(urinalysis showing muddy brown casts, urine sodium >40 meq/l, and FE Na >2%), interstitial nephritis (urinalysis showing leukocytes, sometimes including eosinophils, and sometimes dysmorphic erythrocytes or cellular casts), and rapidly progressive glomerulonephritis (urinalysis showing dysmorphic erythrocytes and frequently red blood cell casts). Postrenal ARF in a child is most commonly due to ureteral obstruction and therefore is best assessed by obtaining renal ultrasound examination in patients at particular risk of stones, or retroperitoneal or pelvic masses.

Referral to a nephrologist should be considered when the etiology of ARF is in doubt and for management of renal causes of ARF. Urology consultation is warranted for postrenal causes of ARF. Patients with developing ARF should have close attention to saline balance, to avoid hypotension (that can exacerbate renal injury) and fluid over-load. Indications for dialysis include hyperkalemia, metabolic acidosis, volume over-load, and severe azotemia.

Drug-induced renal complications

HIV infection requires the use of multiple medications for prolonged periods and the risk of toxicity, including renal toxicity, is high. Renal complications of drugs used commonly in HIV-infected patients are listed in Table 27.2.

Table 27.2. Renal complications of drugs commonly used in HIV patients

Anti-bacterial and anti-protozoal agents	
Aminoglycosides	Acute renal failure, magnesium wasting
Penicillins	Allergic interstitial nephritis
Ciprofloxacin	Allergic interstitial nephritis
Pentamidine	Rhabdomyolysis, azotemia, acute renal failure
Rifampin	Acute renal failure, Fanconi syndrome, renal tubular acidosis, nephrogenic diabetes insipidus, interstitial nephritis, glomerulonephritis.
Sulfa drugs	Azotemia without change in GFR, sulfadiazine crystal-induced obstructive nephropathy, allergic interstitial nephritis
Anti-fungal agents	
Amphotericin	Azotemia, acute renal failure, potassium and magnesium wasting, distal renal tubular acidosis, nephrocalcinosis
Antiviral agents	
Acyclovir	Acyclovir crystal-induced obstructive nephropathy
Dideoxyinosine	Hypokalemia, hyperuricemia, Fanconi syndrome
Indinavir	Nephrolithiasis, flank pain, dysuria, asymptomatic crystalluria, interstitial nephritis, acute renal failure, possibly hypertension
Foscarnet	Acute renal failure, nephrogenic diabetes insipidus
Zidovudine	Rhabdomyolysis,
Several reverse transcriptase inhibitors	Lactic acidosis
Anti-inflammatory agents	
Non-steroid anti-inflammatory drugs	Reduced sodium excretion, interstitial nephritis, nephrotic syndrome

Hematuria

Urinary dipsticks will show a positive test for blood in the presence of intact red blood cells, hemoglobin, and myoglobin. Ingestion of ascorbate will inhibit this test and therefore mask the assessment of hematuria by dipstick, but will not affect the microscopic examination of urine. When occult blood is present in the urine without red blood cells, one must consider hemoglobinuria and myoglobinuria. When red blood cells are present, a careful microscopic inspection using a phase contrast microscope may reveal dysmorphic changes, such as irregular margins and, particularly, surface blebs, which are helpful clues to the presence of glomerular or tubular injury, as distinguished from bleeding originating from lower in the urinary tract. Causes of the latter include stones or crystalluria (e.g., due to indinavir therapy), urothelial malignancy (which has an increased prevalence in HIV-infected adults [9]), and infection.

Table 27.3. Causes of hematuria in HIV-infected patients

Renal causes	Postrenal causes	Other
Dysmorphic erythrocytes on urinalysis	Non-dysmorphic erythrocytes on urinalysis	Erythrocytes absent from urinalysis
Glomerular diseases: glomerulonephritis, nephrotic syndrome	Kidney stone, crystal aggregates	Hemoglobinuria
Interstitial nephritis	Cancer of kidney or bladder Infection in kidney, ureter, bladder, prostate, urethra	Myoglobinuria

Adapted with permission from [1].

Microscopic examination of the urine should be performed in all patients with suspected renal disease, looking for dysmorphic red blood cells (evidence of glomerular or tubular disease), red blood cell casts (evidence of glomerulonephritis or occasionally interstitial nephritis), white blood cell casts (evidence of glomerulonephritis, interstitial nephritis or pyelonephritis), and broad and waxy casts (evidence of chronic renal disease).

Pyuria: infection and interstitial nephritis

Pyuria may be due to infection, drug-induced interstitial nephritis, or glomerulonephritis (Table 27.4). Pyuria is typically defined as more than 2–4 leukocytes per high power field, although the precise range of normal depends on the degree of urinary concentration used to prepare the sample. Allergic interstitial nephritis may be suspected when the patient exhibits eosinophilia, or when eosinophils are present in the urine, although their absence does not exclude the diagnosis. There appears to be no increased risk of bacterial urinary tract infection among HIV-infected children [10]. Other infectious agents which may present with pyuria include the following: *Mycobacterium tuberculosis*, *Mycobacterium avium* complex, the microsporidian of the genus *Encephalitozoon*, cytomegalovirus (CMV), adenovirus, and BK virus (in the polyoma virus family) [11–13]. Adenoviral infection may also present with gross hematuria and ureteric obstruction due to cellular injury and clot. Diagnosis of infection with mycobacterial species, cytomegalovirus, and adenovirus is made by culture. Polyomavirus, typically BK virus, but possibly JC virus or SV40 virus, may be suspected when dysmorphic tubular epithelial cells are present on cytologic examination and this finding is confirmed by immunostaining or PCR. Indinavir therapy is also associated with

Table 27.4. Causes of pyuria in HIV-infected patients

Bacterial infection	Viral infection	Protozoan infection	Other
Gram-negative bacteria: pyelonephritis, cystitis, prostatitis	Cytomegalovirus: interstitial nephritis	Microsporidian Encephalitozoon species: interstitial nephritis	Drug-induced interstitial nephritis
Neisseria gonorrhoeae, Chlamydia species: urethritis	Adenovirus: interstitial nephritis, ureteritis		Stones and crystalluria, including drug (indinavir, acyclovir)
Mycobacterium species: pyelonephritis	Polyomavirus, especially BK virus: interstitial nephritis, ureteritis		Urothelial cancer

Adapted with permission from [1].

interstitial nephritis, associated with normal or elevated BUN and creatinine and with pyuria; characteristic crystals are present in urine and within renal parenchyma and the urine frequently has multinucleated giant cells (histiocytes) [14, 15].

Proteinuria

HIV-associated proteinuria is quite common in children. Thus, of 556 HIV-infected children evaluated over a 12-year period, nearly 13% were found to have persistent urine dipstick findings of 1+ or greater, in the absence of fever or urinary tract infection [16]. All patients with urinary protein on dipstick of 2+ or greater should undergo measurement of 24-hour urine protein and creatinine excretion, or if that is not feasible, should have a random urine protein/creatinine ratio determined [17].

Normal urinary protein is mostly composed of Tamm–Horsfall protein, a product of the distal tubule ($\sim$50%) and low molecular weight serum proteins ($\sim$50%). Normal protein excretion is < 0.3 g/day per/m^2 for full-term babies, < 0.25 g/day per/m^2 for infants and children < 10 years, and < 0.2 g per day/m^2 for children >10 years [18]. Collection of a 24-hour urine can be difficult in children; as an alternative, one can use the protein/creatinine ratio measured on a random urine sample. The urine protein/creatinine ratio is a dimensionless number, obtained by dividing the urine protein in mg/dl by the urine creatinine in mg/dl. Normal values of protein/creatinine ratio are < 0.5 in children < 2 years and < 0.2 in children > 2 years [18]. In patients

Table 27.5. Causes of proteinuria in patients with HIV infection

	Comment
Glomerular proteinuria	Urine albumin >50% urine protein and urine protein typically >2 g/d/1.73 m²
Focal segmental glomerulosclerosis	Especially in black patients
Immune complex glomerulonephritis	Especially in white patients
IgA nephropathy	Especially in white and Asian patients
Thrombotic microangiopathy	
Membranoproliferative glomerulonephritis	Generally associated with hepatitis C
Amyloid nephropathy	Rare
Membranous nephropathy	Rare
Fibrillary/immunotactoid glomerulonephritis	Rare
Histoplasmosis	Rare
Diabetes	Common due to the high prevalence of diabetes in developed countries
Interstitial nephritis	Urine albumin <30% of urine protein and urine protein typically <2 g/d/1.73 m²
Drug (see Table 27.2)	
Mycobacteria, both typical and atypical	Common (at autopsy)
Cryptococcus species	Rare
Polyomavirus (BK, JC, and possibly SV40)	Moderately common
Adenovirus	Rare
Cytomegalovirus	
Microsporidia (*Encephalitozoon* species)	Rare

Adapted with permission from [1].

with nephrotic-range proteinuria, defined as > 3.5 g/day/1.73 m², the random urine protein/creatinine ratio will generally exceed 3.

The degree of pathologic proteinuria provides some clues as to the likely source (Table 27.5). Tubular disease is typically associated with levels of proteinuria of 0.5–2 g/day per/1.73 m². Urinary protein electrophoresis, which identifies and quantitates the major classes of urinary proteins, is also helpful in distinguishing tubular proteinuria (typically with < 20% albumin) from glomerular proteinuria (typically with ~50% albumin). Glomerular disease syndromes include nephritis (hypertension, edema, hematuria, and protein excretion typically 0.5–3 g/day per/1.73 m²) and nephrotic syndrome (edema, hypoalbuminemia, hypercholesterolemia, and protein excretion >3.5 g/day per/1.73 m²). In patients with tubular proteinuria, a careful review of drug history (prescription over the counter and alternative medications) is particularly important.

The management of tubular proteinuria begins with identifying possible infections or offending medications; those with proteinuria >1 g/d per 1.73 m^2 should probably be referred to a nephrologist. Patients with glomerular proteinuria should be referred to a nephrologist, and consideration should be given to the advisability of renal biopsy. Proteinuria >1 g/d per/1.73 m^2 probably merits introduction of angiotensin antagonist therapy to slow the progression of renal injury, although the data to support such a recommendation derives largely from studies of adults.

HIV-associated glomerular diseases

Patients with HIV-associated glomerular disease may present with proteinuria or hematuria on routine urinalysis, or with gross hematuria, edema, hypertension, or elevated blood urea nitrogen (BUN) and creatinine. Since many patients are asymptomatic, routine urinalysis should probably be performed regularly, perhaps semi-annually. The incidence of glomerular disease in children with HIV-1 infection is unknown.

Focal segmental glomerulosclerosis (FSGS) is the most typical glomerular lesion associated with HIV infection and has been termed HIV-associated nephropathy (for recent review see [19]). FSGS is a pathologic syndrome characterized by increased accumulation of glomerular extracellular matrix protein that initially affects some portions (hence segmental) of some glomeruli (hence focal). African-Americans have an increased incidence of FSGS and this is particularly true of HIV-associated FSGS, suggesting a genetic basis. The prevalence of FSGS is estimated at 2%–10% in longitudinal studies of patient populations which are predominantly African-American [20–22]. Children with HIV-associated FSGS typically present with heavy proteinuria, and some may have renal insufficiency at presentation. In patients with vertically acquired HIV infection, the modal time for the appearance of proteinuria is between ages 3 and 5 years [20, 21]. Children with HIV-associated FSGS, like adults, have in past years tended to progress to end stage renal disease (ESRD) fairly rapidly, frequently within a year of the appearance of renal disease [21]. With the advent of highly active antiretroviral therapy (HAART), it appears that the course of progressive renal dysfunction has become more indolent. In some patients the introduction of HAART has been associated with marked improvement in renal function and renal histopathology [23, 24].

A second glomerular lesion, mesangial hypercellularity, has been seen about half as commonly as FSGS in children with HIV infection (and less commonly in adults), and occurs in all racial groups [20–22]. Like patients with FSGS, patients with mesangial hypercellularity typically present with proteinuria or frank nephrotic syndrome. Pediatric patients with mesangial hypercellularity tend to be somewhat older than pediatric patients with HIV-associated FSGS. Mesangial hypercellularity is a diagnosis that represents a subset of minimal change nephrotic syndrome and this disorder is seen chiefly in children (and not in adults), either with or without HIV infection. These patients have slightly increased numbers of mesangial cells and either lack immunoglobulin deposits within the glomerulus or have modest amounts of IgM and/or complement [25]. Patients with mesangial hypercellularity generally appear to have an excellent prognosis, although those with heavy proteinuria may benefit from a trial of prednisone.

A third category of HIV-associated glomerular disease is mesangial proliferative glomerulonephritis, which occurs with a frequency comparable to mesangial hypercellularity [20–22, 26–28]. In pediatric patients, HIV-associated glomerulonephritis has included otherwise uncategorized mesangial glomerulonephritis, IgA glomerulonephritis [27, 28] and crescentic glomerulonephritis [29]. Patients with HIV-associated proliferative glomerulonephritis generally have an excellent prognosis, although this may not be true for the more aggressive lesions.

Finally, a range of other lesions occur in the setting of HIV infection, including minimal change glomerulopathy (nil disease) and lupus nephritis [29]. Atypical hemolytic-uremic syndrome/thrombotic thrombocytopenic purpura (HUS/TTP) may be seen, and has a poor prognosis [30, 31].

Evaluation of glomerular disease

In patients with glomerular proteinuria and in those with suspected glomerular hematuria, it is important to exclude other causes of glomerular disease. A serologic evaluation should include C4, CH50 and a streptococcal antigen panel. In selected patients, where particular diseases are diagnostic considerations, it may also be advisable to order one or more of the following: ANA (to evaluate the possibility of lupus, although false positive tests are common in HIV-infected patients), serologic test for syphilis, antibodies to hepatitis B and hepatitis C, antineutrophil cytoplasmic antibody (to evaluate the possibilty of vasculitis), and antiglomerular basement membrane antibody (to evaluate the possibility of Goodpasture's syndrome). Ultrasound may be performed to assess the renal parenchyma, since enlarged and echogenic kidneys are typical of, but not diagnostic for, FSGS [32]. Referral to a nephrologist should be considered under the following circumstances: unexplained renal insufficiency, proteinuria in excess of 1 g/d per/1.73 m^2 (or a random urine protein/creatinine ratio >1), or unexplained hematuria. Ultimately, renal biopsy may be required to establish the diagnosis and prognosis.

Treatment for glomerular disease

Therapy for chronic glomerular disease associated with HIV infection includes maximizing antiretroviral therapy (on the assumption that pathology may be related to continued high level viral replication), aggressive measures to control hypertension, and the use of angiotensin antagonist therapy (angiotensin converting enzyme (ACE) inhibitors or angiotensin receptor blockers) in patients with proteinuria or declining renal function. Edema may be managed symptomatically with sodium restriction and diuretics. Close consultation with a pediatric nephrologist is recommended.

These treatment recommendations are tentative, since no randomized trials have been reported in adults or children. Prednisone therapy for two months improved serum creatinine and proteinuria in an uncontrolled study of HIV-infected adults [33, 34]. ACE inhibitors have been shown to improve proteinuria and retard progression of renal insufficiency in various renal diseases and may do so in HIV-associated renal disease, although randomized controlled trials are not available [33–36]. To date, there have been no studies of prednisone or angiotensin antagonist therapy inhibitors in children. If angiotensin antagonist therapy is instituted, it is important to be alert for hypotension associated with the first dose of the angiotensin antagonist, particularly when diuretics are used concurrently, and for hyperkalemia. Patients with thrombotic microangiopathy (including hemolytic uremic syndrome and thrombotic thrombocytopenic purpura) are treated with plasmapheresis and/or fresh frozen plasma infusion.

Summary

HIV infection is associated with a surprisingly diverse range of renal disease, including renal disease directly associated with HIV infection, complications due to infections associated with HIV disease, and complications of therapy. With new and more effective antiretroviral therapies and longer patient survival, the nature and distribution of HIV-associated renal syndromes will likely continue to evolve. Careful attention to the diagnosis and management of pediatric HIV-associated renal disease may minimize the impact of acute and chronic renal disease on the growth and development of these children.

Acknowledgments

This work was supported by funding from the Intramural Research Program, NIDDK, NIH.

REFERENCES

1. Kopp, J. B., Renal dysfunction in HIV-1-infected patients. *Curr. Infect. Dis, Rep.* 2002;**4**:449–460.
2. Tolaymat, A., Al-Moushly, F., Sleasman, J., Paryani, S., Neiberger, R. Hyponatremia in pediatric patients with HIV-1 infection. *South. Med. J.* 1995;**88**:1039–1042.
3. Glassock, R. J., Cohen, A. H., Danovitch, G., Parsa, K.P. Human immunodeficiency virus infection and the kidney. *Ann Intern Med* 1990;**112**:35–49.

4. Choi, M. J., Fernandez, P. C., Patnaik, A. *et al.* Brief report: trimethoprim-induced hyperkalemia in a patient with AIDS, 1993; *N. Engl. J. Med.* **328**:703–706.

5. Kleyman, T. R., Roberts, C., Ling, B.N. A mechanism for pentamidine-induced hyperkalemia: inhibition of distal nephron sodium transport. *Ann. Intern. Med.* 1995;**122**:103–106.

6. Zilleruelo, G., Strauss, J. HIV nephropathy in children. *Pediatr. Clin. North Am.* 1995;**42**:1469–1485.

7. Smith, K.Y. Selected metabolic and morphologic complications associated with highly active antiretroviral therapy. *J. Infect. Dis.* 2002; **185** Suppl 2:S123–127.

8. Pardo, V., Strauss, J., Abitbol, C., Zilleruelo, G. Renal disease in children with HIV infection. In Kimmel, P. L., Bens, J.S. Stein, J.H., eds. *Contemporary Issues in Nephrology*, vol 29, New York: Churchill Livingstone, 1995:135–153.

9. Baynham, S., Katner, H., Cleveland, K. Increased prevalence of renal cell carcinoma in patients with HIV infection. *AIDS Patient Care STDs* 1997;**11**:161–165,

10. O'Regan, S., Russo, P., Lapointe, N., Rousseau, E. AIDS and the urinary tract. *J. Acquir. Immune Defic. Syndr.* 1990;**3**:244.

11. Aarons, E. J., Woodrow, D., Hollister, W. S., Canning, E. U., Francis, N., Gazzard, B. G. reversible renal failure caused by a microsporidian infection. *AIDS* 1994;**8**:1119–1121.

12. Shintaku, M., Nasu, K., Ito, M. Necrotizing tubulo-interstitial nephritis induced by adenovirus in an AIDS patient. *Histopathology* 1993;**23**:588–590.

13. Ito, M., Hirabayashi, M., Uno, Y., Nakayam, A., Asai, J. Necrotizing tubulointerstitial nephritis associated with adenovirus infection. *Hum. Pathol.* 1991;**22**:1225–1231.

14. Kopp, J. B., Falloon, J., Filie, A. *et al.* Indinavir-associated interstitial nephritis and urothelial inflammation: clinical and cytologic findings. *Clin. Infect. Dis.* 2002;**34**:1122–1128.

15. van Rossum, A. M., Dieleman, J. P., Fraaij, P. L. *et al.* Persistent sterile leukocyturia is associated with impaired renal function in human immunodeficiency virus type 1-infected children treated with indinavir. *Pediatrics* 2002;**110**:e19.

16. Strauss, J., Zilleruelo, G., Abitbol, C. *et al.* HIV nephropathy (HIVN) in children: Importance of early identification (Abstract). *J. Am. Soc. Nephrol.* 1993;**4**:288.

17. Ginsberg, J., Chang, B., Matarese, R., Garella, S. Use of single voided urine samples to estimate quantitative proteinuria. *N. Engl. J. Med.* 1983;**309**:1543–1546.

18. Makker, S. Proteinuria. In Kher, K. K., Makker, S. P. eds. *Clinical Pediatric Nephrology*, New York: McGraw-Hill, 1992:117–136.

19. Herman, E. S., Klotman, P. E. HIV-associated nephropathy: Epidemiology, pathogenesis, and treatment. *Semin. Nephrol.* 2003; **23**:200–208.

20. Ingulli, E., Tejani, A., Fikrig, S., Nicastri, A., Chen, C., Pomrantz, A. Nephrotic syndrome associated with acquired immunodeficiency syndrome in children. *J. Pediatr.* 1991;**119**:710–716.

21. Strauss, R., Abitbol, C., Zilleruelo, G. *et al.* Renal disease in children with the acquired immunodeficiency syndrome. *N. Engl. J. Med.* 1989;**321**:625–630.

22. Rajpoot, D., Kaupke, M., Vaziri, N., Rao, T., Pomrantz, A., Fikrig, S. Childhood AIDS nephropathy: a 10-year experience. *J. Natl Med. Assoc.* 1997;**88**:493–498.

23. Wali, R. K., Drachenberg, C. I., Papadimitriou, J. C., Keay, S., Ramos, E. HIV-1-associated nephropathy and response to highly-active antiretroviral therapy. *Lancet* 1998;**352**:783–784.

24. Winston, J. A., Bruggeman, L. A., Ross, M. D. *et al.* Nephropathy and establishment of a renal reservoir of HIV type 1 during primary infection. *N. Engl. J. Med.* 2001;**344**:1979–1984.

25. Southwest Pediatric Nephrology Study Group. Childhood nephrotic syndrome associated with diffuse mesangial hypercellularity. *Kidney Int.* 1983;**23**:87–94.

26. Connor, E., Gupta, S., Joshi, V. *et al.* Acquired immunodeficiency syndrome-associated renal disease in children. *J. Pediatr.* 1988;**113**:39–44.

27. Trachtman, H., Gauthier, B., Vinograd, A., Valderrama, E. IgA nephropathy in a child with human immunodeficiency virus type 1 infection. *Pediatr. Nephrol.* 1991;**5**:724–726.

28. Schoeneman, M. J., Ghali, V., Lieberman, K., Reisman, L. IgA nephritis in a child with human immunodeficiency virus: a unique form of human immunodeficiency virus-associated nephropathy? *Pediatr. Nephrol.* 1992;**6**:46–49.

29. Landor, M., Bernstein, L., Rubinstein, A. A steroid-responsive nephropathy in a child with human immunodeficiency virus infection. *Am. J. Dis. Child.* 1993;**147**:261–262.

30. Jorda, M., Rodriques, M. M., Reik, R. A. Thrombotic thrombocytopenic purpura as the cause of death in an HIV-positive child. *Pediatr. Pathol.* 1994;**14**:919–925.

31. Turner, M. E., Kher, K., Rakusan, T. *et al.* Atypical hemolytic uremic syndrome in human immunodeficiency virus-1-infected children. *Pediatr. Nephrol.* 1997;**11**:161–163.

32. Zinn, H. L., Haller, J. O. Renal manifestations of AIDS in children. *Pediatr. Radiol.* 1999;**29**:558–561.

33. Eustace, J. A., Nuermberger, E., Choi, M., Scheel, P. J., Jr., Moore, R., Briggs, W. A. Cohort study of the treatment of severe HIV-associated nephropathy with corticosteroids. *Kidney Int.* 2000;**58**:1253–1260.

34. Smith, M. C., Austen, J. L., Carey, J. T. *et al.* Prednisone improves renal function and proteinuria in human immunodeficiency virus-associated nephropathy. *Am. J. Med.* 1996;**101**:41–48.

35. Burns, G. C., Paul, S. K., Toth, I. R., Sivak, S. L. Effect of angiotensin-converting enzyme inhibition in HIV-associated nephropathy. *J. Am. Soc. Nephrol.* 1997;**8**:1140–1146.

36. Kimmel, P. L., Mishkin, G. J., Umana, W. O. Captopril and renal survival in patients with human immunodeficiency virus nephropathy. *Am. J. Kidney. Dis.* 1996;**28**:202–208.

28 Endocrine disorders

Daina Dreimane, M.D. and Mitchell E. Geffner, M.D.

Childrens Hospital, Los Angeles, CA

Primary endocrinopathies in children with HIV infection are relatively uncommon. Hypothalamic–pituitary function is rarely affected. True endocrine dysfunction in HIV infection usually results from infection or malignancy affecting specific glandular function or from the side effects of pharmacological agents on hormone synthesis or action.

Growth failure and pubertal delay

Growth failure [1–3] occurs in 20%–80% of symptomatic HIV-infected children. Among perinatally infected children, it presents as early as 6 months of age. As the HIV infection becomes more advanced, growth failure may progress to a distinct wasting syndrome.

Proposed mechanisms of growth failure

Mechanisms include the non-specific effects of chronic disease, decreased intake, and enteropathy. Affected children manifest hypermetabolism (increased resting energy expenditure)/catabolism. Hormonal aberrations, while rare, can include deficiencies of growth hormone (GH), sex steroids (during adolescence), and thyroid hormones (see below).

GH/insulin-like growth factor-I (IGF-I) axis

GH deficiency occurs less often than might be predicted, based on the prevalence of AIDS encephalopathy in children. Levels of the GH-dependent surrogates, IGF-I and insulin-like growth factor binding protein-3 (IGFBP-3), even without GH deficiency, are typically low secondary to undernutrition. IGFBP-3 proteolysis also can occur. GH/IGF-I resistance has been documented in vitro [4].

Handbook of Pediatric HIV Care, ed. Steven L. Zeichner and Jennifer S. Read.
Published by Cambridge University Press. © Cambridge University Press 2006.

Sex steroid deficiency

Delayed puberty appears to be common in children with HIV infection [5]. The mechanism remains unknown, but is most likely related to the effects of chronic disease.

Non-hormonal causes of growth failure

Growth failure may result from the effects of chronic disease caused by opportunistic infections, such as infections with *Toxoplasma gondii*, cytomegalovirus (CMV), *Pneumocystis jiroveci*, *Mycobacterium avium intracellulare* (MAI), and *Cryptococcus neoformans*, and tumors such as Kaposi's sarcoma [6, 7]. Drug effects can alter the hormonal regulation of growth. For example, rifampin induces hepatic microsomal enzymes and, thus, increases thyroid hormone clearance. Drug side effects also can alter gonadal function. Ketoconazole inhibits steroidogenesis and thus can prevent the onset or slow the progression of puberty. Megestrol acetate can lower testosterone levels by suppressing LH.

Diagnostic approach

After correction of any associated undernutrition, a bone age X-ray should be ordered which, if significantly delayed, suggests an endocrine cause for growth delay. The pediatrician should screen for hypothyroidism (see below). If thyroid function is normal, provocative GH testing is indicated. Lack of pubertal changes in girls over 13 years old and in boys over 14 years old warrants measurement of random or stimulated gonadotropin (luteinizing hormone (LH) and follicle-stimulating hormone (FSH) by immunochemiluminescent assay (ICMA)) levels to distinguish primary from central forms of hypogonadism.

Treatment

The pediatrician should treat undernutrition, including use of appetite-stimulants such as megestrol acetate [8]. Treatment of HIV infection with highly active antiretroviral therapy (HAART) with protease inhibitors (PI) may improve linear growth [9]. Both approaches tend to stimulate gain of weight out of proportion to that of lean body mass. The endocrinologist may consider non-specific hormonal therapies with anabolic agents, e.g., oxandrolone or human GH. The use of these approaches is associated with preferential gains in lean body mass. Documented GH deficiency is treated with human GH at standard doses (0.15–0.3 mg/kg per week). The GH dose approved for treatment of AIDS wasting in adults is up to 6 mg/day for 3 months [10]. High doses are presumably required to overcome underlying GH/IGF-I resistance. There is no evidence that GH stimulates HIV activity in vivo. Limited studies of GH use in HIV-infected children have been performed to date [11]. Sex steroid deficiency involves replacement of estrogen and progesterone in girls and of testosterone in boys, and should be initiated by the endocrinologist.

Hypothyroidism

Clinically significant derangements of thyroid function in HIV-infected children are infrequent. Symptoms of hypothyroidism include linear growth failure, relative preservation of weight, constipation, cold intolerance, fatigue, and hair loss.

Proposed mechanisms

Primary thyroid failure is rare. Subtle central hypothyroidism can manifest by a lack of rise in nocturnal thyroid-stimulating hormone (TSH). The sick euthyroid syndrome also has been described, as have elevated thyroxine-binding globulin levels.

Diagnostic approach

The pediatrician should screen for hypothyroidism with ultra-sensitive TSH and free thyroxine (T_4) testing. If abnormal, but not absolutely diagnostic, additional thyroid assessments, e.g., thyrotropin-releasing hormone (TRH) testing and nocturnal TSH sampling, by the pediatric endocrinologist may be required.

Treatment

For hypothyroidism, levo-thyroxine ($50-100$ $\mu g/m^2$ per day) is prescribed by the pediatrician under the direction of an endocrinologist.

Metabolic abnormalities related to protease inhibitor therapy

PI therapy in HIV-infected adults has been associated with peripheral fat wasting and truncal obesity (lipodystrophy), hyperlipidemia, and diabetes mellitus, although a similar syndrome may occur in some non-PI-treated individuals. Children treated with PIs have abnormal body fat distribution [14], along with elevated total cholesterol, triglycerides, and low-density lipoprotein (LDL) cholesterol levels [15]. The cause of these lipid derangements is unknown. Although no specific treatment is available, changing to a different PI or a PI-free antiretroviral regimen may be helpful. See Chapter 13 for further information regarding the metabolic complications of antiretroviral therapy.

Adrenocortical insufficiency

Signs and symptoms of HIV infection mimic those of adrenal insufficiency, yet the hypothalamic–pituitary–adrenal (HPA) axis and mineralocorticoid production are normal in ~90% of infected adults. The adrenals are the most common endocrine glands affected by infections and malignancy (49%–92%). Elevated serum cortisol levels may occur as a result of stress, cytokine activation, or, in some cases, cortisol resistance [17].

Lipodystrophy associated with PI therapy has similarities with Cushing's syndrome; however, serum cortisol and urinary free cortisol excretion are not increased [18].

Proposed mechanisms

Opportunistic infections involving the adrenal cortices include infections with CMV, MAI, and *Cryptococcus*. Since glandular destruction rarely exceeds 50% of total adrenal tissue, clinically significant adrenocortical insufficiency is not likely. Tumors, e.g., Kaposi's sarcoma, autoimmune destruction, and cortical lipid depletion, a non-specific finding associated with many severe wasting diseases, have been reported. Ketoconazole inhibits adrenocortical steroidogenesis, megesterol acetate lowers serum cortisol levels and decreases responsiveness to provocative testing, and rifampin increases cortisol metabolism. Theoretically, central adrenocortical insufficiency could occur.

Diagnostic approach

If clinical findings suggest glucocorticoid insufficiency, the pediatrician should screen the integrity of the HPA axis by measuring an 8:00 am serum cortisol level. If over 18 µg/dl at any time, this indicates normal HPA-axis function. If the cortisol result is low or low-normal, further testing by a pediatric endocrinologist is required. Either insulin-induced hypoglycemia or adrenocorticotrophin (ACTH) stimulation is the best test of integrity of the HPA axis. Corticotropin-releasing hormone (CRH) can be used to diagnose mild or partial central adrenal insufficiency. To evaluate mineralocorticoid function, the pediatrician should measure serum electrolytes. If hyponatremia and reciprocal hyperkalemia are found, peripheral renin activity (PRA) and aldosterone should be measured before the electrolytes are corrected and the patient is referred to a pediatric endocrinologist. Hyponatremia without hyperkalemia may occur with isolated glucocorticoid deficiency.

Treatment

If adrenocortical insufficiency is suspected, the pediatrician should consult with an endocrinologist and give intravenous stress doses of hydrocortisone ($50–100$ µg/m^2 per day as a bolus followed by a similar dose given as an infusion over the next few days) as soon as HPA axis testing is completed. If adrenal insufficiency is primary, mineralocorticoid replacement with fludrocortisone ($0.05–0.1$ mg/day orally) also must be given. Although there is no pure parenteral mineralocorticoid available, high-dose hydrocortisone provides significant mineralocorticoid effect. Volume support through fluids and pharmacological agents should be given as needed. After a few days, maintenance glucocorticoid replacement is provided as oral hydrocortisone (15 mg/m^2 per day in three doses with one-half given in the morning and one-quarter given both in the mid-afternoon and at bedtime) and, for cases of primary adrenal insufficiency, maintenance mineralocorticoid continued as oral fludrocortisone (at a dose of between 0.05 and 0.1 mg once daily depending on body size). Principles of stress-dosing of hydrocortisone are taught, including provision of an injectable formulation for home use, and Medic-Alert registration is strongly encouraged.

Abnormal glucose metabolism

Clinically significant hyperglycemia is unusual. In contrast, heightened sensitivity to the metabolic actions of insulin has been described in adults (in contrast to sepsis in which there is insulin resistance).

Proposed mechanisms

Hypoglycemia may result from use of drugs such as pentamidine isothionate, which chronically stimulates unregulated release of insulin in 14%–33% of adults, or from trimethoprim/sulfamethoxazole, which stimulates insulin secretion. Hyperglycemia may result from: opportunistic infections, including CMV (most common), *Cryptococcus, T. gondii*, and *Candida*; tumors, including Kaposi's sarcoma and lymphoma; possible direct pancreatic HIV invasion; and drugs, including pentamidine (which, if used chronically, may destroy β-cells). High-dose glucocorticoids and PIs cause insulin resistance [19].

Diagnostic approach

The pediatrician should check the patient for hypoglycemia by obtaining preprandial blood glucose measurements and for hyperglycemia by obtaining either postprandial blood glucose measurements by bedside blood glucose meter or by checking for urinary glucose. Quarterly glycosylated hemoglobin (hemoglobin A_{1c}) measurements may be ordered.

Treatment

If a derangement in glucose metabolism is drug-induced, the pediatrician should first discontinue the offending agent if possible. For non-acute hypoglycemia, dietary measures should be attempted. If diabetes is found, a pediatric endocrinologist should be consulted promptly. If diabetes is associated with ketoacidosis, insulin will be required, whereas, if diabetes is due to insulin resistance, oral hypoglycemic therapy, such as metformin, may be attempted. These approaches can be used in both adults and children.

Abnormal calcium metabolism

Both hypo- and hypercalcemia have been described in association with HIV infection. Parathyroid gland involvement is rare and, even when CMV and MAI have been found at autopsy, there has usually been no evidence of premortem hypocalcemia.

Proposed mechanisms

Hypocalcemia may result from: critical illness; drugs, including foscarnet, pentamidine, aminoglycosides and amphotericin B (secondary to magnesium depletion), and ketoconazole (by inhibiting renal 1α-hydroxylase activity); and reduced parathyroid hormone (PTH) responsiveness to hypocalcemia. Hypercalcemia has been described with lymphoma and other hematological malignancies as a result of production of $1,25(OH)_2$ vitamin D, PTH-related peptide, or cytokines; and with granulomatous disease, e.g., MAI, as a result of disordered extra-renal synthesis of $1,25(OH)_2$ vitamin D.

Diagnostic approach

If there are symptoms and signs of hypocalcemia or hypercalcemia, the pediatrician should check serum ionized calcium, phosphorus, and magnesium. If the ionized calcium is abnormal, a simultaneous PTH level should be measured.

Treatment

The pediatrician, with the assistance of an endocrinologist, should attempt to eliminate the cause of hypocalcemia if possible, and to normalize the serum calcium with calcium treatment and active vitamin D (calcitriol) if the hypocalcemia is associated with decreased production or action of PTH. Hydration and staged administration of calcium-lowering agents, such as furosemide, prednisone, bisphosphonates, and calcitonin, are used for treatment of hypercalcemia.

Conclusions

If the clinical presentation suggests the presence of an endocrinopathy, the first-line tests outlined above should enable the pediatrician to begin the appropriate evaluation. For assistance with interpretation of initial laboratory data, initiation of second-line hormonal testing (e.g., stimulation tests), and/or introduction of specific hormonal therapies, consultation with a pediatric endocrinologist becomes mandatory.

REFERENCES

1. Geffner, M. E., Van Dop, C., Kovacs, A. A. *et al.* Intrauterine and postnatal growth in children born to women infected with HIV. *Pediatr. AIDS HIV Infect.* 1994;**5**:162–168.
2. Frost, R. A., Lang, C. H., Gelato, M. C. Growth hormone/insulin-like growth factor axis in human immunodeficiency virus-associated disease. *Endocrinologist* 1997;**7**:23–31.
3. Miller, T. L., Easley, K. A., Zhang, W. *et al.* Maternal and infant factors associated with failure to thrive in children with vertically transmitted human immunodeficiency virus-1 infection: the prospective P2C2 human immunodeficiency virus multicenter study. *Pediatrics* 2001;**108**:1287–1296.

4. Geffner, M. E., Yeh, D. Y., Landaw, E. M. *et al*. *In vitro* insulin-like growth factor-I, growth hormone, and insulin resistance occurs in symptomatic human immunodeficiency virus-1-infected children. *Pediatr. Res.* 1993;**34**:66–72.

5. De Martino, M., Tovo, P., Galli, L. *et al*. Puberty in perinatal HIV-1 infection: a multicentre study of 212 children. *AIDS* 2001;**15**:1527–1534.

6. Grinspoon, S. Neuroendocrine manifestations of AIDS. *Endocrinologist* 1997;**7**:32–38.

7. Balter-Seri, J., Ashkenazi, S.. The effects of infectious diseases on the endocrine system. *J. Pediatr. Endocrinol. Metab.* 1997;**10**:245–256.

8. Clarick, R. H., Hanekom, W. A., Yogev, R., Chadwick, E. G. Megestrol acetate treatment of growth failure in children infected with human immunodeficiency virus. *Pediatrics* 1997;**99**:354–357.

9. Dreimane, D., Nielsen, K., Deveikis, A., Bryson, Y. J., Geffner, M. E. Effect of protease inhibitors combined with standard antiretroviral therapy on linear growth and weight gain in human immunodeficiency virus type-1 infected children. *J. Pediatr. Infect. Dis.* 2001;**20**:315–316.

10. Schambelan, M., Mulligan, K., Grunfeld, C. *et al*. Serostim Study Group. Recombinant human growth hormone in patients with HIV-associated wasting. *Ann. Intern. Med.* 1996;**125**:873–882.

11. Hirschfeld, S., Use of human recombinant growth hormone and human recombinant insulin-like growth factor-I in patients with human immunodeficiency virus infection. *Horm. Res.* 1996;**46**:215–221.

12. Hirschfeld, S., Laue, L., Cutler, G. B., Jr, Pizzo, P. A. Thyroid abnormalities in children infected with human immunodeficiency virus. *J. Pediatr.* 1996;**128**:70–74.

13. Heufelder, A. E., Hofbauer, L. C. Human immunodeficiency virus infection and the thyroid gland. *Eur. J. Endocrinol.* 1996;**134**:669–674.

14. Melvin, A. J., Lennon, S., Mohan, K. M., Purnell, J. Q. Metabolic abnormalities in HIV type 1-infected children treated and not treated with protease inhibitors. *AIDS Res. Hum. Retroviruses* 2001;**17**:1117–1123.

15. Danoff, A. Endocrinologic complications of HIV infection. *Med. Clin. North Am.* 1996;**80**:1453–1469.

16. Sellmeyer, D. E., Grunfeld, C. Endocrine and metabolic disturbances in human immunodeficiency virus infection and acquired immune deficiency syndrome. *Endocr. Rev.* 1996;**17**:518–532.

17. Oberfield, S. E., Kairam, R., Bakshi, S. *et al*. Steroid response to adrenocorticotropin stimulation in children with human immunodeficiency virus infection. *J. Clin. Endocrinol. Metab.* 1990;**70**:578–581.

18. Yanovski, J. A., Miller, K. D., Kino, T., Friedman, T. C., Chrousos, G. P., Falloon, J. Endocrine and metabolic evaluation of human immunodeficiency virus infected patients with evidence of protease inhibitor-associated lipodystrophy. *J. Clin. Endocrinol. Metab.* 1999;**84**:1925–1931.

19. Dube, M. P., Johnson, D. L., Currier, J. S., Leedom, J. M. Protease inhibitor-associated hyperglycaemia. *Lancet* 1997;**2**:713–714.

29 Neoplastic disease in pediatric HIV infection

Richard F. Little, M.D.

HIV and AIDS Malignancy Branch, CCR, NCI, National Institutes of Health, Bethesda, MD

Introduction

HIV-infected patients have an increased incidence of malignancies. Three malignancies constitute AIDS-defining diagnoses: Kaposi's sarcoma (KS), non-Hodgkin's lymphoma (NHL), and cervical cancer. There are increased risks for other cancers [1]. Approximately 40% of HIV-infected adults develop cancer [2]. The neoplastic disease risk in HIV-infected children exceeds that of adults, but because of low background incidence, cancers are uncommon in children living in the West. In certain parts of Africa, pediatric neoplastic disease may be more common [3].

Epidemiology of AIDS-related cancers

Kaposi's sarcoma (KS)

In the USA KS primarily affects men who have sex with other men (MSM), and their female partners [4]. In sub-Saharan Africa, it is common among heterosexuals and children [5]. Greater understanding of human herpesvirus 8 (HHV-8) also termed Kaposi's sarcoma-associated herpesvirus (KSHV), helps to explain KS geographic variation [6, 7]. KSHV is a necessary, though insufficient, component in KS etiology.

Approximately 50% of adults infected with HIV and KSHV develop KS within 10 years [8]. Those infected with KSHV before HIV infection have lower risks of KS than those already infected with HIV before KSHV [9]. KSHV may be transmitted sexually and from mother to infant [10]. In Africa, HIV-associated KS is seen in adults and children [11]. Males develop KS more frequently than females. KSHV seroprevalence varies substantially in different regions and in different populations, tracking KS epidemiology. KSHV seroprevalence is <1% in the US blood donor population [7], but 16% of MSM without HIV infection are KSHV-infected [12], and nearly 30% of healthy children without HIV infection in southwest Texas were KSHV positive [13]. KSHV antibodies can be found

Handbook of Pediatric HIV Care, ed. Steven L. Zeichner and Jennifer S. Read.
Published by Cambridge University Press. © Cambridge University Press 2006.

in ~50% of African blood donors [14]. KS is the most common malignancy among men in equatorial Africa [15]. In Africa, boys have a fivefold higher risk than girls, with peak incidence occurring in children <5 years [5].

HIV-related NHL

The overall pediatric incidence of NHL as an initial AIDS-defining diagnosis is 1.7% [16]. This may underestimate true incidence, since HIV-related NHL need not be reported if there is a prior AIDS diagnosis. In patients not treated with highly active antiretroviral therapy (HAART), 15%–18% of NHL will be primary central nervous system lymphoma (PCNSL) [17]. African children with Burkitt's lymphoma are more likely to have HIV infection than children without lymphoma [18]. There has been a threefold increase of Burkitt's attributed to AIDS in Ugandan children [19].

Cervical cancer

Cervical cancer is an important contributor to morbidity and mortality for HIV-infected women, making screening imperative. Cervical dysplasia prevalence in HIV-infected women may reach twice that in women not HIV infected (15% vs. 7%) [20]. CIN has been associated with human papillomaviruses (HPV), especially types 16 and 18. HPV can be found in many sexually active adolescents [21]. The effect of the AIDS epidemic on cervical cancer incidence in Africa appears to be relatively small [19]. See Chapter 8.

Non-AIDS-defining malignancies in HIV-infected patients

Other pediatric HIV infection-associated non-AIDS-defining malignant and premalignant lesions include leiomyosarcoma and leiomyomas [22]. They may be EBV associated [23]. Other cancers are seen in HIV-infected pediatric patients, but not at levels above those seen in the general population[18].

Incidence: HAART and future prospects

It is unclear how HAART will affect the incidence of HIV-related malignancies. There has been a profound decrease in KS incidence among HAART-treated populations [24]. The incidence of HIV-related NHL has also decreased since the advent of HAART [25]. However, as HIV-infected individuals live longer as a result of HAART, and the prevalence of HIV infection consequently increases, there may be more actual cases of malignant complications owing to a larger at-risk population.

Diagnosis and management of HIV-associated malignancies

Kaposi's sarcoma

KS is a highly vascular tumor that can present anywhere on the skin and also involve internal organs, primarily lungs and gastrointestinal tract. Disease can be minimal and

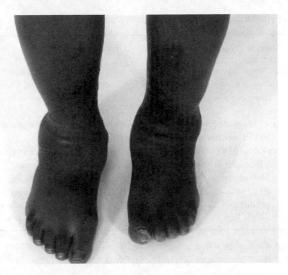

Fig. 29.1. Kaposi's sarcoma involving the skin with associated edema.

indolent, or aggressive, characterized by explosive growth leading to death. The typically violaceous lesions can be flat or nodular, varying in size from a few millimeters to lesions completely circumscribing a limb (see Fig. 29.1). In African children, involvement of lymph nodes, face and oral cavity, and inguinal-genital region is common [11]. KS-associated edema can be severe. Rarely, KS can affect internal organs alone. Chest radiographs are useful in diagnosing pulmonary KS, but without clinical signs or symptoms of organ involvement additional evaluation is generally not indicated. CT scanning is not generally helpful in assessing gastrointestinal KS.

Staging for KS is based on tumor extent (T), immunosuppression severity (I), and history of other systemic HIV-associated illness (S) [26]. Patients are classified as good (subscript 0) or poor risk (subscript 1) (see Table 29.1). Poor risk on any TIS factor is associated with poor prognosis. CD4 cells may not be prognostic if HAART is effective [27].

Pathologic diagnosis is difficult and can be confused with prominent vascularity in lymph nodes or granulomatous conditions. Minimal KS may not require treatment, unless the psychological impact affects the quality of life.

First, antiretroviral therapy (ART) should be optimized [28]. For cases without substantial morbidity, specific anti-KS therapy can be delayed to assess the antitumor effects of ART. Antiretroviral naïve patients who begin HAART and have good responses are more likely to have KS regression.

Depending on presentation, KS may be effectively treated locally (intralesional chemotherapy, cryotherapy, radiation therapy), with systemic interferon-α, or with

Table 29.1. Summary of ACTG staging classification for KS

	Good risk	Poor risk
Tumor	T_0: KS confined to the skin and/or lymph nodes, and/or minimal (non-nodular) oral KS	T_1: ulcerated KS, KS-associated edema, nodular oral KS, or KS involvement of any non-nodal visceral organ
Immune status[a]	I_0: CD4+ lymphocyte count of 150/mm^3 or higher	I_1: CD4+ lymphocyte count less than 150/mm^3
Systemic illness	S_0: Karnofsky performance status $\geq$70; no fever, diarrhea, AIDS-defining opportunistic infections, oropharyngeal candidiasis, or unexplained weight loss	S_1: Karnofsky performance status <70; presence of fever, diarrhea, AIDS-defining opportunistic infections, oropharyngeal candidiasis, or unexplained weight loss

Adapted from the Aids Clinical Trial Group Staging Classification for KS [26].
[a] May not confer prognostic information if HAART effective [27].

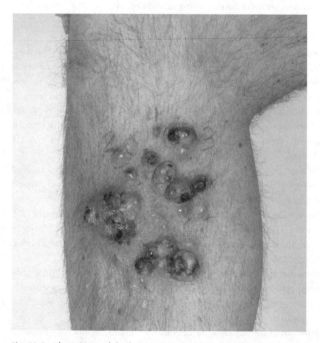

Fig. 29.2. Ulcerating nodular lesions in AIDS–KS.

systemic cytotoxic chemotherapy. Local therapy can be effective if there are few lesions, but cosmetic results can be unsatisfactory due to post-therapy hyperpigmentation. Radiation therapy can be effective when there is severe edema and pain, but the cosmetic outcome is sometimes not acceptable. Interferon-α can be effective, with responses most likely to be seen in patients with over 200 CD4+ cells/mm^3 [29]. Many patients do not tolerate the flu-like symptoms associated with interferon-α.

Monotherapy with liposomal doxorubicin or liposomal daunorubicin is as efficacious as the combination of doxorubicin, bleomycin, and vincristine (or vinblastine) (ABV), with less toxicity (Table 29.2) [30]. Paclitaxel is approved as monotherapy, with response rates of up to 71% [31] but is more toxic than the liposomal anthracyclines. Many oncologists use paclitaxel as first line for particularly severe disease.

Where HAART and liposomal anthracyclines are less available, monotherapy with vincristine or vinblastine is sometimes used palliatively. Alternating vincristine and vinblastine is sometimes useful for palliative care and is well tolerated [32], and has utility in resource-limited settings [33].

NHL

All children who develop NHL should be tested for HIV infection. Among vertically-infected children, the mean age at NHL diagnosis is 35 months (range 6–62 months) [34].

HIV-related NHL staging should include history and physical examination; CT scans of the chest, abdomen and pelvis; head MRI with gadolinium or CT with contrast, if MRI is not available; bilateral bone marrow biopsy, and lumbar puncture with cytological examination. Laboratory evaluation should include complete blood count with differential, T-cell subsets, electrolytes, renal and hepatic function, and LDH.

The World Health Organization lymphoma classification recognizes three main histologic subtypes of AIDS-related lymphoma (ARL): Burkitt's lymphoma, diffuse large B-cell lymphoma (DLBCL), and primary effusion lymphoma (PEL) [35]. AIDS-associated Burkitt's lymphoma peaks in incidence in the first two decades of life (as in non-AIDS patients), whereas DLBCL increases in incidence with age and advancing immune depletion [36]. CNS lymphomas do not appear to be age related. Anaplastic large cell lymphomas represented a higher proportion of cases than expected in a series of NCI pediatric cases and the CDC consistently reports a greater proportion of pediatric AIDS-defining cases as being large cell. The predominant histologic type in this population is not known.

Prognostic features may be similar to those for adults, which include poor outcome with CD4+ lymphocyte count <100 cells/mm^3. Other poor prognostic indicators include prior AIDS-related opportunistic illness, age >40 years, advanced stage disease, elevated LDH, and poor performance status. Since HAART, survival in AIDS-related lymphoma has increased several fold to a median of almost 2 years [25]. Patients who develop their lymphomas while being successfully treated with HAART may have superior outcomes [37].

Table 29.2. Selected chemotherapy regimens for Kaposi's sarcoma, and response rates

Chemotherapy	Dose and schedule	Response	Common toxicity
Liposomal doxorubicin (Doxil®)	20 mg/m² every 2 to 3 weeks	45% [50]	Myelosuppression, palmar plantar erythrodysesthesia
Liposomal daunorubicin (DaunoXome®)	40 mg/m² every 2 weeks	28% [51]	Myelosuppression
Paclitaxel (Taxol®)	135 mg/m² every 3 weeks; 100 mg/m² every 2 weeks; 50 mg/m² weekly	59–71% [31, 52]	Myelosuppression, neurotoxicity, alopecia
ABV (doxorubicin, bleomycin, vinca) alkaloids	ABV every 2–4 weeks: doxorubicin, 10–40 mg/m²; bleomycin 15 U; vincristine 1 mg (OR vinblastine, 6 mg/m²)	24–88% (higher response rates but increased toxicity at higher doxorubicin doses) [51, 53]	Myelosuppression, alopecia, mucositis, neurotoxicity
Vincristine/vinblastine	Vincristine, 1 mg, alternating with vinblastine, 2–4 mg every week	45% [32]	Myelosuppression neurotoxicity

Table 29.3. Low and standard dose m-BACOD for ARL [38]

Drug	Standard-dose	Low-dose
Methotrexate (IV)	200 mg/m^2, day 15	200 mg/m^2, day 15
Bleomycin (IV)	4 U/m^2, day 1	4 U/m^2, day 1
Doxorubicin (IV)	45 mg/m^2, day 1	25 mg/m^2, day 1
Cyclophosphamide (IV)	600 mg/m^2, day 1	300 mg/m^2, day 1
Vincristine (IV)	1.4 mg/m^2, day 1	1.4 mg/m^2, day 1
Dexamethasone (oral)	6 mg/m^2, days 1–5	3 mg/m^2, days 1–5
GM-CSF (SC)	5 mcg/kg days 4–13	5 mcg/kg days 4–13, as needed

Meningeal lymphoma prophylaxis in all patients: Cytarabine 50 mg, IT, days 1, 8, 15, and 22 of cycle 1 only.

Table 29.4. Low and standard dose CHOP in ARL [54]

Drug	Standard dose	Low dose
Cyclophosphamide (IV)	750 mg/m^2 day 1	375 mg/m^2 day 1
Doxorubicin (IV)	50 mg/m^2 day 1	25 mg/m^2 day 1
Vincristine (IV)	1.4 mg/m^2 (2 mg maximum dose)	1.4 mg/m^2 (2 mg maximum dose)
Prednisone (oral)	100 mg days 1–5	100 mg days 1–5
G-CSF (SC)	300–480 mcg/day days 4–13 if needed	

HAART given to all patients (stavudine, lamivudine, indinavir).

Optimal pediatric therapy has not been determined for ARL. These patients should be referred for participation in a clinical trial. Treatment of HIV-related lymphoma should not be based solely on the experience with NHL in the general pediatric population. HIV-associated Burkitt's occurring in a patient with a normal CD4+ lymphocyte count and no history of opportunistic infections should probably be treated like those without HIV infection. Markedly immunosuppressed patients are less likely to tolerate high dose induction regimens effective for NHL, including Burkitt's, in the HIV negative setting. It has not been shown in adults with ARL that dose-intensive regimens are necessary for Burkitt's lymphoma. In advanced HIV infection, the risk of prolonged neutropenia from myelosuppressive therapy may increase the risk of fatal infectious complications; there does not appear to be added survival benefit from intensive regimens [38, 39]. Several combination regimens, including doxorubicin, cyclophosphamide, vincristine, methotrexate, and prednisone, used in a much less intensive fashion than for non-HIV-infected patients, have been explored (Tables 29.3 and 29.4).

Research in adult ARL has focused primarily on combining antiretroviral therapy with combination chemotherapy, which is feasible. Epidemiologic data has shown increased survival since the use of HAART [25]. Adult patients with prior long-term successful HAART receiving combination chemotherapy for ARL have higher response rates versus patients failing HAART [37]. Conventional wisdom has emerged that chemotherapy combined with HAART is required for optimal treatment. However, antiretroviral deferment until completion of EPOCH (infusional etoposide, doxorubicin and vincristine followed by bolus cyclophosphamide with oral prednisone) chemotherapy has yielded disease-free survival in over 90% of cases with over 4 years median follow-up, and strongly suggests that there is no specific therapeutic role of HAART until chemotherapy is completed [40].

Even though there is no consensus on optimal treatment of DLBCL in pediatrics (regardless of HIV status), many patients can be successfully treated. Long-term survival appears to be related to the control of HIV infection provided the lymphoma remains in remission.

Primary central nervous system lymphoma

The outcome for PCNSL is poor. Median survival for adults receiving radiation therapy alone is significantly less for AIDS-related PCNSL (2.6 months) compared to non-AIDS-related PCNSL (16.6 months) [41]. The major differential in diagnosis is CNS *Toxoplasma gondii*, which can be resolved by stereotactic brain biopsy, which is generally safe in HIV-infected patients. However, biopsy is frequently not an option and definitive therapy is often delayed because of diagnostic uncertainty. A frequently employed approach is to initiate empiric anti-toxoplasmosis therapy for 2 to 3 weeks; if there is no response, or rapid progression, a diagnosis of PCNSL is presumed.

Diagnosing PCNSL increasingly relies on the finding that all AIDS-PCNSL contain Epstein–Barr virus (EBV). Combining thallium-201 imaging with qualitative EBV PCR on cerebrospinal fluid accurately identifies lymphoma [42]. With both tests positive, the positive predictive value for lymphoma is 100%. If both tests are negative, the negative predictive value for lymphoma is 100%. If the findings of the two tests are discordant, biopsy remains necessary.

Cervical cancer

Clinical, epidemiologic, and molecular evidence link HPV infection, cervical intraepithelial neoplasia (CIN), and squamous cell cervical carcinomas [20]. HIV patients infected with HPV develop CIN more frequently and at an earlier age than HIV-negative patients with HPV infection [43]. HIV-infected adolescents are at risk for HPV-related atypical squamous metaplasia that can progress to CIN. HIV-infected sexually active adolescents should receive semiannual cervical cytological examination (Papanicolaou smears) with aggressive follow-up for abnormal cytology.

Current standard treatment for CIN is conization of the cervix or hysterectomy. Frank carcinoma of the cervix is treated according to stage. Cervical cancer in HIV-infected women often behaves aggressively, requiring radical hysterectomy and pelvic lymphadenectomy or radiation therapy. In general, clinical outcomes are poor, so preventive care should be emphasized.

Other cancers (not AIDS-defining)

Leiomyosarcoma and leiomyomas

Leiomyoma is a benign smooth muscle tumor mostly of the uterus and gastrointestinal tract, but occasionally also the skin and subcutaneous tissues, probably arising from smooth muscle of small blood vessels. Leiomyosarcomas are malignant neoplasms arising from smooth muscle, and are distinguished by their association with EBV infection in pediatric HIV disease [1]. Leiomyosarcomas commonly arise in the retroperitneum and are highly aggressive. Histological distinction between leiomyoma and leiomyosarcoma is difficult.

Clinical presentation is characterized by fever, radiographic evidence of pulmonary infection unresponsive to antibiotics, bloody diarrhea, abdominal pain, or obstruction. Hepatic and meningeal metastasis has been reported [44].

Therapy consists of complete excision when possible. The role of adjuvant radiation and chemotherapy in children is not defined, but some cases have been treated with infusion doxorubicin, interferon-alpha, and/or radiotherapy, with very limited response [45]. The prognosis is poor, and the malignancy tends to recur.

Lymphoproliferative lesions of mucosa-associated lymphoid tissue (MALT)

Extranodal marginal zone B-cell lymphomas (low grade B-cell lymphoma of MALT type) occur in HIV-infected children, probably with increased frequency [46]. MALT lymphomas have been identified in many extranodal sites, including the gastrointestinal tract (as well as Waldeyer's ring and salivary glands), respiratory tract, thyroid, lung, breast, and skin. They are considered low-grade lymphomas. HIV-related MALT lymphomas are associated with EBV, but less frequently with *Helicobacter pylori* compared to HIV-uninfected patients [46]. MALT lymphomas can be removed surgically, some HIV-uninfected adult cases associated with *H. pylori* have regressed following treatment with appropriate antibiotics [47].

Other non-malignant lymphoproliferative lesions occur in HIV-infected children. Early myoepithelial sialadenitis (MESA) represents a benign reactive lymphoproliferative lesion, which can occasionally progress to MALT [48]. Polyclonal, polymorphic B-cell lymphoproliferative disorder (PBLD) involving the lungs, liver, kidneys, lymph nodes, and spleen may represent an intermediate between benign and malignant lymphoproliferation [49]. Progression from benign polyclonal to malignant clonal lymphoproliferation may involve accumulated genetic changes, which persist due to insufficient immune surveillance.

Lymphoproliferative disorders have been treated with interferon-α, radiation, corticosteroids, cytotoxic chemotherapy or HAART with varying success [46]. It is not clear how often non-malignant lymphoproliferative lesions progress to malignancy.

Antiretroviral therapy and antineoplastic therapy

For a potentially curable malignancy, timely courses of dose-appropriate chemotherapy are necessary to optimize treatment. The impact on survival of concurrently administered HAART and curative intent chemotherapy is unknown. In deciding upon a therapeutic plan, the risks and benefits of combining the two treatments should be considered. Overlapping toxicities may prompt chemotherapy dose reductions or cycle delays, possibly reducing the chances of tumor eradication.

Another important concern is the effect of chemotherapy-associated toxicity on antiretroviral therapy adherence. Most lymphoma chemotherapy regimens are lymphocytotoxic, and such therapy causes CD4+ lymphocyte depletion in patients not HIV-infected. HAART is unlikely to prevent this effect, and thus it can theoretically add to toxicity without achieving the primary therapeutic goal (e.g. maintenance or increase in CD4 cell status). At the very least, physicians should be alert to the potential toxicities and drug interactions of the antiretroviral drugs and the antineoplastic drugs.

For patients receiving palliative therapy, anti-HIV therapy and antineoplastic therapy should optimize control of both processes.

Summary

The pediatric patient with HIV disease and neoplastic complications represents a particular challenge. It remains to be seen whether the recent improvements in anti-HIV therapy and refinements in antineoplastic therapy will translate into substantial therapeutic benefits for pediatric patients with AIDS and cancer.

REFERENCES

1. McClain, K. L., Leach, C. T., Jenson, H. B. *et al.* Association of Epstein–Barr virus with leiomyosarcomas in children with AIDS. *N. Engl. J. Med.* 1995;**332**(1):12–18.

2. Biggar, R. J., Rabkin, C. S. The epidemiology of AIDS-related neoplasms. *Hematol. Oncol. Clin. North. Am.* 1996;**10**(5):997–1010.

3. Banda, L. T., Parkin, D. M., Dzamalala, C. P., Liomba, N. G. Cancer incidence in Blantyre, Malawi 1994–1998. *Trop. Med. Int. Health.* 2001;**6**(4):296–304.

4. Levine, A. M. AIDS-related malignancies: the emerging epidemic. *J. Natl. Cancer. Inst.* 1993;**85**(17):1382–1397.

5. Amir, H., Kaaya, E. E., Manji, K. P., Kwesigabo, G., Biberfeld, P. Kaposi's sarcoma before and during a human immunodeficiency virus epidemic in Tanzanian children. *Pediatr. Infect. Dis. J.* 2001;**20**(5):518–521.

6. Chang, Y., Cesarman, E., Pessin, M. *et al.* Identification of herpesvirus-like DNA sequences in AIDS-associated Kaposi's sarcoma. *Science* 1994;**266**:1865–1869.

7. Gao, S. J., Kingsley, L., Li, M. *et al.* KSHV antibodies among Americans, Italians and Ugandans with and without Kaposi's sarcoma. *Nat. Med.* 1996;**2**(8):925–928.

8. Martin, J. N., Ganem, D. E., Osmond, D. H., Page-Shafer, K. A., Macrae, D., Kedes, D. H. Sexual transmission and the natural history of human herpesvirus 8 infection. *N. Engl. J. Med.* 1998;**338**(14):948–954.

9. Renwick, N., Halaby, T., Weverling, G. J. *et al.* Seroconversion for human herpesvirus 8 during HIV infection is highly predictive of Kaposi's sarcoma. *AIDS* 1998;**12**(18):2481–2488.

10. Whitby, D., Smith, N., Ariyoshi, K. *et al.* Serologic evidence for different routes of transmission of HHV-8 in different populations. Second National AIDS Malignancy Conference, Bethesda, April 6–8, 1998.

11. Ziegler, J. L., Katongole-Mbidde, E. Kaposi's sarcoma in childhood: an analysis of 100 cases from Uganda and relationship to HIV infection. *Int. J. Cancer* 1996;**65**(2):200–203.

12. Casper, C., Wald, A., Pauk, J., Tabet, S. R., Corey, L., Celum, C. L. Correlates of prevalent and incident Kaposi's sarcoma-associated herpesvirus infection in men who have sex with men. *J. Infect. Dis.* 2002;**185**(7):990–993.

13. Baillargeon, J., Leach, C. T., Deng, J. H., Gao, S. J., Jenson, H. B. High prevalence of human herpesvirus 8 (HHV-8) infection in south Texas children. *J. Med. Virol.* 2002;**67**(4):542–548.

14. Enbom, M., Urassa, W., Massambu, C., Thorstensson, R., Mhalu, F., Linde, A. Detection of human herpesvirus 8 DNA in serum from blood donors with HHV-8 antibodies indicates possible bloodborne virus transmission. *J. Med. Virol.* 2002;**68**(2):264–267.

15. Bassett, M. T., Chokunonga, E., Mauchaza, B., Levy, L., Ferlay, J., Parkin, D. M. Cancer in the African population of Harare, Zimbabwe, 1990–1992. *Int. J. Cancer* 1995;**63**(1):29–36.

16. MMWR: US HIV and AIDS cases reported through December 1994 HIV/AIDS Surveillance Report, vol 6. Atlanta: Centers for Disease Control and Prevention, 1995; 1–39.

17. Irwin, D., Kaplan, L. Clinical aspects of HIV-related lymphoma. *Curr. Opin. Oncol.* 1993;**5**(5):852–860.

18. Newton, R., Ziegler, J., Beral, V. *et al.* A case-control study of human immunodeficiency virus infection and cancer in adults and children residing in Kampala, Uganda. *Int. J. Cancer* 2001;**92**(5):622–627.

19. Parkin, D. M., Wabinga, H., Nambooze, S., Wabwire-Mangen, F. AIDS-related cancers in Africa: maturation of the epidemic in Uganda. *AIDS* 1999;**13**(18):2563–2570.

20. Motti, P. G., Dallabetta, G. A., Daniel, R. W. *et al.* Cervical abnormalities, human papillomavirus, and human immunodeficiency virus infections in women in Malawi. *J. Infect. Dis.* 1996;**173**(3):714–717.

21. Carter, J. J., Koutsky, L. A., Wipf, G. C. *et al.* The natural history of human papillomavirus type 16 capsid antibodies among a cohort of university women. *J. Infect. Dis.* 1996;**174**(5):927–936.

22. Chadwick, E. G., Connor, E. J., Hanson, I. C. *et al.* Tumors of smooth-muscle origin in HIV-infected children. *J. Am. Med. Assoc.* 1990;**263**(23):3182–3184.

23. Jenson, H. B., Leach, C. T., McClain, K. L. *et al.* Benign and malignant smooth muscle tumors containing Epstein–Barr virus in children with AIDS. *Leuk. Lymphoma* 1997;**27**(3–4):303–314.

24. Jacobson, L. P., Yamashita, T. E., Detels, R. *et al.* Impact of potent antiretroviral therapy on the incidence of Kaposi's sarcoma and non-Hodgkin's lymphomas among HIV-1-infected individuals. Multicenter AIDS Cohort Study. *J. Acquir. Immune. Defic. Syndr.* 1999;**21** Suppl. 1:S34–S41.

25. Besson, C., Goubar, A., Gabarre, J. *et al.* Changes in AIDS-related lymphoma since the era of highly active antiretroviral therapy. *Blood* 2001;**98**(8):2339–2344.

26. Krown, S. E., Testa, M. A., Huang, J. AIDS-related Kaposi's sarcoma: prospective validation of the AIDS Clinical Trials Group staging classification. AIDS Clinical Trials Group
Oncology Committee. *J. Clin. Oncol.* 1997;**15**(9):3085–3092.

27. Nasti, G., Talamini, R., Antinori, A. *et al.* AIDS-related Kaposi's sarcoma: evaluation of
potential New prognostic factors and assessment of the AIDS Clinical Trial Group staging
system in the HAART era – the Italian Cooperative Group on AIDS and Tumors and the
Italian Cohort of patients naive from antiretrovirals. *J. Clin. Oncol.* 2003;**21**(15):2876–
2882.

28. Yarchoan, R., Little, R.F. Immunosuppression-related malignancies. In DeVita, V. T., Jr.,
Hellman, S., Rosenberg, S. A., eds. *Cancer, Principles and Practice of Oncology*, 6th edn.
Philadelphia: Lippincott Williams and Wilkins, 2001; 2575–2597.

29. Krown, S.E. Interferon and other biologic agents for the treatment of Kaposi's sarcoma.
Hematol. Oncol. Clin. North Am. 1991: **5**(2): 311–322.

30. Northfelt, D. W., Dezube, B. J., Thommes, J. A. *et al.* Efficacy of pegylated-liposomal
doxorubicin in the treatment of AIDS-related Kaposi's sarcoma after failure of standard
chemotherapy. *J. Clin. Oncol.* 1997;**15**(2):653–659.

31. Welles, L., Saville, M. W., Lietzau, J. *et al.* Phase II trial with dose titration of paclitaxel
for the therapy of human immunodeficiency virus-associated Kaposi's sarcoma. *J. Clin.
Oncol.* 1998;**16**(3):1112–1121.

32. Kaplan, L., Abrams, D., Volberding, P. Treatment of Kaposi's sarcoma in acquired immunodeficiency syndrome with an alternating vincristine–vinblastine regimen. *Cancer Treat.
Rep.* 1986;**70**(9):1121–1122.

33. Stein, M. E., Spencer, D., Ruff, P., Lakier, R., MacPhail, P., Bezwoda, W. R. Endemic African
Kaposi's sarcoma: clinical and therapeutic implications. 10-year experience in the Johannesburg Hospital (1980–1990). *Oncology* 1994;**51**(1):63–69.

34. Mueller, B. U., Shad, A. T., Magrath, I. T. *et al.* Malignancies in children with HIV infection, In Pizzo, P. A., Wilfert, C. M., eds. *Pediatric AIDS: The Challenge of HIV Infection in
Infants, Children, and Adolescents.* 2nd edn. Baltimore: Williams & Wilkins, 1994.

35. Jaffe, E. S., Harris, N. L., Stein, H., Vardiman, J. W., *World Health Organization Classification of Tumors: Pathology and Genetics: Tumors of Haematopoietic and Lymphoid Tissues.*
Lyon: IARC Press, 2001; 351.

36. Beral, V., Peterman, T., Berkelman, R., Jaffe, H. AIDS-associated non-Hodgkin lymphoma.
Lancet 1991;**337**:805–809.

37. Antinori, A., Cingolani, A., Alba, L. *et al.* Better response to chemotherapy and prolonged
survival in AIDS-related lymphomas responding to highly active antiretroviral therapy.
AIDS 2001;**15**(12):1483–1491.

38. Kaplan, L. D., Straus, D. J., Testa, M. A. *et al.* Low-dose compared with standard-dose m-
BACOD chemotherapy for non-Hodgkin's lymphoma associated with human immun-
odeficiency virus infection. National Institute of Allergy and Infectious Diseases AIDS
Clinical Trials Group. *N. Engl. J. Med.* 1997;**336**(23):1641–1648.

39. Walsh, C., Wernz, J. C., Levine, A. *et al.* Phase I trial of m-BACOD and granulocyte
macrophage colony stimulating factor in HIV-associated non-Hodgkin's lymphoma.
J. Acquir. Immune Defic. Syndr. 1993;**6**(3):265–271.

40. Little, R. F., Pittaluga, S., Grant, N. *et al.* Highly effective treatment of acquired immunodeficiency syndrome-related lymphoma with dose-adjusted EPOCH: impact of antiretroviral therapy suspension and tumor biology. *Blood* 2003;**101**(12):4653–4659.

41. Forsyth, P. A., Yahalom, J., DeAngelis, L. M. Combined-modality therapy in the treatment of primary central nervous system lymphoma in AIDS. *Neurology* 1994;**44**(8):1473–1479.

42. Antinori, A., De Rossi, G., Ammassari, A. *et al.* Value of combined approach with thallium-201 single-photon emission computed tomography and Epstein–Barr virus DNA polymerase chain reaction in CSF for the diagnosis of AIDS-related primary CNS lymphoma. *J. Clin. Oncol.* 1999;**17**(2):554–560.

43. Northfelt, D. W. Cervical and anal neoplasia and HPV infection in persons with HIV infection. *Oncology* (Huntingt) 1994;**8**(1):33–37; discussion 38–40.

44. Morgello, S., Kotsianti, A., Gumprecht, J. P., Moore, F. Epstein–Barr virus-associated dural leiomyosarcoma in a man infected with human immunodeficiency virus. Case report. *J. Neurosurg.* 1997;**86**(5):883–887.

45. McClain, K. L., Joshi, V. V., Murphy, S. B. Cancers in children with HIV infection. *Hematol. Oncol. Clin. North. Am.* 1996;**10**(5):1189–1201.

46. Joshi, V. V., Gagnon, G. A., Chadwick, E. G. *et al.* The spectrum of mucosa-associated lymphoid tissue lesions in pediatric patients infected with HIV: a clinicopathologic study of six cases. *Am. J. Clin. Pathol.* 1997;**107**(5):592–600.

47. Montalban, C., Manzanal, A., Boixeda, D. *et al. Helicobacter pylori* eradication for the treatment of low-grade gastric MALT lymphoma: follow-up together with sequential molecular studies. *Ann. Oncol.* 1997; 8 Suppl **2**:37–39.

48. Isaacson, P. G., Gastrointestinal lymphoma. *Hum. Pathol.* 1994;**25**(10):1020–1029.

49. Joshi, V. V., Kauffman, S., Oleske, J. M. *et al.* Polyclonal polymorphic B-cell lymphoproliferative disorder with prominent pulmonary involvement in children with acquired immune deficiency syndrome. *Cancer* 1987;**59**(8):1455–1462.

50. Northfelt, D. W., Dezube, B. J., Thommes, J. A. *et al.* Pegylated-liposomal doxorubicin versus doxorubicin, bleomycin, and vincristine in the treatment of AIDS-related Kaposi's sarcoma: results of a randomized phase III clinical trial. *J. Clin. Oncol.* 1998;**16**(7):2445–2451.

51. Gill, P. S., Wernz, J., Scadden, D. T. *et al.* Randomized phase III trial of liposomal daunorubicin versus doxorubicin, bleomycin, and vincristine in AIDS-related Kaposi's sarcoma. *J. Clin. Oncol.* 1996;**14**(8):2353–2364.

52. Gill, P. S., Tulpule, A., Espina, B. M. *et al.* Paclitaxel is safe and effective in the treatment of advanced AIDS-related Kaposi's sarcoma. *J. Clin. Oncol.* 1999;**17**(6):1876–1883.

53. Gill, P. S., Rarick, M., McCutchan, J. A. *et al.* Systemic treatment of AIDS-related Kaposi's sarcoma: results of a randomized trial. *Am. J. Med.* 1991;**90**:427–433.

54. Ratner, L., Lee, J., Tang, S. *et al.* Chemotherapy for human immunodeficiency virus-associated non-Hodgkin's lymphoma in combination with highly active antiretroviral therapy. *J. Clin. Oncol.* 2001;**19**(8):2171–2178.

Part V

Infectious problems in pediatric HIV disease

30 Serious infections caused by typical bacteria

Shirley Jankelevich, M.D.

Pediatric Medicine Branch, National Institute of Allergy and Infectious Diseases, NIH,
Bethesda, MD

Introduction

Bacterial infections in HIV-infected children often present in a manner similar to that seen in non-HIV-infected children although these infections occur more frequently, persist longer, have more frequent recurrences and disseminate more readily than in non-HIV-infected children. Because of this increased risk, the US Center for Disease Control and Prevention (CDC) added a new category of invasive bacterial infections to the list of pediatric AIDS-defining illnesses in 1987 [1]. When HIV-infected children present with a suspected bacterial infection, the differential diagnosis is large because the illnesses can be due to opportunistic and endemic infections. These infections include those due to viruses, fungi, mycobacteria, and parasites and can mimic the presentations typically associated with bacterial infections. In addition, bacteria that are unusual in the immunocompetent host may cause significant disease in immunosuppressed HIV-infected children.

Multiple immunologic abnormalities in HIV-infected children and additional factors in resource-poor countries that include malnutrition, micronutrient deficiencies and lack of adequate medical care result in increased susceptibility to infection. Furthermore, certain vaccines against bacterial agents or their toxins administered to HIV+ children often produce antibody titers that are lower and less persistent than that seen in non-HIV-infected children.

The antimicrobial regimens used in the treatment of many bacterial infections in HIV-infected children are often the same as for HIV-uninfected children. Suggested empiric regimens are listed in Table 30.1. The duration of therapy may need to be greater than that used for non-HIV-infected, especially in HIV-infected children with neutropenia and should be based, in part, on the clinical course of the child. Lack of response to an antibiotic regimen appropriate for the antibiotic susceptibility of the isolated bacteria and of sufficient duration should prompt a re-evaluation of the child since co-infection with several different pathogens including mycobacteria, fungus,

Handbook of Pediatric HIV Care, ed. Steven L. Zeichner and Jennifer S. Read.
Published by Cambridge University Press. © Cambridge University Press 2006.

Table 30.1. Clinical syndromes, bacterial and non-bacterial pathogens and empiric treatment

Clinical syndrome	[1] Commonly isolated bacteria / Less commonly isolated bacteria	[2] Non-bacterial pathogens	[3,4] Empiric treatment targeted at most commonly isolated bacteria
Meningitis/meningo-encephalitis syndrome	*Streptococcus pneumoniae* *Haemophilus influenzae* type b *Neisseria meningitidis* *Salmonella* spp. *Listeria monocytogenes* Group B streptococcus *Treponema pallidum* Other aerobic bacteria and anaerobic bacteria	**Viruses** Enterovirus HSV VZV CMV Measles EBV JC virus **Mycobacteria** *Mycobacterium tuberculosis* *Mycobacterium avium* complex **Parasites** *Acanthamoeba* spp. *Naegleria fowleri* *Malaria falciparum* *Toxoplasma gondii* *Trypanosoma cruzi* **Fungi** *Cryptococcus neoformans* *Coccidioides immitis*	For children > 1 month old: (a) Vancomycin plus cefotaxime or ceftriaxone if: • strains with intermediate-level or high-level resistance to both penicillins and cephalosporins are present in the geographic area (b) cefotaxime or ceftriaxone alone if no intermediate-level or high-level resistance to both penicillins and cephalosporins is present in the geographic area or (b) Vancomycin and ceftazidime if: • CSF shunt present

Pneumonia	*Streptococcus pneumoniae*		(a) Cefuroxime or cefotaxime or ceftriaxone
	Haemophilus influenzae type B		(b) Ceftazidime if neutropenia
	Staphylococcus aureus		Start TMP/SMX for patients at risk for
	Viridans streptococci		PCP until PCP ruled out if patient is:
	Streptococcus pyogenes		• less than 12 months old regardless of
	Listeria monocytogenes		CD4 count
	Haemophilus influenzae		• 1–5 years old with < 500 CD4
	Pseudomonas spp.		cells/mm^3
	Bordetella pertussis		• >5 years old with < 200 CD4
	Salmonella spp.		cells/mm^3
	Escherichia coli		
	Klebsiella pneumoniae		
	Moraxella catarrhalis		
	Nocardia spp.		
	Other aerobic bacteria and		
	anaerobic bacteria		
		Viruses	
		CMV	
		RSV	
		Influenza A and B	
		Parainfluenza	
		Adenovirus	
		Atypical bacteria	
		Mycoplasma pneumoniae	
		Chlamydia pneumoniae	
		Legionella spp.	
		Mycobacteria	
		Mycobacterium tuberculosis	
		Mycobacterium avium complex, other	
		atypical mycobacterial spp.	
		Fungi	
		Pneumocystis carinii	
		Aspergillus spp.	
		Cryptococcus neoformans	
		Histoplasma capsulatum	
		Coccidioides immitis	
		Parasites	
		Strongyloides stercoralis	
		Malaria	

(cont.)

Table 30.1. (cont.)

Clinical syndrome	[1]Commonly isolated bacteria / Less commonly isolated bacteria	[2]Non-bacterial pathogens	[3,4]Empiric treatment targeted at most commonly isolated bacteria
Suspected bacteremia/sepsis syndrome (no CVC present)	*Streptococcus pneumoniae* *Staphylococcus aureus* *Haemophilus influenzae* type b Non-typhoidal *Salmonella* spp. *Campylobacter jejuni* Viridans streptococci *Streptococcus pyogenes* *Escherichia coli* *Listeria monocytogenes* *Enterococcus* spp. *Neisseria meningitidis* *Klebsiella pneumoniae* *Enterobacter* spp. *Proteus mirabilis* *Citrobacter freundii* *Rhodococcus equii* *Actinomyces isrealii* Other aerobic bacteria and anaerobic bacteria In patient with CD4 count <50 cells/mm^3 or ANC < 500 cells/mm^3, consider: • *Pseudomonas* spp.	**Viruses** HSV VZV CMV Influenza A and B Adenovirus Enterovirus **Mycobacteria** *Mycobacterium tuberculosis* *Mycobacterium avium* complex, other atypical mycobacterial spp. **Fungi** *Candida* spp. **Parasites** Malaria	(a) Ceftriaxone (cefotaxime) if: • CD4 count > 200 cells/mm^3 and an ANC > 500, +/−presence of CVC (b) Ceftazidime or other antipseudomonal drug if: • CD4 count < 50 cells/mm^3 and ANC < 500 cells/mm^3 Add vancomycin to above if: (1) CVC plus high prevalence of oxacillin-R *S. aureus* or (2) the child is toxic-appearing and the geographic region has substantial numbers of penicillin-resistant and cephalosporin-resistant pneumococci

Bacteremia (CVC present)	*Staphylococcus aureus* *Staphylococcus epidermidis* *Pseudomonas* spp. *Acinetobacter* spp. Other Gram-negative rods *Bacillus cereus* *Enterococcus* spp. Other aerobic and anaerobic bacteria **Fungi** *Candida* spp.	(1) Vancomycin plus (a) Ceftriaxone (cefotaxime) if: • CD4 count > 200 cells/mm^3 and an ANC > 500, +/− removal of CVC or (b) Ceftazidime or other antipseudomonal drug if: • CD4 count < 50 cells/mm^3 or • ANC < 500 cells/mm^3
Urinary tract infections	*Escherichia coli* *Klebsiella* spp. *Enterobacter* spp *Enterococcus* spp. *Pseudomonas* spp. *Proteus* spp. *Morganella* spp. Other aerobic and anaerobic bacteria **Viruses** Adenovirus CMV Polyoma virus **Mycobacteria** *Mycobacterium tuberculosis*	Ampicillin and gentamicin or Cefotaxime (ceftriaxone)

(*cont.*)

Table 30.1. (*cont.*)

Clinical syndrome	[1] Commonly isolated bacteria Less commonly isolated bacteria	[2] Non-bacterial pathogens	[3,4] Empiric treatment targeted at most commonly isolated bacteria
Cellulitis	*Staphylococcus aureus* Group A streptococcus *Haemophilus influenzae type b* Group B streptococcus *Pseudomonas aeruginosa* Other aerobic and anaerobic bacteria		(1) First generation cephalosporin or an antistaphylococcal penicillin if: • infection on extremity and • patient is well appearing (2) Ceftriaxone (cefotaxime) if: • facial cellulitis or • patient is ill-appearing or • cellulitic area has a purplish hue (3) Add: Ceftazidime (or other antipseudomonal drugs) to above regimen if: • Severely immunocompromised or • gravely ill patients
Central catheter-related soft tissue infections	*Staphylococcus aureus* *Staphylococcus epidermidis* Other aerobic bacteria		Regimen should include vancomycin Catheter removal is necessary for bacterial eradication in cases of catheter tunnel infections.

Ecthyma gangrenosum	*Pseudomonas aeruginosa*	Two antipseudomonal antibiotics
Lymphadenitis	*Staphylococcus aureus* group A streptococci Viridans streptococci *Enterobacter* spp. *Staphylococcus epidermidis* Other aerobic and anaerobic bacteria *Bartonella henselae* **Fungi** *Aspergillus* spp. **Mycobacteria** MAI and other atypical mycobacteria *Mycobacterium tuberculosis*	Nafcillin (oxacillin)
Perirectal abscesses	*Bacteroides* spp. *Prevotella melaninogenica* *Peptostreptococcus* spp. *Escherichia coli* *Klebsiella pneumoniae* *Staphylococcus aureus.* *Enterococcus* spp. *Acinetobacter* spp. Other aerobic and anaerobic bacteria	Clindamycin or metronidazole plus an aminoglycoside, ceftriaxone (cefotaxime)
Septic arthritis	*Streptococcus pneumoniae* *Staphylococcus aureus* Viridans streptococci *Streptococcus pyogenes* *Haemophilus influenzae* type b *Salmonella* spp. *Klebsiella* spp Other aerobic and anaerobic bacteria.	Nafcillin (oxacillin) or ceftriaxone (cefotaxime)

(cont.)

Table 30.1. (cont.)

Clinical syndrome	[1]Commonly isolated bacteria Less commonly isolated bacteria	[2]Non-bacterial pathogens	[3,4]Empiric treatment targeted at most commonly isolated bacterial bacteria
Osteomyelitis	*S. aureus* *Streptococcus pyogenes* Non-typhoidal *Salmonella* spp. *Haemophilus influenzae* type b *Moraxella catarrhalis* Other aerobic and anaerobic bacteria	**Mycobacteria** *Mycobacterium tuberculosis* MAI, other atypical mycobacteria BCG **Fungi** *Candida* spp.	Nafcillin (oxacillin) or ceftriaxone (cefotaxime)
Syphilis – congenital or acquired			Aqueous crystalline penicillin G

Note:

1. Bacterial species predominance and resistance patterns may vary with geographic locations.

2. The differential diagnosis for infectious and non-infectious causes of these syndromes is broad; unusual and endemic infections must be considered in the diagnosis.

3. Empiric treatment recommended is targeted at the most commonly isolated bacteria. See text for treatment for specific organisms. All antibiotics should be IV.

4. Following isolation of an organism or if an unusual pathogen is suspected, antibiotic therapy should be modified appropriately.

viruses and parasites may be present. The Integrated Management of Childhood Illness (IMCI) strategy developed by WHO is currently being used as a guideline for the care and treatment of many diseases affecting children less than 5 years of age in some resource-poor countries but is often not specific for HIV-infected children in resource-poor countries. This chapter recommends diagnostic procedures and antibiotic therapies based on current practices in healthcare institutions in resource-rich countries. These procedures and strategies may not be appropriate in other settings. The management strategy employed anywhere must consider the local needs and resources, the local prevalence of the suspect pathogens, and the local patterns of antibiotic resistance.

While this chapter generally addresses bacterial infections, it is important for the practitioner to have a low threshold for consulting experts in the care of immunosuppressed patients and for expanding the differential diagnosis, the diagnostic work-up, and therapeutic coverage to include other less likely potential pathogens. All HIV-infected children with constitutional symptoms and suspected severe bacterial infection should have blood cultures drawn in addition to other appropriate diagnostic tests.

Resistance of numerous bacterial pathogens to many antibacterial agents, including those that cause serious bacterial infections (SBIs), continues to increase globally. Differing frequencies, patterns, and distributions of resistant bacteria vary significantly with geographic regions. Increases in bacterial resistance hinder treatment of bacterial infections in HIV-infected patients, especially in resource-poor countries, because expensive, complicated therapeutics may then be needed for appropriate treatment. Resistance to trimethoprim-sulfamethoxazole (TMP/SMX) is of particular concern because it is the least expensive and most useful prophylactic antimicrobial agent for *Pneumocystis carinii* pneumonia (PCP) and bacterial infections. The widespread use of TMP/SMX and increasing bacterial resistance may lead to decreased effectiveness of TMP/SMX prophylaxis for the prevention of SBIs globally.

Bacteria most commonly associated with serious infections in HIV-infected children

Streptococcus pneumoniae

Streptococcus pneumoniae is responsible for the majority of SBI in HIV-infected children. Invasive pneumococcal disease may occur in HIV-infected children despite active immunization with the pneumococcal polysaccharide vaccine or passive immunization and chemoprophylaxis [2]. Treatment is becoming more problematic because of continually increasing resistance globally to many available antibiotics. Isolates with resistance to penicillin, cefotaxime/ceftriaxone, carbapenems, erythromycin, TMP/SMX and chloramphenicol have been identified. Penicillin-resistant strains of pneumococci often have some degree of cross-resistance to other antibiotics. A new property termed vancomycin tolerance, the ability of *Streptococcus pneumoniae* to escape lysis and killing by vancomycin, has recently been identified (3). Such resistance may result in treatment failure, particularly in cases of pneumococcal meningitis in which bactericidal activity is critical for eradication. *S. pneumoniae* with resistance to ceftriaxone, cefotaxime and cefuroxime (MIC >2 µg/ml) is also increasing. Antibiotic resistance of *S. pneumoniae* to penicillin is characterized as intermediate resistance, with MICs of 0.1 to 1 µg/ml, and high resistance, with MICs of ≥ 2 µg/ml. High doses of penicillin and related beta-lactam antibiotics provide antibiotic levels that are sufficient to overcome intermediate resistance of *S. pneumoniae* in serum and in all tissue except for that in the central nervous system. While invasive, non-meningeal infections with intermediately resistant *S. pneumoniae* can be treated with higher doses of penicillins, such a strategy cannot be used for any invasive infections with *S. pneumoniae* with high-level resistance.

Non-typhoidal *Salmonella* spp.

Salmonella may be particularly severe in HIV-infected children, with a very high incidence of disseminated infection, resulting in bacteremia, pneumonia, osteomyelitis and meningitis, as well as relapses despite antibiotic treatment [4, 5]. Antibiotic resistance in non-typhoidal *Salmonella* spp. to ampicillin, chloramphenicol, streptomycin, sulfamethoxazole and tetracycline. Isolates that are multidrug resistant to five different antibiotics are being observed worldwide.

Campylobacter spp.

Campylobacter spp., especially *jejuni*, can cause gastroenteritis that may disseminate and cause widespread serious infection, including bacteremia, in HIV-infected patients. If *Campylobacter jejuni* is suspected, both blood and stool cultures should be obtained. *Campylobacter* spp. with resistance to tetracycline, ampicillin and quinolones in various geographic regions and multidrug resistance has been reported [7]. No studies have established the optimal treatment of *Campylobacter* bacteremia.

Pseudomonas spp.

HIV-infected persons have an increased frequency of *Pseudomonas* infections, most often *P. aeruginosa*, due to the underlying immunodeficiency and invasive procedures, such as placement of a central venous catheter [8, 9]. Infections caused by *Pseudomonas* spp. include bacteremia, pneumonia, urinary tract infections, otitis media and externa, skin and soft tissue infections, sinusitis and epiglottitis. Bacteremia due to *Pseudomonas* carries a high mortality [10]. Many isolates of *Pseudomonas* are resistant to multiple antibiotics, including beta-lactam antibiotics and aminoglycosides, with some isolates now resistant to several quinolones and imipenem-cilastatin [10]. In addition, antibacterial resistance in *Pseudomonas* may develop in patients while on treatment with appropriate antipseudomonal antibiotics.

Staphylococcus aureus

S. aureus is a common cause of bacterial skin infections in HIV-infected patients [11], but is also associated with catheter-related infections, bacteremia, pneumonia and sinusitis. Most strains of hospital-acquired *S. aureus* are resistant to penicillin. Methicillin/oxacillin-resistant strains have been appearing in hospitals at an alarming rate. Methicillin-resistant *S. aureus* (MRSA) is significantly increased in frequency in S. Africa relative to that found in the USA (50% vs. 23%). Vancomycin often remains the only active antibiotic against these strains, although vancomycin tolerance has been observed.

Staphylococcus epidermidis

S. epidermidis is often associated with central venous catheter-related infections, but occasionally may cause more invasive infections. Because most strains of *S. epidermidis* are resistant to penicillin and methicillin/oxacillin, vancomycin remains the treatment of choice.

Haemophilus influenzae

H. influenzae type b is responsible for severe invasive infection in children including meningitis, bacteremia, pneumonia, epiglottitis, septic arthritis, cellulitis and empyema. HIV-infected children are still at risk for these infections despite vaccination since immune responses to immunogens may be blunted in HIV-infected children, particularly those with advanced disease. Resistance to beta-lactams, chloramphenicol, TMP/SMX and erythromycin as well as multidrug resistance is being seen globally. Depending on the local resistance patterns, treatment with cefotaxime, ceftriaxone, or ampicillin in combination with chloramphenicol for invasive infections may need to be used until the resistance pattern of the isolate is known. Duration of therapy for 7 to 10 days, or longer in complicated cases, is needed. Chemoprophylaxis with rifampin should be considered for the index case and household contacts [6].

Clinical syndromes and treatment

Bacteremia

Bacteremia often occurs following infection of the lung, gastrointestinal tract, vascular catheters, ears and skin and soft tissue (for review see [12]). Often, no source of bacteremia can be identified, especially in cases of *S. pneumoniae*. Patients may have more than one episode of bacteremia or polymicrobial bacteremia, especially in children with low CD4 T-cell counts and advanced disease. The bacteria species most often associated with bacteremia in HIV-infected children are shown in Table 30.1. Complications and mortality are high in HIV-1 infected children and include septic shock and disseminated intravascular coagulation.

Blood cultures should be obtained before treatment whenever possible and a source for the bacteremia should be sought and specifically treated. In a patient with a central venous catheter (CVC), both peripheral and CVC cultures should be obtained. If the CVC is removed, the catheter tip should be sent to the microbiology laboratory for culture. Empiric treatment of suspected bacteremia is shown in Table 30.1.

Streptococcus pneumoniae

For pneumococcal non-meningeal infections, antibiotics that may be used include penicillin G, cefotaxime or ceftriaxone, vancomycin, chloramphenicol, clindamycin, or meropenem or imipenem/cilastatin [6]. The antibiotic chosen should be based on the local resistance patterns, the susceptibility of the isolate, and the severity of illness. In areas with significant amounts of penicillin-resistance or for patients who are severely ill, initial treatment should be cefotaxime or ceftriaxone plus vancomycin until the resistance patterns are determined. Vancomycin should be discontinued once the isolate is shown to be susceptible to penicillin or a cephalosporin. Ten to fourteen days of treatment with appropriate antibiotics is generally sufficient.

Non-typhoidal Salmonella

HIV-1 infected patients, including children, have an increased risk of development of Salmonella bacteremia. Very high rates of relapse occur following completion of short courses of antibiotic treatment [4, 12, 13]. Metastatic complications may occur and result in osteomyelitis, meningitis, pneumonia, endocarditis and pyelonephritis [12]. Treatment with ceftriaxone or cefotaxime should be instituted until susceptibility is known. Ampicillin or TMP-SMX should be used for susceptible isolates. Treatment for 4–6 weeks is necessary to prevent relapse.

Staphylococcus aureus

Staphylococcus aureus is a frequent cause of bacteremia in HIV-infected children [12] and frequently results in metastatic disease with infection at multiple sites. Clinicians should have a low threshold for suspecting metastatic disease. Methicillin or oxacillin should be used for susceptible strains. First- or second-generation cephalosporins or clindamycin may also be used [6]. Vancomycin should be reserved only for methicillin-resistant S. aureus. The length of treatment without metastatic foci may need to be as long as 21 days [6]. If the patient remains bacteremic for more than approximately three days after beginning adequate therapy, a thorough evaluation for sites of dissemination, such as lungs, heart valves, bones, and CNS, should be considered.

Pseudomonas spp.

Factors that predispose to Pseudomonas bacteremia are a low CD4+ lymphocyte count, neutropenia, and the presence of a CVC, although Pseudomonas bacteremia may occur even without these risk factors. Bacteremia with Pseudomonas may be associated with several different types of skin lesions that include tender, red papular lesions and ecthyma grangrenosum. Treatment includes intensive clinical support and a combination of two antipseudomonal agents [14], such as ceftazidime or imipenem/cilastatin plus an aminoglycoside or quinolone. Susceptibility must be determined because of the high frequency of multiply drug-resistant strains [10]; antibiotics therapy should be adjusted based on the results of the susceptibility tests. The sources of infection must be determined (lungs, skin infection, UTI, sinuses, CVC) and treated surgically when appropriate. If a CVC is infected, it may be possible to eradicate the infection without catheter removal in approximately 65% of cases [12]. If infection persists or recurs, catheter removal will be necessary.

Campylobacter jejuni

Campylobacter jejuni bacteremia occurs more frequently in adults and children with advanced HIV disease than in the non-immunocompromised population [15]. Bacteremia follows *Campylobacter* gastroenteritis, which often presents with severe, usually bloody diarrhea, cramping, nausea, and fever. Both blood and stool cultures should be obtained. No studies have established the optimal treatment of *Campylobacter* bacteremia. Two weeks of intravenous therapy with cefotaxime, imipenem/cilastatin or meropenem, ampicillin/sulbactam, gentamicin, chloramphenicol or erythromycin, will most likely provide adequate treatment. The specific antibiotic used should be based on the antibiotic susceptibility pattern of the bacterial isolate.

Catheter-associated bacteremia

The presence of a CVC increases the frequency of bacterial infections in HIV-1 infected children. Bacteria involved in CVC infections include *Staphylococcus aureus, Staphylococcus epidermidis, Enterococcus* spp., *Pseudomonas* spp. and other gram-negative rods [8], as well as *Bacillus cereus* [16]. For certain species of bacteria (e.g., *Staphylococcus epidermidis*), catheter-associated bacteremia can often be treated with antibiotics alone without catheter removal, if the patient is stable and the blood cultures rapidly become sterile [8]. Treatment involves approximately 14 days of appropriate antibiotics, followed by observation for recurrence. Certain bacteria, such as *Bacillus* spp., often cannot be eradicated without catheter removal [16]. In these cases, a shorter course of approximately 7 days of antibiotics should be given following catheter removal.

Pneumonia

Bacterial pneumonia is increased in frequency and severity in HIV-infected children. Many patients have multilobar involvement and a slower response to antibiotic treatment [17]. The spectrum of bacteria associated with pneumonia in HIV-infected children, shown in Table 30.1, is wide, although the most common pathogens seen include *S. pneumoniae, H. influenzae* type b, *S. aureus* and *E. coli*. Other pathogens less commonly observed are viridans streptococci, *S. pyogenes, M. catarrhalis, B. pertussis, K. pneumoniae, Salmonella* spp., *P. aeruginosa, Legionella* spp. and *Nocardia* spp.

The differential diagnosis of an HIV-infected child with fever, tachypnea and hypoxia is extensive and includes bacterial, viral, fungal and parasitic pneumonias, LIP, *M. tuberculosis* pneumonia and malaria (Table 30.1). Patients without neutropenia will often have leukocytosis and their clinical presentation is similar to that seen in normal children. A chest radiograph, blood cultures, and sputum gram stain and cultures should be obtained. If a good specimen cannot be obtained from expectorated sputum, sputum specimens representative of the lower respiratory tract may be obtained from induced sputum. The most sensitive diagnostic techniques are bronchoscopy and lung biopsy [19]. If empyema is present, a specimen should be obtained for microbiologic evaluation. In addition to bacterial studies, respiratory specimens should be evaluated for *Pneumocystis carinii* and for mycobacterial, fungal, and viral causes of pneumonia.

Pneumococcal pneumonia usually appears on chest X-ray as localized segmental or lobar consolidation and may be complicated by effusion, empyema, or abscesses and is often associated with bacteremia. Children with *H. influenzae* (type b and nontypeable) may also have consolidated areas on chest X-ray although diffuse bilateral infiltrates similar to that seen with PCP may also be seen. The chest X-ray in a child with *Pseudomonas* pneumonia usually shows a lobar infiltrate, or, less commonly, diffuse interstitial disease. Cavitary lesions may also be present [18].

Because of the high prevalence of penicillin resistance in *S. pneumoniae* and many other respiratory pathogens, the initial antibiotic regimen should consist of a second generation cephalosporin, e.g., cefuroxime, or a third generation cephalosporin, e.g., cefotaxime or ceftriaxone. Neutropenic patients should be treated with an antipseudomonal drug such as ceftazidime to provide activity against *Pseudomonas*. The bacteria isolated and the antibiotic susceptibility pattern should then guide changes in the antibiotic regimen. Suggested regimens for empiric therapy are shown in Table 30.1. Because slower responses to antibiotic treatment or relapses may occur in HIV+ children [18], careful monitoring and prolonged antibiotic therapy may be necessary in certain cases.

Streptococcus pneumoniae

S. pneumoniae presents in a similar manner to that in non-immunocompromised patients, although relapses are more common and often associated with bacteremia. The chest radiographic appearance of pneumococcal pneumonia is described above. The treatment for pneumonia without meningitis is the same as for bacteremia.

Haemophilus influenzae (type b and non-typeable)

H. influenzae is a common cause of pneumonia in HIV-infected adults and children. Chest X-ray findings are described above. Cefotaxime or ceftriaxone or ampicillin plus chloramphenicol [6] should be used initially, but may be changed to ampicillin if the isolate is susceptible.

Pseudomonas spp.

Pneumonia due to *Pseudomonas spp.* is infrequent but particularly problematic because it results in a necrotizing infection and may be poorly responsive to antibiotic treatment [9]. It may present as a fulminant infection with bacteremia or may have a chronic or subacute course. Unlike pneumonia due to *S. pneumoniae, Pseudomonas* infection is usually associated with a CD4 cell count <50 cells/µl. Multiple relapses are common and may occur despite an intravenous (IV) antibiotic course of 14 days [20]. Chest X-ray findings are described above. Patients should be treated for minimum of 14 days of treatment with two synergistic antibiotics, such as ceftazidime plus an aminoglycoside [20].

Meningitis/meningoencephalitis

Streptococcus pneumoniae is the most common cause of acute bacterial meningitis. Pathogens responsible for meningitis and meningoencephalitis are shown in Table 30.1. CSF should be obtained and appropriate studies, including stains and cultures for bacteria, fungus and AFB, and rapid antigen tests for bacteria and cryptococcus, should be performed. When appropriate, additional studies to determine if the patient has a CNS infection due to unusual or endemic pathogens should be performed. If purulent CSF is obtained upon lumbar puncture (LP) or if an etiologic agent cannot be identified, empiric treatment should be instituted immediately (shown in Table 30.1). Dexamethasone may be used if *S. pneumoniae* or *H. influenzae* is suspected although concomitant administration of dexamethasone decreases the penetration of vancomycin into the cerebrospinal fluid in animal studies [21]. Following isolation of an organism, treatment should be modified depending on the bacteria identified and the antibiotic susceptibility pattern. Repeat LP may need to be performed in some children if the response is not satisfactory, the etiologic agent is penicillin-resistant *S. pneumoniae* and results from cefotaxime and ceftriaxone resistance testing are not yet available, dexamethasone was administered [6], or gram-negative organisms are isolated. Therapy may need to be prolonged, depending on the response and the resistance pattern of the bacterial isolates.

Streptococcus pneumoniae

Treatment of pneumococcal meningitis has become complex because of extensive antibiotic resistance of *S. pneumococcus*. Meningitis due to penicillin-susceptible pneumococcus can be treated with meningitis doses of penicillin, ampicillin, cefotaxime, or ceftriaxone. However, treatment of penicillin-resistant pneumococcus is problematic mainly because concentrations of penicillins and cephalosporins in the cerebrospinal fluid are usually unable to achieve prompt eradication of some intermediately resistant and most highly resistant pneumococcal strains. Strains of penicillin-resistant pneumococci that remain susceptible to cephalosporins can be treated with cefotaxime and ceftriaxone [6].

Meningitis due to strains with intermediate-level or high-level resistance to both penicillins and cephalosporins should be treated with a combination of vancomycin and either ceftriaxone or cefotaxime. For meningitis due to penicillin-resistant and cephalosporin-resistant pneumococcus, a combination of vancomycin plus a third-generation cephalosporin should be used and rifampin added after 24–48 hours if the isolate is susceptible to rifampin, the patient has clinical deterioration, repeat LP fails to show eradication of the bacteria or the isolate has high-level resistance to ceftriaxone or cefotaxime (MIC≥4 µg/ml) [6].

Meropenem is not recommended for the treatment of meningitis caused by intermediate- or high-level penicillin-resistant pneumococcus, because a recent study revealed that 49% of 59 isolates with either intermediate-level or high-level resistance to penicillin also had meropenem resistance [21], unless sensitivity to meropenem is specifically demonstrated.

Other bacterial pathogens

Meningitis due to *Salmonella* spp. should be treated with ceftriaxone or cefotaxime for at least 4 to 6 weeks to prevent relapse [6]. *H. influenzae* meningitis can be treated with ceftriaxone or cefotaxime or the combination of ampicillin and chloramphenicol [6] for at least 10 days along with initial doses of dexamethasone.

Urinary tract infection

HIV-infected children have an increased incidence of urinary tract infection (UTI) [8, 22, 23]. The most common pathogens causing UTI are listed in Table 30.1. An appropriate urine specimen should be examined for white cells and bacteria, and cultured. Blood cultures and appropriate renal studies should be obtained on patients with fever or pyelonephritis. Because of the elevated relative risk of bacteremia, aggressive IV antibiotic treatment is required in patients with suspected pyelonephritis or constitutional symptoms [24] as indicated in Table 30.1. Unlike cystitis, which can often be treated with a relatively short course of therapy, pyelonephritis usually requires 10 to 14 days of therapy. Resistance among uropathogenic *Escherichia coli* to TMP-SMX is increasing and must be taken into account if a patient receiving treatment with TMP-SMX is not improving clinically [25].

Skin and soft tissue infections

Bacterial skin and soft tissue infections are frequently seen in HIV-infected children and include cellulitis, catheter-related soft tissue infections, skin lesions caused by *P. aeruginosa*, lymphadenitis and perirectal abscesses. A variety of other organisms may cause skin and soft tissue infections in certain clinical situations (Table 30.1). Micro-biologic evaluation (Gram stain and culture) of infected material should be performed and blood cultures should be obtained if the child is ill appearing. If lesions are thought to be due to disseminated infection, a thorough work-up for other sites of infection should be performed. Suggested regimens for empiric treatment for these infections is shown in Table 30.1.

It is important to recognize the two distinct types of central catheter-related soft tissue infections, exit site infections and tunnel infections, as they require different therapeutic approaches. Exit site infections are superficial infections around the catheter site with erythema and tenderness, and, occasionally, discharge. A tunnel infection is an infection that extends along the subcutaneous tunnel through which the CVC runs. In tunnel infections, erythema at the exit site, tenderness on palpation over the entire catheter tunnel and discharge that can be expressed from the exit site is often found. Bacteria causing these two types of infections and empiric therapy are shown in Table 30.1. If *S. aureus* and *S. epidermidis* are isolated and are shown to be susceptible to oxacillin, vancomycin should be stopped and oxacillin or nafcillin therapy instituted. Exit site infections may often be treated with antibiotic therapy alone for 7 to 14 days. Catheter removal is necessary for bacterial eradication in cases of catheter tunnel infection. Since the infection is deep-seated, antibiotic treatment often must be continued for at least 7 days following catheter removal.

Skin lesions caused by *P. aeruginosa* infection are more common in children in the late stages of HIV infection than in children who are uninfected or in the early stages of HIV-infection and include ecthyma gangrenosum, erythematous macular or maculo-papular lesions and violaceous nodules [26]. *P. aeruginosa* can be cultured from these lesions. Ecthyma gangrenosum is a painless, round, indurated, ulcerated lesion containing a central black eschar. It usually occurs during *P. aeruginosa* bacteremia, but may occur following infection of hair follicles. The erythematous and macular, maculopapular, or nodular lesions occur following disseminated *P. aeruginosa* infection [26]. Treatment with two antipseudomonal antibiotics for 10 to 14 days should be instituted.

Perirectal abscesses are seen more frequently in immunosuppressed patients, especially those with neutropenia [27]. Rectal exam is usually sufficient to detect a perianal abscess, although CT imaging may be needed in systemically ill children who are thought to have deep abscesses. Material obtained from drainage or aspiration of the abscesses should be sent for Gram stain and aerobic and anaerobic culture. Empiric regimens are shown in Table 30.1. In the non-neutropenic child, consideration should be given to surgical drainage or aspiration of the abscess even if local fluctuance is not palpable [27, 28]. In an HIV-infected child with severe neutropenia, drainage is often not attempted because of the lack of pus formation. In these cases, IV antibiotics are given for 2 to 3 weeks, and surgical drainage or aspiration performed if there is disease progression with abscess formation [27, 28].

Septic arthritis

Septic arthritis is thought to occur following bleeding into a joint with secondary seeding of bacteria from another site [29] and may account for the larger number of cases of septic arthritis that have been reported in patients with both hemophilia and HIV infection [29]. Although fever, increased leukocyte counts and elevated erythrocyte sedimentation rates are often present, the classic signs of joint swelling, pain, redness and warmth are usually modified. Joint aspiration with appropriate chemistries, hematologic and microbiologic studies should be performed. The predominant bacteria are given in Table 30.1. Treatment consists of intravenous antibiotics targeted against the isolated bacteria for 3 weeks. Arthrotomy, arthroscopic lavage or repeated aspiration is needed as adjunctive therapy to decrease joint cartilage destruction by proteolytic enzymes that accumulate in the infected joint.

Osteomyelitis

Osteomyelitis is seen less frequently than other serious bacterial infections in HIV-infected patients and is associated with many organisms (Table 30.1). Occasionally, mixed infection may be seen. Diagnosis involves appropriate radiographic studies and culture of blood and material obtained from infected bone by needle aspirate or biopsy. Treatment requires prolonged IV therapy with antibiotics that achieve high bone penetration and are directed against the identified or presumed causative bacteria. If *Salmonella* spp. has been isolated, therapy may be required for 4 to 6 weeks [6]. In some instances, blood and/or bone cultures may not identify an organism. In such cases, patients are treated with empirically chosen antibiotics in consultation with an infectious diseases specialist.

Congenital syphilis

Co-infection of syphilis and HIV has major implications for both the mother and the fetus with respect to diagnosis, progression of disease and response to treatment. Altered serologic responses may result in a delay in diagnosis [30]. There may also be rapid progression of disease, resulting in neurosyphilis and uveitis. Treatment failures in HIV-infected patients may occur with single dose intramuscular penicillin in early primary syphilis and with erythromycin in secondary syphilis.

Evaluation of newborn infants for congenital syphilis [6] should be performed in all neonates whose mother has positive non-treponemal tests (VDRL and RPR tests) or a history of syphilis and (a) no or inadequate treatment, (b) lack of serologic response or information regarding serologic response following therapy, (c) syphilis during pregnancy and lack of serologic response following treatment with penicillin or treatment with a non-penicillin antibiotic or treatment instituted within the month before delivery, or (d) HIV-infection with lesions suggestive of syphilis, even without a positive non-treponemal test.

Evaluation of the infant for congenital syphilis includes appropriate physical examination and standard blood tests including complete blood count (CBC), liver function tests, a non-treponemal serologic test of neonatal serum [6], CSF cell count, protein concentration and VDRL on CSF, and long-bone radiographs. Neonatal serum for IgM against treponemal antigens may also be determined by the Centers for Disease Control and Prevention (CDC) [6]. The interpretation of serologic tests in infants co-infected with *T. pallidum* and HIV may be difficult since they may have delayed, elevated or absent treponemal (FTA-ABS) and non-treponemal serologic tests [30]. All syphilis serologic tests should be performed on neonate serum rather than cord blood since non-treponemal screening on cord blood may be yield false-negative results. All positive non-treponemal tests should always be confirmed with a treponemal test [30].

Evaluation of neonates for neurosyphilis may be difficult. Neonatal CSF may have a positive VDRL test because of transfer of maternal VDRL antibodies into the neonate's CSF. There is a broad range of normal CSF cell counts and protein concentrations in neonates and the CSF may have increased cell counts and protein concentrations even in the absence neurosyphilis. Furthermore, neurosyphilis cannot be excluded even if the CSF VDRL or CSF FTA-ABS tests are negative [6].

Infants with proven or probable congenital syphilis, or infants who have required a work-up for congenital syphilis but in whom the diagnosis can not be excluded, should be treated with the following: aqueous crystalline penicillin G, 100 000 to 150 000 U/kg per day given q12h for the first 7 days of life and then q8h thereafter for 10 days or procaine penicillin G 50 000 U/kg per dose intramuscular in a single dose for 10 days [6]. Aqueous crystalline penicillin is preferred because of its high penetration into the CSF. It is essential that these infants have good follow-up because of the potential failure of even the most effective antibiotic therapy in eradicating syphilis in HIV-infected patients.

Summary

HIV-infected children are at increased risk for a wide variety of typical and usual bacterial pathogens. Increasing resistance of these bacteria worldwide to commonly used agents as well as other more expensive antibiotics presents greater challenges to the treatment of these children, especially in resource-poor nations. Repeated infections often occur, especially in those children who are more severely immunosuppressed. Many of the typical bacterial infections have common presentations but may require prolonged antibiotic treatment. Prompt recognition and treatment of these infections often result in a successful outcome.

REFERENCES

1. Center for Disease Control and Prevention. Revised classification system for human immunodeficiency virus infection in children less than 13 years of age: CDC; 1994 September 30, 1994. Vol. **43**, RR-12.

2. Krasinski, K. Bacterial infections. In Pizzo, P. A., ed. *Pediatric AIDS*. Baltimore: Williams & Wilkins; 1994: 241–253.

3. Henriques Normark, B., Novak, R., Ortqvist, A., Kallenius, G., Tuomanen, E., Normark, S. Clinical isolates of *Streptococcus pneumoniae* that exhibit tolerance of vancomycin. *Clin. Infect. Dis.* 2001;**32**(4):552–558.

4. Rubinstein, A. Pediatric AIDS. *Curr. Probl. Pediatr.* 1986;**16**(7):361–409.

5. Jacobs, J. L., Gold, J. W., Murray, H. W., Roberts, R. B., Armstrong, D. Salmonella infections in patients with the acquired immunodeficiency syndrome. *Ann. Intern. Med.* 1985;**102**(2):186–188.

6. Committee on Infectious Diseases. *Red Book 2000*, 25th edn. Elk Grove Village: American Academy of Pediatrics; 2000.

7. Tee, W., Mijch, A., Wright, E., Yung, A. Emergence of multidrug resistance in *Campylobacter jejuni* isolates from three patients infected with human immunodeficiency virus. *Clin. Infect. Dis.* 1995;**21**:634–638.

8. Roilides, E., Marshall, D., Venzon, D., Butler, K., Husson, R., Pizzo, P. A. Bacterial infections in human immunodeficiency virus type 1-infected children: the impact of central venous catheters and antiretroviral agents. *Pediatr. Infect. Dis. J.* 1991;**10**(11):813–819.

9. Roilides, E., Butler, K. M., Husson, R. N., Mueller, B. U., Lewis, L. L., Pizzo, P. A. *Pseudomonas* infections in children with human immunodeficiency virus infection. *Pediatr. Infect. Dis. J.* 1992;**11**(7):547–553.

10. Tacconelli, E., Tumbarello, M., Ventura, G., Lucia, M. B., Caponera, S., Cauda, R. Drug resistant *Pseudomonas aeruginosa* bacteremia in HIV-infected patients. *J. Chemother.* 1995;7 Suppl **4**:180–183.

11. Geusau, A., Tschacler, E. HIV-related skin disease. *J. Roy. Coll. Phys. Lond.* 1997;**31**:374–379.

12. Kovacs, A., Leaf, H. L., Simberkoff, M. S. Bacterial infections. *Med. Clin. North Am.* 1997;**81**(2):319–343.

13. Chaisson, R. E. Infections due to encapsulated bacteria, *Salmonella*, *Shigella*, and *Campylobacter*. *Infect. Dis. Clin. North Am.* 1988;**2**(2):475–484.

14. Johann-Liang, R., Cervia, J. S., Noel, G. J. Characteristics of human immunodeficiency virus-infected children at the time of death: an experience in the 1990s. *Pediatr. Infect. Dis. J.* 1997;**16**:1145–1150.

15. Ruiz-Contreras, J., Ramos, J. T., Hernandez-Sampelayo, T., de Jose, M., Clemente, J., Gurbindo, M. D. *Campylobacter* sepsis in human immunodeficiency virus-infected children. The Madrid HIV Pediatric Infection Collaborative Study Group. *Pediatr. Infect. Dis. J.* 1997;**16**(2):251–253.

16. Cotton, D. J., Gill, V. J., Marshall, D. J., Gress, J., Thaler, M., Pizzo, P. A. Clinical features and therapeutic interventions in 17 cases of *Bacillus* bacteremia in an immunosuppressed patient population. *J. Clin. Microbiol.* 1987;**25**(4):672–674.

17. Huovinen, P., Resistance to trimethoprim-sulfamethoxazole. *Clin. Infect. Dis.* 2001;**32**(11):1608–1614.

18. Gallant, J. E., Ko, A. H. Cavitary pulmonary lesions in patients infected with human immunodeficiency virus. *Clin. Infect. Dis.* 1996;**22**(4):671–682.

19. Izraeli, S., Mueller, B. U., Ling, A., *et al.* Role of tissue diagnosis in pulmonary involvement in pediatric human immunodeficiency virus infection. *Pediatr. Infect. Dis. J.* 1996;**15**:112–116.

20. Baron, A. D., Hollander, H. *Pseudomonas aeruginosa* bronchopulmonary infection in late human immunodeficiency virus disease. *Am. Rev. Respir. Dis.* 1993;**148**(4 Pt 1):992–996.

21. Spach, D. H., Jackson, L. A. Bacterial meningitis. *Neurol. Clin.* 1999;**17**(4):711–735.

22. Bernstein, L. J., Krieger, B. Z., Novick, B., Sicklick, M. J., Rubinstein, A. Bacterial infection in the acquired immunodeficiency syndrome of children. *Pediatr. Infect. Dis.* 1985;**4**(5):472–475.

23. Krasinski, K., Borkowsky, W., Bonk, S., Lawrence, R., Chandwani, S. Bacterial infections in human immunodeficiency virus-infected children. *Pediatr. Infect. Dis. J.* 1988;**7**(5):323–328.

24. Ruiz-Contreras, J., Ramos, J. T., Hernandez-Sampelayo, T., *et al.* Sepsis in children with human immunodeficiency virus infection. The Madrid HIV Pediatric Infection Collaborative Study Group. *Pediatr. Infect. Dis. J.* 1995;**14**(6):522–526.

25. Brown, P. D., Freeman, A., Foxman, B. Prevalence and predictors of trimethoprim-sulfamethoxazole resistance among uropathogenic *Escherichia coli* isolates in Michigan. *Clin. Infect. Dis.* 2002;**34**(8):1061–1066.

26. Flores, G., Stavola, J. J., Noel, G. J. Bacteremia due to *Pseudomonas aeruginosa* in children with AIDS. *Clin. Infect. Dis.* 1993;**16**(5):706–708.

27. Arditi, M., Yogev, R. Perirectal abscess in infants and children: report of 52 cases and review of literature. *Pediatr. Infect. Dis. J.* 1990;**9**:411–415.

28. Shaked, A., Shinar, E., Fruend, H. Managing the granulocytopenic patient with acute perianal inflammatory disease. *Am. J. Surg.* 1986;**152**:510–512.

29. Gilbert, M. S., Aledort, L. M., Seremetis, S., Needleman, B., Oloumi, G., Forster, A. Long term evaluation of septic arthritis in hemophilic patients. *Clin. Orthop.* 1996:54–59.

30. Lambert, J. S., Stephens, I., Christy, C., Abramowicz, J. S., Woodin, K. A. HIV and syphilis: maternal and fetal considerations. *Pediatr. AIDS HIV Infec.: Fetus to Adolesc.* 1995;**6**:138–144.

31 Tuberculosis

Rohan Hazra, M.D.

HIV and AIDS Malignancy Branch, NIH, Bethesda, MD

The HIV/AIDS epidemic has led to a resurgence in the rates of tuberculosis in the developed world. In the developing world, co-infection with HIV and tuberculosis is extremely common and a major cause of morbidity and mortality. Tuberculosis in HIV-infected children can be more severe than disease in HIV-uninfected children, and treatment is complicated by drug–drug interactions between antiretrovirals and tuberculosis medications. Nevertheless, effective treatment of tuberculosis in the HIV-infected child is critically important for prolonged survival, even in the absence of antiretroviral therapy.

Epidemiology

Mycobacterium tuberculosis is the etiologic agent of tuberculosis. Humans are the only reservoir for the organism. In the USA the number of cases of tuberculosis has been declining, but the global burden of disease is staggering. World Health Organization (WHO) data for 1997 estimated almost 8 million new cases that year, 16.2 million existing cases, 1.87 million deaths attributable to tuberculosis, and global prevalence of infection of 32% [1]. WHO estimates that the worldwide prevalence of tuberculosis and HIV co-infection is 0.18%, with 8% of new cases of tuberculosis occurring in patients who are HIV seropositive. This rate of HIV seropositivity among incident tuberculosis cases is as high as 65% in some African nations.

In an adult, a case of tuberculosis can result from either reactivation of endogenous latent infection or exogenous primary infection or reinfection [2]. A case of tuberculosis in a child should be considered a public health emergency, because it represents recent infection and thus is indicative of ongoing transmission in the community. Limited data in the USA demonstrate that 12% of children diagnosed with tuberculosis are HIV-infected [3].

Handbook of Pediatric HIV Care, ed. Steven L. Zeichner and Jennifer S. Read.
Published by Cambridge University Press. © Cambridge University Press 2006.

Pathogenesis

Tuberculosis is spread from person to person via airborne droplet nuclei. These particles of 1 to 5 microns in diameter are produced when patients with pulmonary or laryngeal tuberculosis cough, sneeze, or speak. They can also be released by procedures to induce sputum and during bronchoscopy. Droplet nuclei are small enough to reach the terminal alveoli, where tuberculosis organisms then replicate. Alveolar macrophages ingest the organisms but are unable to kill them. After infection begins in the alveoli, the infection can disseminate rapidly to regional lymph nodes, the bloodstream and to sites throughout the body, before cellular immunity develops.

Bacterial replication can continue at the primary site of infection and at metastatic foci until cellular immunity develops 2–12 weeks after infection, when bacteria are contained and walled-off within granulomas. The development of immunity is marked by a positive tuberculin skin test (TST). With the onset of cellular immunity, most adults are able to control their infection. Although necrosis of the initial pulmonary focus can occur with subsequent calcification evident on chest radiograph, in most cases infection controlled by cellular immunity is clinically and radiographically inapparent. Patients such as these are considered to have latent tuberculosis infection, and approximately 5%–10% of them will develop active disease during their lifetime in the absence of therapy. The pathophysiologic basis of latent tuberculosis infection is poorly understood. Organisms can remain in this state, walled-off within granulomas, for decades without causing disease or invoking an immune response capable of eradicating the organisms, but can then re-emerge when cellular immunity decreases, secondary to HIV infection, steroid treatment, or old age.

Children less than 4 years of age are more likely to develop active disease after tuberculosis infection and are more likely to have a negative TST at the time of diagnosis than older children and adults [3]. The age distribution for pediatric tuberculosis has two peaks, at less than 4 years of age and in late adolescence. Most children with tuberculosis in the USA live in households in which other members have risk factors for tuberculosis, including recent immigration, history of tuberculosis treatment, TST positivity, occupations in healthcare, incarceration, HIV infection, intravenous drug use, alcoholism, homelessness, and diabetes [4].

HIV infection greatly increases susceptibility to tuberculosis. The annual risk of developing tuberculosis in an HIV-infected adult can be as high as 8%–12% [5], and the risk for progressive disease after newly acquired infection is up to 50% [6]. The impact of tuberculosis on HIV infection is also significant. Various studies have shown that tuberculosis leads to immune activation, increased viral replication, decreased CD4 counts, increased risk of opportunistic infections and increased risk of death [7, 8].

Clinical presentations

Clinical manifestations at the time of initial infection vary according to the age of the patient and the immune response. In general, the clinical features of tuberculosis in HIV-infected children are very similar to those in immunocompetent children, although disease is usually more severe. Pulmonary disease is evident in most cases, but rapidly progressive disseminated disease, including meningitis, can be seen without obvious pulmonary findings. HIV infection and young age both increase the risk for miliary disease and tuberculous meningitis. Therefore, tuberculosis should be considered in the HIV-infected child with meningitis, and disseminated disease should be considered in the HIV-infected child diagnosed with tuberculosis.

Disease in children less than 5 years of age is marked by pneumonitis, hilar and mediastinal adenopathy, bronchial collapse secondary to compression by lymph nodes, and subsequent atelectasis. The primary complex consists of a relatively small area of alveolar consolidation, lymphangitis, and regional lymphadenitis. HIV-infected children are more likely to be symptomatic, with fever and cough, and to have atypical findings, such as hilar lymphadenopathy, multilobar infiltrates, and diffuse interstitial disease. As hypersensitivity develops, hilar and mediastinal lymphadenopathy greatly increase and often cause compression of bronchi, resulting in a segmental lesion. This lesion can consist of both atelectasis and consolidation. A less frequent result of the enlarging lymphadenopathy is hyperaeration of a segment, lobe, or entire lung. Pleural effusion is uncommon in children. Pulmonary tuberculosis in adolescents can resemble primary disease in young children, but the more common clinical scenario in this population is that of chronic upper lobe disease with cavitation.

Lymphohematogenous spread of *M. tuberculosis* probably occurs in all cases of tuberculosis. In adults the most common result is occult infection, or extrapulmonary disease years later, such as renal tuberculosis. Young children and HIV-infected adults are at increased risk of hematogenous spread resulting in miliary tuberculosis. In the absence of treatment, meningitis usually ensues several weeks after hematogenous spread.

Approximately 25% of pediatric tuberculosis cases are complicated by extrapulmonary disease. HIV-infected children seem to have an even higher rate of extrapulmonary disease, with an increased risk of tuberculous meningitis. Other forms of extrapulmonary disease include tuberculosis infection of the bones and joints, and rarely disease of the eye, middle ear, GI tract, and kidney.

Diagnosis

The cornerstone of diagnostic methods for tuberculosis is the tuberculin skin test (TST). The test consists of the intradermal injection of 5 tuberculin units of purified protein derivative and measurement of induration 48–72 hours after placement. Multiple puncture tests (e.g., Tine) and other PPD strengths (e.g., 250 tuberculin units) should not be used as they are not accurate [9]. The cutoff size for a positive result depends upon the immune status of the person tested and epidemiologic factors. For HIV-infected children and adults, ≥5 mm is considered positive and indicative of infection. Because up to 30%–40% of HIV-infected children with tuberculosis will have a negative TST, an HIV-infected child with exposure to an infectious contact should receive treatment even if the child's TST is negative. Despite widespread use for decades and extensive experience, the TST has several serious drawbacks, including false-positive responses secondary to exposure to non-tuberculous mycobacteria or prior vaccination with BCG, the necessity for two patient visits, false-negative responses secondary to HIV or other immunosuppression, and variability in the interpretation of the test.

Diagnostic microbiology for tuberculosis consists of microscopic visualization of acid-fast bacilli (AFB) from clinical specimens, the isolation in culture of the organism, and drug susceptibility testing. Because *M. tuberculosis* replicates very slowly, with a generation time of 15–20 hours, visible growth on solid media emerges only after 3–6 weeks. Fortunately, more rapid liquid culture detection methods have been developed. The yield for detecting AFB and culturing *M. tuberculosis* from pediatric samples, from sputum or gastric aspirates, is <50%, but appears higher in HIV-infected children and HIV-uninfected infants. Obtaining early morning gastric aspirates for AFB stain and culture is the method of choice when attempting to diagnose tuberculosis in young children who are often unable to produce sputum. A standardized protocol for obtaining the gastric aspirates can improve the yield from these specimens to 50%, and the yield is maximized with the culture of three samples obtained separately [10]. Often, the diagnosis is based upon history of close contact with an adolescent or adult with tuberculosis, and clinical and radiographic findings compatible with tuberculosis.

Two nucleic acid amplification tests can identify *M. tuberculosis* from clinical specimens within 24 hours [11]. The amplified *Mycobacterium tuberculosis* direct test (MTD, Gen-Probe, San Diego, CA) is approved by the FDA for detection of *M. tuberculosis* ribosomal RNA from both AFB positive and negative respiratory specimens. The AMPLICOR® *Mycobacterium tuberculosis* Test (Roche Molecular Systems, Branchburg, NJ) is approved for detection of *M. tuberculosis* ribosomal DNA from AFB positive respiratory specimens. The US Centers for Disease Control and Prevention (CDC) has published an algorithm for the use of the two tests [12]. These tests have shown limited ability to detect *M. tuberculosis* in gastric aspirates, and thus are of limited value in children [4, 13].

Treatment

Latent tuberculosis

No studies of latent tuberculosis therapy in HIV-infected children have been reported, so recommendations about this population are derived from the guidelines for HIV-uninfected children and HIV-infected adults. See Table 31.1 for recommended pediatric doses. Isoniazid (INH) given to adults for the treatment of latent tuberculosis

Table 31.1. Commonly used drugs for the prevention and treatment of tuberculosis in children [17]

Drug	Dosage forms (USA)	Doses in mg/kg (maximum dose)[a]	Adverse reactions	Drug interactions[a]
Isoniazid (INH)	50 mg/5 ml susp. 100 mg tablet 300 mg tablet	Daily: 10–20 (300 mg) Two times/week: 20–40 (900 mg) Three times/week: 20–40 (900 mg)	Rash, hepatic enzyme elevation, peripheral neuropathy	Increases levels of phenytoin and disulfiram
Rifampin	150 mg capsule 300 mg capsule Suspension can be formulated from capsule contents	Daily: 10–20 (600 mg) Two times/week: 10–20 (600 mg) Three times/week: 10–20 (600 mg)	Rash, hepatitis, fever, orange-colored body fluids	Major effects on PIs and NNRTIs. Refer to reference [18] for dose adjustments
Rifabutin	150 mg capsule	Daily: 10–20 (300 mg) Two times/week: 10–20 (300 mg)	Leukopenia, gastrointestinal upset, anterior uveitis, arthralgias, rash, hepatic enzyme elevation, orange-colored body fluids	Major effects with PIs and NNRTIs. Refer to reference 42 for dose adjustments
Pyrazinamide	500 mg tablet	Daily: 15–30 (2.0 g) Two times/week: 50–70 (3.5 g) Three times/week: 50–70 (2.5 g) 15 mg/kg/dose qd, max. 2.5 g qd (treatment only)	Gastrointestinal upset, hepatitis, rash, arthralgias, hyperuricemia	Might make glucose control more difficult in patients with diabetes
Ethambutol	100 mg tablet 400 mg tablet	Daily: 15–25 (1600 mg) Two times/week: 50 (4000 mg) Three times/week: 25–30 (2000 mg)	Optic neuritis, decreased red–green color vision, rash	No known important interactions.
Streptomycin	1 g vial (IM or IV only)	Daily: 20–40 (1 g) Two times/week: 25–30 (1.5 g) Three times/week: 25–30 (1.5 g)	Ototoxicity, nephrotoxicity	

[a] Life-threatening drug interactions may occur with these and other drugs that affect hepatic metabolism – review all potential interactions before adding these or other drugs to a patient's regimen.

for 9–12 months decreases the risk of active disease by approximately 80%; results in children are similar [9]. For children who are HIV-infected and TST-positive, the recommended regimen is INH daily or twice-a-week for 9 months, with monitoring of liver function tests [9]. Factors to consider when choosing the frequency of dosing include expected adherence to the regimen and need for directly observed therapy. Some experts recommend at least 12 months for children who are HIV-infected [14]. INH is also recommended for HIV-infected children with recent contact with an adult with tuberculosis, even if the child's TST is negative.

In HIV-infected adults a 2-month regimen of daily rifampin and pyrazinamide (PZA) is as effective as 12 months of INH for latent tuberculosis treatment, but this regimen is more toxic and has been associated with cases of severe and fatal hepatitis [15]. It has not been studied in children, and therefore, is not recommended for the pediatric population. In the UK, a 3-month regimen of rifampin and INH or a 6-month regimen of INH alone are the recommended regimens for latent tuberculosis in both adults and children [16]. If INH resistance is known or expected in the contact, the recommendation is treatment with rifampin for 6 months. As detailed below, the use of rifampin with certain non-nucleoside reverse transcriptase inhibitors (NNRTIs) and protease inhibitors (PIs) is contraindicated.

Tuberculosis disease

For an HIV-infected child not receiving treatment with NNRTIs or PIs an initial 4-drug regimen, consisting of INH, rifampin, PZA, and a fourth drug, either ethambutol or streptomycin, for 2 months and INH and rifampin for an additional 4 months is recommended. In the USA, ethambutol is preferred, even for children too young to have visual acuity and red–green color perception evaluated, because these toxicities are exceedingly rare in children at the recommended dose. Nevertheless, renal function, ophthalmoscopy and, if possible visual acuity, should be determined prior to initiation of therapy with ethambutol and monitored regularly during treatment with ethambutol. If renal function is abnormal, dose modification is essential. Use of streptomycin is hampered by the need for injection, which can be especially problematic in children with low body mass, and the potential for ototoxicity and nephrotoxicity. If the isolate from the adult contact is known to be drug susceptible, the ethambutol can be excluded. Therapy should include ongoing assessment of response, and be administered as directly observed therapy (DOT), if possible. Daily administration of the drugs for the first 2 weeks to 2 months followed by daily, twice (as long as CD4 count is not low – see below) or three times per week therapy to complete 6 months is acceptable. Some experts recommend a longer course of treatment, up to 9 months total [14].

Treatment for active tuberculosis in an HIV-infected child receiving treatment with NNRTIs or PIs is more complicated. Overall, as outlined below, the options include the use of rifampin in some circumstances, the use of rifabutin with altered doses, or discontinuing HAART while treating tuberculosis.

The use of rifampin with the PIs and NNRTIs was initially contraindicated, because rifampin is a potent inducer of the hepatic cytochrome CYP450 enzyme system and thus drastically decreases the levels of the drugs metabolized by that system, such as the PIs and NNRTIs [17]. Additional data, which led to the revision of these guidelines in March 2000, suggested that rifampin can be administered in patients receiving the following [17, 18]:

- efavirenz and two NRTIs
- ritonavir and one or more NRTIs
- ritonavir-boosted saquinavir therapy.

It is important to note that these revised guidelines are based upon limited data in adults, and thus their applicability to children is questionable. Given that data on HIV-infected children treated with ritonavir-boosted saquinavir are limited, and the fact that drug–drug interactions are amplified with the addition of rifampin, the use of rifampin in HIV-infected children also receiving efavirenz, ritonavir, or ritonavir-boosted saquinavir therapy should only be undertaken with great caution, and potentially with the aid of therapeutic drug monitoring of antiretrovirals and rifampin.

A related rifamycin, rifabutin, is a much less potent inducer of the CYP450 system and thus can be used with some CYP450-metabolized drugs with dose adjustments. Rifapentine, a new, long-acting rifamycin, is not recommended as a substitute for rifampin because its safety and effectiveness have not been established for the treatment of patients with HIV-related tuberculosis. Specific guidelines about the replacement of rifampin with rifabutin have been published [17, 18]. In summary, they include the following points:

- dose of rifabutin should be halved in the presence of amprenavir, nelfinavir, or indinavir
- dose of rifabutin should be halved and administered two to three times per week in the presence of ritonavir (including situations in which ritonavir is used as a pharmacokinetic enhancer of another PI, such as combination lopinavir/ritonavir (Kaletra);
- dose of indinavir co-administered with rifabutin should be increased 25%;
- dose of nelfinavir co-administered with rifabutin should probably be increased 33%;
- dose of rifabutin co-administered with efavirenz should be increased 50–100%;
- it is unknown whether dose of rifabutin should be decreased in the presence of nevirapine or saquinavir;
- rifabutin should not be administered with delavirdine (because of the marked decrease in delavirdine concentrations when administered with rifabutin).

While the guidelines endorse use of rifampin- or rifabutin-based regimens for the treatment of tuberculosis with co-administration of HAART, some have argued that the effect of the rifamycins on PI drug levels is too unpredictable, and the subsequent risk of HIV resistance too great, and therefore recommend the deferral of HAART until rifampin-based tuberculosis treatment is completed [19]. Another alternative is to use a rifamycin-sparing regimen of INH, streptomycin, PZA, and ethambutol for 8 weeks, followed by intermittent INH, streptomycin, and PZA for an additional 7 months [17].

Tuberculosis resistant to standard antibiotics has become a major problem in many areas. Patients with HIV infection and tuberculosis are at increased risk of having INH resistance, rifampin resistance, and multidrug resistance. The recommendation for the treatment of rifampin resistance alone is INH, streptomycin, PZA, and ethambutol for 2 months, followed by an additional 7 months of INH, streptomycin, and PZA. The recommendation for the treatment of INH resistance alone is a rifamycin, PZA, and ethambutol for 6–9 months [17]. For the treatment of multidrug-resistant tuberculosis, referral should be made, if possible, to an expert in HIV and tuberculosis treatment. Use of an aminoglycoside and quinolone should be considered, and treatment should continue until 24 months after conversion to negative culture and always be administered as directly observed therapy (DOT).

Directly observed therapy

The WHO's goals for global tuberculosis control by 2005 are to detect 70% of all AFB smear-positive cases and treat 85% of them successfully [20]. The strategy utilizes directly observed therapy, known as DOT, or DOTS, with the "S" referring to short course therapy. The five elements of DOTS are (a) government commitment, (b) diagnosis by sputum smear microscopy, (c) standardized short-course therapy, (d) adequate and reliable drug supply, and (e) reporting and recording system that allows for data collection and treatment evaluation. The strategy has been successful in many parts of the world, but logistical issues have hampered implementation in some areas. The WHO has highlighted that the lack of collaboration between tuberculosis and HIV programs is one reason for the lack of success with DOTS.

Bacillus of Calmette and Guerin (BCG)

Bacillus of Calmette and Guerin (BCG) is a live, attenuated vaccine for controlling tuberculosis. It was derived from *M. bovis* in 1921, and has been administered to more people in the world than any other vaccine (see also Chapter 5). The recommendations regarding the use of the vaccine differ around the world, based upon local rates of tuberculosis incidence and prevalence, divergent results of studies conducted in different areas of the world, local practice, and custom. Differences about the particular strain that is used, the recommended age at vaccination, and the need for booster doses of vaccine also exist.

A meta-analysis of 18 studies showed a protective effect of 75%–86% for the prevention of meningeal and miliary tuberculosis, but did not calculate a protective effect against pulmonary disease because of the great heterogeneity of results [21]. The protective efficacy of BCG against pulmonary tuberculosis varies greatly (0%–80%), but another meta-analysis of 26 studies concluded that the average efficacy is 50% [22].

Data on BCG vaccination of HIV-infected children are limited, but in one study of Haitian children, the complication rates after a higher than normal dose of BCG vaccination were 9.6% in infants born to HIV-negative women, 13.3% in HIV-uninfected infants born to HIV-infected women, and 30.8% in HIV-infected infants [23]. In this study, and in others cited by the authors, the reactions were usually mild. The authors' review of BCG complications in HIV-infected children revealed only four reported cases of disseminated BCG infection among 431 HIV-infected or exposed children who received BCG.

The USA and the Netherlands are the only countries to have never adopted a program of universal vaccination with BCG. In the USA, where the overall risk of tuberculosis is low, the primary strategy for controlling tuberculosis is to minimize the risk of transmission by early identification and treatment of patients with active disease, and by identifying and treating those with latent tuberculosis infection. Therefore, in the USA, BCG is rarely indicated, and is not recommended for HIV-infected children or adults.

In contrast, because of the consistent protection demonstrated against tuberculosis meningitis and miliary disease in children, BCG was incorporated into the WHO's Expanded Program on Immunization in 1974. The WHO recommends BCG at birth for infants born in areas of high tuberculosis prevalence, including asymptomatic, HIV-infected or exposed infants. Infants or children with AIDS, and infants or children in areas of low tuberculosis prevalence should not receive BCG.

Summary

Tuberculosis is a major cause of morbidity and mortality among HIV-infected children worldwide. The clinical manifestations among HIV-infected children are similar to those seen in uninfected children, although disease can be more severe. Treatment is complicated by the potential drug–drug interactions between the antituberculous therapy and the NNRTIs and PIs. Effective treatment of tuberculosis in the HIV-infected child is critically important for prolonged survival. Improved understanding of the molecular basis of tuberculosis pathogenesis should lead to new ways to prevent, diagnose, and to treat this disease.

REFERENCES

1. Dye, C., Scheele, S., Dolin, P., Pathania, V., Raviglione, M. C. Consensus statement. Global burden of tuberculosis: estimated incidence, prevalence, and mortality by country. WHO Global Surveillance and Monitoring Project. *J. Am. Med. Assoc.* 1999;**282**(7):677–686.

2. van Rie, A., Warren, R., Richardson, M. *et al.* Exogenous reinfection as a cause of recurrent tuberculosis after curative treatment. *N. Engl. J. Med.* 1999;**341**(16):1174–1179.

3. Ussery, X., Valway, S., McKenna, M., Cauthen, G., McCray, E., Onorato, I. Epidemiology of tuberculosis among children in the United States: 1985 to 1994. *Pediatr. Infect. Dis.* 1996;**15**:697–704.

4. Starke, J. R., Smith, M. H. D. Tuberculosis. In Feigin, R. D., Cherry, J. D., eds. *Textbook of Pediatric Infectious Diseases*. 4th edn. W.B. Saunders Co.; 1998:1196–1239.

5. Selwyn, P., Hartel, D., Lewis, V. *et al*. A prospective study of the risk of tuberculosis among intravenous drug users with human immunodeficiency virus infection. *N. Engl. J. Med.* 1989;**320**:545–550.

6. Daley, C., Small, P., Schecter, G. *et al*. An outbreak of tuberculosis with accelerated progression among persons infected with the human immunodeficiency virus. An analysis using restriction-fragment-length polymorphisms. *N. Engl. J. Med.* 1992;**326**:231–235.

7. Braun, M. M., Badi, N., Ryder, R. W. *et al*. A retrospective cohort study of the risk of tuberculosis among women of childbearing age with HIV infection in Zaire. *Am. Rev. Respir. Dis.* 1991;**143**(3):501–504.

8. Whalen, C., Horsburgh, C. R., Hom, D., Lahart, C., Simberkoff, M., Ellner, J. Accelerated course of human immunodeficiency virus infection after tuberculosis. *Am. J. Respir. Crit. Care Med.* 1995;**151**(1):129–135.

9. CDC. Targeted tuberculin testing and treatment of latent tuberculosis infection. *Morb. Mortal. Wkly Rep.* 2000;**49** (RR-6).

10. Pomputius, W. F., 3rd, Rost, J., Dennehy, P. H., Carter, E.J. Standardization of gastric aspirate technique improves yield in the diagnosis of tuberculosis in children. *Pediatr. Infect. Dis. J.* 1997;**16**(2):222–226.

11. Havlir, D. V., Barnes, P. F. Tuberculosis in patients with human immunodeficiency virus infection. *N. Engl. J. Med.* 1999;**340**(5):367–373.

12. CDC. Update: nucleic acid amplification tests for tuberculosis. *Morb. Mortal. Wkly Rep.* 2000;**49** (No. 26).

13. Neu, N., Saiman, L., San Gabriel, P. *et al*. Diagnosis of pediatric tuberculosis in the modern era. *Pediatr. Infect. Dis. J.* 1999;**18**(2):122–126.

14. American Acadedmy of Pediatrics. Tuberculosis. In Pickering, L. K., ed. *Red Book: Report of the Committee on Infectious Diseases*. 25th edn. Elk Grove Village, IL: American Academy of Pediatrics; 2000.

15. CDC. Update: fatal and severe liver injuries associated with rifampin and pyrazinamide for latent tuberculosis infection, and revisions in American Thoracic Society/CDC recommendations – United States, 2001. *Morb. Mortal. Wkly Rep.* 2001;**50** (No. 34).

16. Chemotherapy and management of tuberculosis in the United Kingdom: recommendations 1998. Joint Tuberculosis Committee of the British Thoracic Society. *Thorax* 1998;**53**(7):536–548.

17. CDC. Prevention and treatment of tuberculosis among patients infected with human immunodeficiency virus: principles of therapy and revised recommendations. *Morb. Mortal. Wkly Rep.* 1998;**47** (RR-20).

18. CDC. Updated guidelines for the use of rifabutin or rifampin for the treatment and prevention of tuberculosis among HIV-infected patients taking protease inhibitors or nonnucleoside reverse trancriptase inhibitors. *Morb. Mortal. Wkly Rep.* 2000;**49** (No. 9).

19. Jenny-Avital, ER. Protease inhibitors and rifabutin: isn't the jury still out? *Clin. Infect. Dis.* 2001;**32**(2):322–323.

20. WHO. *Global Tuberculosis Control Surveillance, Planning, Financing*. World Health Organization; 2002.

21. Rodrigues, L. C., Diwan, V. K., Wheeler, J. G. Protective effect of BCG vaccine against tuberculous meningitis and miliary tuberculosis: a meta-analysis. *Int. J. Epidemiol.* 1993;**22**:1154–1158.

22. Colditz, G. A., Brewer, T. F., Berkey, C. S. *et al.* Efficacy of BCG vaccine in the prevention of tuberculosis. Meta-analysis of the published literature. *J. Am. Med. Assoc.* 1994;**271**:698–702.

23. O'Brien, K. L., Ruff, A. J., Louis, M. A. *et al.* Bacillus Calmette–Guerin complications in children born to HIV-1-infected women with a review of the literature. *Pediatrics* 1995;**95**(3):414–418.

32 Disseminated *Mycobacterium avium* complex infection

Robert N. Husson, M.D.

Children's Hospital, Division of Infectious Diseases, Boston, MA

Non-tuberculous mycobacteria are major opportunistic pathogens of HIV-infected children and adults who have severe immunosuppression. Organisms of the *Mycobacterium avium* complex are the predominant pathogens, typically causing systemic infection, (referred to as disseminated *M. avium* complex infection or DMAC). With the advent of highly active antiretroviral therapy (HAART) and the resulting improved preservation of immune competence, DMAC infection has become less common [1]. Among HIV-infected children with advanced disease, however, DMAC infection remains an important cause of morbidity and mortality, so that prevention and management of non-tuberculous mycobacterial infection are important aspects of the care of children with AIDS.

Epidemiology

Mycobacterium avium and many of the other non-tuberculous mycobacteria are widely distributed in the environment. They are found in water and soil in nature and have been identified in food and in institutional water systems [2, 3]. These organisms are uncommon causes of infection in normal hosts, and thus are opportunistic pathogens in patients with depressed cell-mediated immunity, including those with HIV infection.

While DMAC infection is a major opportunistic infection in North America and Western Europe, it is uncommonly identified in persons with AIDS in Africa or other less-developed areas of the world. It is not known whether this difference reflects differences in distribution of pathogenic strains of MAC in the environment. Almost certainly, part of this difference is the result of lack of blood culture testing to identify DMAC infection in these settings. In addition, earlier mortality, resulting from high rates of infection with *M. tuberculosis* and other more virulent pathogens, limits the population of survivors with advanced immune suppression who are at risk for DMAC infection [4].

Handbook of Pediatric HIV Care, ed. Steven L. Zeichner and Jennifer S. Read.
Published by Cambridge University Press. © Cambridge University Press 2006.

Microbiology and pathogenesis

M. avium and most other mycobacteria that cause disease in persons with AIDS are typically slow-growing and require two to several weeks to grow in culture [5]. Some of the less commonly identified mycobacteria grow poorly in culture or require specially supplemented growth media so that it may be difficult to document the presence of infection despite obtaining multiple cultures. The use of broth culture methods with radiometric or other methods of growth detection give positive results more quickly than traditional agar plate-based methods. These have come into widespread use, and have been adapted to determine susceptibility to some of the more commonly used anti-mycobacterial agents. Nucleic acid probes are available to provide rapid identification of members of the *M. avium* complex (*M. avium*, *M. intracellulare*, and other uncommon closely related species) and the *M. tuberculosis* complex. Other species must be identified using traditional methods, which may require several additional weeks. Because of the need for special expertise, media and equipment, many clinical microbiology laboratories do not perform mycobacterial cultures, and send out samples to reference laboratories. Susceptibility testing of non-tuberculous mycobacteria is not standardized, and is recommended only for determining susceptibility to clarithromycin (which also defines susceptibility to azithromycin) [6].

Relatively little is known about the pathogenesis of DMAC infection in children or adults with AIDS. DMAC infection is rare in adults with more than 100 CD4+ lymphocytes/mm^3 and typically occurs in individuals who have <50 CD4+ lymphocytes/mm^3. In children, DMAC infection also occurs primarily in those with severe immune deficiency. Data from a large cohort of HIV-infected children treated with antiretroviral therapy in the pre-HAART era indicate that DMAC infection can occur in children < 6 years of age at higher levels of CD4+ lymphocytes than in older children or adults [7]. This age dependence of CD4+ lymphocyte count and degree of immunosuppression has led to the development of guidelines that incorporate age-specific CD4+ lymphocyte counts at which prophylactic therapy should be introduced to prevent DMAC infection [8].

The mode of acquisition of *M. avium* infection is not clearly established. Gastrointestinal and respiratory colonization are thought to be primary portals of entry that can then lead to disseminated infection. Person-to-person transmission has not been documented and is not believed to be a significant mode of infection. When DMAC infection occurs, mycobacteria may be found in blood, bone marrow, lymph nodes (especially abdominal lymph nodes), bone, and solid organs including liver and spleen.

In DMAC infection the mycobacteria are typically found within macrophages. In the absence of effective cell-mediated immunity the infected macrophages are unable to kill the organisms, resulting in large numbers of intracellular bacilli that may be seen on acid-fast staining of pathologic specimens. Granulomas are typically absent or poorly formed. In the absence of treatment, ongoing bacterial replication results in an extremely large systemic organism burden, making subsequent treatment more difficult.

Clinical presentation and diagnosis

Clinical and laboratory findings in patients with DMAC are non-specific. The most common symptoms associated with DMAC infection include weight loss or failure to gain weight, persistent diarrhea, abdominal pain, fever, sweats and fatigue [9–11]. Laboratory abnormalities may include anemia, leukopenia and thrombocytopenia. Serum chemistries are generally not markedly abnormal, although some patients may have elevations of alkaline phosphatase or lactate dehydrogenase.

In some patients, a "reconstitution syndrome" has occurred within weeks to months of starting HAART. This syndrome, with new onset of constitutional symptoms, especially fever or abdominal pain, often occurs in association with focal lymphadenopathy. In these patients, immune reconstitution in response to HAART appears to have generated a more vigorous immune response to mycobacterial infection that was previously asymptomatic, with the resulting signs and symptoms of infection.

DMAC infection is diagnosed by blood culture or culture of a normally sterile site, e.g., lymph node or bone marrow. Bone marrow culture has been shown to contain higher numbers of organisms than blood, but is not commonly performed [12]. In settings where tuberculosis is not common, histology demonstrating macrophages containing acid fast bacilli strongly suggests the diagnosis of DMAC in a patient with typical signs and symptoms. Culture is essential however, to distinguish non-tuberculous mycobacteria from *M. tuberculosis* and, when *M. tuberculosis* is not present, to determine which species of non-tuberculous mycobacterium is the cause of infection.

In a patient with less than 100 CD4+ lymphocytes, with suggestive clinical findings or laboratory abnormalities, a blood culture for *M. avium* infection should be obtained. As noted above, symptoms, signs and laboratory abnormalities associated with DMAC infection are non-specific, so that a patient with advanced immunosuppression based on age-specific CD4+ lymphocyte counts who has persistent fever, weight loss or other symptoms should be evaluated for DMAC infection. Symptoms caused by DMAC infection may precede the onset of bacteremia, so that several mycobacterial cultures over time may be required to yield a positive result [11]. Cultures from stool or respiratory specimens do not indicate disseminated infection *per se*, although cultures from these non-sterile sites should prompt evaluation for disseminated infection, and may be a precursor to disseminated infection.

Because of the potential toxicity of the treatment regimens and the possibility of alternative causes of symptoms, empiric therapy of DMAC infection based on persistent symptoms despite negative cultures or diagnostic histopahology is rarely warranted. DMAC infection in HIV-infected children is associated with abdominal and chest lymphadenopathy; CT scan may be valuable in identifying these abnormalities, but biopsy is required to determine whether the enlarged nodes are caused by DMAC infection, tuberculosis, or other infectious or non-infectious etiologies.

Prevention

The most effective strategy for the prevention of DMAC infection in children with HIV infection is to preserve the child's immune system through early diagnosis and effective anti-retroviral treatment. Despite the major decline in the incidence of DMAC infection that was associated with introduction of HAART, DMAC remains among the most common opportunistic infections in HIV-infected individuals [1]. In adults receiving HAART, the risk of infection remains strongly correlated with low CD4+ lymphocyte counts; the risk of DMAC infection in persons whose counts have recovered above threshold values for the initiation of prophylaxis is comparable to the risk among persons whose counts never fell to this level [13]. Viral load appears to be an independent, though less strong, risk factor for several opportunistic infections including DMAC in persons receiving HAART [14].

The most recent US Public Health Service/Infectious Disease Society of America guidelines for the prevention of opportunistic infections were published in November 2001 [8]. These guidelines specifically address initiation of primary prophylaxis and discontinuation of primary and secondary prophylaxis for DMAC in adults and adolescents. In children, age-specific CD4+ lymphocyte criteria are used to decide when to initiate primary prophylaxis. It is likely that, in children with a sustained response to HAART with CD4+ lymphocyte counts above these cutoffs, primary prophylaxis can be discontinued, although data to support this approach are lacking. Discontinuation of secondary prophylaxis in children with prior DMAC infection is not recommended at present. Specific prophylactic strategies for prevention of DMAC infection are described in Chapter 5.

Treatment

Treatment has been shown to decrease symptoms and prolong survival in persons with AIDS and DMAC infection [15–17]. As is the case for preventive therapy, the treatment of established DMAC infection in HIV-infected children is based on inference from adult data, limited published pediatric information and experience of clinicians who treat HIV-infected children. While treatment has been shown to be clinically beneficial and to decrease mycobacteremia, effective therapy of DMAC infection is often limited by toxicities and drug interactions. In addition, when DMAC infection occurs in a patient who has had prophylaxis with azithromycin or clarithromycin, a substantial minority of the breakthrough MAC strains will be resistant to these agents. When this occurs, effective treatment is much more difficult because these agents are the cornerstone of effective therapy against DMAC.

When DMAC infection is documented by a positive culture of blood or other sterile site, multidrug therapy should be initiated (Table 32.1). Monotherapy with a macrolide has been shown to result in the emergence of high level resistance to these agents in most children in a matter of weeks [16]. The addition of ethambutol decreases the rate of relapse so that initial therapy should include clarithromycin or azithromycin plus ethambutol [18]. Most experts initiate therapy with clarithromycin if possible, because of its greater potency in vitro and one study demonstrating bacteriologic superiority of clarithromycin plus ethamubtol vs. azithromycin plus ethambutol, although a separate study did not identify significant differences between these regimens [19, 20].

Ethambutol is not available as a liquid preparation and is not approved for use in children because of concern for optic nerve toxicity that may be difficult to recognize. It has been used in children, however, without a high incidence of toxicity, so long as renal function is normal. Because of the rapid occurrence of relapse with bacteriologic resistance when macrolide monotherapy is used, DMAC infection in children should always be treated with combination therapy that includes clarithromycin or azithromycin plus ethambutol. Renal function, ophthalmoscopy and, if possible, visual acuity and color discrimination, should be determined prior to initiation of therapy. If renal function is abnormal, ethambutol should be used with caution, dose modification and regular monitoring of renal function is essential. Monitoring of vision, including visual acuity, peripheral vision, and color discrimination should be performed regularly in patients receiving ethambutol. Rifabutin may be included as a third drug, although the benefit of adding this drug to the two-drug regimen is less clear and its use may be limited by drug interactions and toxicity [21]. Though not available in a liquid preparation, a rifabutin suspension can be formulated from the contents of the capsules.

Nearly all isolates from patients not receiving clarithromycin or azithromycin as prophylaxis are susceptible to these agents, and a majority from those who have received prophylaxis are susceptible. Susceptibility testing of isolates from patients who have not been receiving macrolide prophylaxis prior to the diagnosis of DMAC infection is generally not necessary. For patients who develop DMAC infection despite prophylactic therapy, testing of the initial isolate for susceptibility to clarithromycin should be performed. Susceptibility testing should also be performed on isolates from patients who fail to respond to therapy, or who have recurrent symptoms and new positive cultures following an initial response macrolide-based therapy for DMAC [6]. Susceptibility to clarithromycin predicts susceptibility to azithromycin so that testing for azithromycin susceptibility is not necessary.

Among other available drugs with antimycobacterial activity, correlation between susceptibility in vitro and clinical response has not been clearly demonstrated. Clofazamine is active in vitro against most MAC strains from AIDS patients. This agent does not appear to impact mycobacterial clearance in patients receiving macrolide-containing regimens, however, and use of clofazamine has been associated with

Table 32.1. Commonly used drugs for the prevention and treatment of DMAC infection in children with HIV infection

Drug	Dosage forms	Doses[a]	Major toxicities	Drug interactions[b]
Clarithromycin	125 mg/5ml susp. 250 mg/5ml susp. 250 mg tablet 500 mg tablet	7.5–12.5 mg/kg/dose bid, max. 500 mg bid (treatment or prophylaxis – use lower dose for prophylaxis)	Nausea, diarrhea, abdominal pain Uncommon: headache, leukopenia, elevation of transaminases, altered taste	Decreases hepatic metabolism of many drugs. Protease inhibitors may increase clarithromycin concentration; efavirenz may reduce clarithromycin concentration.
Azithromycin	100 mg/5ml susp. 200 mg/5ml susp. 250 mg capsule 600 mg tablet 1000 mg packet for single dose susp.	5–10 mg/kg/dose qd, max. 500 mg qd (treatment or prophylaxis – use lower dose for prophylaxis) or 20–25 mg/kg/dose q week, max 1200 mg q week (prophylaxis only)	Nausea, diarrhea, abdominal pain, possible ototoxicity Uncommon: headache, leukopenia, elevation of transaminases	Minor effect on hepatic metabolism
Rifabutin[c,d]	150 mg capsule	5–6 mg/kg/dose qd, max. 300 mg qd (treatment or prophylaxis)	Leukopenia, gastrointestinal upset, anterior uveitis, arthralgias, rash, elevation of transaminases, skin discoloration, secretion discoloration	Increases hepatic metabolism of many drugs. Drugs that slow hepatic metabolism may increase rifabutin concentration and toxicity and may require dose adjustment or discontinuation. Should not be used with saquinavir or delavirdine; major dose adjustment required for other protease inhibitors and NNRTIs.

Table 32.1. (cont.)

Drug	Dosage forms	Doses[a]	Major toxicities	Drug interactions[b]
Ethambutol[c]	100 mg tablet 400 mg tablet	15–25 mg/kg/dose qd, max. 2.5 g qd (treatment only)	Optic neuritis (rare at 15 mg/kg – monitor visual acuity and red–green color vision monthly); headache, peripheral neuropathy, rash, hyperuricemia	No known important interactions. Drug is cleared by renal excretion; check baseline renal function and do not use in patients with significant renal impairment.

[a] Limited data from clinical trials are available to support the doses of these agents for the prevention and treatment of DMAC infection in children. Doses provided in this table are those that have been used by persons expert in the care of HIV-infected children. Azithromycin or clarithromycin are first choice agents for prophylaxis; established infection is treated with clarithromycin (first choice) or azithromycin (alternative) plus ethambutol, with or without rifabutin (see text).

[b] Life-threatening drug interactions may occur with these and other drugs that affect hepatic metabolism – review all potential interactions before adding these or other drugs to a patient's regimen. See [23] and Chapter 12 for specific dose adjustments and contraindications for these drugs.

[c] Not approved for children under 13 years of age.

[d] Rifabutin is a second line agent for the prevention of DMAC infection in children who cannot receive clarithromycin or azithromycin.

increased mortality in clinical trials of DMAC therapy in adults, so its use is not recommended [22]. Streptomycin and amikacin are active against some strains and may be useful as a second-line agent, but are available only for intramuscular or intravenous administration. Quinolones including ciprofloxacin and ofloxacin may also have a role as second-line agents against strains that are susceptible. Linezolid, a relatively new antimicrobial agent, is active against some MAC strains in vitro, though its utility as a therapeutic agent against DMAC has not been studied.

Treatment options for a patient who has relapsed while receiving a macrolide-based treatment regimen, or who cannot tolerate clarithromycin or azithromycin are severely limited. No regimen that does not contain clarithromycin or azithromycin has been shown to be of clinical benefit. Combinations of rifabutin, ethambutol, amikacin and a quinolone may be tried, but the risk of toxicities must be weighed against the low likelihood of substantial clinical benefit. Whether or not there is a role for linezolid in this setting is not known.

The major limitations to therapy for DMAC infection are toxicities and drug interactions. The major toxicities of the drugs commonly used for treatment and prophylaxis are shown in Table 32.1. The important drug interactions for each of these drugs result from their effect on the hepatic metabolism of other agents, including many of the protease inhibitors and non-nucleoside reverse transcriptase inhibitors (NNRTIs), and are shown in Table 32.1 [8, 23, 24]. Clarithromycin, though not azithromycin, decreases the clearance of many drugs that are eliminated by hepatic metabolism. Drug interactions are also discussed in Chapter 12. Rifabutin induces the metabolism of many of these same drugs. Conversely, concentrations of clarithromycin and rifabutin may be altered significantly in patients receiving other drugs that affect hepatic metabolism. For example, major dose reductions of rifabutin or use of an alternative are required in patients receiving many of the currently available protease inhibitors and NNRTI's, in order to avoid toxicity. Specific contraindications and dose adjustment recommendations resulting from drug interactions of clarithromycin and rifabutin with specific antiretroviral agents are addressed in detail in the US Public Health Service/Infectious Disease Society of America guidelines [8].

Management of immune reconstitution syndrome associated with focal MAC infection is not well established. Antiretroviral therapy should be maintained and anti-DMAC therapy should be initiated. Corticosteroids have been used in some patients and may be beneficial when the symptoms or pathologic consequences associated with the focal inflammatory response are significant.

Several other non-tuberculous mycobacterial species can cause infection in AIDS patients. The appropriate treatment for these infections depends on the species causing the infection; in some cases no effective regimen has been defined. Therapy of these infections should be designed in consultation with an expert in the treatment of such infections.

REFERENCES

1. Palella, F. J., Jr., Delaney, K. M., Moorman, A. C. *et al.* Declining morbidity and mortality among patients with advanced human immunodeficiency virus infection. HIV Outpatient Study Investigators. *N. Engl. J. Med.* 1998;**338**(13):853–860.

2. von Reyn, C. F., Waddell, R. D., Eaton, T. *et al.* Isolation of *Mycobacterium avium* complex from water in the United States, Finland, Zaire, and Kenya. *J. Clin. Microbiol.* 1993;**31**(12):3227–3230.

3. von Reyn, C., Maslow, J., Barber, T., Falkinham, J., III, Arbeit, R. Persistent colonisation of potable water as a source of *Mycobacterium avium* infection in AIDS. *Lancet* 1994;**343**:1137–1141.

4. Pettipher, C. A., Karstaedt, A. S., Hopley, M. Prevalence and clinical manifestations of disseminated *Mycobacterium avium* complex infection in South Africans with acquired immunodeficiency syndrome. *Clin. Infect. Dis.* 2001;**33**(12):2068–2071.

5. Inderlied, C., Kemper, C., Bermudez, L. The *Mycobacterium avium* complex. *Clin. Microbiol. Rev.* 1993;**6**:266–310.

6. Woods, G.L. Susceptibility testing for mycobacteria. *Clin. Infect. Dis.* 2000;**31**(5):1209–1215.

7. Dankner, W. M., Lindsey, J. C., Levin, M. J. Correlates of opportunistic infections in children infected with the human immunodeficiency virus managed before highly active antiretroviral therapy. *Pediatr. Infect. Dis. J.* 2001;**20**(1):40–48.

8. USPHS/IDSA Prevention of Opportunistic Infections Working Group. 2001 USPHS/IDSA Guidelines for the Prevention of Opportunistic Infections in Persons Infected with Human Immunodeficiency *Virus* 2001:1–65.

9. Hoyt, L., Oleske, J., Holland, B., Connor, E. Nontuberculous mycobacteria in children with acquired immunodeficiency syndrome. *Pediatr. Infect. Dis. J.* 1992;**11**:354–360.

10. Lewis, L., Butler, K., Husson, R. *et al.* Defining the population of human immunodeficiency virus-infected children at risk for *Mycobacterium avium-intracellulare*. *J. Pediatr.* 1992;**121**:677–683.

11. Gordin, F., Cohn, D., Sullam, P., Schoenfelder, J., Wynne, P., Horsburgh, C. J. Early manifestations of disseminated *Mycobacterium avium* complex disease: a prospective evaluation. *J. Infect. Dis.* 1997;**176**:126–132.

12. Hafner, R., Inderlied, C. B., Peterson, D. M. *et al.* Correlation of quantitative bone marrow and blood cultures in AIDS patients with disseminated *Mycobacterium avium* complex infection. *J. Infect. Dis.* 1999;**180**(2):438–447.

13. Kaplan, J. E., Hanson, D., Dworkin, M. S. *et al.* Epidemiology of human immunodeficiency virus-associated opportunistic infections in the United States in the era of highly active antiretroviral therapy. *Clin. Infect. Dis.* 2000;**30** Suppl. 1:S5–S14.

14. Kaplan, J. E., Hanson, D. L., Jones, J. L., Dworkin, M. S. Viral load as an independent risk factor for opportunistic infections in HIV-infected adults and adolescents. *AIDS* 2001;**15**(14):1831–1836.

15. Horsburgh, C., Jr., Havlik, J., Ellis, D. *et al.* Survival of patients with acquired immune deficiency syndrome and disseminated *Mycobacterium avium* complex infection with and without antimycobacterial chemotherapy. *Am. Rev. Respir. Dis.* 1991;**144**:557–559.

16. Husson, R., Ross, L., Inderlied, C. *et al.* Orally administered clarithromycin for the treatment of systemic *Mycobacterium avium* complex infection in children with acquired immunodeficiency syndrome. *J. Pediatr.* 1994;**124**:807–814.

17. Shafran, S. D., Singer, J., Zarowny, D. P. *et al.* A comparison of two regimens for the treatment of *Mycobacterium avium* complex bacteremia in AIDS: rifabutin, ethambutol, and clarithromycin versus rifampin, ethambutol, clofazamine and ciprofloxacin. *N. Engl. J. Med.* 1996;**335**:377–383.

18. Dube, M., Sattler, F., Torriani, F. *et al.* A randomized evaluation of ethambutol for prevention of relapse and drug resistance during treatment of *Mycobacterium avium* complex bacteremia with clarithromycin-based combination therapy. *J. Infect. Dis.* 1997;**176**:1225–1232.

19. Ward, T. T., Rimland, D., Kauffman, C., Huycke, M., Evans, T. G., Heifets, L. Randomized, open-label trial of azithromycin plus ethambutol vs. clarithromycin plus ethambutol as therapy for *Mycobacterium avium* complex bacteremia in patients with human immunodeficiency virus infection. Veterans Affairs HIV Research Consortium. *Clin. Infect. Dis.* 1998;**27**(5):1278–1285.

20. Dunne, M., Fessel, J., Kumar, P. *et al.* A randomized, double-blind trial comparing azithromycin and clarithromycin in the treatment of disseminated *Mycobacterium avium* infection in patients with human immunodeficiency virus. *Clin. Infect. Dis.* 2000;**31**(5):1245–1252.

21. Gordin, F. M., Sullam, P. M., Shafran, S. D. *et al.* A randomized, placebo-controlled study of rifabutin added to a regimen of clarithromycin and ethambutol for treatment of disseminated infection with *Mycobacterium avium* complex. *Clin. Infect. Dis.* 1999;**28**(5):1080–1085.

22. Chaisson, R. E., Keiser, P., Pierce, M. *et al.* Clarithromycin and ethambutol with or without clofazimine for the treatment of bacteremic *Mycobacterium avium* complex disease in patients with HIV infection. *AIDS* 1997;**11**(3):311–317.

23. Piscitelli, S., Flexner, C., Minor, J., Polis, M., Masur, H. Drug interactions in patients infected with human immunodeficiency virus. *Clin. Infect. Dis.* 1996;**23**:685–691.

24. Tseng, A., Foisy, M. Management of drug interactions in patients with HIV. *Ann. Pharmacother.* 1997;**31**:1040–1058.

33 Fungal infections

Corina E. Gonzalez, M.D.

Division of Pediatric Hematology/Oncology, Georgetown University Hospital, Washington DC

Introduction

Fungal infections represent an important cause of morbidity and mortality in HIV-infected children [1] (Table 33.1). Most children with low CD4+ lymphocyte counts develop mucosal candidiasis that increases in severity with worsening immunosuppression [2]. Invasive fungal infections due to primary pathogens such as *Cryptococcus neoformans*, *Coccidioides immitis*, *Histoplasma capsulatum*, *Penicillium marneffei*, and others occur less frequently in pediatric than in adult patients with the acquired immunodeficiency syndrome (AIDS), probably because children are less likely to be exposed to these agents. More recently, invasive pulmonary aspergillosis has emerged as an HIV-associated complication.

Fungal infections may present with atypical clinical manifestations making their recognition a challenge. When fungal cultures or serologic or antigenic markers are negative, biopsies of affected sites can help in making a diagnosis [3].

Recently, the therapeutic options for invasive fungal infections have broadened with the introduction of the triazole compounds fluconazole and itraconazole, the lipid formulations of amphotericin B, the allilamine terbinafine, and, the echinocandin caspofungin [4–7]. These antifungals have different pharmacological properties and clinically important drug interactions that must be considered (Tables 33.2 and 33.3) [7–9]. Despite these advances, there are still a limited number of effective and safe antifungal agents (Table 33.4).

Cutaneous infections

Cutaneous candidiasis

Cutaneous candidiasis may develop as diaper dermatitis or as a more generalized eruption [10]. Candida diaper dermatitis is characterized by erythema bordered by scales,

Handbook of Pediatric HIV Care, ed. Steven L. Zeichner and Jennifer S. Read.
Published by Cambridge University Press. © Cambridge University Press 2006.

Table 33.1. Diagnosis and physical findings of selected mycoses complicating pediatric HIV infection

Fungal infection	Physical findings	Diagnosic methods
Oral candidiasis	Mucosal erythema, white-beige plaques	KOH preparation, culture
Esophageal candidiasis	Dysphagia, odynophagia, retrosternal pain	Barium swallow: evidences of plaques and ulceration "moth-eaten" appearance. These findings are suggestive but not diagnostic. Endoscopy: mucosal erythema, white-beige plaques. Culture and biopsy of the lesions.
Disseminated candidiasis	Fever, endophthalmitis, and cutaneous lesions	Blood cultures, biopsy of skin lesions.
Cryptococcosis	Fever, headaches, pulmonary infiltrates, alteration of mental status, and septic shock	Cryptococcal antigen titers in serum and CSF. Sputum and BAL direct examination and culture. Blood and CSF culture.
Histoplasmosis	Fever, pulmonary infiltrates, hepato-splenomegaly, lymphadenopathy, cutaneous lesions, and septic shock	Antigen detection in serum and urine. Sputum, BAL, and bone marrow direct examination and culture. Blood culture. Bone marrow, skin or pulmonary biopsy.
Coccidioidomycosis	Fever, headaches, pulmonary infiltrates,confusion, and cutaneous lesions	Sputum and BAL direct examination and culture. Skin or pulmonary biopsy Galactomanan antigen in serum and BAL.
Aspergillosis	Fever, pulmonary infiltrates	Sputum and BAL direct examination and culture. Pulmonary biopsy.
Penicillinosis	Fever, pulmonary infiltrates, hepatospleno megaly, lymphadenopathy and cutaneous lesions	Skin biopsy direct examination and culture. Blood culture. Lymph node biopsy. Sputum and BAL direct examination and culture.

KOH: potassium hydroxide; BAL: bronchoalveolar lavage; CSF: cerebrospinal fluid.

Table 33.2. Systemic antifungal agents used for treatment of fungal infections

Antifungal polyenes

Mechanism of Action: polyenes bind to membrane ergosterol and appear to form pores which increase membrane permeability and leakage of cell molecules. An additional mechanism of action may include oxidative damage of the fungal cell.

Spectrum of activity: *Candida* spp., *Cryptococcus neoformans*, *Torulopsis glabrata*, *Blastomyces dermatitides*, *Histoplasma capsulatum*, *Coccidioides immi Paracoccidioides brasilensis*, *Aspergillus* spp., *Penicillium marneffei*, and the agents of zygomycosis.

	Administration	Pharmacokinetic profile	Toxicity
Deoxycholate Amphotericin B (AMB) (Fungizone) 100 mg vial	AMB is a colloidal suspension that must be prepared in electrolyte free D5W at 0.1 mg/mL to avoid precipitation. There is no need to protect the suspension from the light. The duration of the IV infusion can range from 1 to 6 hrs depending on patient tolerance to acute adverse reactions. Manufacturer recommends a test dose of 1 mg, but its value predicting the occurrence of side effects is unknown.	Oral bioavailability is negligible. At recommended dosages, peak concentrations of AMB are higher than the MICs reported for most fungi. AMB appears to accumulate extensively in tissues. Little drug penetrates into CSF, vitreous humor or amniotic fluid. Elimination and metabolism of the drug is not well understood. Because of its tissue binding, release is very slow with a terminal phase half life is about 15 days. Requires dose adjustment with renal insufficiency.	Infusion related adverse reactions are common (~70–90%) and include fever and rigors, which may also be accompanied by headaches, nausea, vomiting, hyperpnea, hypo or hypertension, and arrhytmias. Phlebitis is associated with the peripheral administration of AMB. A reduction in the infusion rate and premedication with acetaminophen or hydrocortisone, may decrease the incidence of these side effects. Rigors respond to meperidine. Toxicity of major concern is nephrotoxicity (~80%) which may manifest as a tubulopathy by kaliuresis, hypokalemia, hypomagnesemia, or RTA type II, or as a decrease in GFR with rising BUN and serum creatinine. Normal saline loading pre or post infusion may restore GFR to normal. Avoid use of concomitant nephrotoxic drugs (e.g. aminoglycosides), if possible. Less common adverse reactions include anemia, thrombocytopenia and anaphylaxis.

(cont.)

Table 33.2. (cont.)

	Administration	Pharmacokinetic profile	Toxicity
Amphotericin B lipid complex (ABLC) (Abelcet) 100 mg vial	ABLC must be administered at a rate of 2.5 mg/kg/hr usually over 1–2 hrs. If the infusion time exceeds 2 hrs, mix the suspension by shaking the infusion bag. Do not dilute with saline solutions or mix with electrolytes or other drugs. Do not use in-line filters	Compared to AMB, it has a larger volume of distribution, rapid blood clearance and higher tissue concentrations particularly in the RES.	Fever and rigors ∼20%; increased creatinine ∼15%; anemia 4%.
Amphotericin B colloidal dispersion (ABCD) (Amphocil) 100 mg vial	ABCD must be diluted in D5W and infuse at 1 mg/kg/hr. Do not use in-line filter.	Compared to AMB, it has a larger volume of distribution, and higher tissue concentrations particularly in the RES	Fever and rigors ∼50%; increased creatinine ∼20%.
Amphotericin B liposome (Ambisome) 50 mg vial	Ambisome must be diluted with D5W and infused over a period of 1 to 2 hrs. Only approved for empirical use during neutropenia at 3 mg/kg/day.	Compared to AMB, it achieves higher peak plasma concentrations this may translate into better penetration into tissue sites, such as CSF.	Fever and rigors 8–20%; nausea ∼10%; vomiting ∼5%; increased creatinine ∼20%
Nystatin (*Mycotastin*) 30 gm cream 500, 000U tabs	Topical and oral	Very minimal gastrointestinal absorption	Virtually no side effects. Bitter taste.

The lipid formulations of AMB enable AMB to be administered in higher doses (2 to 10 mg/kg/d) with less nephrotoxicity and acute side effects. Lipid formulations of AMB are appropriate alternatives to conventional AMB and may represent an advance in antifungal therapy. They are as efficacious and have a more favorable safety profile than AMB. While some would restrict the use of these lipid formulations as a secondary alternative to AMB because of their high costs and lack of data showing superior efficacy, consideration for their use as initial therapy should be given on a case-by-case basis. Their use is warranted on patients with renal impairment, with unacceptable toxicity associated with AMB, or in patients with fungal infections refractory to AMB.

Table 33.2. (cont.)

Antifungal azoles

Mechanism of action: inhibit the cytochrome P 450-dependent enzyme involved in the conversion of lanosterol to ergosterol, a major component of the fungal cell wall. Azoles may also inhibit the cytochrome c oxidative and peroxidative enzymes, with the resultant increase in intracellular peroxide generation, which may contribute to the degeneration of subcellular structures.

Spectrum of activity: Dermatophytes, *Blastomyces dermatitides*, *Histoplasma capsulatum*, *Coccidioides immitis*, *Paracoccidioides brasilensis*, *Penicillium marneffei*, and *Sporotrix schenckii*. One notable exception is the lack of activity of miconazole against *B. dermatitides*. In addition, all azoles are active against *Candida albicans* but somewhat less active against many of the non-*albicans* spp of *Candida*. Ketoconazole, fluconazole and itraconazole are active against *Cryptococcus neoformans*. Itraconazole is the only azole with substantial activity against *Aspergillus* ssp.

	Administration	Pharmacokinetic profile	Toxicity
Ketoconazole (Nizoral) 200 mg tablets 2% topical cream 1% shampoo	Topical and oral. Absorption can be improved when the drug is administered with a high lipid content meal or orange juice.	Oral bioavailability of ketoconazole is variable among individuals. In normal subjects can be as high as 75%. Reduced gastric acidity due to achlorhydria, AIDS, antacids, or the ingestion of a high carbohydrate meal decrease its absorption. It is widely distributed in the body but penetrates poorly into the CSF. Ketoconazole is extensively metabolized in the liver with a terminal half life of 7–9 hrs.	GI: nausea and vomiting are the most frequent dose dependent side effects, 10–40%. Less frequent are abdominal pain, and anorexia. Skin: pruritus and rash, 2–4%. Liver: asymptomatic elevations of transaminases, 2–10%, hepatitis. Endocrine system: adrenal insufficiency (rare), decreased libido, impotence, gynecomastia, menstrual irregularities. Other: disulfiram-like reactions, fever, chills, photophobia (rare). Safety during pregnancy has not been established.

(*cont.*)

Table 33.2. (*cont.*)

	Administration	Pharmacokinetic profile	Toxicity
Fluconazole (Diflucan) 50, 100, and 200 mg tablets, 350 and 1400 mg oral suspension, and 2 mg/mL intravenous formulation	Oral and intravenous. Intravenous infusion is well tolerated. It is recommended that fluconazole be dosed twice daily in children with severe fungal infections. A 72 hr dosing interval seems appropriate for premature infants.	Fluconazole is rapidly and completely absorbed from the gastrointestinal tract. It is widely distributed in the body. In contrast to other systemic azoles, has low protein binding and penetrates well into virtually all tissue sites, including into the CSF. Steady-state plasma concentrations are achieved after several days, but can be rapidly attained by doubling the dose on the first day of therapy. It is eliminated primarily by renal excretion. Dose modification is recommended in individuals with renal impairment. Terminal half-life is 27–37 hrs in adults, 14–17 hrs in children, and 55–88 hrs in premature infants.	GI: nausea and vomiting 5%. Skin: rash, possible exfoliative (Stevens-Johnson syndrome), alopecia in scalp or pubic area. Liver: asymptomatic elevations of plasma transaminases 1–7%, hepatitis (rare). Other: headache, seizures Few cases of craniofacial and skeletal abnormalities following prolonged in-utero exposure to fluconazole have been reported.

| *Itraconazole* (*Sporanox*) 100 mg capsules 10 mg/ml Oral solution with cyclodextrin | Oral and intravenous. Absorption of capsules can be improved when the drug is administered with a high lipid content meal or orange juice. The drug is poorly absorbed in patients with hypo or achlor-hydria. By comparison, the oral solution of the drug does not need to be administered with food and its absorption is not affected by the level of gastric acidity. | Oral bioavailability of itraconazole is variable among individuals. In normal subjects can be as high as 70%. Reduced gastric acidity decreases its absorption. It is widely distributed in the body but penetrates poorly into the CSF or vitreous humor. However, tissue concentrations, including nervous tissue, are 2 to 5 times higher than those of plasma. Steady state plasma concentrations are achieved after 14 days, thus a loading dose during the first 3 days of therapy is recommended for treatment of serious infections. Itraconazole is extensively metabolized in the liver with a terminal half-life of 30 hrs. Itraconazole in cyclodextrin solution has improved bioavailability of the drug by as much as 30%, when administered to healthy volunteers. Children <than 12 yrs with neoplastic disease may require higher doses on a mg/kg basis (>5mg/kg/d) than adults for equivalent therapeutic benefits. Because the pharmacokinetics of the drug are related nonlinearly to dose, monitoring serum levels is recommended when treating severe fungal infections, plasma concentrations of at least 250–500 ng/ml are desirable. | GI: nausea and vomiting 5%, abdominal pain diarrhea Skin: pruritus, rash. Liver: asymptomatic elevations of plasma transaminases (1–5%), hepatitis (rare). Other: headache, dizziness, hypokalemia, hypertension, edema, impotence (rare). Safety during pregnancy has not been established. |

Table 33.2. (cont.)

	Administration	Pharmacokinetic profile	Toxicity
Voriconazole (*Vfend*) 50 and 200 mg tablets 40mg/mL. Oral suspension 200 mg vials for intravenous use	Oral and intravenous. Tablets should be taken at least 1 hour before or 1 hour after meals	Oral bioavailability of voriconazole is estimated to be 96%. It is widely distributed in the body and penetrates well into tissues. Steady state plasma concentrations are achieved within one day after a loading dose on first day of therapy. It is eliminated via hepatic metabolism via cytochrome P450 enzymes with less than 2% of the dose eliminated unchanged in the urine. The CYP2C19 is significantly involved in its metabolism. This enzyme exhibits genetic polymorphism. For example, 15–20% of Asians may be expected to be poor metabolizers and may require dose reduction. The pharmacokinetics of voriconazole are non-linear due to saturation of its metabolism. Dose modification is recommended in individuals with mild to moderate cirrhosis; after the standard loading dose, patients should receive 50% of the maintenance dose. No adjustments are needed for patients with renal impairment. Voriconazole is dialyzed but a 4 hour session does not removed sufficient amount to warrant dose adjustment.	Visual disturbances: approximately 30% of patients have experience altered or enhanced visual perception, blurred vision, color vision change, and/or photophobia. These disturbances are generally mild, occur within 30 to 60 minutes from administration, and attenuate with repeated doses. Rarely resulted in the discontinuation of the drug. Skin: rash 6%, photosensitivity usually associated with long-term treatment. GI: anorexia, nausea, vomiting, dry mouth. Liver: asymptomatic elevations of the transaminases 1–2%, hepatitis rare. Other (< 1%): fever, chills, headaches, and chest pain most likely associated with IV therapy. Tachycardia, hyper/hypotension, vasodilation, hallucination, dizziness. Safety during pregnancy has not been established.

| *Miconazole (Monistat IV)* Ampoule 200 mg Only indicated for invasive infections due to Pseudallescheria boydii | Intravenous route of administration. The drug should be diluted in D5W of 0.9% NS and infused over a period of 60–120 minutes per ampoule. | Miconazole is widely distributed to body tissues. It also penetrates well into infected joints and vitreous humor, but only relatively low concentrations are reached in the CSF. The drug is extensively metabolized in the liver with a terminal half life of 20–25hrs. | GI: nausea and vomiting ~15%. Skin: pruritus 30%, rash 10%. Hematologic: anemia 45%, leucopenia thrombocytosis or thrombocytopenia. Other: phlebitis, fever, psychosis, hyperlipidemia, hyponatremia. Rapid infusion of the drug has been associated with transient tachycardia, cardiac arrhytmias, anaphylaxis and cardiac and respiratory arrest. Initial dose requires careful observation. |

Table 33.2. (cont.)

	Miscellaneous systemic antifungal agents			
	Mechanism of action/ Spectrum of activity	Administration	Pharmacokinetic profile	Toxicity
Griseofulvin (Fulvicin, Grifulvin, Grisactin) 250–500 mg tabs 125 mg/5 ml suspension	Inhibits fungal mitosis by disrupting the mitotic spindle. Effective against all dermatophytes	Oral, administer after a high fat content meals.	Oral bioavailability varies among the individuals. Griseofulvin is metabolized in the liver with serum half life of 24–36 hrs. Increases warfarin metabolism. Barbiturates depress its activity.	GI: nausea, vomiting, abdominal pain, diarrhea. Skin: photosensitivity, urticaria, and rarely angioneurotic edema Other: leucopenia, fatigue, dizziness, headache, mental confusion, disulfram-like reaction (rare). Increases blood and urine porphyrins, should not be used in patients with porphyria.
Flucytosine (Ancobon) 250–500 mg tabs	Flucytosine is the fluorine analogue of cytosine, inhibits synthesis of both DNA and RNA. Effective against *Cryptococcus neoformans* and *Candida spp*	Oral	Is rapidly and virtually completely absorbed after oral administration. It is widely distributed in the body and achieves significant concentrations in the CSF. It is eliminated primarily by renal excretion with a serum half life of 3–5 hrs. Dose modification is recommended in individuals with renal impairment. Antifungal synergism between flucytosine and amphotericin B, has been reported.	GI (6%) diarrhea, anorexia, nausea, vomiting. Hematologic (22%): leucopenia, thrombocytopenia, when serum level >70 μg/mL. Aplastic anemia (very rare). Liver: asymptomatic increase in transaminases. Skin (7%): rash

Drug	Mechanism / Spectrum	Route	Pharmacokinetics	Adverse effects
Terbinafine (Lamisil) 250 mg tabs	Interferes with the ergosterol biosynthetic pathway in the fungal cell wall, inhibiting the enzyme squalene epoxidase. Effective against all dermatophytes, *Malassezia furfur* and *Candida albicans*. Its MICs and MFCs against dermatophytes are the lowest of all currently available systemic antifungal agents.	Oral	Good oral bioavailability. Steady state concentrations occur after 10–14 days of treatment with skin, stratum corneum and nailplate concentrations above the MFC for dermatophytes. Therapeutic levels persist for a considerable period after cessation of therapy, also favoring short duration therapy.	GI (5%): anorexia, abdominal pain, diarrhea Skin (2%): rash Liver: asymptomatic increase of transaminases Other: malaise, exacerbation of SLE.
Caspofungin (Cancidas) 50 mg vials for intravenous use	Inhibits the synthesis of (β 1–3)-glucan in the fungal cell wall. Effective against *Candida* and *Aspergillus* spp.	IV	The drug is highly protein bound (97%), has a plasma elimination half-life of 9–10 hrs, and is metabolized to inactive metabolites in the liver. Dose adjustment in moderate hepatic failure appears to be necessary. No dose modification is needed in renal failure.	GI: nausea, vomiting Fever Headacke Liver: asymptomatic increase in transaminases Infusion related reactions, histamine-type reactions.
Micafungin (Mycamine) 50 mg vials for intravenous use	Inhibits the synthesis of (β 1–3)-glucan in the fungal cell wall. Effective against *Candida* and *Aspergillus* spp.	IV	The drug is highly protein bound (99%). The primary protein is albumin, however, the drug does not competitively displace bilirubin binding to albumin. It is metabolized to inactive metabolites in the liver. The cytochrome P450 enzymes are not a major pathway for micafungin metabolism. No dose modification is needed in renal failure or moderate hepatic insufficiency.	GI: nausea, vomiting Headache Liver: asymptomatic increase in transaminases infusion related reactions, histamine-type reactions

MIC: minimal inhibitory concentration; CSF: cerebrospinal fluid; RTA: renal tubular acidosis; GFR: glomerular filtration rate; RES: reticulo-endothelial system; MFC: minimal fungicidal concentration; GI: gastrointestinal

Table 33.3. Drug interactions involving azole antifungal drugs

Effect and drug involved	Clinically important interaction	Potentially important interaction[a]
Decrease plasma concentration of the azole		
– Decrease absorption		
Antacids	Ketoconazole, Itraconazole	
H2-receptor antagonist drugs	Ketoconazole, Itraconazole	
Sucralfate		Ketoconazole
– Increase metabolism		
Isoniazid	Ketoconazole	
Phenytoin	Ketoconazole, Itraconazole, Voriconazole	
Lond acting barbiturates, Carbamazepine		Voriconazole
Rifampin, Rifabutin	Ketoconazole, Itraconazole, Voriconazole[h]	Fluconazole
Efavirenz, Ritonavir	Voriconazole[h]	
Increase plasma concentration of the azole		
Ritonavir, Indinavir	Itraconazole	Ketoconazole, Miconazole
Clarithromycin, Erythromycin	Itraconazole	
Increase plasma concentration of the coadministered drug		
Cyclosporine, Tacrolimus, Sirolimus	Ketoconazole, Fluconazole, Itraconazole Voriconazole[h]	
Methylprednisolone		Itraconazole
Digoxin		Itraconazole
Nifedipine, Amlodipine, Felodipine	Itraconazole	Voriconazole
Lovastatin, Simvastatin	Itraconazole	Voriconazole
Phenytoin	Ketoconazole, Fluconazole, Voriconazole	Itraconazole
Carbamazepine	Itraconazole	
Sulfonilurea drugs, specially Tolbutamide		Ketoconazole, Itraconazole, Fluconazole, Voriconazole
Terfenadine and Aztemizole[b]	Ketoconazole, Itraconazole, Fluconazole	Voriconazole
Cisapride[b]	Ketoconazole, Itraconazole, Fluconazole	Voriconazole
Midazolam, Triazolam, Alprazolam[c]	Ketoconazole, Itraconazole	Fluconazole, Voriconazole

Table 33.3. (*cont.*)

Effect and drug involved	Clinically important interaction	Potentially important interaction[a]
Rifabutin	Itraconazole	
Sildenafil citrate	Itraconazole, Fluconazole	
Buspirone	Itraconazole	
Busulfan, Vinca alkaloids	Itraconazole, Voriconazole	
Oxibutinin	Itraconazole	
Quinidine	Itraconazole	
Theophilline		Itraconazole, Fluconazole
Warfarine	Itraconazole, Voriconazole, Fluconazole	Ketoconazole
Zidovudine		Fluconazole
Saquinavir[d]		Fluconazole
Indinavir, Ritonavir[e]	Itraconazole	Ketoconazole, Itraconazole
Omeprazole	Voriconazole	
Decrease plasma concentration of the coadministered drug		
Theophylline	Ketoconazole	
Didanosine[f]	Ketoconazole, Itraconazole	

[a.] This information is based on results of controlled studies or limited observations in patients. Monitoring of plasma concentrations and an adjustment in the dose may be indicated.

[b.] Elevated plasma levels of their metabolites may prolong QT intervals on EKG and cause cardiac arrhytmias. Therefore, administration of these drugs with ketoconazole, itraconazole, and voriconazole is contraindicated.

[c.] Elevated plasma levels of both drugs may prolong hypnotic and sedative effects.

[d.] No dose adjustment of saquinavir is required.

[e.] A dose reduction of Indinavir should be considered when coadministered with ketoconazole.

[f.] Give at least two hours between administration of didanosine and azoles.

[h.] Voriconazole is contraindicated when co-administered with sirolimus, rifabutin, efavirenz, and ritonavir.

with satellite papules and pustules. In HIV-infected infants, this condition tends to recur, requiring protracted therapy. Treatment includes attentive local care with frequent diaper changes and good hygiene, and antifungal therapy. Initial treatment often consists of topical nystatin, with clotrimazole or miconazole cream used for further treatment. Simultaneous administration of oral antifungal agents, such as nystatin, may further reduce colonization. Treatment may require one to three weeks. Persistence of dermatitis during nystatin treatment, may indicate dermatophytosis [10, 11].

Table 33.4. Drugs of choice for selected fungal infections

Infection	Drug of choice	Dosage	Alternative Therapy
Aspergillosis	Amphotericin B or	1–1.5 mg/kg/d, IV	Itraconazole [a,b,c] 5–12 mg/kg/d, PO/IV
	Lipid formulations	5–8 mg/kg/d, IV	Caspofungin 70 mg/m2 day 1 and 50 mg/m2/d IV, thereafter
	Voriconazole	6 mg/kg IV/PO q 12h day 1 and 4mg/kd IV/PO q 12h thereafter if > 40 kg 200 mg q 12h.	Voriconazole + Caspofungin (same dosages)
Blastomycosis	Amphotericin B	0.5–1 mg/kg/d, IV	Itraconazole [a,b] 5–12 mg/kg/d, PO/IV
			Ketoconazole 5–10 mg/kg/d, PO
Candidiasis			
Oropharyngeal	Nystatin or	200–600.000 U q6h, PO	Itraconazole [a,b] 5–12 mg/kg/d, PO
	Clotrimazole (trouches)	10 mg 5 times a day, PO	Amphotericin B 100 mg qid, PO
Esophageal	Fluconazole	3–12 mg/kg/d, PO	Amphotericin B 0.5–1 mg/kg/d, IV
	Fluconazole	3–12 mg/kg/d, PO/IV	Ketoconazole 5–10 mg/kg/d, PO
	Amphotericin B	0.5–1 mg/kg/d, IV	Itraconazole [a,b] 5–12 mg/kg/d PO/IV
	Caspofungin	50 mg/m2/d IV	Ketoconazole 5–10 mg/kg/d, PO
	Fluconazole [e]	3–12 mg/kg/d, PO	
Chronic suppression [d]			Itraconazole [a,b] 5–12 mg/kg/d, PO
			Ketoconazole 5–10 mg/kg/d, PO.
Vaginal	Topical azole formulation		
	Fluconazole	150 mg/d, PO	
Disseminated	Amphotericin B or	0.6 – 1.5 mg/kg/d, IV	Voriconazole 6 mg/kg IV/PO q 12h day 1 and 4 mg/ kd IV/PO q 12h thereafter if > 40 kg 200 mg q 12h.
	Lipid formulations±	5 mg/kg/d, IV	
	Fluocytosine [f,g]	100–150 mg/kg/d ÷ q6h, PO	
	Fluconazole [h]	8–12 mg/kg/d, IV	
	Caspofungin	70 mg/m2 day 1 and 50 mg/m2/d IV, thereafter	
Coccidioidomycosis	Amphotericin B	0.5–1mg/kg/d, IV j	Fluconazole 8–12 mg/kg/d PO/IV [i]
			Itraconazole [a,b] 5–12 mg/kg/d, PO/IV
Chronic suppression [d]	Fluconazole	8–12 mg/kg/d PO	Amphotericin B 0.5–1 mg/kg/weekly, IV
			Itraconazole [a,b] 5–12 mg/kg/d, PO/IV
Cryptococcosis	Amphotericin B +	0.7–1 mg/kg/d, IV [a]	Fluconazole 12 mg/kd/d, PO/IV [i]
	Fluocytosine [g]	100–150 mg/kg/d ÷ q6h, PO	
Chronic suppression [d]	Fluconazole	12 mg/kg/d, PO/IV	Amphotericin B 0.5–1 mg/kg weekly, IV
			Itraconazole [a,b] 5–12 mg/kg/d, PO
Histoplasmosis	Amphotericin B or	0.5–1 mg/kg/d, IV	Itraconazole [a,b] 5–12 mg/kg/d, PO/IV
	Lipid formulations [i]	3–5 mg/kg/d, IV	Ketoconazole 5–10 mg/kg/d, PO
	Itraconazole [a,b]	5–12 mg/kg/d, PO	Amphotericin B 0.5–0.8 mg/kg per weekly, IV
Chronic suppression [d]			

(cont.)

	Drug of choice	Dose	Alternative(s) / Dose
Paracoccidioidomycosis	Amphotericin B	0.5 mg/kg/d, IV	Itraconazole[a,b] 5–12 mg/kg qd or bid, PO
Chronic suppression[d]	Fluconazole	12 mg/kg/d, PO/IV	Ketoconazole 5–10 mg/kg qd or bid, PO or a sulfonamide[k] Amphotericin B 0.5–1 mg/kg weekly, IV
Penicilliosis	Amphotericin B	0.5–1 mg/kg/d, IV	Itraconazole[a,b] 5–12 mg/kg/d, PO
Chronic suppression[d]	Itraconazole[a,b]	5–12 mg/kg	Itraconazole[a,b] 12 mg/kg/d, IV/PO
Phaeohyphomycosis	Amphotericin B ± Flucytosine[g]	1–1.5 mg/kg/d, IV 100–150 mg/kg/d, PO	Itraconazole[a,b] 12 mg/kg/d, IV/PO Voriconazole 6 mg/kg IV/PO q 12h day 1 and 4 mg/kd IV/PO q 12h thereafter. If > 40 kg 200mg q 12h for *S. prolificans* infection
Pseudoallescheriasis	Voriconazole	6 mg/kg IV/PO q 12h day 1 and 4 mg/kg IV/PO q 12h thereafter 200 mg q 12 h	Ketoconazole 5–10 mg/kg/d, PO
	Itraconazole	5–12 mg/kg/d, IV/PO	
Sporotrichosis Cutaneous	Itraconazole[a,b]	5–12 mg/kg/d, IV/PO	Potassium iodide 1–5 ml tid, PO Fluconazole 3–6 mg/kg/d
Systemic	Amphotericin B	0.5–1 mg/kg/d, IV	Itraconazole[a,b] 12 mg/kg/d, IV/PO
Trichosporonosis Systemic	Amphotericin B + Fluconazole + Flucytosine	1–1.5 mg/kg/d, IV 8–12 mg/kg/d, IV 100–150 mg/kg/d ÷ q6h, PO	
Zygomycosis	Amphotericin B Lipid formulation	1–1.5 mg/kg/d, IV 5–10 mg/kg/d, IV	No dependable alternative

a. Dosage adjustment required if absorption impaired by reduced gastric acidity.
b. For life-threatening infections require a loading dose; 4 mg/kg tid for 3 days is sufficient.
c. For aspergillosis, itraconazole is appropriate after completion of a course of amphotericin B, in stable patients
d. There are no data on which to base specific recommendations in children, but lifelong suppressive therapy is appropriate.
e. Recommended only if subsequent episodes are frequent or severe.
f. Flucytosine may be useful in combination with amphotericin B when there is a deep seated infection, particularly in the central nervous system.
g. To minimize bone marrow suppression, peak plasma concentrations should be maintained between 40–60 μg/mL. Monitoring serum levels is required.
h. Only in uncomplicated candidemia.
i. For life-threatening or severe infections in children, higher doses are recommended, 10–12 mg/kg in two divided doses. Loading dose is twice the target dose on first day therapy.
j. Recent findings indicate that fluconazole is effective against coccidioidal meningitis in adults. Thus, a trial of fluconazole appears warranted before starting intrathecal amphotericin B. Intraventricular, intralumbar, or intracisternal injection has been recommended in addition to IV amphotericin B for coccidioidal meningitis, the initial dos of 0.1 mg three times a week is increased gradually to a maximum of 0.5 mg, with hydrocortisone (10–15 mg) added as required to relieve headache.
k. Sulfadiazine 4–6 grams/day, or a long term sulfonamide such as sulfamethoxypyridazine 1–2 grams/day.
l. Ambisome, Amphotericin B colloidal dispersion, and Amphotericin B lipid complex.

Dermatophyte Infections

Dermatophytosis is caused by *Microsporum* spp., *Trichophyton* spp., and *Epidermophyton floccosum*. Common dermatophyte infections are tinea capitis, tinea corporis, and tinea fascialis. Tinea capitis is highly infectious. It may present with a variety of lesions, including gray patch scaling, conditions mimicking seborrheic dermatitis, black dot alopecia, folliculitis, pustules, and kerion [10]. Tinea facialis and corporis appear as scaling macular eruptions on the face, hairline, or body. Potassium hydroxide (KOH) direct examination, or calcofluor examination, and culture can be used to verify the diagnosis. The treatment of choice for tinea capitis remains griseofulvin, administered twice daily with a fatty meal, ideally accompanied by 2.5% selenium sulfide, 4% povidone iodine, or ketoconazole shampoos [10–13]. Either shampoo will decrease transmission of infection to households [13]. Treatment duration is guided clinically and by negative hair cultures. Relapses are managed with systemic azoles or terbinafine. Treatment of tinea facialis or corporis includes topical azoles or terbinafine [11].

Other superficial fungal infections

Tinea versicolor (*Malassezia furfur*) presents with hyper- or hypopigmented macules on the shoulders, neck and upper chest. Infectious folliculitis is another manifestation of *M. furfur* infection of the skin. Both conditions can be treated with topical azoles, but recurrence is common. An alternative is a short course of an oral azole for 2 weeks [10]. Onychomycosis may be managed with grisofulvin or oral azoles, but long duration therapy is required. Terbinafine is an effective alternative for onychomycosis [10, 11].

Mucosal infections

Oropharyngeal candidiasis

Oropharyngeal candidiasis is the most common opportunistic infection in HIV-infected children. Manifestations of oral candidiasis can include punctate or diffuse mucosal erythema, angular cheilitis, and white–beige plaques on the oropharyngeal mucosa. These lesions may become confluent, involving extensive regions of the oral mucosa. The plaques can be removed with difficulty to reveal a granular base that bleeds easily. Severe oropharyngeal candidiasis may impair alimentation. The diagnosis is based on clinical signs and symptoms and confirmed by the response to antifungals. Definite diagnosis requires direct microscopic examination and culture confirmation.

Topical antifungals usually control oropharyngeal candidiasis and are recommended for initial therapy. Nystatin has limited activity in moderate to advanced forms in immunocompromised hosts [14]. Clotrimazole, administered four to five times per day, appears to be more active than nystatin, but clotrimazole troches must be retained in the mouth until completely dissolved, a difficulty in younger children. Children with oropharyngeal candidiasis refractory to topical therapy can be treated with oral fluconazole, a triazole usually effective for treatment of oropharyngeal and esophageal candidiasis [14–16]. However, an increasing number of reports describe *Candida* infections refractory to fluconazole [2, 17–19]. These cases usually occur in children with severely depressed cell-mediated immunity and involve *Candida* strains with demonstrated resistance to fluconazole [20]. Such patients may respond well to short and intermittent courses of amphotericin B. Cyclodextrin itraconazole, an itraconazole formulation with improved bioavailability, has been successfully used in children and adults with fluconazole-refractory oropharyngeal candidiasis [21].

Esophageal candidiasis

Esophageal candidiasis can occur with or without oropharyngeal candidiasis, or other infections of the esophagus such as herpes simplex, cytomegalovirus, and bacterial infections. Symptoms can include substernal pain, dysphagia, and odynophagia [22, 23]. Some patients may be asymptomatic. Esophagoscopy with mucosal biopsy is the most definitive method for establishing a diagnosis (Fig. 33.1). However, this practice may not be feasible or safe in many children and an empirical approach based on clinical presentation and a positive barium swallow with the typical moth-eaten appearance (Fig. 33.2) is often warranted. Children with HIV infection may initially receive therapy, depending upon severity of symptoms and level of immunosuppression, with oral or intravenous triazoles, caspofungin or amphotericin B. Nystatin is ineffective.

Vulvovaginal candidiasis

Vulvovaginal candidiasis is a common infection in HIV-infected adolescents [24]. Recurrent episodes of vulvovaginal candidiasis often precede the oropharyngeal infection. Symptoms include vulvar pruritus, burning or pain, thick and curdy vaginal discharge, and external dysuria. Rapid microscopic examination of a fresh wet mount is the recommended method for confirmation of vaginal candidiasis [24]. Treatment includes topical azoles or short courses of oral fluconazole.

Other mucosal fungal infections

Laryngeal candidiasis or *Candida* epiglottitis typically occurs in the setting of oropharyngeal candidiasis. Patients may develop hoarseness, laryngeal stridor and respiratory compromise [25]. Treatment includes amphotericin B or intravenous fluconazole.

Invasive fungal infections

Infections due to opportunistic fungi
Disseminated candidiasis

Disseminated candidiasis is unusual in HIV-infected children [26, 27]. It may arise from the gastrointestinal tract, particularly when herpes simplex or cytomegalovirus infections disrupt mucosal barriers, but more typically it occurs in association with indwelling central venous catheters [26–28]. It may develop as isolated candidemia or as a disseminated disease with deep organ involvement. Common complications

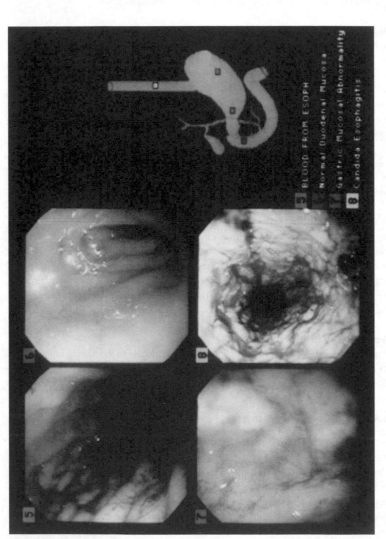

Fig. 33.1. Upper gastrointestinal endoscopy showing confluent white–beige plaques on the esophageal mucosa due to *Candida albicans*.

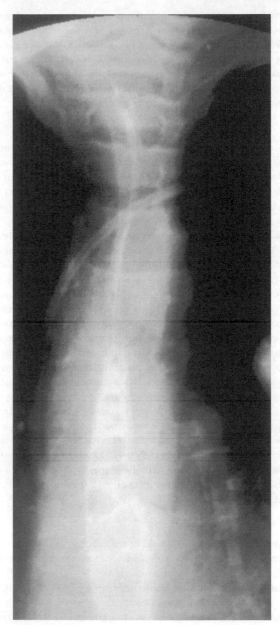

Fig. 33.2. Esophagogram of a patient with esophageal candidiasis; typical moth-eaten appearance.

include endophthalmitis, renal candidiasis, arthritis, and osteomyelitis. About half of all reported cases of fungemia in HIV-infected children have been due to non-*albicans* *Candida* species [27]. Successful management of candidemia or disseminated candidiasis depends on early detection by blood cultures, removal of the central venous catheter, and rapid institution of antifungal treatment for an average duration of two to three weeks. Since non-*albicans* species of *Candida* are frequently involved, fluconazole is not recommended as a first-line therapy.

Cryptococcosis

Cryptococcus usually enters via the respiratory tract, but pulmonary involvement usually remains clinically silent while the organism seeds the central nervous system and causes meningoencephalitis. Mortality has been associated with fulminant cryptococcemia and disseminated disease. Clinical manifestations can range from fever of unknown origin, to chronic meningitis, to septic shock [29, 30]. Meningitis is probably the most common manifestation of cryptococcosis in children. Fever, headache, and altered mental status are frequent symptoms. These can be indolent, evolving over weeks. Such subtle manifestations, as well as the benefit of early treatment on outcome, clearly justify a low threshold for initiating appropriate diagnostic investigations in symptomatic HIV-infected children. Diagnosis is established by lumbar puncture, direct examination of CSF with India ink stain, and culture. Latex agglutination cryptococcal polysaccharide antigen titers in serum and cerebrospinal fluid correlate with the tissue burden of *C. neoformans* and are an important tool in the diagnosis and evaluation of the therapeutic response [31]. The choice of antifungal drugs and duration of treatment are not well defined in children. Data from the adult population indicate that induction therapy with the combination of amphotericin B plus flucytosine results in earlier cerebrospinal fluid clearance and fewer relapses than amphotericin B alone [32]. Lipid formulations of amphotericin B also are effective for induction therapy of cryptococcosis [33–35]. Induction therapy can be limited to the period of clinical response (2–6 weeks). Fluconazole plus flucytosine is a potent oral antifungal regimen in adults, however little is known about this combination in children [36, 37]. HIV-infected children with cryptococcosis must be treated indefinitely. Fluconazole is typically used for long-term suppressive therapy [15, 38–40]. In the presence of hydrocephalus, reduction of high intracranial pressures by serial lumbar punctures or by shunting of ventricular fluid is recommended.

Aspergillosis

Aspergillosis is an infrequent, but often lethal, fungal infection in children with AIDS [41, 42]. Invasive pulmonary and sinus aspergillosis are most common; cutaneous and disseminated infections have also been reported in HIV-infected children [42]. Clinical manifestations may be subtle, and include intermittent fever, headache, cough, dyspnea, and pleuritic pain. Hemoptysis and epistaxis are usually associated with advanced disease. Neutropenia was observed in about 70% of the HIV-infected children reported with invasive aspergillosis. The chest radiographic pattern is non-specific and includes subpleural infiltrates, bronchopneumonia, or cavitary lesions. The need for establishing a specific diagnosis is essential in the management of aspergillosis. Thus, induced sputum or brochoalveolar lavage should be performed. Recovery of *Aspergillus* species from a respiratory site in an HIV-infected patient with pulmonary infiltrates not responsive to broad-spectrum antibiotics should be considered a significant indication of true infection and treatment should be initiated immediately. In the case of negative results, fine needle aspiration or open lung biopsy are indicated. Therapy for aspergillosis consists of high-dose amphotericin B or voriconazole resection. Surgical removal of the affected area should be strongly considered. Particularly in the setting of neutropenia, granulocyte colony-stimulating factor or granulocyte macrophage colony-stimulating factor may be used as adjunctive therapy. Even if complete resolution is achieved, long-term suppressive therapy with itraconazole is required. The new oral formulation in cyclodextrin is preferable because of its improved bioavailability.

Infections due to dimorphic fungi
Histoplasmosis
Histoplasmosis in pediatric AIDS patients generally progresses from a primary pulmonary focus to widespread dissemination [43–45]. The infection is often fatal if untreated. Clinical manifestations may include recurrent fevers, weight loss, generalized malaise, respiratory symptoms, hepatosplenomegaly, and lymphadenopathy. A distinctive syndrome of severe disseminated histoplasmosis consists of fever, cutaneous lesions, pulmonary infiltrates, and thrombocytopenia or pancytopenia, and may progress to septic shock [43, 44]. The chest radiograph may demonstrate a variety of patterns, including reticulonodular, miliary, and lobar infiltrates. Histoplasmosis can be diagnosed by direct microscopic examination of fluid or tissue samples, culture, and antigen detection. Blood cultures and culture and examination of bone marrow aspirate and biopsy can be used for rapid and reliable diagnosis in case of disseminated infection. Biopsy may demonstrate non-caseating and caseating granulomas with small 2–4 %μ diameter yeast-like cells within the cytoplasm of macrophages. Organisms may also be identified on bronchoalveolar lavage or lung biopsy. Differentiating non-budding yeast cells of *H. capsulatum* from the cysts of *Pneumocystis carinii* may be difficult; the use of calcofluor white and monoclonal antibodies may facilitate this differential diagnosis. Importantly, diagnosis of histoplasmosis can be achieved by antigen detection in serum and urine [46]. With lower diagnostic yields, antigen detection can also be applied to CSF or bronchoalveolar lavage. *H. capsulatum* antigen detection offers a non-invasive mean, for monitoring disease response to anti-fungal therapy [47, 48]. Circulating antibodies against *H. capsulatum* can be detected by complement fixation. However, this test relies on antibody production by the host, which is often impaired in the setting of HIV infection. The treatment of choice for histoplasmosis in children with AIDS is amphotericin B. It has been demonstrated in adults with AIDS and histoplasmosis that amphotericin B, particularly liposomal

amphotericin B, induces a more rapid clearance of fungal burden than itraconazole [47]. Itraconazole has been used for treatment of histoplasmosis in pediatric patients. However, no efficacy data is available. Chronic suppressive therapy with itraconazole is necessary and has been effective in maintaining long-term remissions of the disease [43, 49].

Coccidioidomycosis

Coccidioides immitis is found in semiarid areas of the southwestern United States, Mexico, and Central and South America. Children with HIV infection residing in endemic areas for *C. immitis* appear to be at risk for development of infection, which can present as a progressive pneumonia or as a disseminated infection. The most common symptoms include fever, chills, weight loss, cough, chest pain, headache, altered sensorium, and skin rashes, corresponding to involvement of lungs, brain, skin, and other tissue sites [50, 51]. Diagnosis can be established by direct examination and culture of respiratory secretions, or by biopsy. Serological tests are important in both diagnosis and monitoring of patients with coccidioidomycosis. Amphotericin B is the treatment of choice. Coccidioidomycosis has a high potential for relapse, thus chronic suppressive therapy with oral fluconazole or itraconazole is necessary [52, 53].

Penicillinosis

Penicillium marneffei has been recognized increasingly as a cause of systemic infection in HIV-infected children in Southeast Asia, where this dimorphic fungus is endemic. In northern Thailand, penicillinosis is the third most common opportunistic infection in patients with AIDS, exceeded only by tuberculosis and cryptococcosis. *P. marneffei* infection resembles disseminated histoplasmosis in HIV-infected children, but skin involvement is more common in penicillinosis. The most common presenting manifestations include fever, weight loss or failure to thrive, anemia, hepatosplenomegaly, pulmonary infiltrates, and generalized papular rash [45, 54]. Rash is present in about 60% of the cases, often consisting of papules with or without central umbilication or acne-like pustules. Microscopic examination of Wright's stained skin lesion smears is a simple and rapid diagnostic technique. *P. marneffei* also can be isolated from blood cultures and bone marrow or lymph node biopsy. The diagnosis is confirmed by visualizing the characteristic features of the yeast in tissue sections and by culture and final identification of the fungus. Both antigen and antibody detection are also available. Limited data in children and recent prospective studies in adults with AIDS suggest that an initial course of amphotericin B is effective. Those studies revealed that amphotericin B induction therapy cleared infection from blood faster than itraconazole [55]. Chronic suppression therapy is needed after the discontinuation of induction therapy. In vitro sensitivity studies showed that *P. marneffei* is sensitive to miconazole, itraconazole, and ketoconazole; fluconazole is less active [56]. Itraconazole can prevent relapse of penicillinosis; ketoconazole is a less expensive alternative [15, 56, 57].

Paracoccidioidosis

There have been few reported cases of paracoccidioidomycosis, infection with a fungus endemic to Latin America, in HIV-infected patients. This may be due to the use of co-trimoxazole, a drug that is effective against *Paracoccidioides brasiliensis*, for *Pneumocystis carinii* pneumonia prophylaxis. Paracoccidioidomycosis presents as an acute or subacute disease; clinical manifestations evolve within a few weeks and include fever, weight loss, fatigue, cough, lymphadenopathy, and skin lesions. A few patients had central nervous system disease [45].

Summary

Fungal infections are a significant cause of morbidity and mortality in children with AIDS. Recognition and diagnosis of the majority of these infections remains challenging. Despite the recent advances in antifungal drug development, therapeutic management options remain constrained by the limited number of safe and effective antifungal agents.

REFERENCES

1. Walsh, T. J., Mueller, F. M. C., Groll, A., Gonzalez, C. E., Roilides, E. Fungal infections in children with human immunodeficiency virus infection. In Pizzo, P. A., Wilfert, C. M., eds. *Pediatric AIDS. The Challenge of HIV Infection in Infants, Children, and Adolescents*, 3rd edn. Baltimore, MD: Williams & Wilkins; 1998:183–204.

2. Sangeorzan, J. A., Bradley, S. F., He, X., Zarins, L. T., Ridenour, G. L. Epidemiology of oral candidiasis in HIV-infected patients: colonization, infection, treatment, and emergence of fluconazole resistance. *Am. J. Med.* 1994;**97**:339–346.

3. Muller, F. M. C., Groll, A. H., Walsh, T. J. Current approaches to diagnosis and treatment of fungal infections in children infected with human immunodeficiency virus. *Eur. J. Pediatr.* 1999;**158**:187–199.

4. Cartledge, J. D., Midgely, J., Gazzard, B. G. Itraconazole solution: higher serum drug concentrations and better clinical response rates than the capsule formulation in acquired immunodeficiency syndrome patients with candidosis. *J. Clin. Pathol.*, 1997;**50**:477–480.

5. Groll, A. H., Walsh, T. J. Caspofungin: pharmacology, safety and therapeutic potential in superficial and invasive fungal infections. *Expert Opin. Investig. Drugs.* 2001;**10**:1545–1558.

6. O'Sullivan, D. P. Terbinafine: tolerability in general medicine. *Br. J. Dermatol.* 1999;**141** (Suppl. 56):21–25.

7. Willems, L., van der Geest, R., de Beule, K. Itraconazole oral solution and intravenous formulations: a review of pharmacokinetics and pharmacodynamics. *J. Clin. Pharm. Ther.*, 2001;**26**:159–169.

8. Gupta, A. K., Katz, H. I., Shear, N. H. Drug interactions with itraconazole, fluconazole, and terbinafine and their management. *J. Am. Acad. Dermatol.* 1999;**41**:237–249.

9. Piscitelli, S. C., Flexner, C., Minor, J. R., Polis, M. A., Masur, H. Drug interactions in patients infected with human immunodeficiency virus. *Clin. Infect. Dis.* 1996;**23**:685–693.

10. Aly, R., Berger, T. Common superficial fungal infections in patients with AIDS. *Clin. Infect. Dis.*, 1996;**22**:(Suppl 2):128–132.

11. Millikan, L. E. Role of antifungal agents for the treatment of superficial fungal infections in immunocompromised patients. *Cutis*, 2001;**68** (Suppl. 1): 6–14.

12. Bennett, M. L., Fleischer, A. B., Jr, Loveless, J. W., Feldman, S. R. Oral griseofulvin remains the treatment of choice for tinea capitis in children. *Pediatr. Dermatol.*, 2000;**17**:304–309.

13. Neil, G., Hanslo, D., Buccimazza, S., Kibel, M. Control of the carrier state of scalp dermatophytes. *Pediatr. Infect. Dis. J.* 1990;**9**:57–58.

14. Flynn, P. M., Cunningham, C. K., Kerkering, T. *et al.* Oropharyngeal candidiasis in immnocompromised children: a randomized, multicenter study of orally administered fluconazole suspension versus nystatin. *J. Pediatr.* 1995;**127**:322–328.

15. Centers for Disease Control and Prevention. USPHS/IDSA guidelines for the prevention of opportunistic infections in persons infected with human immunodeficiency virus. *Morb. Mortal. Wkly. Rep.*, 2002;**51**:RR 8.

16. Patton, L. L., Bonito, A. J., Shugars, D. A. A systematic review of the effectiveness of antifungal drugs for the treatment of oropharyngeal candidiasis in HIV-positive patients. *Oral. Surg. Oral. Med. Oral. Pathol. Oral. Radiol. Endodermatol.* 2001;**92**:170–179.

17. Lopez-Ribot, J. L., McAtee, R. K., Perea, S., Kirkpatrick, W. R., Rinaldi, M. G., Patterson, T. F. Multiple resistant phenotypes of *Candida albicans* coexist during episodes of oropharyngeal candidiasis in human immunodeficiency virus-infected patients. *Antimicrob. Agents. Chemother.*, 1999;**43**:1621–1630.

18. Maenza, J. R., Keruly, J. C., Moore, R. D., Chaisson, R. E., Merz, W. G., Gallant, J. E. Risk factors for fluconazole-resistant candidiasis in human immunodeficiency virus-infected patients. *J. Infect. Dis.* 1996;**173**:219–225.

19. Maenza, J. R., Merz, W. G., Romagnoli, M. J., Keruly, J. C., Moore, R. D., Gallant, J. E. Infection due to fluconazole-resistant *Candida* in patients with AIDS: prevalence and microbiology. *Clin. Infect. Dis.* 1997;**24**:28–34.

20. Walsh, T. J., Gonzalez, C. E., Piscitelli, S. *et al.* Correlation between in vitro and in vivo antifungal activities in experimental fluconazole-resistant oropharyngeal and esophageal candidiasis. *J. Clin. Microbiol.* 2000;**38**:2369–2373.

21. Saag, M. S., Fessel, W. J., Kaufman, C. A. Treatment of fluconazole-refractory oropharyngeal candidiasis with itraconazole oral solution in HIV-positive patients. *AIDS Res. Hum. Retroviruses.* 1999;**15**:1413–1417.

22. Chiou, C. C., Groll, A., Gonzalez, C. E. *et al.* Esophageal candidiasis in pediatric acquired immunodeficiency syndrome: clinical manifestations and risk factors. *Pediatr Infect. Dis. J.* 2000;**19**:729–734.

23. Kodsi, B. E., Wickremesinghe, P. C., Kozinn, P. J., Iswara, K., Goldberg, P. K. Candida esophagitis: a prospective study of 27 cases. *Gastroenterology* 1976;**71**:715–719.

24. Eckert, L. O., Hawes, S. E., Stevens, C. E., Koutsky, L. A., Eschenbach, D. A., Holmes, K. K. Vulvovaginal candidiasis: clinical manifestations, risk factors, management algorithm. *Obstet. Gynecol.* 1998;**92**:757–765.

25. Balsam, D., Sorrano, D., Barax, C. Candida epiglottitis presenting as stridor in a child with HIV infection. *Pediatr. Radiol.* 1992;**22**:235–236.

26. Gonzalez, C. E., Venzon, D., Lee, S., Mueller, B. U., Pizzo, P. A., Walsh, T. J. Risk factors for fungemia in pediatric HIV-infection: a case control study. *Clin. Infect. Dis.* 1996;**23**:515–552.

27. Walsh, T. J., Gonzalez, C. E., Roilides, E. Fungemia in children infected with the human immunodeficiency virus: new epidemiologic patterns, emerging pathogens, and improved outcome with antifungal therapy. *Clin. Infect. Dis.* 1995;**20**:900–906.

28. Leibovitz, E., Rigaud, M., Chandwani, S. Disseminated fungal infections in children infected with human immunodeficiency virus. *Pediatr. Infect. Dis. J.* 1991;**10**:888–894.

29. Gonzalez, C. E., Shetty, D., Lewis, L. L., Mueller, B. U., Pizzo, P. A., Walsh, T. J. Cryptococcosis in HIV-infected children. *Pediatr. Infect. Dis. J.* 1996;**15**:796–800.

30. Leggiadro, R. J., Kline, M. W., Hughes, W. T. Extrapulmonary cryptococcosis in children with acquired immunodeficiency syndrome. *Pediatr. Infect. Dis. J.* 1991;**10**:658–662.

31. Powderly, W. G., Cloud, G. A., Dismukes, W. E., Saag, M. S. Measurement of cryptococcal antigen in serum and cerebrospinal fluid: value in the management of AIDS-associated cryptococcal meningitis. *Clin. Infect. Dis.* 1994;**18**:789–792.

32. Van der, Horst C. M., Saag, M. S., Cloud, G. A. Treatment of cryptococcal meningitis associated with the acquired immunodeficiency syndrome. *N. Engl. J. Med.* 1997;**337**: 15–21.

33. Coker, R. J., Viviani, M., Gazzard, B. G. Treatment of cryptococcosis with liposomal amphotericin B (Ambisome) in 23 patients with AIDS. *AIDS* 1993;**7**:829–835.

34. Leenders, A. C., Reiss, P., Portegies, P. *et al.* Liposomal amphotericin B (AmBisome) compared with amphotericin B followed by oral fluconazole in the treatment of AIDS-associated cryptococcal meningitis. *AIDS* 1997;**11**:1463–1471.

35. Sharkey, P. K., Graybill, J. R., Johnson, E. S. *et al.* Amphotericin B lipid complex compared with amphotericin B in the treatment of cryptococcal meningitis in patients with AIDS. *Clin. Infect. Dis.* 1996;**22**:315–321.

36. Larsen, R. A., Bozzette, S. A., Jones, B. E. *et al.* Fluconazole combined with flucytosine for treatment of cryptococcal meningitis in patients with AIDS. *Clin. Infect. Dis.*, 1994;**19**:741–745.

37. Larsen, R. A., Leal, M. A., Chan, L. S. Fluconazole compared with amphotericin B plus flucytosine for cryptococcal meningitis in AIDS. A randomized trial. *Ann. Intern. Med.* 1990;**113**:183–187.

38. Bozzette, S. A., Larsen, R. A., Chiu, J. *et al.* A placebo controlled trial of maintenance therapy with fluconazole after treatment of cryptococcal meningitis in the acquired immunodeficiency syndrome. *N. Engl. J. Med.*, 1991;**324**:580–584.

39. Powderly, W. G., Saag, M. S., Cloud, G. A. *et al.* A controlled trial of fluconazole or amphotericin B to prevent relapse of cryptococcal meningitis in patients with the acquired immunodeficiency syndrome. *N. Engl. J. Med.*, 1992;**326**:793–798.

40. Saag, M. S., Cloud, G. A., Graybill, J. R. A comparison of itraconazole versus fluconazole as maintenance therapy for AIDS-associated cryptococcal meningitis. *Clin. Infect. Dis.*, 1999;**28**:291–296.

41. Holding, K. J., Dworkin, M. S., Wan, P. C. Aspergillosis among people infected with human immunodeficiency virus: incidence and survival. Adult and adolescent spectrum of HIV disease project. *Clin. Infect. Dis.* 2000;**31**:1253–1257.

42. Shetty, D., Giri, N., Gonzalez, C. E., Pizzo, P. A., Walsh, T. J. Invasive aspergillosis in HIV-infected children. *Pediatr. Infect. Dis. J.*, 1997;**16**:216–221.

43. Byers, M., Feldman, S., Edwards, J. Disseminated histoplasmosis as the acquired immunodeficiency syndrome defining illness in an infant. *Pediatr. Infect. Dis. J.* 1992;**11**:127–128.

44. Leggiadro, R. J., Barrett, F. F., Hughes, W. T. Disseminated histoplasmosis of infancy. *Pediatr. Infect. Dis. J.* 1988;**7**:799–805.

45. Marques, S. A., Robles, A. M., Tortorano, A. M., Tuculet, M. A., Negroni, R., Mendes, R. P. Mycoses associated with AIDS in the third world. *Med. Mycol.* 2000;**38**:269–279.

46. Fojtasek, M. F., Kleiman, M. B., Connolly-Stringfield, P., Blair, R., Wheat, L. J. The *Histoplasma capsulatum* antigen assay in disseminated histoplasmosis in children. *Pediatr. Infect. Dis. J.* 1994;**13**:801–805.

47. Wheat, L. J., Cloud, G., Johnson, P. C. *et al.* Clearance of fungal burden during treatment of disseminated histoplasmosis with liposomal amphotericin B versus itraconazole. *Antimicrob. Agents Chemother.* 2001;**45**:2354–2357.

48. Wheat, L. J., Connolly, P., Haddad, N., Le Monte, A., Brizendine, E., Hafner, R. Antigen clearance during treatment of disseminated histoplasmosis with itraconazole versus fluconazole in patients with AIDS. *Antimicrob. Agents Chemother.* 2002;**46**:248–250.

49. Wheat, L. J., Hafner, R., Wulfsohn, M. *et al.* Prevention of relapse of histoplasmosis with itraconazole in patients with the acquired immunodeficiency syndrome. *Ann. Intern. Med.* 1993;**118**:610–616.

50. MacDonald, N., Steinhoff, M. C., Powell, K. R. Review of coccidiodomycosis in immunocompromised children. *Am. J. Dis. Child.*, 1981;**135**:553–556.

51. Stevens, D. A. Coccidiodomycosis. *N. Engl. J. Med.* 1995;**332**:1077–1082.

52. Galgiani, J. N., Catanzaro, A., Cloud, G. A. *et al.* Fluconazole therapy for coccidioidal meningitis. The NIAID-Mycoses Study Group. *Ann. Intern. Med.* 1993;**119**:28–35.

53. Shehab, Z. M., Britton, H., Dunn, J. H. Imidazole therapy in coccidioidal meningitis in children. *Pediatr. Infect. Dis. J.*, 1988;**7**:440–444.

54. Sirisanthana, V., Sirisanthana, T. Disseminated *Penicillium marneffei* infection in human immunodeficiency virus infected children. *Pediatr. Infect. Dis. J.* 1995;**14**:935–940.

55. Sirisanthana, T., Supparatpinyo, K., Perriens, J., Nelson, K. E. Amphotericin B and itraconazole for the treatment of disseminated *Penicillium marneffei* infection in human immunodeficiency virus-infected patients. *Clin. Infect. Dis.* 1998;**26**:1107–1110.

56. Supparatpinyo, K., Nelson, K. E., Merz, W. G. *et al.* Response to antifungal therapy by human immunodeficiency virus-infected patients with disseminated *Penicillium marneffei* infections and *in vitro* susceptibilities of isolates from clinical specimens. *Antimicrob. Agents. Chemother.* 1993;**37**:2407–2411.

57. Supparatpinyo, K., Perriens, J., Nelson, K., Sirisanthana, T. A controlled trial of itraconazole to prevent relapse of *Penicillium marneffei* infection in patients with the human immunodeficiency virus. *N. Engl. J. Med.* 1998;**339**:1739–1743.

34 Herpesvirus infections

Richard M. Rutstein, M.D.

Division of General Pediatrics, Children's Hospital of Philadelphia, Philadelphia, PA

Stuart E. Starr, M.D.

(Formerly): Division of Allergy, Immunologic and Infectious Diseases, Children's Hospital of Philadelphia, Philadelphia, PA

Introduction

Herpesviruses share a common structure: double-stranded DNA, surrounded by a protein capsid and a lipid and glycoprotein envelope. Primary infection typically occurs during childhood or early adult years. Beyond neonates, infection rarely results in serious illness in immunocompetent hosts. Herpesvirus infections are usually controlled by the cellular immune system (see Chapter 1): immunocompromised patients can develop serious, life-threatening herpesvirus infections. In normal hosts herpesviruses establish lifelong, latent infection, which may reactivate. Sites harboring latent infection are sensory autonomic ganglia, for herpes simplex virus (HSV) and varicella-zoster virus (VZV); for cytomegalovirus (CMV), Epstein–Barr virus (EBV) and human herpesvirus 6 (HHV-6), lymphocytes are latent reservoirs. A complex interplay exists between herpesviruses and HIV [1]. In some in vitro systems, infection with CMV or HSV may increase susceptibility of cells to HIV infection. In HIV-infected cells, infection with CMV or HSV can upregulate HIV expression. Co-infection with HIV and CMV enhances CMV replication.

In immunocompromised hosts, primary herpesvirus infections may be more severe than in healthy children. Reactivation infections occur more frequently and severely in HIV-infected children. CMV, HSV, VZV, and Epstein–Barr virus (EBV), HHV-6, and human herpesvirus-8 (HHV-8 or Kaposi's sarcoma-associated herpesvirus, KSHV) cause significant morbidity in HIV-infected individuals.

Cytomegalovirus (CMV)

Epidemiology

CMV is transmitted via blood, urine, saliva, tears, breast milk, stool, and genital secretions. CMV may be transmitted in utero, perinatally, or postnatally. In children, infection

Handbook of Pediatric HIV Care, ed. Steven L. Zeichner and Jennifer S. Read.
Published by Cambridge University Press. © Cambridge University Press 2006.

usually occurs through saliva or urine. In young adulthood, CMV seropositivity rates rise secondary to sexual activity.

In developed countries, 10%–15% of children are infected by early adolescence, with increased rates among lower socioeconomic groups. In developing countries CMV is frequently acquired in infancy. Prevalence increases to ~50% in women of childbearing age. Seropositivity increases with advancing age; virtually all individuals seroconvert eventually.

Congenital CMV infection is the most common intrauterine infection in the USA, affecting 1%–2% of all infants, 5%–10% of whom are symptomatic, with associated mental retardation, sensorineural hearing loss, chorioretinitis, and neurologic defects [2]. Transmission from mother to fetus results from primary and recurrent maternal infection, though symptomatic infection is more likely with primary infection.

Perinatal CMV infection (acquired intrapartum, or via breast feeding) occurs in 25%–50% of neonates exposed to CMV in the birth canal [3]. Infection occurs in up to 40%–60% of infants breastfed for >1 month by seropositive mothers [2]. Beyond the neonatal period, CMV infection is typically asymptomatic, although an EBV-negative mononucleosis syndrome can occur.

The rate of CMV seropositivity is higher among adults with lifestyles associated with high risk for HIV infection, 85%–90% in healthy, gay adults. HIV-infected infants have an increased incidence of congenital/perinatal CMV infection [4–7].

Possible influence of CMV infection on rate of progression of HIV infection

In HIV-infected adults and children, co-infection with CMV results in more rapid HIV disease progression, shortened survival, and worse immunological parameters [7, 8]. However, since severely immunocompromised HIV-infected patients are more likely to have CMV viremia, CMV co-infection may be associated with HIV disease progression, but not cause it.

Clinical manifestations

CMV is the most frequent severe viral opportunistic infection in HIV-infected persons. CMV infection is implicated in 10% of deaths in adults with AIDS; evidence of CMV disease is found at autopsy in 50%–75% of HIV-infected adults. While pneumonitis is the most common CMV disease in bone marrow transplant recipients, retinal and gastrointestinal manifestations of CMV are the primary syndromes in adults with AIDS [9, 10].

CMV-related clinical syndromes include retinitis, colitis, esophagitis, gastritis, encephalitis, polyradiculitis, hepatitis, and adrenalitis. In adults, retinitis is the most common manifestation of CMV disease (50%–80% of cases), followed by colitis and pneumonitis. CMV disease clinical manifestations generally do not occur until the CD4+ lymphocyte count falls below $100/mm^3$. The risk of developing retinitis over 24 months is 20% and 40%, for adults with CD4 counts of $<100/mm^3$ and $<50/mm^3$, respectively. The median CD4+ lymphocyte count at diagnosis of retinopathy is <50 cells/mm^3 [9, 10]. In children, CMV causes 8%–10% of AIDS-defining illness; retinitis accounts for 25%. CMV end organ disease of the liver, colon, lung, or brain accounts for 75%. The overall lifetime incidence of CMV-related disease in HIV-infected children before HAART is 30%–60%. Through 2001, CMV-end organ disease occured in ~10% of children with AIDS in the USA. About 25% of children with a CMV positive blood or urine culture had autopsy evidence of CMV disease [4–7].

The incidence of CMV infection and excretion increases with HIV disease progression. Symptomatic HIV-infected children have a higher rate of CMV viruria than asymptomatic HIV-infected children and HIV-exposed children (46% vs. 14%). Once CMV shedding begins, it generally continues. One-third of HIV-infected children (60% of children with AIDS), 15%–20% of HIV-exposed, uninfected children, and <15% of unexposed infants shed CMV [4–8].

Specific organ systems

Retinitis

CMV retinitis (see Chapter 20) occurs in 10%–20% of adult AIDS patients, up to 30% have evidence of CMV retinitis at autopsy. Disease typically begins unilaterally, but often progresses to bilateral disease. Symptoms include loss of vision, visual field cuts, and floaters. In children, the disease is frequently asymptomatic, discovered on ophthalmologic examination. Fever and irritability may be the only signs of CMV retinitis in infancy.

The CMV-diseased retina has large yellowish-white, granular areas with perivascular exudates and hemorrhage. Histological findings include coagulation necrosis and microvascular abnormalities. CMV retinits must be differentiated from HIV-related retinopathy. In the latter condition, cotton wool spots, representing areas of ischemic atrophy, appear on the retina (See Chapter 20).

Gastrointestinal manifestations

The incidence of CMV gastrointestinal disease in adults with AIDS ranges from 4%–52% [11]. Gastrointestinal CMV disease is the most common condition leading to abdominal surgery in HIV-infected adults. Patients presenting with sudden severe abdominal pain must be evaluated for CMV-related gastrointestinal perforation and/or hemorrhage.

Many gastrointestinal tract cell types can be infected with CMV, most commonly vascular endothelial cells, but also fibroblasts, smooth muscle cells, and glandular epithelium. The most common GI manifestation, CMV colitis, occurs in 5%–10% of adults with AIDS. Presenting symptoms are non-specific and include diarrhea, abdominal pain, weight loss, hematochezia, anorexia, and fever. Other possible causes of colitis in an HIV-infected patient include common bacterial pathogens (*Mycobacterium avium* complex, *Giardia lamblia*, *Cryptosporidium parvum*, *Clostridium difficile*) and primary HIV colitis. Massive acute bleeding from CMV colitis and perforation can occur; toxic megacolon may be a complication. CMV may mimic Crohn's disease or cause pseudomembranous colitis.

CMV can also cause oral and esophageal ulcers, and esophagitis. Symptoms may include substernal pain, dysphagia, odynophagia, and decreased appetite, with or without fever [12].

Hepatic involvement with CMV is common, but generally mild. Histologic evidence of CMV hepatitis is seen in 25%–33% of patients with end-organ CMV disease. Liver enzymes and alkaline phosphatase may be elevated; bilirubin levels are usually normal. Ascending cholangiopathy has also been associated with CMV infection. The disease presents with fever, right upper quadrant abdominal pain, and elevated serum alkaline phosphatase levels. CMV gastric infection produces epigastric pain, nausea, and vomiting. Infection can progress to overt gastric ulcers, with or without bleeding, gastric outlet obstruction, and perforation. Rarely, CMV has been implicated as the etiology of pancreatitis.

Pulmonary disease

CMV is an infrequent pulmonary pathogen in HIV-infected individuals. Even when CMV is isolated from lung secretions or tissue, its role in causing lung disease may be difficult to assess. Patients with CMV lung infection may have disease caused by another pathogen, for example *Pneumocystis* [13, 14].

CMV pneumonia is generally interstitial, with gradual onset of shortness of breath and a dry, non-productive cough. Auscultatory findings are minimal. CMV pneumonia is more common in adults with other end-organ CMV disease, and severe immunosuppression (CD4 $< 25/\text{mm}^3$). Median survival after diagnosis is less than 30 days [15].

Central nervous system

Autopsy series report central nervous system (CNS) CMV infection in 20%–50% of AIDS patients [16]. Some cases of CMV-related encephalopathy and ventriculitis have been reported. Both HIV- and CMV-related encephalopathy are characterized by diffuse increased white matter signal density on magnetic resonance imaging studies. CMV culture of the CSF often remains negative, even in proven cases of CMV encephalopathy. CMV has been implicated in axonal polyradiculopathy in adults. This disease presents much like Guillain–Barré syndrome, with painful, ascending muscle weakness, loss of deep tendon reflexes, and loss of bladder/bowel control.

Diagnosis

The distinction between CMV infection and CMV disease is difficult. In children >12 months, detection of CMV antibody indicates prior infection, but not necessarily disease. A positive CMV urine culture or detection of CMV antigen in shell vial cultures indicates CMV infection, but since HIV-infected children may excrete virus for prolonged periods, a positive urine culture does not define the time of primary infection, except when urine culture had previously been negative.

Isolation of virus in cultured cells remains the standard for diagnosing CMV infection. Classic culture methods require 1 to 3 weeks for isolation of CMV; using centrifugation-assisted shell vial culture amplification techniques, CMV may be detected within 24 hours. CMV can be isolated from only one-third of patients with known CMV and from oropharyngeal secretions of only one-third of patients with esophageal lesions with histologic evidence of CMV [12]. Several diagnostic methods, including detection of pp65 antigenemia, qualitative and quantitative PCR, and DNA hybridization can detect CMV infection 3–6 months prior to the development of clinically recognized disease.

Detection of CMV antigenemia involves staining neutrophils with monoclonal antibody directed against the viral matrix protein, pp65. Cells are counted by flow cytometry and results reported as the number of stain-positive cells per 50 000 or 200 000 counted cells. Plasma DNA PCR is more sensitive than urine or blood cultures and may be the most sensitive test for identifying patients at high risk for CMV disease, including CMV retinitis (plasma DNA PCR > 100–1000 copies/ul). Detection of CMV by DNA PCR and/or antigenemia accurately predicts short-term risk of developing CMV-related end-organ disease. Patients who convert from positive to negative CMV PCR DNA while on anti-CMV therapy have better outcomes. Effective therapy also decreases pp65 antigenemia [17, 18]. While fundoscopic examination can usually make the diagnosis of CMV retinitis, diagnosis of other end-organ CMV disease is based on isolation of CMV and/or characteristic histopathologic findings (pathognomonic "owl's eye" intranuclear and smaller intracytoplasmic inclusions).

With CMV-related colitis, sigmoidoscopy reveals diffuse areas of erythema, submucosal hemorrhage, and diffuse mucosal ulcerations, which may be indistinguishable from ulcerative colitis. With esophagitis the most frequent finding is a large, solitary distal ulcer. Histopathologic changes in the GI tract include vasculitis, neutrophil infiltration, and non-specific inflammation. CMV inclusions and/or positive cultures help confirm the diagnosis.

Diagnosis of CMV-related pneumonia is based on the exclusion of other pathogens, and isolation of CMV from lung tissue or bronchial fluid, with histologic evidence of CMV disease (pathognomonic cells with intranuclear inclusions). Treatment should be limited to patients with histopathologic changes at lung biopsy or, if too ill for biopsy, those with worsening pulmonary disease in the absence of other pathogens.

In CMV CNS disease, examination of the CSF reveals pleocytosis in ~50% of cases, frequently with a polymorphonuclear predominance; the protein concentration is elevated in 75%, and hypoglycorrhachia occurs in 30%. Up to 20% of patients may have completely normal CSF findings. Detection of CMV DNA in CSF by PCR is highly sensitive and specific [16].

Treatment

Three drugs are available to treat CMV, ganciclovir, cidofovir, and foscarnet. Ganciclovir and cidofovir, nucleoside and nucleotide analogues, have mechanisms of action

Table 34.1. Clinical syndromes caused by herpesviruses in HIV-infected children

CMV	HSV	VZV
Retinitis	Gingivostomatitis	Chicken pox (varicella)
Pneumonitis	Labial/genital	Herpes zoster
Colitis	Esophageal ulcers	Persistent skin infection
Esophageal ulcers	Encephalitis	Encephalitis
Hepatitis		
Pancreatitis		
Encephalitis		
Polyradiculopathy		

that closely resemble the nucleoside analogue antiretroviral reverse transcriptase inhibitors. Treatment for CMV disease and other herpesvirus infections is outlined in Table 34.2.

The drug used as first-line therapy for CMV end-organ disease is intravenous ganciclovir, since the others have significant toxicities. (Oral valganciclovir, a ganciclovir prodrug, may have an increasing role in therapy, see below.) Ganciclovir, a guanosine nucleoside analogue, is converted in vivo to ganciclovir triphosphate, the intracellularly active form of the drug. Ganciclovir is phosphorylated first to the monophosphate by CMV gene product ORF (open reading frame) UL97. Since the phosphorylase is only expressed in CMV-infected cells, phosphorylation of ganciclovir by UL97 helps to selectively target the effects of ganciclovir to infected cells. After initial phosphorylation, the monophosphate is phosphorylated to the active triphosphate form by cellular enzymes. Ganciclovir triphosphate competitively inhibits native deoxyguanosine triphosphate from interacting with viral DNA polymerase, inhibiting viral DNA replication. Futhermore, it acts as chain terminator (see also Chapter 1).

Two mechanisms cause ganciclovir resistance, mutations in UL97 phosphorylase and in CMV DNA polymerase. Certain UL97 point mutations block ganciclovir phosphorylation and demonstrate low-level resistance. Mutations in CMV DNA polymerase gene (UL54) confer high-level resistance. Patients with high-level ganciclovir resistance frequently have mutations in both genes. Less than 2%–5% of newly diagnosed CMV retinitis patients have resistance mutations before therapy. On therapy, 10%–25% develop resistance-related mutations.

The ganciclovir starting dose is 5 mg/kg twice a day for 2 weeks, followed by 5 mg/kg/day, 5–7 days per week. The major side effect is myelosuppression. Dosage reduction or use of filgrastim (G-CSF) frequently is necessary.

Cidofovir is a cytodine nucleotide analogue. Thus, it does not require phosphorylation by CMV UL97. Cidofovir is further phosphorylated to the triphosphate by cellular phosphorylases. Phosphorylated cidofovir competitively inhibits native cytosine

Table 34.2. Treatment of herpesvirus infection in HIV-infected children

Virus	Syndrome	Drug	Dose/route	Common side effects
CMV	Retinitis induction	Ganciclovir	iv:5 mg/kg, BID for 14 days	Myelosuppression
	Alternative drugs:	Foscarnet	iv:90 mg/kg, BID or 60 mg/kg/TID for 14 days	Nephrotoxicity
		Cidofovir	iv:5 mg/kg qwk for 2 doses, pretreat with probenicid and saline loading	Nephrotoxicity
	Maintenance	Ganciclovir	iv:5 mg/kg/day	
	Alternative drugs:	Ganciclovir, foscarnet	po:1 gm TID IV:90–120 mg/kg per day	
		Cidofovir	5 mg/kg q2 wks, pretreat with probenicid and saline loading	
	GI/Pulmonary	Valganciclovir same as for retinitis induction	Adult: 900 mg bid	Neutropenia
HSV 1, 2	primary oral/genital	Acyclovir	iv:750 mg/m^2 per day in 3 doses po:1200 mg/m^2 per day, in 3 doses	Phlebitis, nephrotoxicity, nausea, vomiting, rash
	Alternative drugs:	Famciclovir	Adults:125–500 mg bid	GI upset
		Valacyclovir	Adults:0.5–1 gram bid	
	For acyclovir resistance	Foscarnet		
	Recurrent encephalitis	Acyclovir	same as above	
		Acyclovir	iv: 1500 mg/m^2 per day or 30 mg/kg per day in 3 divided doses	
Varicella-zoster virus	Varicella	Acyclovir	iv-1500 mg/m^2 per day in 3 doses PO-80 mg/kg per day in 4 divided doses	Phlebitis, nephrotoxicity, nausea, vomiting, rash
		Famciclovir	Adults: 500 mg tid	
		Valacyclovir	Adults:1 gram tid	
	Zoster	Same as for varicella		
	Acyclovir resistant virus	Foscarnet		

binding to the viral DNA polymerase, and causes chain termination. Since cidofovir does not require UL97-mediated phosphorylation, CMVs resistant to ganciclovir due to UL97 mutations retain cidofovir sensitivity. However, mutants in the viral DNA polymerase can confer resistance against both ganciclovir and cidofovir. If virus demonstrates high level resistance to ganciclovir, it will likely be resistant to cidofovir.

Cidofovir has a significant and potentially difficult to manage set of toxicities, including potentially severe proximal tubular injuries producing proteinuria, glycosuria, and bicarbonate and phosphate wasting. A substantial incidence of neutropenia also occurs. Renal function should be carefully monitored with cidofovir therapy. Cidofovir is dosed at 5 mg/kg intravenously every week for 2 weeks as induction therapy, then every other week for maintenance. Cidofovir must be given with oral probenecid and saline loading.

Foscarnet is another drug for CMV infection. Foscarnet is a structurally simple pyrophosphate analogue. Foscarnet inhibits viral DNA polymerase. Foscarnet does not require phosphorylation to an active form. Ganciclovir-resistant UL97 CMV mutants can be foscarnet sensitive. Mutations in UL97 exist that confer resistance to foscarnet. Some of these may be distinct from mutations conferring resistance to ganciclovir and cidofovir. Some viruses are resistant to all three approved CMV antivirals. Foscarnet also appears to have some degree of antiviral activity against HIV.

Foscarnet can produce significant, severe toxicities. The main foscarnet toxicity is decreased renal function, leading to serious electrolyte and calcium imbalances, with secondary seizures. Foscarnet renal toxicity may be increased when coadministered with other nephrotoxic agents, particularly amphotericin B, pentamidine, and aminoglycosides. Electrolytes should be carefully monitored in patients. Renal side effects may be minimized by infusing foscarnet over 1 hour, with saline fluid loading.

Approximately 80%–90% of CMV retinitis cases respond initially to treatment, but relapse invariably occurs if therapy is discontinued. Relapses are delayed if maintenance therapy is given with ganciclovir or foscarnet. Dual therapy with ganciclovir and foscarnet has been used successfully for some cases of rapidly progressive CMV disease or disease not responsive to monotherapy.

The difficulty of continuing daily intravenous therapy, and the potential for drug toxicity, has made the development of alternative maintenance therapies for CMV disease a high priority. Strategies tested to date for prevention of recurrent retinitis include: oral ganciclovir, intravitreal administration of medication (as with implants impregnated with either ganciclovir or cidofovir, see Chapter 20), or cidofovir, an agent with a longer half-life [19, 20].

There have been two main problems with local therapy: risk of ophthalmologic side effects, such as retinal detachment, and development of extraocular CMV disease. One study comparing treatment options for CMV retinitis maintenance therapy found a breakthrough rate at 6 months of 44.3% for patients treated with ganciclovir implants, 24.3% for patients treated with the implant plus oral ganciclovir, and 19.6%

for intravenous ganciclovir treatment. Local treatment of CMV retinitis has no effect on other, systemic CMV disease. Patients treated with protease inhibitor-containing HAART regimens had low rates of new CMV disease, regardless of treatment group.

Valganciclovir (VCG) is an orally administered prodrug of ganciclovir. A randomized trial in HIV-infected adults with newly diagnosed CMV retinitis found oral VGC as effective as intravenous ganciclovir in treating the first episode and delaying progression of illness [21, 22].

There may be a role for using VGC in a pre-emptive manner, in patients with low CD4 counts despite HAART, and evidence of CMV infection, prior to the development of end-organ disease.

The necessity of maintenance therapy for CMV-related hepatitis, pneumonia or colitis has not been firmly established. Therapy with ganciclovir or foscarnet results in symptomatic improvement, but maintenance therapy may not prevent relapse or development of CMV disease in other organs [23].

Agents under development for the treatment of CMV-related disease include intravitreous fomivirsen for CMV retinitis, which appears to have considerable activity when injected every 2–4 weeks (after an induction period) for patients with eye disease that progressed or relapsed on other anti-CMV therapies. Other potential agents, not yet in advanced clinical trials, include maribavir (a protein kinase inhibitor), and inhibitors of the terminase complex that cleaves viral DNA(tomeglovir and GW-275175X).

Limited options are available for treatment of HIV-infected children. Use of intravitreal ganciclovir and intravenous cidofovir is still investigational in children. Intravenously-administered ganciclovir or foscarnet is available.

CMV in patients treated with highly active antiretroviral therapy (HAART)

Since the advent of highly active antiretroviral therapy (HAART), the incidence of opportunistic infections among HIV-infected adults has dropped markedly. Overall, the incidence of CMV end-organ disease has declined from 15–20/100 patient-years to 1–5/100 patient-years [19]. Clearing of CMV viremia has been reported following immunologic improvement with HAART [24, 25].

Since the advent of HAART, some patients have developed an inflammatory vitritis related to quiesent or subclinical CMV retinitis with immune recovery, which may be severe and may respond to intraocular steroid therapy [26].

Certain CMV patients receiving HAART may be able to discontinue maintenance ganciclovir therapy without experiencing CMV disease recurrence. Such patients should be treated with HAART for >6 months, with CD4 counts increasing to >100–150 cells/mm^3, and have negative CMV antigenemia before discontinuing anti-CMV therapy [21]. Even with decreasing CMV, close surveillance must continue as CMV disease in patients on HAART now occurs at CD4 levels once thought protective. It is too early to know if the incidence of CMV disease in HIV-infected children will be affected by HAART.

Herpes simplex virus (HSV)

Epidemiology

HSV-1 and HSV-2 affect all populations. HSV-1 is transmitted by contact with infected oral secretions, HSV-2 through infected genital secretions. Primary HSV-1 infection may be asymptomatic. Primary oral infections or recurrences may be accompanied by high fever, extensive mucosal ulceration, drooling, and anorexia. In immunocompetent hosts, the disease lasts 10–14 days. The most common symptom of reactivation is herpes labialis, estimated to occur in 25%–50% of infected individuals, frequently in association with febrile illness, local trauma, or sun exposure. Painful vesicles appear at the vermilion border, progress to ulcers and then crust over 2–4 days.

Primary infection in young adults has been associated with pharyngitis and, less commonly, a mononucleosis-like syndrome. Children of lower socioeconomic class acquire HSV-1 earlier than children of higher classes. Only 30%–40% of individuals from middle and upper socioeconomic classes are seropositive by the second decade of life, compared to 75%–90% of individuals from lower socioeconomic classes.

HSV-2 is generally acquired through contact with genital lesions. The seroprevalence is low until late adolescence, when it increases to 20%–30%.

After primary infection with HSV, the virus remains latent within sensory ganglia. Reactivation of latent virus occurs more frequently in hosts with immune compromise, typically involving mucocutaneous areas near the original entry site, the lips or face for HSV-1, genital areas for HSV-2. In severely immunocompromised patients, recurrent infection may spread, including viremic spread to distant sites [27].

Clinical manifestations

Orolabial herpes

Primary infection with HSV usually occurs in the perioral, ocular, or genital areas, but any skin site may be involved. Lesions can be extensive; they can mimic dermatomal herpes zoster, although pain usually is less severe.

Reactivation occurs more frequently and tends to be more severe in immunosuppressed hosts. Both adults and children with HIV infection may develop chronic, severe, or recurrent orolabial herpes. In some patients, chronic ulcerative lesions and virus shedding persists for weeks. From 5%–10% of children with AIDS and primary gingivostomatitis subsequently develop symptomatic frequent recurrences with severe ulcerative lesions.

Esophagitis

HSV causes up to 25% of autopsy-proven esophagitis in HIV-infected adults; 25%–50% have evidence of HSV infection elsewhere. Though rarely reported in normal children, esophageal HSV disease infection is relatively common in immunocompromised children. Symptoms include retrosternal pain and odynophagia. Herpetic lesions usually are not seen in the oral cavity. Definitive diagnosis requires endoscopy with biopsy and viral culture. In HIV-infected children with esophagitis symptoms, endoscopic evaluation and biopsy is recommended for those with a low probability of candidal esophagitis (without thrush at the time of presentation and not responding to initial anticandidal therapy).

Nervous system

HSV causes infrequent, but life-threatening, necrotizing hemorrhagic encephalitis in immunocompetent hosts, notably involving the temporal lobe. Though HSV-1 is the primary etiologic agent, HSV-2 may also cause encephalitis, particularly in the newborn. With HIV infection, herpes encephalitis may not present with a classic localization, and may be complicated by infection with other agents, such as CMV.

The usual symptoms are those associated with acute encephalitis: headache, fever, behavior changes, and seizures. EEG and CAT scan reveal changes consistent with HSV encephalitis in 35%–45% of cases. MRI is the imaging procedure of choice, and reveals localized edema in the temporal and orbital surfaces of the frontal lobes. CSF findings are non-specific and resemble those found with other viral encephalitides.

Genital disease

Primary genital herpes rarely occurs in immunocompetent infants, unless a caregiver inoculates the area via contaminated hands, or due to sexual abuse. In adolescents, symptoms of primary genital herpes are similar to those in adults, with fever, pain, itching, dysuria, discharge, and regional adenopathy. Vesicular lesions or ulcers may be noted in the perineal/vaginal/anal area. Lesions tend to last 2–3 weeks. In HIV-infected patients, the frequency and severity of recurrences of genital herpes increase as immunodeficiency worsens. Chronic deep necrotic ulcers secondary to HSV infection have been described in some severely immunodeficient, HIV-infected adults.

Disseminated disease

HSV-1 and, rarely, HSV-2 cause disseminated disease, with involvement of liver, adrenals, lungs, kidney, spleen, and brain in severely immunocompromised hosts. Patients may develop a hemorrhagic shock syndrome, with hemorrhage, evidence of intravascular coagulation, seizures, renal failure, and death, despite antiviral therapy.

Diagnosis

The diagnosis of HSV infection may be suspected clinically based on the typical appearance of vesicles and ulcers. Viral isolation remains the definitive diagnostic test. HSV grows rapidly, and is usually detected in tissue culture cells within 1–3 days. New methodologies (shell vial culture, enzyme-linked culture system) may further decrease time to detection. Definitive diagnosis of esophageal disease requires endoscopy with biopsy and culture.

Cells collected from scrapings of skin lesions, conjunctiva, or mucosa can be examined for HSV antigens by direct immunofluorescence, allowing for quick virus identification, which can distinguish between VZV and HSV. Histologic examination reveals intranuclear inclusions and multinucleated giant cells.

MRI is the initial imaging study of choice to evaluate possible HSV encephalitis. Detection of HSV DNA in CSF by PCR has replaced brain biopsy as the diagnostic test of choice. Infectious virus is rarely present in the CSF, but HSV DNA usually is detected by PCR. In one adult study, HSV PCR on cerebrospinal fluid had 100% sensitivity and 99.6% specificity for autopsy-confirmed HSV encephalitis [28]. As early institution of treatment is critical, immunocompromised patients presenting with acute neurologic symptoms consistent with possible HSV encephalitis should be considered for empiric acyclovir therapy.

Treatment

The drug of choice for HSV infections is acyclovir. Acyclovir is an acyclic purine nucleoside analogue. It is phosphorylated by viral kinase, and then further phosphorylated by the host cell kinases into an active drug, which inhibits viral DNA polymerase by competing with native guanosine triphosphate and by chain termination of the replicating viral genomic DNA. Acyclovir has a good therapeutic index in part because it has very high affinity for HSV thymidine kinase. Acyclovir penetrates well into tissues, including the brain and CSF.

Symptomatic HIV-infected children with primary gingivostomatitis should be treated with intravenous acyclovir at a dose of 750 mg/m^2/per day, in three divided doses, or oral acyclovir at a dose of 12 000 mg/m^2/per day in three divided doses. For disseminated disease or encephalitis, a higher parenteral dose, 15 000 mg/m^2/per day or 300 mg/kg/per day in three divided doses is recommended.

Severe oral recurrences should be treated with oral acyclovir. Daily suppressive therapy is recommended for children with more than three to six recurrences per year. Acyclovir-resistant HSV infection has been reported, generally in patients who have received multiple courses or who receive chronic suppressive therapy. The most common basis for resistance is a mutation affecting viral thymidine kinase. In addition, some acyclovir-resistant isolates have mutant viral DNA polymerase.

For patients with acyclovir-resistant HSV infections, foscarnet is a reasonable alternative, since it inhibits most acyclovir-resistant strains in vitro. Foscarnet is given at a dose of 40 mg/kg every 8 hours, but has significant toxicities, including renal toxicities (see above) [29].

Valacyclovir and famciclovir are oral drugs that have activity against HSV and better bioavailability than acyclovir. Both are effective in reducing the duration of symptoms and viral shredding in adults with recurrent genital herpes. Neither of these newer agents has been well studied in children. Neither is active against acyclovir-resistant HSV.

Varicella-zoster virus

Epidemiology

Primary infection with VZV causes chickenpox. Following primary infection, VZV establishes latent infection in peripheral and cranial sensory ganglia. Latency may persist for life. VZV may reactivate to cause herpes zoster (shingles). Herpes zoster occurs primarily in the elderly, and in younger, immunocompromised individuals. Transmission of VZV is thought to occur by the respiratory route through droplet inhalation of viral particles from skin lesions and respiratory tract. Humans are the only known VZV reservoir. Infected individuals can transmit infection from 1–2 days before rash appears until all lesions are crusted. Individuals with chickenpox are more likely to transmit infection than individuals with herpes zoster. Close contact increases the risk of acquiring infection. Immunosuppressed patients should take care to avoid exposure to both chickenpox and shingles.

Before immunization (see Chapter 5) became available, most individuals acquired chickenpox during childhood. The incubation period is usually 14–16 days (range of 10–21 days). Administration of varicella-zoster immuno globulin (VZIG) may lengthen the incubation period to 28 days. HIV-infected children are probably as likely to be exposed to VZV infection and to develop chickenpox as non-infected children. HIV-infected are more likely to develop recurrent VZV infection (see below).

Clinical manifestations

Varicella

In healthy children, chickenpox is relatively benign; complications, including skin infections, pneumonia, and encephalitis occur in a small percentage. Less common, life-threatening complications include bacterial sepsis, toxic-shock syndrome and Reye's syndrome.

In developed countries, before the availability of HAART and acyclovir, chickenpox in the HIV-infected child was often severe and prolonged, frequently complicated lung or liver involvement, with occasional widespread dissemination to lung, liver, brain, and pancreas [30]. More recently, most chickenpox cases in HIV-infected children have been uncomplicated [31,32].

Herpes zoster

In HIV-infected adults, the zoster incidence is 2.5–4 cases/100 patient-years. An increased incidence of zoster may occur within the first 6 months of beginning HAART, suggesting that zoster may represent an "immunoreconstitution syndrome" [33,34]. Zoster is much more common among HIV-infected children than among non-infected children. The zoster incidence in immunocompetent children <10 years is <1/1000; HIV-infected children have a 10%–70% cumulative risk. Zoster occurs more frequently in association with low CD4 cell counts [35]. Recurrent VZV infection may present as disseminated rash typical of chickenpox, rather than as a dermatomally limited zoster-like rash [35]. HIV-infected children may have multiple episodes of recurrent disease. Those with low CD4 cell counts are more likely to develop multiple recurrences.

Persistent VZV infection

HIV-infected children, particularly those with low CD4 counts, may develop persistent skin lesions despite treatment. The lesions may have an atypical, sometimes hyper-keratotic appearance [31]. Some children may become infected with acyclovir-resistant strains of VZV, with resistance more likely in children receiving chronic therapy with multiple courses of acyclovir [35].

VZV-related retinal disease
Is described in Chapter 20.

Nervous system
In severely immunocompromised patients, VZV can cause encephalitis, myelitis, or meningitis. Adults typically presented with rash (71%) and fever (60%), mild CSF pleo-cytosis (mean WBC 126/mm^3) and elevated protein; 12% have acute retinal necrosis. A small number of patients (9%) had no distinctive presentation [36].

Diagnosis
A clinical diagnosis of VZV infection can often be made based on physical findings. Typical VZV skin lesions look alike in HIV-infected children and healthy children. The differential diagnosis of VZV infection includes insect bites, other viruses associated with vesicular rashes (including HSV and certain enteroviruses), and contact dermatitis. HSV infection can present with vesicular lesions in a dermatomal distribution.

Several methods are available for laboratory diagnosis of VZV infection. Detection of multinucleated giant cells with intranuclear inclusions in Tzanck smears of scrapings from vesicular lesions would be consistent with the diagnosis of VZV infection, but other viruses, including HSV, can produce similar changes. Immunofluorescent staining of scrapings from lesions provides a specific diagnosis. Cells scraped from the bases of lesions and allowed to adhere to glass slides are incubated with fluorescein-conjugated antibodies that react with antigens of VZV or HSV. Cells containing VZV or HSV antigens can then be visualized by fluorescence microscopy. Using this method, VZV and HSV infections can be diagnosed rapidly and with great accuracy,

VZV also can be isolated from vesicular fluid or from swabs of ulcers. PCR methods also can be used to detect VZV DNA in vesicular lesions, but such tests are available only in a small number of research laboratories and false positive results can occur.

Serologic assays also may be useful for diagnosis of VZV infection, particularly if viral isolation and PCR assays are not available or yield negative results. Acute and con-valescent sera, the latter collected 2 to 3 weeks after onset of illness, should be tested simultaneously. Detection of a fourfold or higher rise in antibody titer in the fluorescent antibody membrane antigen (FAMA) test, or seroconversion (initial negative titer with subsequent positive titer) provides strong evidence of a recent VZV infection. FAMA assays are technically demanding and generally are not available in clinical laboratories. Commercially available enzyme-linked immunoabsorbent and latex agglutination assays are useful for detecting seroconversion, but are less reliable for detecting rises in antibody titer.

ARN generally is diagnosed by its classic appearance on ophthalmologic examination. Neurologic complications of VZV infection are diagnosed, based on symptoms and a clinical exam consistent with VZV and a positive CSF VZV PCR assay.

Treatment

Acyclovir is the drug of choice for VZV infections in HIV-infected children. Since severe disease may develop, all HIV-infected children should be treated with acyclovir, in most cases with intravenous therapy, since plasma levels following oral administration are significantly lower than with intravenous administration. The recommended dose of intravenous acyclovir for VZV infections is 1500 mg/m^2/per day in three divided doses. Oral administration may be considered for HIV-infected children with normal or only slightly decreased CD4 cell counts. An oral dose of 80 mg/kg/per day should be used. Lower doses are unlikely to be efficacious, and higher doses have not been studied. Acyclovir also is the drug of choice for herpes zoster in HIV-infected children. For zoster, acyclovir can often be given orally, since herpes zoster is less likely than chickenpox to disseminate and cause life-threatening disease. Patients with very low CD4 cell counts, trigeminal or ocular involvement, or extensive herpes zoster should be treated, at least initially, with intravenous acyclovir. Two newer antivirals, famciclovir (prodrug of penciclovir) and valacyclovir (prodrug of acyclovir) are well absorbed orally, and both are effective for herpes zoster in adults. Neither has been tested for safety and efficacy in children.

After acyclovir is started, new lesions may continue to appear for up to 72 hours. Crusting of all lesions may take considerably longer, 5–7 days. Patients who continue to develop new lesions, or whose lesions fail to heal, despite therapy with acyclovir, could be infected with an acyclovir-resistant strain. Resistance appears to result from viral thymidine kinase mutations. Occasional resistant isolates have viral DNA polymerase mutations. Isolates resistant to acyclovir are also resistant to famciclovir and valacyclovir.

Patients who fail to respond clinically to acyclovir, including those with acyclovir-resistant strains, may be switched to foscarnet, which has activity against most acyclovir-resistant strains. Foscarnet can cause severe nephrotoxicity (see above) and therefore should be used only for acyclovir-resistant virus. Foscarnet-resistant VZV is uncommon, but has been reported.

Prophylaxis

VZIG should be given to susceptible HIV-infected children within 72 hours after a significant exposure to VZV infection.

A trial of varicella vaccine in asymptomatic HIV-infected children with normal CD4 counts has led to the recommendation that such children should receive the vaccine [37]. Patients with severe immunocompromise may be at risk of developing disseminated disease due to VZV vaccine [38].

Epstein–Barr virus (EBV)

EBV infection is worldwide. Transmission occurs through close interpersonal contact, in less developed countries, almost all school-age children have evidence of EBV infection. In more developed countries acquisition of EBV occurs later. Primary infection in infants or young children may be inapparent, or may result in a short febrile illness. In older children and adults, EBV infection may cause the infectious mononucleosis syndrome (fever, pharyngitis, adenopathy, and hepatic or splenic enlargement).

EBV is a potent B-cell stimulator and has been associated with lymphoproliferative syndromes in immunosuppressed hosts. EBV has been linked to HIV-related lymphoproliferative syndromes. The most common EBV-related syndromes in HIV-infected children are lymphocytic interstitial pneumonitis (LIP, see Chapter 24) and non-Hodgkin's lymphoma (discussed in Chapter 29).

Human herpesvirus 6

HHV-6 is a member of the *Roseolovirus* genus of herpesviruses. It is the causative agent for most cases of roseola, a febrile illness of early childhood associated with a distinctive rash and, occassionally, febrile seizures. Many cases of primary infections are asymptomatic. Primary infection generally occurs before the age of two. During latency, cellular reservoirs include CD4+ lymphocytes and possibly epithelial cells of the salivary glands.

The CD4+ lymphocyte is the primary target of HHV-6. In cell cultures HHV-6 can infect HIV-infected CD4+ lymphocytes. In vitro experiments indicate that HHV-6 can upregulate HIV expression in co-infected cells, possibly through transactivation of the HIV promotor [39]. Differential effects of HHV-6 in dually infected cell cultures have been described, based on the variants of HHV-6 and HIV used. Preliminary data suggests that HHV-6 infection may play a role in progression of HIV infection in children [40].

Kaposi's sarcoma-associated herpesvirus (KSHV)
(human herpesvirus-8, HHV-8)

KSHV has been linked to Kaposi's sarcoma, primary effusion lymphomas, and multicentric Castleman's disease and is discussed in more detail in Chapter 29.

Summary

With the introduction of HAART and improved immunologic reconstitution, herpesvirus infections may become a less challenging feature of pediatric HIV disease management. Nevertheless, careful attention to the diagnosis, assessment, and management of herpesvirus infections in children with HIV can significantly enhance survival and the quality of life. Development of more effective, less toxic antivirals and vaccines against herpesviruses remains an important goal.

REFERENCES

1. Heng, M. C., Heng, S. Y., Allen, S. G. Co-infection and synergy of human immunodeficiency virus-1 and herpes simplex virus-1. *Lancet* 1994;**343**:255–258.

2. Alford, C. A., Stagno, S., Pass, R. F. *et al.* Congenital and perinatal cytomegalovirus infections. *Rev. Infect. Dis.* 1990;**12**:S745–753.

3. Stagno, S., Reynold, D., Tsiantos, A. *et al.* Cervical cytomegalovirus excretion in pregnant and nonpregnant women: suppression in early gestation. *J. Infect. Dis.* 1975;**131**:522–527.

4. Doyle, M., Atkins, J. T., Rivera-Matos, I. R. Congenital cytomegalovirus infection in infants infected with human immunodeficiency virus type. *Pediatr. Infect. Dis J.* 1996;**15**:1102–1106.

5. Frenkel, L. D., Gaur, S., Tsolia, M. *et al.* Cytomegalovirus infection in children with AIDS. *Rev. Infect. Dis.* 1990;**12**:S820–S821.

6. Kitchen, B. J., Engler, H. D., Gill, V. J. *et al.* Cytomegalovirus infection in children with human immunodeficiency virus infection. *Pediatr. Infect. Dis. J.* 1997;**16**:358–363.

7. Chandwani, S., Kaul, A., Bebenroth, D. *et al.* Cytomegalovirus infection in human immunodeficiency virus type 1-infected children. *Pediatr. Infect. Dis. J.* 1996;**15**:310–314.

8. Nigro, G., Krzysztofiak, A., Gattinara, G. C. *et al.* Rapid progression of HIV disease in children with cytomegalovirus DNAemia. *AIDS* 1996;**10**:1127–1133.

9. Ives, D. V. Cytomegalovirus disease in AIDS. *AIDS* 1997;**11**:1791–1797.

10. De Jung, M. D., Galasso, G. J., Gazzard, B. *et al.* Summary of the II International Symposium on cytomegalovirus. *Antiviral Res.* 1998;**39**:141–162.

11. Goodgame, R. W. Gastrointestinal cytomegalovirus disease. *Ann. Intern. Med.* 1993;**119**:924–935.

12. Wilcox, C. M., Diehl, D. L., Cello, J. M. *et al.* Cytomegalovirus esophagitis in patients with AIDS: a clinical, endoscopic, and pathologic correlation. *Ann. Intern. Med.* 1990;**113**:589–593.

13. Bozzette, S. A., Arcia, J., Bartok, A. E. *et al.* Impact of *Pneumocystis carinii* and cytomegalovirus on the course and outcome of atypical pneumonia in advanced human immunodeficiency virus disease. *J. Infect. Dis.* 1992;**165**:93–98.

14. Jacobson, M. A., Mills, J., Rush, J. *et. al.* Morbidity and mortality of patients with AIDS and first episode *Pneumocystis carinii* pneumonia unaffected by concomitant pulmonary cytomegalovirus infection. *Am. Rev. Respir. Dis.* 1991;**144**:6–9.

15. Salomon, N., Gomez, T., Perlman, D. C., Laya, L., Eber, C., Mildvan, D. Clinical features and outcome of HIV-related cytomegalovirus pneumonia. *AIDS* 1997;**11**:319–324.

16. Cinque, P., Vago, L., Brytting, M. *et al.* Cytomegalovirus infection of the central nervous system in patients with AIDS: diagnosis by DNA amplification from cerebrospinal fluid. *J. Infect. Dis.* 1992;**166**:1408–1411.

17. De Jung, M. D., Galasso, G. J., Gazzard, B. *et al.* Summary of the II International Symposium on cytomegalovirus. *Antiviral Res.* 1998;**39**:141–162.

18. Spector, S. A., Hsia, K., Crager, M. *et al.* Cytomegalovirus (CMV) DNA load is an independent predictor of CMV disease and survival in advanced AIDS. *J. Virol.* 1999;**73**:7027–7030.

19. The Studies of Ocular Complications of AIDS Research Group, in Collaboration With The AIDS Clinical Trials Group. The ganciclovir implant plus oral ganciclovir versus parenteral cidofovir for the treatment of cytomegalovirus retinitis in patients with acquired immunodeficiency syndrome: the ganciclovir cidofovir cytomegalovirus retinitis trial. *Am. J. Opthalmol.* 2001;**131**:457–467.

20. Drew, W. L., Ives, D., Lalezari, J. P. *et al.* Oral ganciclovir as maintenance for cytomegalovirus retinitis in patients with AIDS. *N. Engl. J. Med.* 1995;**333**:615–620.

21. Martin, D. F., Sierra-Madero, J., Walmsley, S. *et al.* A controlled trial of valganciclovir as induction therapy for cytomegalovirus retinitis. *N. Engl. J. Med.* 2002;**346**:1119–1126.

22. Segarra-Newnham, M., Salazar, M.I. Valganciclovir: a new oral alternative for cytomegalovirus retinitis in human immunodeficiency virus-seropositive individuals. *Pharma* 2002;**22**:1124–1128.

23. Blanshard, C., Benhamou, Y., Dohin, E. *et al.* Treatment of AIDS-associated gastrointestinal cytomegalovirus infection with foscarnet and ganciclovir: a randomized comparison. *J. Infect. Dis.* 1995;**172**:622–628.

24. Pallela, F. J., Delaney, K. M., Moorman, A. C. *et al.* Declining morbidity and mortality among patients with advanced human immunodeficiency virus infection. *N. Eng. J. Med.* 1998;**338**:853–860.

25. Casado, J. L., Arrizabalage, J., Montes, M. *et al.* Incidence and risk factors for developing cytomegalovirus retinitis in HIV-infected patients receiving protease inhibitor therapy. *AIDS* 1999;**13**:1497–1501.

26. Salmon-Ceron, D. Cytomegalovirus infection: the point in 2001. *HIV Med.* 2001;**2**:255–259.

27. Cavert, W. Viral infections in human immunodefiency virus disease. *Med. Clin. North Am.* 1997;**81**:411–427.

28. Cinque, P., Vago, L., Marenz, R. *et al.* Herpes simplex virus infections of the central nervous system in human immunodeficiency virus-infected patients: clinical management by polymerase chain reaction assay of cerebrospinal fluid. *Clin. Infect. Dis.* 1998;**27**:303–309.

29. Hardy, W. D. Foscarnet treatment of acyclovir-resistant herpes simplex virus infection in patients with acquired immunodeficiency syndrome: preliminary results of a controlled, randomized, regimen-comparative trial. *Am. J. Med.* 1992;**92**:30S–35S.

30. Jura, E., Chadwick, E. G., Josephs, S. H. *et al.* Varicella-zoster virus infections in children infected with human immunodeficiency virus. *Pediatr. Infect. Dis. J.* 1989;**8**:586–590.

31. Kelley, R., Mancao, M., Lee, F., Sawyer, M., Nahmias, A., Nesheim, S. Varicella in children with perinatally acquired human immunodeficiency virus infection. *J. Pediatr.* 1994;**124**:271–273.

32. Gershon, A. A., Mervish, N., LaRussa, P. *et al.* Varicella-zoster virus infection in children with underlying human immunodeficiency virus infection. *J. Infect. Dis.* 1997;**176**:1496–1500.

33. Aldeen, T., Hay, P., Davidson, F., Lau, R. Herpes zoster infection in HIV-seropositive patients associated with highly active antiretroviral therapy. *AIDS* 1998;**12**:1719–1720.

34. Martinez, E., Gatell, J., Moran, Y. *et al.* High incidence of herpes zoster in patients with AIDS soon after therapy with protease inhibitors. *Clin. Infect. Dis.* 1998;**27**:1510–1513.

35. Von Seidlein, L., Gillette, S. G., Bryson, Y. *et al.* Frequent recurrence and persistence of varicella-zoster virus infections in children infected with human immunodeficiency virus type 1. *J. Pediatr.*, 1996;**128**:52–57.

36. Blanchardiere, A. D. L., Rozenberg, F., Caumes, E. *et al.* Neurologic complications of Varicella-zoster virus infection in adults with human immunodeficiency virus infection. *Scand. J. Infect. Dis.* 2000;**32**:263–269.

37. Levin, M. J., Gershon, A. A., Weinberg, A. *et al.* Immunization of HIV-infected children with varicella vaccine. *J. Pediat.* 2001;**139**:305–310.

38. Kramer, J. M., LaRussa, P., Tsai, W. C. *et al.* Disseminated vaccine strain varicella as the acquired immunodeficiency syndrome-defining illness in a previously undiagnosed child. *Pediatrics* 2001;**108**. URL:http://www.pediatrics.org/cgi/content/full/108/2/e39.

39. Horvat, R. T., Wood, C., Josephs, S. F., Balachandran, N. Transactivation of the human immunodeficiency virus promoter by human herpesvirus 6 (HHV-6) strains GS and Z-29 in primary human T lymphocytes and identification of transactivating HHV-6 (GS) gene fragments. *J. Virol.* 1991;**65**:2895–2902.

40. Kositanont, U., Wasi, C., Wanprapar, N. *et al.* Primary infection of human herpesvirus 6 in children with vertical infection of human immunodeficiency virus type 1. *J. Infect. Dis.* 1999;**180**:50–55.

35 Pneumocystis jiroveci pneumonia

Leslie K. Serchuck, M.D.

Pediatric, Adolescent & Maternal AIDS Branch, NICHD/NIH, Rockville, MD

Introduction

In developed countries, *Pneumocystis jiroveci* pneumonia (PCP) is the most common AIDS-defining condition and the most life-threatening infection in children infected with HIV. The incidence of PCP in developed countries has decreased dramatically with the introduction of highly active antiretroviral therapy (HAART) and routine use of prophylaxis.

Biology and taxonomy

Pneumocystis has now been identified as a fungus by genetic analysis, enzyme characterization, and the presence of a translation elongation factor 3 gene found exclusively in fungi [1, 2]. It is not, however, susceptibe to polyenes and azole antifungal agents since it lacks ergosterol, a characteristic of fungal cell membranes and the target of these drugs.

Pneumocystis, a unicellular eukaryotic organism, exists in three morphologic forms: sporozoite, trophozoite, and cyst. Trophozoites (2–5 μm) adhere to alveolar epithelium where they multiply and mature into cysts (5–8 μm). These cysts are round or crescent-shaped thick-walled structures that contain up to eight sporozoites (1–2 μm) which, when released, mature to become trophozoites. The cyst and trophozoite forms are found in lung and pleural fluid.

Epidemiology

Serum antibodies to *Pneumocystis* can be found in greater than 80% of all children by age 2 to 4 years, suggesting that primary asymptomatic infection occurs commonly in immunocompetent hosts [3, 4]. Since the 1980s, patients most at risk for PCP remain those with advanced HIV disease and impaired cell-mediated immunity. HIV-infected

Handbook of Pediatric HIV Care, ed. Steven L. Zeichner and Jennifer S. Read.
Published by Cambridge University Press. © Cambridge University Press 2006.

infants are at increased risk of developing PCP, but at much higher CD4+ lymphocyte cell counts than older children or adults. Additionally, the CD4+ lymphocyte count can fall precipitously in HIV-infected infants. Therefore, all HIV-exposed infants should receive prophylaxis for PCP from the age of 6 weeks. Prophylaxis may subsequently be discontinued for infants definitely found not to be infected.

PCP is the most common AIDS-defining illness in children in developed countries. As of December 2000, it had been reported in 33% of all pediatric AIDS cases in the USA, with the greatest percentage of those cases occurring in children <1 year old, peaking between ages 3 and 6 months [5]. An analysis of 3300 HIV-infected children participating in Pediatric AIDS Clinical Trials Group studies from 1988–98 reported a PCP event rate of 1.3 per 100 person-years [6].

The epidemiology of PCP in HIV-infected infants and children is similar worldwide. The incidence of PCP in HIV-infected African children hospitalized with severe pneumonia ranges from 10 to 48% depending on diagnostic technique [7, 8]. The incidence was less at institutions where a negative induced sputum was not followed by an additional attempt at diagnosis using bronchoscopy with alveolar lavage (BAL), a technique with superior sensitivity. In Bangkok, PCP is responsible for at least one-third of all severe pneumonias in HIV-infected children; presumptive PCP was the most common AIDS-defining condition in Thai children during 1988–1995 [9]. On the Caribbean island of Barbados, PCP was identified in greater than 37% of HIV-infected children presenting for clinical care. It was the primary cause of death in 65% of children with AIDS [10]. Reports from South Africa and the United Kingdom suggest that co-infection with cytomegalovirus occurs commonly in children with pneumonia and that survival is significantly worse in these infants [11, 12].

In some African studies, mortality due to PCP occurs in greater than 60% of pediatric patients treated with trimethoprim-sulfamethoxazole and prednisone. In the USA, mortality ranges from 38–62% and median survival time from time of diagnosis is 9–19 months [13–15]. The mortality rate in untreated cases approaches 100%.

Pathogenesis

The organism is ubiquitous in nature and strains are species specific. The environmental reservoir of *Pneumocystis* is unknown, although *Pneumocystis* DNA has been identified in pond water and air samples from hospital rooms of patients with PCP [16, 17]. Persons most likely become infected by inhalation of the organism. Since most immunocompetent persons have antibodies to *Pneumocystis*, illness in immunocompromised hosts may represent reactivation of latent infection. However, there have been clusters of cases reported among immunosuppressed patients, suggesting the possibility of common source infection or person-to-person transmission, and molecular epidemiology studies suggest that new acquisition of infection can also occur [18, 19]. CD4+ lymphocytes are necessary for effective host resistance to *Pneumocystis*. Thus, patients with impaired cell-mediated immunity (i.e., infants; patients infected with HIV or immunosuppressed due to malnutrition, cytotoxic agents, or corticosteroids) are at highest risk of developing PCP.

PCP impairs lung function by causing alveolar erosion when the *Pneumocystis* trophozoite adheres to the type I pneumocyte. Cellular infiltration, interstitial fibrosis, and increased inflammation characterize the ensuing alveolar damage. An accumulation of interstitial edema and mononuclear cell infiltration occurs as infection progresses (20). Increased alveolar-capillary permeability leads to decreased lung compliance, total lung capacity, and vital capacity [21]. The host inflammatory response may further impair lung function.

Clinical features

Pulmonary disease

The onset of illness is usually abrupt in children with AIDS, though it may be insidious, developing over a period of weeks. The classic presentation includes high-grade fever (> 40 °C), tachypnea, dyspnea, and non-productive cough. Physical examination often reveals an acutely ill child with bibasilar rales and evidence of respiratory distress and hypoxia. Cyanosis may be present or rapidly develop. Rarely, children may present without fever [22] or with increasing lethargy and weight loss. One case report reported chest pain as the only presenting clinical symptom in a young child [23]. HIV-infected patients with extrapulmonary pneumocystosis (EP) may present with symptoms that are referable only to the affected organ or tissue, such as hearing loss, abdominal pain, and ascites with either absent or clinically insignificant pulmonary involvement [24, 25].

Extrapulmonary pneumocystosis

Extrapulmonary pneumocystosis (EP) may be the initial presentation of *Pneumocystis* infection even without concurrent PCP [24]. In adult series in HIV patients, EP represents between 0.06 to 2.5% of *Pneumocystis* infections. EP has been reported to occur in the ear, eye, thyroid, spleen, and GI tract, including peritoneum, stomach, duodenum, small intestine, transverse colon, liver, and pancreas. It may occur in the adrenal glands, bone marrow, heart, kidney and ureter, lymph nodes, meninges and cerebral cortex, and muscle. EP may occur at any one of these sites alone or at numerous, non-contiguous sites simultaneously and should be considered in the differential of unexplained hearing loss, visual field loss, thyroiditis, new onset ascites or clinical signs consistent with colitis.

PCP – Laboratory features

Hypoxemia and alveolar–arterial oxygen gradient greater than 30 mm Hg are found characteristically in PCP. Arterial oxygen tension (PaO_2) is often between 34 and

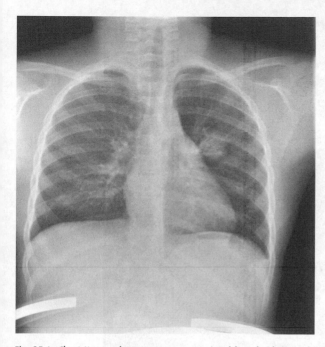

Fig. 35.1. Chest X-ray pulmonary mucosa-associated lymphoid tissue (MALT): left upper lobe anterior pulmonary mass projected over the left hilum.

73 mm Hg. Respiratory alkalosis may occur as PCP worsens. Lactate dehydrogenase is often increased but is not specific for PCP [26]. Serum total protein and albumin concentrations are frequently depressed.

PCP – Radiography

Chest radiographs show hyperinflation or bilateral diffuse parenchymal infiltrates with a "ground glass" or reticulogranular appearance but may be normal. A diffuse reticular pattern with alveolar densities, air bronchograms, and pneumothoraces may be present [27, 28] (Figs. 35.1 and 35.2). Patients receiving aerosolized pentamidine prophylaxis may present with upper lobe disease. Localized nodular densities in the periphery, lobar infiltrates, pulmonary air cysts, and pleural effusions may occur in severe disease. High-resolution computed tomography (HRCT) may reveal abnormalities despite a normal radiograph (Fig. 35.3). Ground-glass attenuation, consolidation, nodules, thickening of interlobular septa and thin-walled cysts are seen [29]. Radionuclide gallium scans often show increased gallium uptake but are not specific for PCP [30].

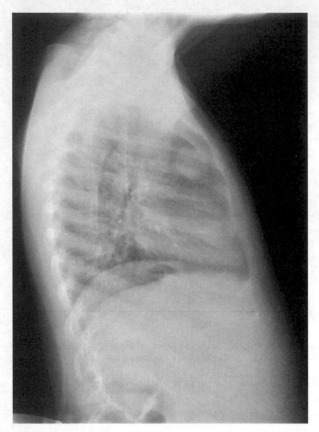

Fig. 35.2. Corresponding lateral chest X-ray of Fig. 35.1.

PCP – Diagnosis

The differential diagnosis of PCP includes bacterial, viral, and fungal pneumonias, including Epstein–Barr virus; cytomegalovirus pneumonitis (may be indistinguishable on HRCT); *Mycobacterium avium intracellulare* pulmonary infection; and lymphoid interstitial pneumonitis (pulmonary lymphoid hyperplasia – also presents with multiple, small widespread nodules). In addition, co-infection with *Candida albicans, Mycobacterium tuberculosis, Aspergillus fumigatus* and *Streptococcus pneumoniae* can also occur.

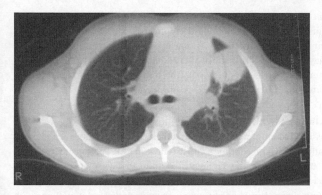

Fig. 35.3. Chest computed tomography pulmonary mucosa-associated lymphoid tissue (MALT): Left upper lobe mass adjacent to the mediastinum with a bronchus traversing the lesion.

Diagnostic procedures

Since it is not possible to culture *Pneumocystis* in vitro, the diagnosis of *Pneumocystis* infection in both pulmonary and extrapulmonary sites relies on a variety of direct staining, histologic, and molecular diagnostic techniques.

Nasopharyngeal aspirate (NPA)

NPA has been used in some African countries to diagnosis PCP in infants and young children with severe pneumonia when BAL is not available. It is performed using a modified feeding catheter attached to a 5-ml syringe containing 3–5 ml of normal saline. The catheter is passed through either nostril into the nasopharynx, saline flushed and immediately aspirated [8]. Cysts are identified using a direct monoclonal antibody immunofluorescent stain. PCR might be used for rapid diagnosis and increased sensitivity in NPA [31].

Induced sputum analysis (ISA)

ISA is an easy, non-invasive test wherein a patient produces sputum after inhalation of nebulized 3% hypertonic saline. Sensitivity ranges from 25–90% and depends on specimen collection, preparation, and analysis by experienced personnel [32]. The negative predictive value is only 48%, however, and BAL should follow a negative ISA. Complications of ISA include nausea, vomiting and bronchospasm.

Fiberoptic bronchoscopy with bronchoalveolar lavage (BAL)

BAL is the diagnostic procedure of choice in hospitals where prevalence of PCP is low or where ISA is difficult to obtain, or to confirm a negative ISA. Sensitivity of BAL (which requires at least 15–25 ml of lavage fluid) ranges from 55%–97% and is not affected by previous aerosolized pentamidine prophylaxis [32, 33]. Importantly, BAL may be positive for at least 72 hours after PCP treatment has been instituted. Treatment should not be delayed while awaiting the results of the procedure [34]. Complications of BAL include transient increase in pulmonary infiltrates at the lavage site, transient hypoxemia, pneumothorax, hemoptysis, and postbronchoscopy fever.

Fiberoptic bronchoscopy with transbronchial biopsy (TBB)

This procedure is not recommended routinely unless the BAL is negative or non-diagnostic in a patient with a presentation consistent with PCP. The sensitivity of TBB ranges from 87%–95% and cysts may be identified up to 10 days after treatment has begun (up to 4–6 weeks in some patients) [35]. Complications of TBB include pneumothorax and hemorrhage. This procedure may be contraindicated in patients with severe thrombocytopenia.

Non-bronchoscopic bronchoalveolar lavage.

This technique has been used with infants and children in whom bronchoscopy is technically difficult. Although a larger specimen can be obtained using this procedure than through ISA, the procedure carries a significant risk of aspiration because the catheter is placed blindly.

Open lung biopsy

This diagnostic procedure is the most sensitive for PCP but is seldom used today, as it requires thoracotomy and chest tube drainage. Complications include pneumothorax, pneumomediastinum, and hemorrhage.

Diagnostic methods

Diagnostic stains and histology

There are three different stains used in the diagnosis of *Pneumocystis* organisms in specimens. These include: Gomori-methenamine-silver stain, which stains the cyst wall brown or black; toluidine blue stain, which stains the cyst wall blue or lavender and also stains fungal elements; and Giemsa and/or Wright's stain, which stains *Pneumocystis* trophozoites and intracystic sporozoites pale blue with a punctate red nucleus. This stain does not stain the cyst wall. Many laboratories are currently diagnosing *Pneumocystis* with monoclonal fluorescent antibodies, which stain the cyst wall of *Pneumocystis*.

Polymerase chain reaction (PCR)

It is possible to amplify *P. carinii* DNA sequences by PCR directly from blood or serum samples as well as from nasopharyngeal aspirates and BAL specimens [36]. This is currently a research tool and is not available at most institutions.

Treatment (see Table 35.1)

Children with known or suspected HIV infection who present with a clinical picture consistent with PCP, and CD4 counts or age that place them at risk for PCP infection, should be treated presumptively without delay, and without waiting for confirmation by diagnostic examinations. Intravenous trimethoprim–sulfamethoxazole (TMP/SMX) should be initiated (unless patient is known to be allergic) regardless of the patient's prior prophylactic regimen. TMP/SMX at full treatment doses remains the first-line treatment of choice in patients who develop PCP while on TMP/SMX prophylaxis. Improvement occurs usually within 4 to 7 days, although initial worsening on effective treatment may also occur due to the lysis of organisms. The recommended duration of treatment is a minimum of 21 days. Secondary prophylaxis to prevent recurrence should be instituted for all children once treatment for confirmed PCP has been completed.

Treatment failure is defined as a clinical deterioration, with worsening respiratory status and arterial blood gases after at least 4 days of appropriate treatment. Alternative etiologies or confirmation of co-infections with cytomegalovirus (CMV) pneumonitis, *Candida albicans*, *Mycobacterium avium intracellulare* complex (MAC), *Mycobacterium tuberculosis*, *Aspergillus fumigatus* or *Streptococcus pneumoniae* should be pursued. If additional diagnoses are not confirmed, treatment failure should be considered and a change in PCP therapy may be warranted. Treatment with intravenous pentamidine should be considered in such cases. Alternatively, studies in adults and limited pediatric data suggest that therapy with clindamycin with primaquine, atovaquone, trimetrexate glucuronate with leucovorin, or dapsone with trimethoprim may be appropriate in such cases or in patients when TMP/SMX is not tolerated due to allergy or toxicity.

Supportive measures

Oxygen should be given to maintain PaO_2 >70 mm Hg. Assisted ventilation should be initiated when PaO_2 ≤60 mm Hg with ≥50% FiO_2. Continuous positive airway pressure (CPAP) by facemask may improve oxygenation in cases with tachypnea and desaturation refractory to standard masks, thereby mitigating the need for mechanical ventilation.

Therapy for PCP

Trimethoprim/sulfamethoxazole (TMP/SMX)

TMP/SMX is preferred for initial treatment of PCP because of its excellent tissue penetration, oral bioavailability, rapid in vivo activity, and wide availability [37, 38]. It blocks the *Pneumocystis* organism's folic acid biosynthesis by inhibiting sequential steps in the biosynthetic pathway.

Table 35.1. Treatment of *Pneumocystis* infection

Drug	Dosage	Mode of action	Adverse effects	Comments
Trimethoprim/ sulfamethoxazole (TMP/SMX)	15–20 mg/kg per day TMP + 75–100 mg/kg per day SMX IV every 6 hrs 20 mg/kg per day TMP + 100 mg/kg per day PO every 6–8 hrs Duration: 21 days	Blocks sequential steps in folic acid metabolism	Rash – erythematous maculopapular, Stevens–Johnson; neutropenia; thrombocytopenia; megaloblastic or aplastic anemia; increased liver function tests	– Use only in children > 4–6 weeks. – May consider change to oral therapy to complete 21 days in mild-moderate disease
Pentamidine isothionate	4 mg/kg per day IV/IM every 24 hrs (infused over 60–90 min.) Duration: 21 days	Mechanism unknown May interfere with nucleic acid synthesis	Hypotension; pancreatitis; renal failure; insulin-dependent diabetes; fever; neutropenia; hypo/hyperglycemia; torsades de pointe (prolonged QT interval)	– For patients who can't tolerate TMP/SMX or are not responding after 5–7 days. – Do not give with didanosine. – Rx may be complicated by toxicities in 80% patients
Clindamycin / primaquine	Clindaymycin: 10 mg/kg IV or PO every 6 hrs Primaquine 0.5 mg/kg (30 mg base) PO every 24 hrs Duration: 21 days	Mechanism unknown	Skin rashes; nausea, neutropenia, hemolytic anemia (in G6PD), diarrhea (*C. difficile*)	– Effective in mild-moderate PCP in adults – Contraindicated in G6PD deficiency

Drug	Dosage	Mechanism	Adverse effects	Comments
Atovaquone	3–24 m: 45 mg/kg per day susp. PO every 24 hrs 2–13 yr: 30–40 mg/kg per day susp. PO every 12 hrs 13–16 yrs: 750 mg/day (5 ml) PO every 12 hrs Duration 21 days	Mechanism unknown May interrupt pyrimidine synthesis.	Diarrhea; nausea skin rashs (after first week) transaminitis	– Effective in mild to moderate PCP – May be used in patients with G6PD – Bioavailability significantly increased by administration with fatty food
Trimetrexate / leucovorin	Trimetrexate: 45 mg/m² IV every 24 hrs for 21 days Leucovorin: 20 mg/m² IV every 6 hrs for 24 d (72 hrs after trimetrexate discontinuation)	1500 x more potent than TMP for dihydrofolate reductase	Reversible neutropenia; skin rashes; stomatitis; transaminitis; anemia; thrombocytopenia	– Most effective as salvage therapy in patients who fail TMP/SMX – Must use with Leucovorin which protects host cells from disruption of dihydrofolate reductase pathway
Dapsone/ trimethoprim	Dapsone: 2 mg/kg PO every 24 hrs (maximum 100 mg) T: 5 mg/kg PO every 8 hrs Duration: 21 days	Inhibitor of dihydropteroate synthase	Methemoglobinemia; hemolytic anemia; neutropenia; thrombocytopenia	– Effective in mild-moderate PCP in adults – Contraindicated in G6PD

Dosage and administration

TMP/SMX should only be used in children who are older than 4–6 weeks of age because the drug can displace bilirubin bound to albumin and increase the risk of kernicterus in young infants. The dose is 15–20 mg/kg per day (of TMP component) given intravenously in four divided doses (dose infused over 1 hour). Oral treatment (20 mg/kg per day of TMP component in three or four divided doses) to complete a 21-day course may be considered once pneumonitis has resolved, or in the case of mild disease.

Adverse reactions

Patients with AIDS appear to have an increased incidence of adverse reactions such as rash (including Stevens–Johnson syndrome), neutropenia, thrombocytopenia, megaloblastic or aplastic anemia. Between 15% and 35% of HIV-infected children may experience some toxicity. In children with cutaneous reactions, oral or intravenous desensitization with TMP/SMX has been found to be useful in allowing children to restart TMP/SMX therapy without significant allergic sequelae. Desensitization should be performed in a pediatric intensive care unit whenever possible.

Pentamidine isothionate (PI)

PI is the drug of choice for patients unable to tolerate TMP/SMX or who have not shown improvement after 4–7 days of TMP–SMX therapy. Combination therapy with TMP/SMX and PI does not appear to be more beneficial than PI alone and is potentially more toxic [39]. In patients with clinical improvement after 7–10 days of intravenous PI, an oral regimen (i.e., atovaquone) to complete a 21-day course may be considered.

Dosage and administration

PI should be administered at a dose of 4 mg/kg per day given intravenously or intramuscularly (IV given over 60–90 minutes to reduce incidence of hypotension).

Adverse reactions

The most common adverse drug reaction is renal toxicity, which usually occurs in the second week of treatment. Severe hypotension, prolonged QT interval (torsades de pointe), and cardiac arrhythmias may occur. Hypoglycemia (usually occurs after 5–7 days of therapy) or hyperglycemia, hypercalcemia, hyperkalemia, pancreatitis, and insulin-dependent diabetes mellitus have also been reported. Many patients complain of a metallic and/or bitter taste.

Clindamycin/primaquine

This combination has shown efficacy in the treatment of mild-to-moderate PCP in adults [37]. There is also evidence suggesting it may be the most beneficial alternative for patients not responding to TMP/SMX or pentamidine [40]. Its mechanism of action against *Pneumocystis* is unknown.

Dosage and administration

Dosing of this combination has not been studied in children with PCP. Drug doses are extrapolated from approved pediatric dosing for other indications. Children should receive clindamycin 10 mg/kg (to a maximum of 600 mg) intravenously every 6 hours for 21 days. Primaquine should be administered as 0.3 mg/kg (30 mg base) orally once daily for 21 days.

Adverse reactions

Adverse reactions can include skin rashes, nausea, and diarrhea, neutropenia, anemia, and *Clostridium difficile*-associated colitis.

Atovaquone

This drug is recommended for mild to moderately severe PCP for patients who cannot tolerate TMP/SMX. Bioavailability of atovaquone is greatly increased by administration with fatty foods. Its mechanism of action against *Pneumocystis* is unknown although it may interrupt pyrimidine synthesis.

Dosage and administration

Infants 3 to 24 months require 45 mg/kg/per day suspension while children 2 through 12 years old may receive 30 mg/kg/per day suspension given orally in two divided doses with fatty foods. For 13- to 16-year-olds the recommended dose is 750 mg (5 ml) suspension administered orally with meals twice daily for 21 days (total daily dose 1500 mg) [41].

Adverse reactions

Most adverse reactions appear after the first week of therapy. Skin rashes, nausea, anemia, neutropenia, and diarrhea have been reported. Patients may develop elevated liver transaminase concentrations.

Drug interactions

Fluconazole and prednisone increase the concentration of atovaquone, whereas acyclovir, opiates, cephalosporins, rifampin and benzodiazepines decrease its plasma concentration.

Trimetrexate glucuronate/leucovorin

Trimetrexate is effective as initial and salvage therapy in severe PCP in adults. There is limited pediatric data [42]. Trimetrexate is an extremely potent inhibitor of *Pneumocystis* dihydrofolate reductase (DHFR). To prevent adverse hematological effects it must be used in conjunction with leucovorin, a reduced folate.

Dosage and administration

Based on limited pediatric data available for this agent, trimetrexate should be administered at 45 mg/m^2 per day intravenously for 21 days with leucovorin 20 mg/m^2 intravenously every 6 hours for 24 days or for 72 hours after the last dose of trimetrexate.

Adverse reactions

Reversible neutropenia is the primary adverse event with this agent. Skin rashes, stomatitis, transaminitis, anemia, and thrombocytopenia may occur, as well as an elevation of serum transaminases. Most events are reversible even with continued drug administration at reduced dose.

Dapsone/trimethoprim

This combination has been shown to be effective in the treatment of mild-to-moderate PCP in adults [37]. Data regarding its toxicity and efficacy in children with PCP is lacking. It is contraindicated in patients with glucose-6-phosphate dehydrogenase (G-6-PD) deficiency due to the risk of hemolytic anemia. Dapsone/trimethoprim is an inhibitor of *Pneumocystis* dihydropteroate synthesis.

Dosage and administration

Based on limited available pediatric data, dapsone should be administered 2 mg/kg by mouth once daily (maximum 100 mg) for 21 days. Trimethoprim is administered 5 mg/kg by mouth three times daily for 21 days.

Adverse reactions

Adverse reactions include methemoglobinemia, transaminitis, anemia, neutropenia, and thrombocytopenia.

Adjunctive therapies

Corticosteroids

An inflammatory response due to dying organisms may cause a worsening of respiratory status after therapy initiation [43]. Corticosteroids are recommended for adults with moderate to severe PCP [44]. Several small pediatric studies have shown a reduction in acute respiratory failure, decrease in requirement of ventilatory support and significant decrease in mortality with early use of adjunctive corticosteroids [45–47]. However, steroids should be used with caution in patients who may be co-infected with *Pneumocystis* and CMV because corticosteroids may adversely affect the course of the CMV disease [12, 48]. The dosage of corticosteroids used in children varies among studies. Alternatives include: (1) prednisone: Day 1–5 = 40 mg twice daily, Day 6–10 = 40 mg daily, Day 11–21 = 20 mg daily; (2) Prednisone (or methylprednisolone sodium): Day 1–5 = 1 mg/kg twice daily, Day 6–10 = 0.5 mg/kg per dose twice daily; Day

11–18 = 0.5 mg/kg once a day; (3) Methylprednisolone intravenously: Day 1–7 = 1 mg/kg every 6 hours, Day 8–9 = 1 mg/kg twice a day, Day 10–11 = 0.5 mg/kg twice a day; Day 12–16 = 1 mg/kg once a day.

Surfactant

A few case reports have shown that patients with PCP have decreased amounts of pulmonary surfactant. Surfactant therapy has been beneficial in improving pulmonary function in case reports of infants with confirmed PCP accompanied by ARDS and respiratory failure requiring assisted ventilation [49–51]. Surfactant offers a possible treatment strategy in desperately ill infants. It should be used in consultation with a pediatric infectious disease specialist.

Summary

The incidence of PCP is decreasing in developed countries with improved identification of HIV-infected pregnant women and their infants, primary PCP prophylaxis, and use of highly active antiretroviral therapy. Disease continues to be prevalent in developing countries in children with severe pneumonia. *Pneumocystis* remains a significant cause of morbidity and mortality in immunocompromised children throughout the world. Transmission may occur through reactivation of latent infection; environmental sources via the airborne route, or potentially from human to human. The treatment of choice for established PCP is high dose trimethoprim/sulfamethoxazole with corticosteroids in moderate to severe disease. Alternatives to trimethoprim/sulfamethoxazole for the intolerant or failing patient include intravenous pentamidine, clindamycin with primaquine, atovaquone, trimetrexate glucuronate with leucovorin, or dapsone with trimethoprim.

REFERENCES

1. Edman, J. C., Kovacs, J. A., Masur, H., Santi, D. V., Elwood, H. J., Sogin, M. L., Ribosomal RNA sequence shows *Pneumocystis carinii* to be a member of the fungi. *Nature* 1988;**334**(6182):519–522.

2. Stringer, J. R., *Pneumocystis carinii*: what is it, exactly? *Clin. Microbiol. Rev.* 1996;**9**(4):489–498.

3. Vargas, S. L. Hughes, W. T., Santolaya, M. E. Search for primary infection by *Pneumocystis carinii* in a cohort of normal, healthy infants. *Clin. Infect. Dis.* 2001;**32**(6):855–861.

4. Sheldon, W. Subclinical *Pneumocystis* pneumonitis. *Am. J. Dis. Child.* 1959;97:287–297.

5. CDC, Prevention DoHA. Pediatric HIV/AIDS Surveillance: Slide Series L262. In CDC; 2001.

6. Dankner, W. M., Lindsey, J. C., Levin, M. J. Correlates of opportunistic infections in children infected with the human immunodeficiency virus managed before highly active antiretroviral therapy. *Pediatr. Infect. Dis. J.*, 2001;**20**(1):40–48.

7. Zar, H. J., Dechaboon, A., Hanslo, D., Apolles, P., Magnus, K. G., Hussey, G. *Pneumocystis carinii* pneumonia in South African children infected with human immunodeficiency virus. *Pediatr. Infect. Dis. J.* 2000;**19**(7):603–607.

8. Ruffini, D. D., Madhi, S. A. The high burden of *Pneumocystis carinii* pneumonia in African HIV-1-infected children hospitalized for severe pneumonia. *AIDS* 2002;**16**(1):105–112.

9. Chokephaibulkit, K., Wanachiwanawin, D., Chearskul, S. *et al. Pneumocystis carinii* severe pneumonia among human immunodeficiency virus-infected children in Thailand: the effect of a primary prophylaxis strategy. *Pediatr. Infect. Dis. J.* 1999;**18**(2):147–152.

10. Kumar, A., St John, M. A. HIV infection among children in Barbados. *West Indian Med. J.* 2000;**49**(1):43–46.

11. Jeena, P. M., Coovadia, H. M., Chrystal, V. *Pneumocystis carinii* and cytomegalovirus infections in severely ill, HIV-infected African infants. *Ann. Trop. Paediatr.* 1996;**16**(4):361–368.

12. Williams A. J., Duong, T., McNally, L. M., Tookey, P. A., Masters, J., Miller, R. *et al. Pneumocystis carinii* pneumonia and cytomegalovirus infection in children with vertically acquired HIV infection. *AIDS* 2001;**15**(3):335–339.

13. Graham, S. M., Mtitimila, E. I., Kamanga, H. S., Walsh, A. L., Hart, C. A., Molyneux, M. E. Clinical presentation and outcome of *Pneumocystis carinii* pneumonia in Malawian children. *Lancet* 2000;**355**(9201):369–373.

14. Simond, R. J., Oxtoby, M. I., Caldwell, M. B., Gwinn, M. L., Rogers, M. F. *Pneumocystis carinii* pueumonia among US children with perinatally acquired HIV infection. *J. Am. Med. Assoc.* 1993;**270**(4):470–474.

15. Sheikh, S., Bakshi, S. S., Pahwa, S. G. Outcome and survival in HIV-infected infants with *Pneumocystis carinii* pneumonia and respiratory failure. *Pediatr. AIDS HIV Infect.* 1996;**7**(3):155–163.

16. Casanova-Cardiel, L., Leibowitz, M. J. Presence of *Pneumocystis carinii* DNA in pond water. *J. Eukaryot. Microbiol.* 1997;**44**(6):28S.

17. Olsson, M., Lidman. Latouche. S. *et al.* Identification of *Pneumocystis carinii f. sp. hominis* gene sequences in filtered air in hospital environments. *J. Clin. Microbiol.* 1998;**36**(6):1737–1740.

18. Beck, J. M. *Pneumocystis carinii* and geographic clustering: evidence for transmission of infection. *Am. J. Respir. Crit. Care Med.* 2000;**162**(5):1605–1606.

19. Helweg-Larsen, J., Tsolaki, A. G., Miller, R. F., Lundgren, B., Wakefield, A. E. Clusters of *Pneumocystis carinii* pneumonia: analysis of person-to-person transmission by genotyping. *Quart. J. Med.* 1998;**91**(12):813–820.

20. Benfield, T. L., Prento, P., Junge, J., Vestbo, J., Lundgren, J. D. Alveolar damage in AIDS-related *Pneumocystis carinii* pneumonia. *Chest* 1997;**111**(5):1193–1199.

21. Coleman, D. L., Dodek, P. M., Golden, J. A. *et al.* Correlation between serial pulmonary function tests and fiberoptic bronchoscopy in patients with *Pneumocystis carinii* pneumonia and the acquired immune deficiency syndrome. *Am. Rev. Respir. Dis.* 1984;**129**(3):491–493.

22. Hughes, W. T. *Pneumocystis carinii* pneumonia: new approaches to diagnosis, treatment and prevention. *Pediatr. Infect. Dis. J.* 1991;**10**(5):391–399.

23. Mueller, B. U., Butler, K. M., Husson, R. N., Pizzo, P. A. *Pneumocystis carinii* pneumonia despite prophylaxis in children with human immunodeficiency virus infection. *J. Pediatr.* 1991;**119**(6):992–994.

24. Ng, V. L., Yajko, D. M., Hadley, W. K. Extrapulmonary pneumocystosis. *Clin. Microbiol. Rev.* 1997;**10**(3):401–418.

25. Hagmann, S., Merali, S., Sitnitskaya, Y., Fefferman, N., Pollack, H. *Pneumocystis carinii* infection presenting as an intra-abdominal cystic mass in a child with acquired immunodeficiency syndrome. *Clin. Infect. Dis.* 2001;**33**(8):1424–1426.

26. Boldt, M. J., Bai, T. R. Utility of lactate dehydrogenase vs radiographic severity in the differential diagnosis of *Pneumocystis carinii* pneumonia. *Chest* 1997;**111**(5):1187–1192.

27. Sivit, C. J., Miller, C. R., Rakusan, T. A., Ellaurie, M., Kushner, D. C. Spectrum of chest radiographic abnormalities in children with AIDS and *Pneumocystis carinii* pneumonia. *Pediatr. Radiol.* 1995;**25**(5):389–392.

28. Solomon, K. S., Levin, T. L., Berdon, W. E., Romney, B., Ruzal-Shapiro, C., Bye, M. R. Pneumothorax as the presenting sign of *Pneumocystis carinii* infection in an HIV-positive child with prior lymphocytic interstitial pneumonitis. *Pediatr. Radiol.* 1996;**26**(8):559–562.

29. Ambrosino, M. M., Roche, K. J., Genieser, N. B., Kaul, A., Lawrence, R. M. Application of thin section low-dose chest CT (TSCT) in the management of *pediatric AIDS. Pediatr. Radiol.* 1995;**25**(5):393–400.

30. Coleman, D. L., Hattner, R. S., Luce J. M., Dodek, P. M., Golden, J. A., Murray, J. F. Correlation between gallium lung scans and fiberoptic bronchoscopy in patients with suspected *Pneumocystis carinii* pneumonia and the acquired immune deficiency syndrome. *Am. Rev. Respir. Dis.* 1984;**130**(6):1166–1169.

31. Kamiya, Y., Mtitimila, E., Graham, S. M., Broadhead, R. L., Brabin, B., Hart, C. A. *Pneumocystis carinii* pneumonia in Malawian children. *Ann. Trop. Paediatr.* 1997;**17**(2):121–126.

32. Kroe, D. M., Kirsch, C. M., Jensen, W. A. Diagnostic strategies for *Pneumocystis carinii* pneumonia. *Semin. Respir. Infect.* 1997;**12**(2):70–78.

33. Levine, S. J., Masur, H., Gill, V. J. *et al.* Effect of aerosolized pentamidine prophylaxis on the diagnosis of *Pneumocystis carinii* pneumonia by induced sputum examination in patients infected with the human immunodeficiency virus. *Am. Rev. Respir. Dis.* 1991;**144**(4):760–764.

34. de Blic, J., McKelvie, P., Le Bourgeois, M., Blanche, S., Benoist, M. R., Scheinmann, P. Value of bronchoalveolar lavage in the management of severe acute pneumonia and interstitial pneumonitis in the immunocompromised child. *Thorax* 1987;**42**(10):759–765.

35. Shelhamer, J. H., Ognibene, F. P., Macher, A. M. *et al.* Persistence of *Pneumocystis carinii* in lung tissue of acquired immunodeficiency syndrome patients treated for pneumocystis pneumonia. *Am. Rev. Respir. Dis.* 1984;**130**(6):1161–1165.

36. Weig, M., Klinker, H., Bogner, B. H., Meier, A., Gross, U. Usefulness of PCR for diagnosis of *Pneumocystis carinii* pneumonia in different patient groups. *J. Clin. Microbiol.* 1997;**35**(6):1445–1449.

37. Warren, E., George, S., You, J., Kazanjian, P. Advances in the treatment and prophylaxis of *Pneumocystis carinii* pneumonia. *Pharmacotherapy* 1997;**17**(5):900–916.

38. Hughes, W. T. Current issues in the epidemiology, transmission, and reactivation of *Pneumocystis carinii. Semin. Respir. Infect.* 1998;**13**(4):283–288.

39. Walzer, P. D. *Pneumocystis carinii.* In Mandell, G. D. R., Benett, J. ed. *Principles and Practices of Infectious Diseases.*, New York: Churchill Livingstone; 1990:2103–2210.

40. Smego, R. A., Jr., Nagar, S., Maloba, B., Popara, M. A meta-analysis of salvage therapy for *Pneumocystis carinii* pneumonia. *Arch. Intern. Med.* 2001;**161**(12):1529–1533.

41. Hughes, W, Dorenbaum, A, Yogev, R. *et al.* Phase I safety and pharmacokinetics study of micronized atovaquone in human immunodeficiency virus-infected infants and children. Pediatric AIDS Clinical Trials Group. *Antimicrob. Agents Chemother.* 1998;**42**(6):1315–1318.

42. Smit, M. I., De Groot, R., Van Dongen, J. J., Van der Voort, E., Neijens, H. J., Whitfield, L. R. Trimetrexate efficacy and pharmacokinetics during treatment of refractory *Pneumocystis carinii* pneumonia in an infant with severe combined immunodeficiency disease. *Pediatr. Infect. Dis. J.* 1990;**9**(3):212–214; discussion 215.

43. Masur, H. Prevention and treatment of *Pneumocystis* pneumonia. *N. Engl. J. Med.* 1992;**327**(26):1853–1860.

44. NIH Panel. Consensus statement on the use of corticosteroids as adjunctive therapy for *Pneumocystis* pneumonia in the acquired immunodeficiency syndrome. The National Institutes of Health-University of California Expert Panel for corticosteroids as adjunctive therapy for *Pneumocystis* Pneumonia. *N. Engl. J. Med.* 1990;**323**(21):1500–1504.

45. Bye, M. R., Cairns-Bazarian, A. M., Ewig, J. M. Markedly reduced mortality associated with corticosteroid therapy of *Pneumocystis carinii* pneumonia in children with acquired immunodeficiency syndrome. *Arch. Pediatr. Adolesc. Med.* 1994;**148**(6):638–641.

46. McLaughlin, G. E., Virdee, S. S., Schleien, C. L., Holzman, B. H., Scott, G. B. Effect of corticosteroids on survival of children with acquired immunodeficiency syndrome and *Pneumocystis carinii* related respiratory failure. *J. Pediatr.* 1995;**126**(5 Pt 1):821–824.

47. Sleasman, J. W., Hemenway, C., Klein, A. S., Barrett, D. J. Corticosteroids improve survival of children with AIDS and *Pneumocystis carinii* pneumonia. *Am. J. Dis. Child.* 1993;**147**(1):30–34.

48. Jensen, A. M., Lundgren, J. D., Benfield, T., Nielsen, T. L., Vestbo, J. Does cytomegalovirus predict a poor prognosis in *Pneumocystis carinii* pneumonia treated with corticosteroids? A note for caution. *Chest* 1995;**108**(2):411–414.

49. Creery, W. D., Hashmj, A., Hutchison, J. S., Singh, R. N. Surfactant therapy improves pulmonary function in infants with *Pneumocystis carinii* pneumonia and acquired immunodeficiency syndrome. *Pediatr. Pulmonol* 1997;**24**(5):370–373.

50. Hughes, W. L., Sillos, E. M., LaFon, S. *et al.* Effects of aerosolized synthetic surfactant, atovaquone, and the combination of these on murine *Pneumocystis carinii* pneumonia. *J. Infect. Dis.* 1998;**177**(4):1046–1056.

51. Marriage, S. C., Underhill, H., Nadel, S. Use of natural surfactant in an HIV-infected infant with *Pneumocystis carinii* pneumonia. *Intens. Care Med.* 1996;**22**(6):611–612.

Part VI

Medical, social, and legal issues

36 Medical issues related to the care of HIV-infected children in the home, daycare, school, and community

Stephen J. Chanock, M.D.

Pediatric Oncology Branch, National Cancer Institute, NIH, Bethesda, MD

Introduction

Children with HIV infection spend very little time in hospital; they live, learn, grow and play in different settings in the community. Despite significant advances in the understanding of HIV infection, misconceptions continue to harm children with HIV infection. These misunderstandings have led to ostracism in situations which present no risk to others. A major challenge for those caring for children with HIV infection is to promote acceptance of HIV-infected children in the community. Healthcare providers bear an important responsibility to educate children, their caretakers, and the community at large on the risk of transmission of HIV and other infections. Recommended practices for reducing the risk for transmission should be implemented without exaggeration of risk for transmission. Every effort should be made to promote understanding and compassion, and to maintain confidentiality for children with HIV infection [1–3].

Transmission of HIV

Transmission of HIV requires a sufficient quantity of virus. The risk for transmission of HIV is directly related to exposure to contaminated body fluids [1]. HIV has been isolated from many body fluids (see Table 36.1), but HIV transmission is most commonly associated with exposure to blood or semen, which are rich in lymphocytes and monocytes [1]. There are four major modes of HIV transmission: (a) between sex partners; (b) from an HIV-infected mother to her child during pregnancy, delivery, or breastfeeding; (c) by direct inoculation of infected blood or blood-containing tissues, including transfusion, transplantation, reuse of contaminated needles, or penetrating injuries with contaminated needles; (d) splattering or spraying of mucous membranes

Handbook of Pediatric HIV Care, ed. Steven L. Zeichner and Jennifer S. Read.
Published by Cambridge University Press. © Cambridge University Press 2006.

Table 36.1. Body fluids from which HIV has been isolated (in general order of frequency of recovery)[a]

Blood
Semen
Vaginal and cervical secretions
Amniotic fluid
Breast milk
Saliva
Tears
Throat swabs
Cerebrospinal fluid
Synovial, pleural, peritoneal, and pericardial fluid

[a] HIV has not been routinely isolated from stool or vomitus; however, these fluids theoretically may contain HIV if contaminated with blood.

Table 36.2. Risk for transmission of HIV is dependent upon

Volume of exposed blood or contaminated body fluid
Concentration of HIV in source person's blood or body fluid (related to the stage of infection)
Antiretroviral therapy
Route of exposure (in order of decreasingly efficient transmission)
Intravenous
Mucosal (broken $\gg$ intact)
Percutaneous (non-intact $\gg$ intact skin)
Pathogenic features of the source's virus
Underlying health of exposed individual

or non-intact skin with infected blood [4]. The risk of HIV transmission by one of these four modes depends upon a number of factors listed in Table 36.2. Inhalation of aerosols, bites from bloodsucking insects, or ingestion of food prepared or served by an infected person have not been associated with transmission of HIV. Estimates of the risks posed by different exposures are provided in Chapter 17, which also describes interventions aimed at reducing the chance of infection.

The risk for HIV transmission to and from children

Existing data do not support casual contact as a risk factor for transmission. Body fluids visibly contaminated with blood pose a risk for transmission; casual contact does not. Accidental spilling or splattering of contaminated body secretions is a less efficient mode of transmission than the four listed above. HIV transmission in household settings has only been reported in individuals exposed to blood or secretions known to be

Table 36.3. Appropriate precautions outside the hospital environment[a]

Education

Prevention of exposure

Recognition of exposure

Knowledge that HIV is only transmitted via intimate contact (intimate sexual contact or inoculation of contaminated material)

Proper clean-up procedure/use of standard precautions

Appreciation of importance of good handwashing technique between contacts

Need to remain calm

Access to medical advice (if needed)

Materials

Gloves and gowns for anticipated exposure to any body fluid

Masks and goggles only if splattering or spraying of material is likely

Bleach (for 1:10 or 1:100 dilution in water)

Disposable vessel for cleaning fluid

Disposal bags or container

[a] Standard precautions [7] were designed for hospital-based conditions but should be applied to any location where exposure to body fluids is anticipated.

highly contaminated with HIV through percutaneous inoculation or via contact with non-intact skin or mucous membranes [1].

The HIV virion is labile and highly susceptible to disinfectants, making the risk of transmission from contaminated environmental surfaces very low. Still, in the event of a spill, the recommended solution for cleaning a spill is diluted bleach (at 1:10 to 1:100 concentration) [5–7]. Gloves, suitable material to clean the spill, and adequate disposal containers (Table 36.3) should be available where children play, learn or rest [1].

In horizontal household exposure studies, transmission via casual contact is exceptionally rare, if it occurs at all [1, 4]. Biting is common among children but rarely results in exposure to blood. Transmission following a bite is unlikely unless blood is inoculated percutaneously. In prospective studies of individuals bitten by HIV-infected patients, no seroconversions have been reported. In a handful of reported cases, individuals have seroconverted following a severe, bloody human bite. Data do not support HIV transmission by kissing, particularly non-romantic kissing between children and loved ones. In the two cases of possible transmission following passionate or deep kissing, at least one of the partners was noted to have bleeding gums and blood-stained saliva, which probably accounted for transmission [1].

The risk of HIV transmission from contact among children in households, schools, daycare centers, and other out-of-home childcare settings is extremely small. Sequence analysis has pinpointed the household source of infection, exposure to blood or bloody material through non-intact skin or mucous membranes. Nearly 20 studies, including more than 1300 household contacts, have shown that, within households, new cases

Table 36.4. Household contact activities not associated with transmission of HIV infection

Sharing the same bed
Bathing together
Kissing on lips
Sharing comb
Sharing toilet
Sharing eating utensil
Giving injection
Sharing toothbrush[a]

[a] Sharing of toothbrush or razor is not recommended.

of HIV only occurred in individuals with other, major risk factors for acquisition of infection [1]. Many of these studies have specifically demonstrated the absence of transmission associated even with household activities that might involve contact with blood or other potentially infected body fluids, such as sharing razors or tooth brushes (see Table 36.4) [4].

Reported cases of HIV transmission have been associated with the provision of home healthcare, typically via needle stick or splattering of contaminated material onto non-intact skin or mucosal membranes [8]. Prospective studies of health care workers following needle-stick injuries indicate the estimated the risk of HIV transmission following a single percutaneous exposure to HIV-infected blood is about 0.3% [8]. Deep penetrating injury, visible blood on the contaminated device, a high viral load in the source individual, recent placement of the catheter in a blood vessel, or death of the source patient within 60 days after exposure increase the likelihood of transmission [3, 8, 9]. HIV transmission following exposure of non-intact skin or mucous membranes to HIV-infected blood has rarely been reported. The estimated risk for this exposure is less than 0.1% [1]. These rare cases have resulted from extensive exposure to concentrated HIV-contaminated body fluids, splashed into an open wound or onto mucous membranes.

Precautions and HIV transmission

Guidelines for universal precautions were developed to curtail the risk for transmission of all blood-borne pathogens [1, 5]. Other blood-borne infectious agents, including hepatitis B and C are transmitted more efficiently than HIV [3]. The guidelines are known as "standard precautions" [7] and should always be observed for every patient, with or without a known infection. They mandate safe practices in all settings and barrier precautions when contact with blood or body fluids is anticipated (Tables 36.3 and 36.5) [5, 7]. Gloves should be used for handling blood, body fluids, excretions, secretions, mucous membranes, and non-intact skin. Gowns and gloves should be worn if extensive or uncontrolled contact with blood or potentially infected materials is

Table 36.5. Techniques of standard precautions that should be practiced outside of hospital

Handwashing	Before and after contact with body fluids. Always after removing gloves.
Gloves	Worn if contact with virus-containing body fluid is anticipated
Masks/eye wear	If splattering of body fluid is likely
Non-sterile gown	Protect skin/clothing from splashes
	Dispose of properly for cleaning
Patient equipment	Handle carefully to avoid splattering
Linen	Change and dispose of without exposure to others
Surface cleaning	Thorough cleaning of exposed surface
	Removal of fluid
	Disinfect with bleach solution (see Table 36.3)

anticipated. Masks, protective eyewear, face shields, and gowns should be used if there is a chance of splattering infected material onto the face or body, a type of exposure that would typically be a concern in a hospital. Gloves should be removed and hands washed immediately after contact with blood or body fluids. For the care of children, gloves are not recommended for routine diaper changes and cleaning of nasal secretions [2], and when feeding a child, including breast milk. However, some experts have argued that standard precautions be used when preparing or offering breast milk, if the HIV infection status of the mother or breast milk donor is unknown.

With children, the cornerstone of preventing transmission by needle-stick or exposure to contaminated sharp items is avoidance. Tamper-proof infectious waste disposals must be kept out of reach of children [10]. Homecare providers should receive proper education in standard precautions. Only non-recapping equipment should be used out of hospital. Under no circumstances should needles, syringes, or other such equipment be used for more than one person without sterilization. Blood or potentially infected body fluids spilled on environmental surfaces should be promptly removed and disposed of properly. Contaminated surfaces must be cleaned with a bleach solution after the liquid material has been absorbed and disposed of properly [5, 7].

Appropriate infection control practices should be rigorously followed in all health care settings, such as clinics, offices, or homes. Common play areas on pediatric wards, in clinics, and in offices need to be supervised by staff trained to handle situations, such as bleeding episodes, that may pose a risk of disease transmission. Toys should be cleaned and disinfected before being used by another child if they are contaminated by blood. Otherwise, there should be no restriction on availability of toys.

General principles for HIV infection control outside the hospital

An approach to HIV infection control must be developed that protects both the HIV-infected child and others (Table 36.6). First, confidentiality must be protected at all times. Knowledge of HIV infection status should be restricted to only those who are

Table 36.6. HIV infection in the home: what to say and do

Assurance that transmission of HIV results from inoculation of contaminated blood only
Home transmission only results from accidental inoculation
   Need to have intimate contact with infected material
Casual or physical contact has never been associated with transmission
   Sharing and casual contact are to be encouraged
Use barrier protection for anticipated contact with blood or blood-tinged material
Avoid exposure to blood or blood-contaminated materials
   Prevent access to medical supplies and drugs
Immediately report blood spillage
Clean up spills with appropriate materials
   Keep children away during clean-up
Protect confidentiality of family unit

---

responsible for medical decisions. There is no indication for public disclosure of HIV infection status unless the child's parents and healthcare providers believe it suitable. Mandatory HIV testing is not indicated for attendance at schools, nor for participation in athletics and daycare. Education of lay people (e.g., coaches, daycare providers, foster parents and teachers) who may supervise HIV-infected children is essential. Blood exposures from fights, unintentional injuries, nosebleeds, shed teeth, menstruation, and other causes can occur in many different venues. All institutions that care for and educate children should educate staff about safe practices, establish policies for protecting confidentiality, provide suitable cleaning materials, and use appropriate infection control practices, including standard precautions, for all children (Tables 36.3 and 36.5).

Because of the advances in antiretroviral therapy, many children are living longer and attending activities outside of the home. Many choose to disclose their HIV infection status. Educational programs should be available in all settings, and in addition, support systems are needed to counsel and advise infected children. Appropriate infection control practices should be reviewed in all settings where children play, learn, or rest [2, 11]. Although HIV-infected children pose only a trivial risk to their uninfected peers, they may acquire secondary infections from HIV-uninfected children that can be life threatening. Concern for acquisition of a serious, secondary infections will most likely determine activity restrictions [12, 13]. Table 36.7 reviews the recommended precautions for contagious diseases that may be particularly dangerous to children with HIV infection.

Specific issues pertaining to children outside the hospital environment
Schools
In the past, children with HIV infection have been discriminated against in schools and, on occasion, barred from attendance. These instances have galvanized public

attention, but more importantly have propagated the unfounded notion that HIV is likely to be transmitted in schools. An educational program directed at staff and the student body can help create an accepting environment for children with HIV infection. Many HIV-infected children have chosen to disclose their HIV infection. They attend school with the full support of their teachers and peers and have an extremely positive experience (see Chapter 38).

Children with HIV infection can participate in all school activities to the extent that their health permits [14, 15]. Coordinating a child's medical and educational needs requires ongoing communication among the family, healthcare providers, and school health staff. Like other children with special health needs, children with HIV infection benefit from educational programs that provide needed medical services, such as management of emergencies and administration of medications. All educational institutions should have a policy regarding students and staff who have HIV infection.

In the school, confidentiality is a particularly important issue; privacy rights must be protected at all times. A child's HIV infection status should be disclosed only with the informed consent of the parents or other legal guardians and, when age appropriate, assent of the child. School personnel aware of the child's HIV infection should be limited to the school medical advisor, school nurse, and teacher. The administration of HIV-related medications in school may compromise confidentiality; an infected child should be encouraged to self-administer most medications.

Athletic activities

Children naturally engage in physical play and athletic competition. Physical play and sports present a theoretical possibility of HIV transmission. These fears are generally unfounded because HIV transmission in the setting of supervised athletics has not been reported. Suitable first-aid training and kits should be available wherever children engage in active play and athletics (Tables 36.3 and 36.5) [7, 16]. HIV testing of athletes should not be a prerequisite for participation in sports.

Generally, athletes with HIV infection should be permitted to participate in competitive sports at all levels, at least those not involving close and intense potentially violent contact. It may be advisable to restrict participation in sports due to concerns for HIV transmission, for example if a patient has an increased likelihood of having poorly controlled bleeding due to thrombocytopenia or has skin lesions that cannot be adequately covered. The American Academy of Pediatrics recommends that an HIV-infected athlete considering a sport such as football or wrestling be encouraged to consider an alternative sport after discussing the risk factors for transmission of HIV [2, 16]. Finally, many coaches may be particularly effective educators about the risks of HIV transmission through unprotected sex, and through the sharing of needles or syringes for injection of anabolic steroids or other drugs.

Table 36.7. Appropriate precautions for common childhood infections[a]

Special organism	Precautions in			Comments
	Hospital[b]	School	Daycare	
Candida	None	No	No	Ubiquitous
Cytomegalovirus	None	No	No	Ubiquitous
Coccidioidomycosis	None	No	No	No person-to-person transmission
Cryptococcus	None	No	No	No person-to-person transmission
Cryptosporidia	Contact	No	Yes	Child with diarrhea should be excluded from daycare
Epstein–Barr virus	None	No	No	Ubiquitous
Haemophilus influenza type b	Droplet	No	No	Prophylaxis of contacts[e]
Hepatitis B	None	No	Yes	Avoid biting and blood contact[e]
Histoplasmosis	None	No	No	No person-to-person transmission
Herpes simplex	Contact	No	Yes	Exclude child with mouth sores and drooling
Influenza	Droplet	No	No	Common in winter
Isospora hominis	Contact	No	Yes	Pathogenicity negligible in immunocompetent children
Mycobacterium avium intracellulare	None	No	No	No person-to-person transmission
Measles	Airborne	Yes	Yes	Exclude child until resolved[e]

Pertussis	Droplet	Yes[c]	Yes[c]	Exclude child until treated[e]
Pneumococcus	None	No	No	Ubiquitous in normal children
Pneumocystis carinii	None	No	No	Ubiquitous
Respiratory syncytial virus	Contact	No	No	Common in winter/spring
Rotavirus	Contact	No	Yes	Child with diarrhea should be excluded from daycare
Salmonella	Contact	No	Yes	Infected child should be excluded until three stools negative
Staphylococcus	Contact	Yes[c]	Yes[c]	Exclude child until resolved
Streptococcus	Contact	Yes[c]	Yes[c]	High rate of carriage among children
Syphilis	Contact	No	No	Should have been treated in infancy
Toxoplasma	None	No	No	No person-to-person transmission
Tuberculosis	Airborne	Yes	Yes	Until treated[d]
Varicella-zoster	Airborne + contact	Yes	Yes	Exclude child until lesions scabbed

[a] Adapted from [1].

[b] Based upon standard precautions recommendations [7].

[c] Precautions can be discontinued once the patient has been on therapy for at least 24 hours.

[d] Consultation with physician recommended, particularly in area with high prevalence of resistant strains of tuberculosis.

[e] Immunization recommended for all children.

Daycare centers

Transmission of HIV in childcare is theoretically possible, but very unlikely. The CDC, AAP, and the American Public Health Association have recommended that children with HIV infection be allowed to attend childcare [10, 17]. Exceptional circumstances that argue against attendance at daycare include a strong propensity for aggressive biting, the likelihood of having uncontrollable bleeding episodes, the presence of oozing skin lesions that cannot be covered (e.g., on the face), or a degree of immunosuppression which would place the patient at risk in the day care setting [1]. The child's physician should participate in the decision to enroll a child in daycare.

In some communities, daycare centers designed to meet the special medical, developmental, and other needs of children with HIV infection exist, but HIV-infected children need not be restricted to such specialized programs. Most experts agree that infected children benefit greatly from participation in normal activities with other children.

Adoption

Adoption of an HIV-infected child entails responsibilities for medical care that can be far more demanding than the responsibilities involved in caring for well children. Prospective adoptive or foster parents of HIV-infected children and children at risk for whom the diagnosis has not been excluded should be aware of the diagnosis, treatment plan, and prognosis of the child [1]. This should include education concerning appropriate infection control measures [18]. Children born to infected mothers should be tested with permission of the biologic mother, when possible. Because nearly all HIV-infected children who are to be adopted or placed in foster care have acquired infection perinatally, great care should be taken to protect the confidentiality of the biologic mother's HIV infection status.

Summer camp and other recreational activities

A range of camping opportunities have become available to children with HIV infection. Some are restricted to children with HIV infection, while others mainstream children with others not infected with HIV. Family camps offer a nurturing environment for children and families together. Proper training in the management of blood and potentially infectious fluid spills is required of all staff. Generally, medical, and nursing support should be available to handle both standard emergencies and serious illnesses. Suitability for attendance should be based upon the condition of the child. In the camp environment, children should not be restricted in their activities on the basis of their HIV status. However, secondary conditions, such as diarrhea or cryptosporidiosis, may preclude specific activities such as swimming in an enclosed public pool. Some activities that could pose a risk to more severely immunosuppressed children or to children with additional problems such as bleeding disorders may need to be limited.

Management of exposure to HIV

By definition, children are at risk for accidental exposure to HIV outside the hospital environment [1]. If a child is exposed to HIV-infected body fluids, a knowledgeable physician should be contacted immediately for assessment and intervention. Post-exposure prophylaxis for HIV is described in Chapter 17.

Recommended management of an accidental exposure to HIV includes reporting exposures promptly, evaluating the nature of the exposure, counseling the exposed person regarding management, and testing the source person (with consent) for hepatitis B surface antigen and HIV antibody. During the follow-up period, the exposed child should seek medical evaluation for any acute illness. Updated information on HIV postexposure prophylaxis is available from the Internet at CDC's home page (http://www.cdc.gov) and the National AIDS Clearinghouse (1-800-458-5231). Policy statements from the American Academy of Pediatrics can be found on their website (http://www.aap.org).

Precautions for other infections

HIV-infected children are more susceptible to severe complications of both opportunistic and common pediatric infections. Opportunistic infections are generally not transmitted by person-to-person exposure, since they are usually present in the environment or carried by the at-risk host [12]. Common pediatric infections (such as varicella or measles), or other infections seen in both adults and children, such as tuberculosis, are transmitted and can represent serious risks to the HIV-infected child. Prophylaxis for opportunistic infections is discussed in Chapter 5. Because the consequences of selected infections, such as varicella or measles, can be so severe in HIV-infected children, providers must be vigilant and knowledgeable about ongoing outbreaks in the community. Restricting a child from participation in school, daycare or athletics should only be recommended if documented cases have been reported.

Strategies to prevent acquisition of a secondary infection include immunization (both passive and active), protecting a child from exposure (which may be unrealistic), and prophylaxis with antimicrobial agents [12]. While prophylaxis is effective in decreasing the risk of infection, it is not fully protective; prolonged usage leads to selection of resistant organisms.

Standard precautions should be followed for all patients, regardless of their presumed infection status [7]. Recommendations for isolation have been streamlined into three categories, based upon the mode of transmission: droplet, contact, and airborne [7]. Recommendations have also been generated for specific clinical syndromes highly suspicious for infection that require temporary implementation of precautions until a definitive diagnosis is confirmed. Standard precautions have only been recommended for hospital-based practice, but their application is appropriate for care of children outside the hospital. Recommendations concerning attendance in school or daycare should be based upon these precautions and can easily be applied to other settings, such as family gatherings, athletic events, summer camps or recreational programs (14, 15, 18).

Conclusions

The presence of HIV infection, *per se*, should not restrict children from participating in athletics, daycare and school unless an exceptional circumstance intervenes. Children with HIV infection should enjoy full access to healthcare, privacy, education, and social interactions. Management of children with HIV infection outside of the hospital environment should be viewed as routine as long as the proper guidelines for infection control practices and confidentiality are followed. The activities of children with HIV can be restricted if there is a possible debilitating complication or the risk of a secondary infection is high. Only unusual circumstances should result in the restriction of HIV-infected children due to concerns of HIV transmission. Because of the evolving nature of the HIV epidemic, updated recommendations will most likely continue to be issued by organizations including the American Academy of Pediatrics and the Centers for Disease Control and Prevention and other national and international bodies.

REFERENCES

1. Chanock, S. J., Donowitz, L., Simonds, R. J. Medical issues related to provision of care for the HIV-infected child in the hospital, home, day care, school and community. In Pizzo, P. A., Wilfert, C., eds *Pediatric AIDS*, 3rd edn, 1998:645–662.

2. American Academy of Pediatrics Committee on Pediatric AIDS and Committee on Infectious Diseases. Issues related to human immunodeficiency virus transmission in schools, child care, medical settings, the home and community. *Pediatrics* 1999;**104**:318–324.

3. American Academy of Pediatrics. In Peter, G. ed. *2000 Red Book: Report of the Committee on Infectious Diseases*, 25th edn, Elk Grove, IL: American Academy of Pediatrics, 2000.

4. Simonds, R. J., Chanock, S. J. Medical issues related to caring for HIV-infected children in and out of the home. *J. Pediatr. Infect. Dis.* 1993;**12**:845–852.

5. Centers for Disease Control. Recommendations for prevention of HIV transmission in health-care settings. *Morb. Mortal. Wkly. Rep.* 1987;36(suppl. 2S):1–18S.

6. Occupational Safety and Health Administration. Occupational exposure to bloodborne pathogens. *Fed. Regist.* 1991;**56**:64175–64182.

7. Hospital Infection Control Practices Advisory Committee. Guidelines for isolation precautions in hospitals. *Infect. Control Hosp. Epidemiol.* 1996;**17**:53–80.

8. Tokars J. I., Bell, D. M., Culver, D. H. *et al.* Percutaneous injuries during surgical procedures. *J. Am. Med. Assoc.* 1992;**267**:2899–2904.

9. Henderson, D. K. Post-exposure treatment of HIV – taking some risk for safety's sake. *N. Engl. J. Med.* 1997;**337**:1542–1543.

10. Simmons, B., Trusler, M., Roccaforte, J., Smoth, P., Scott, R. Infection control for home health. *Infect. Control Hosp. Epidemiol.* 1990;**11**:362–370.

11. American Academy of Pediatrics Committee on Pediatric AIDS and Committee on Adolescence. Adolescents and human immunodeficiency virus infection: the role of the pediatrician in prevention and intervention. *Pediatrics* 2001;**107**:188–190.

12. Centers for Disease Control and Prevention. 1997 USPHS/IDSA Guidelines for the prevention of opportunistic infections in persons infected with human immunodeficiency virus. *Morb. Mortal. Wkly Rep.* 1997;**46**: RR-12,1–46.

13. Centers for Disease Control. Guidelines for preventing the transmission of tuberculosis in health-care settings, with special focus on HIV-related issues. *Mob. Mortal. Wkly Rep.* 1990;**39** (No. RR-17):1–29.

14. American Academy of Pediatrics Task Force on Pediatric AIDS. Education of children with human immunodeficiency virus infection. *Pediatrics* 1991;**88**:645–648.

15. Centers for Disease Control. Education and foster care of children infected with human T-lymphotrophic virus type III/lymphadenopathy-associated virus. *Morb. Mortal. Wkly Rep.* 1985;**34**:517–521.

16. American Academy of Pediatrics, Committee on Sports Medicine and Fitness. Human immunodeficiency virus [acquired immunodeficiency syndrome (AIDS) virus] in the athletic setting. *Pediatrics* 1991;**88**:640–641.

17. American Academy of Pediatrics Committee on Infectious Diseases. Health guidelines for the attendance in day-care and foster care settings of children infected with human immunodeficiency virus. *Pediatrics* 1987;**79**:466–471.

18. American Academy of Pediatrics Task Force on Pediatric AIDS. Guidelines for human immunodeficiency virus (HIV)-infected children and their foster families. *Pediatrics* 1992;**89**:681–683.

37 Contact with social service agencies

Sandra Y. Lewis, Psy.D.

Montclair State University and François-Xavier Bagnoud Center
UMDNJ – New Jersey Medical School, Newark, NJ

Heidi J. Haiken, M.S.W., L.C.S.W.

François-Xavier Bagnoud Center, UMDNJ – School of Nursing, Newark, NJ

Introduction/overview

Though a cure for HIV disease remains elusive, in many patients virus in the blood can be reduced to undectable levels and disease progression can be significantly slowed. The use of antiretroviral prophylaxis and cesarian section reduces the rate of perinatal transmission of HIV infection, thus increasing the likelihood that a child born to a mother with HIV infection will not be infected. Medical advances, nutritional support, psychosocial support, coordination of key services, and attention to quality of life issues have contributed to improved treatment and prevention outcomes for HIV-exposed and HIV-infected children. Children with HIV infection are living well into their teen years and beyond. Parents living with HIV who have access to HIV care are able to be primary caregivers for their children for a longer period of time. Although this chapter is primarily oriented to the experience of patients living in the USA, some of the information, particularly the information concerning broader psychological and social concerns should be helpful to patients in other parts of the world.

Psychosocial concerns

Amidst the notable successes in HIV care, there continue to be a number of salient psychosocial issues. Prominent among these are the following.

1. Children growing into teenagers with HIV are facing adolescent developmental challenges. The developmental problems faced by children and families have changed, producing new challenges in parenting and planning for the future. As children grow older, issues such as disclosure, development of intimacy, career and school choices, and the usual tasks of adolescence may offer overwhelming challenges for parents and require support from health and mental health professionals.

Handbook of Pediatric HIV Care, ed. Steven L. Zeichner and Jennifer S. Read.
Published by Cambridge University Press. © Cambridge University Press 2006.

2. HIV-negative children living with family members who are infected have significant psychosocial needs. Forehand *et al.* [1] note that children of HIV-infected mothers evidenced greater psychosocial adjustment difficulties when compared to their peers whose mothers are HIV-uninfected. It is important that affected children have access to services such as healthcare, mental healthcare, recreation, and other services that help to normalize their lives. In many cases, such services are available through HIV care programs being accessed by infected family members.

3. The decrease in perinatal HIV transmission makes it more likely that children may be orphaned because uninfected children may lose parents to HIV disease. While parents are living longer, healthier lives, permanency planning is an urgent issue. Within the USA, parents have a number of options for permanency planning and can get assistance through HIV care facilities. In some states, providers and legislators are developing programs such as the Kinship Navigator Program in New Jersey that aim to keep children in the care of extended family (website: http://www.state.nj.us/humanservices/sp8i/html).

Like other chronic illnesses, HIV infection can disrupt the child's ability to engage in normal daily activities such as school, cause serious psychological and emotional problems, and may lead to premature death [2]. Distinctive psychosocial issues set HIV disease apart from other chronic illnesses. These include: stigma, family secrecy about diagnosis, lack of social support, isolation, interaction between HIV and other family problems such as drug abuse and poverty, the multigenerational nature of HIV among women and children, and the multiple losses due to HIV, which can increase the psychosocial burden and emotional distress experienced by many families living with HIV/AIDS [3–5]. Families living with HIV are often required to interface with numerous agencies because they are coping with social, psychological, and medical issues.

Assessing family needs

Families living with HIV infection can have widely varying compositions, ranging from the nuclear family, consisting of parents and children, to grandparents caring for their ill adult children and grandchildren, to foster families. Determining how the family provides key elements of care for HIV-infected children is essential for the effective management of health care. The limits of foster parents' legal rights to make medical and other decisions may vary from state to state and must be evaluated with each family.

Many families affected by HIV disease are also poor, so healthcare providers must assess whether basic needs, such as food and shelter, are being satisfied. When a family comes for a medical visit, their perceptions regarding the primary needs of the day must be assessed, which may not be obvious. Healthcare providers should ask families explicitly what their concerns are for the day, including both medical and social concerns. Providers should keep available a list of community resources that provide support with basic needs such as housing and food.

Other, more basic, concerns may arise. For example, the possibility that the child may be in danger because the basic needs for food and shelter are not being met or because the child is at risk of being physically abused. Providers should compile lists of organizations that can provide resources and treatment facilities where troubled parents can seek help. Providers may also need to help families establish a good working relationship with a social service agency so that they can receive proper assistance.

Families with HIV-infected members face many challenges. They often live under significant stress and may be fragile. However, they also have strengths that have helped them manage previous difficult situations. Past coping strategies provide clues for developing effective plans for families.

Managed care and other insurance coverage

In the USA, the complicated system of medical insurance and reimbursement present a specific set of challenges to those who would deliver excellent care to the HIV-infected child. Managed care is a system in which a primary healthcare provider (PCP) is considered the gatekeeper of medical services needed by the client. The PCP will make referrals to specialists if the PCP determines that a referral is needed. Health Maintenance Organizations (HMOs) are one type of managed care program. Another option is the traditional health insurance plan, also known as "fee for service," in which each physician who sees the client charges the client for the service or bills the insurance company directly. Each plan varies, and families should talk with their insurance company or benefits specialist about which plan is appropriate for them

HIV infection can exert extreme stresses on many families. Specialists and generalists, social workers, and case managers who provide care for HIV-infected children must be aware of some of the key features of the medical insurance system. Recommendations that providers caring for patients with HIV may want to consider include the following.

1. Maintain an automated list of your clients, their health insurance plan, their primary care provider (PCP), and the number of referrals that have already been made to specialists, since insurance companies may limit such referrals.
2. Determination of the relationship between each client and their PCP, and the establishment of a working relationship with their PCP. The insurance company may need to be consulted to determine the extent of services they can provide or reimburse.
3. Assess whether the family can obtain their own referrals. If not, determine who from your office is responsible for calling the PCP when a referral is needed, if the insurance company requires that referrals be made through the PCP.
4. Evaluate if families can obtain their own referrals. Assist with skill training as needed.

5. Have readily accessible the telephone numbers for the most commonly used insurance companies, and their complaint lines. Some states require that patients whose health insurance is provided through Medicaid use a Medcaid HMO, which may not offer access to needed specialists or other kinds of care. It is helpful to have information for families using Medicaid HMOs, regarding how to change or be exempted from the HMO, if possible.
6. Determine insurance company policies regarding pre-existing conditions and the type of services they will reimburse.
7. Maintain good communication with insurers.

Social Security and Medicaid

In the USA, Social Security and Medicaid Programs are also available for patients. The regulations for Social Security can change frequently, based upon the current federal and state legislation and funding levels, and changing laws and regulations. Supplemental Security Income (SSI) is available for children with AIDS if they meet certain requirements [6]. The Social Security Administration publishes this information at: http://www.ssa.gov/OPHome/handbook/ssa-hbk.htm. The requirements include "marked and severe functional limitations," the duration of the disability and "inability to have gainful activity due to a physical or mental impairment." Patients and families may not be eligible for SSI if their income exceeds certain limits, calculated based on a complicated formula. In most states, children eligible for SSI are eligible for Medicaid. States can contribute or match federal entitlements, so that the eligibility and funding levels can vary significantly from state to state. (Further information can also be found in Chapter 39.)

In certain circumstances, presumptive SSI is available to eligible clients with HIV infection while long-term eligibility is assessed. This means that they are given SSI for 6 months based on minimal documentation substantiating a diagnosis of AIDS or HIV infection with low CD4 count, and/or certain opportunistic infections, and other medical or functional criteria. To expedite this process, it may be helpful to have the presumptive SSI applications in your office. To determine the level of physical and cognitive functioning of the child as well as their financial eligibility for the program, advise clients to take items such as medical reports, medical bills, social security cards, rent receipts, and bank account information to the Social Security office. Social Security officials recommend that you inform clients of the basic eligibility requirements before they apply. The Social Security Administration has guides available for clients on Social Security and HIV infection.

Changes in SSI eligibility may result in the loss of Medicaid benefits. Resources need to be found without delay to prevent a lapse in the clients' medication regimen. Programs such as the AIDS Drug Distribution Program (ADDP) can often provide resources for

Table 37.1. Alternative sources for resources

Organization	Services/grants offered
The Elisabeth Glaser Pediatric AIDS Foundation Association François-Xavier Bagnoud	➤ Educational grants for student interns and research ➤ Projects in Africa aimed at reduction of perinatal HIV transmission ➤ Orphan projects ➤ Human rights ➤ HIV/AIDS prevention and treatment programs ➤ Training for providers
Children Affected by AIDS	➤ Emergency direct service grants ➤ Direct service grants ➤ Education grants ➤ Administration grants
M.A.C. Cosmetics	➤ Donations to pediatric HIV/AIDS programs through their ➤ Profits from Viva Glam lipsticks support AIDS organizations

HIV-associated related medications. Another alternative is to seek medications through the indigent assistance programs from the pharmaceutical companies.

Medicaid model waivers

Model waivers are federally funded and state administered funds available for medical services. The most common waiver for children with AIDS is the AIDS Community Care Alternatives waiver, commonly known as ACCAP. To apply for this waiver, the child must be HIV-infected and under the age of 13 years, or have the disability diagnosis of AIDS if they are 13 years and older and need homecare services. ACCAP does have a financial cap on the services provided to a child. However, there are no financial criteria for children to be eligible for ACCAP.

Alternative sources for resources

As listed in Table 37.1 there are other sources of private funding. This table is not exhaustive, but includes some key resources, services, and sources for grants.

Discharge planning

Often, upon discharge, professionals find it difficult to offer the care that they believe a patient needs because of the constraints imposed by insurance companies and government programs. Social work involvement in discharge planning at the beginning of an admission can reduce the length of stay [7]. Social workers can assist the medical team in defining and addressing the physical, social, and emotional needs of the family during a hospital stay, and can help make plans so the plan for the patient's care continues effectively after discharge. Discharge resources may include a visiting nurse, health aides, providing needed medical equipment, and training for adult caregivers to help them utilize the equipment properly at home. Upon discharge, the parent should receive specific instructions regarding filling prescriptions, the follow-up appointment, and contingency plans if a problem occurs.

Interacting with multiple agencies

Patients and their families are often uncertain what information and documentation they will be expected to provide to insurance companies and government agencies. It is helpful to recommend that clients keep a folder with copies of:

- Social Security cards
- Income tax returns
- Proof of address (This can be two items mailed to the patient.)
- Birth certificates
- Legal guardianship papers
- Standby guardianship papers
- Insurance/Medicaid cards
- Rent and utility receipts

Clients can also be educated about interviewing with various agencies. Some clients do not receive services because they are unable to ask for services in the way that they agency expects them to ask. Basics of service referrals include the following.

- Make sure that the services are available prior to referring clients. (Funding cuts may be sudden.)
- Locate a contact person within frequently used agencies.
- Establish a rapport with frequently used agencies.
- Assess if ongoing meetings would be useful with certain agencies to prevent duplication of services.

Working with child welfare agencies

Boyd-Franklin and Boland [8] highlight the role child welfare agencies can play in the care of HIV-infected children. First, child welfare workers provide a source of support to foster families who may be overwhelmed negotiating the many medical and social services agencies. Their services can range from concrete assistance with transportation to support with community reactions to caring for an HIV-infected child.

Child welfare agencies can be helpful in placing children when parents become unable to provide care due to the parent's deteriorating health, substance abuse, or social issues such as homelessness or inadequate housing. It is important that providers collaborate with parents around using child welfare services so that these interventions are not utilized in a punitive way. Even in situations where abuse or neglect is suspected, these concerns must be discussed with the parent and a plan developed in consultation with the parent. It may be that a respite placement or foster placement of a parent and child are viable options for a family.

Global issues in accessing care and treatment

A number of agencies and organizations are involved in addressing the global AIDS epidemic. Among these are UNICEF, WHO, HHS, the Centers for Disease Control and Prevention Global AIDS Program (CDC-GAP), United States Agency for International Development (USAID), UNAIDS, the International Partnership Against AIDS in Africa (IPAA), Association François-Xavier Bagnoud (AFXB), and the Elizabeth Glaser Pediatric AIDS Foundation (EGPAF). Each agency has a variety of global programs. In sub-Saharan Africa, prevention of mother-to-child transmission (PMTCT) and care for AIDS orphans represents a major focus in pediatric and family HIV. Efforts are under way in some countries to extend PMTCT programs so that HIV-positive mothers and infants can receive care. It is important that providers learn about the variety of resources available to families in their area.

Putting it all together

HIV in women and children is a multigenerational family disease distinguished by a number of emotional and social issues. Many families affected by HIV/AIDS face many other severe challenges, such as poverty, homelessness, limited access to health-care and health information, and discrimination. Coping with HIV often requires the involving of numerous social service and healthcare systems. The multisystems model provides a much-needed framework for healthcare providers to facilitate this coordination, limit duplication of service, and clarify the roles of various providers [8, 9].

Empowering families is the guiding principle of the multisystems approach. Families are coached to understand how various service systems can meet their needs and how to negotiate those systems. Families become active participants in developing a plan and deciding how to utilize the various services available. When a number of service systems, healthcare providers, or other professionals are involved with a family, it is crucial that representatives from each of those programs meet regularly to update each other and clarify their roles.

The advantage of the multisystems approach is a coordinated response to the myriad of socio-environmental, emotional, and medical issues faced by families living with HIV. Various needs are addressed and the family builds a strong support network. Both families and providers are empowered when service systems complement each other and all the pieces of the puzzle come together for the family. The information and resources outlined in this chapter are offered as a map guiding professionals and families through the maze of social issues, managed care, funding sources, discharge planning, and other complexities of meeting social service needs.

Handy websites

Africare – www.africare.org
AFXB – www.afxb.org
CD C Global Aids Program World Health Organization – www.whoint/hiv/aboutdept/en; www.cdc.gov/nchsstplod/gap
Children Affected by AIDS Foundation – www.caaf4kids.org – UNAIDS
The Elizabeth Glaser Pediatric AIDS Foundation – www.pedaids.org
FXB Center – www.fxbcenter.org
MAC Aids Fund. www.macaidsfund.org
Medicaid – www.hcfa.gov/
Social Security – www.ssa.gov
Various information – www.hivpositive.com; www.thebody.com; www.hivatis.org; www.hivfiles.org; www.aidsetc.org; www.aidsinfo.nih.gov; www.womenchildrenhiv

Handy phone numbers

The Elizabeth Glaser Pediatric AIDS Foundation 1- 310 314–1459
Children Affected by AIDS 1-310-258-0850
Children's Hope Foundation 1-212-233-5133
M.A.C. Cosmetics 1-646-613 -6478
Social Security Administration 1-800-772-1213
François-Xavier Bagnoud Center, Newark NJ 1-973-972-0400, e-mail info@fxb center.org

REFERENCES
1. Forehand. R., Steele, R., Armistead, L., Morse, E., Simon, P., Clark, L. The Family Health Project: psychosocial adjustment of children whose mothers are HIV infected. *J. Consult. Clin. Psychol.* 1998;**66**(3):513–520.
2. Boland, M., Czarniecki, L., Haiken, H. Providing care for HIV-infected children. In Stuber, M., ed. *Children and AIDS*. Washington, DC: American Psychiatric Press, Inc, 1992:165–181.

3. Lewis, S., Haiken, H., Hoyt, L. A psychocial perspective on long-term survivors of pediatric immunodeficiency virus infection. *J. Dev. Behav. Pediat.* 1994;**15**:S12–S17.
4. Sherwen, L., Storm, D. Looking toward the twenty-first century: The role of nursing research in care of children and families affected by HIV. *Nursing Clin. North Am.* 1996;**31**:165–178.
5. Steiner, G., Boyd-Franklin, N., Boland, M. Rational and overview of the book. In Boyd-Franklin, N., Steiner, G., Boland, M., eds. *Children, Families, and HIV/AIDS: Psychosocial and Therapeutic Issues*. New York: Guilford Press, 1995.
6. Social Security Administration. Supplemental security income; determining disability for a child under age 18; interim final rules with request for comments. *Fed. Register (USA)* 1997;**68**:6407–6432.
7. Boone, C., Coulton, C., Keller, S. The impact of early and comprehensive social services on length of stay. *Social Work Health Care* 1981;**7**:1–9.
8. Boyd-Franklin, N., Boland M. A mulitsystems approach to service delivery for HIV/AIDS families. In Boyd-Franklin, N., Steiner, G., Boland, M., eds. *Children, Families, and HIV/AIDS*: *Psychosocial and Therapeutic Issues*. New York: Guilford Press, 1995:199–215.
9. Boyd-Franklin, N. *Black Families in Therapy: A Multisystems Approach*. New York: Guilford Press, 1989.

38 Psychosocial factors associated with childhood bereavement and grief

Lori S. Wiener, Ph.D.

HIV and AIDS Malignancy Branch, National Cancer Institute, NIH, Bethesda, MD

The tragedy of HIV/AIDS grows more profound as time passes [1]. The AIDS pandemic will cause a decline in life expectancy in 51 countries over the next two decades [2]. For each individual infected with the disease, many more are affected by the loss, including children, their parents, siblings, and caregivers. Disruptions to work patterns caused by absenteeism due to illness and funerals, the lack of physical space in morgues and burial grounds reach deep into everyday life, are a constant reminder of the fatal nature of this disease [3]. Populations are trying to exist in a state of daily and ongoing loss.

Bereavement, one of the most frequent life stressors impacting individuals infected with or affected by HIV [4], differs from grief related to other chronic illnesses. Those affected by HIV are typically exposed to multiple losses over a relatively short period of time, decreasing the likelihood that there will be adequate time to process and mourn each loss prior to the next death. One of the most potent barriers to successful mourning is the social stigma related to this disease [5]. The burden of secrecy further complicates the bereavement and subsequent healing process.

The grieving process may begin at the time of HIV diagnosis and is referred to as anticipatory grief [6]. People with HIV experience a wide range of losses other the imminence of death [7], including the loss of certainty, hopes for the future, relationships, health, control, sexual desirability and body image, status, dignity, privacy, and security. AIDS-related deaths are further complicated by the legal, financial, stigmatizing, and emotional factors that surround the disease.

There is no single portrait of a grieving child from an HIV-infected family. Children living in HIV-infected families are of all ages, cultural and ethnic backgrounds [8]. The majority of these children have already experienced the burdens of poverty, seen the effects of substance abuse and violence, and endured many other types of loss and trauma in their families [9]. Death of a family member is often one more destabilizing factor.

Handbook of Pediatric HIV Care, ed. Steven L. Zeichner and Jennifer S. Read.
Published by Cambridge University Press. © Cambridge University Press 2006.

Loss in childhood

Each year, millions of children throughout the world experience the death of close family member [10]. Often, adults strive to hide their true feelings about death to protect their children, mainly because they do not know how to assist their child with the emotional impact of death.

Each child's experience with grief varies dramatically, based on the developmental stage and the information shared with the child. Children should be made aware of family illnesses; hiding an illness is often more frightening for children than the truth, and may complicate the grieving process. However, AIDS-related grieving presents unique challenges, especially concerning issues surrounding disclosure. After a parent discloses the HIV/AIDS diagnosis, children will begin to struggle with fears about a parent's or their own death. This is an appropriate time to begin discussions about the fatal nature of the disease in a developmentally appropriate way. Pennells and Smith [9] review age-related grief reactions that are summarized in Table 38.1.

Social and emotional development as a factor

Young children experience the loss of a loved one, but do not understand the permanence of that loss, and continue to seek the presence of the deceased. The experience of death may cause feelings of insecurity and instability. A child may cry, yearn for the deceased, become clingy, and make attempts at reunion with the deceased through playing [11]. Parents or elders mistakenly substantiate this belief/misconception by explaining death in terms of sleeping or another temporary state. For children between the ages of 5 and 9, death often elicits fear and fantasy behaviors. Feelings of guilt or responsibility for their loved one's death are common. At this age, children manifest an almost morbid curiosity about rituals surrounding death and about the function of dead bodies. For children between the ages of 9 and 12, the finality and irreversibility of death is understood and they begin to fear their own death. Children grieve in a manner similar to adults at this stage, and may attempt to deny their overwhelming feelings of loss in an effort to "get on with life." Adolescents are capable of grieving as adults do, with appropriate crying, feelings of remorse and loss, anger, and depression. They may question their own identity and the meaning of life. Periods of social isolation can occur, as peers are uncertain how to respond to a grieving friend. The death may cause an adolescent to feel painfully different from his/her peers. Role changes may occur as well, as the adolescent assumes increased responsibility around the home. A journal in which the adolescent can record memories, feelings, and hopes for the future, is almost always beneficial to the grieving process.

Table 38.1. When children grieve: developmental considerations

0–2 years
- The child will seek the presence of the deceased person and will experience a loss, but does not have the capabilities to understand the permanence of that loss. They cannot comprehend the word "forever."

2–5 years
- Experience of death at this age may cause the child's world to feel unsafe and unpredictable.
- Reactions may include tearfulness, temper tantrums, clinginess, bed-wetting, and sleep problems.
- In play, they may make attempts to reunite with the deceased person.
- Child may still believe that death is reversible . . . simple, repeated explanations that the deceased person cannot come back to life are needed.
- If they are terminally ill, their greatest fears are associated with separation from their loved ones.

5–9 years
- Children have a wider social network at this point and consequently, children are more sensitive to other people's reactions, remarks from peers, etc.
- Children are learning who they can trust with their feelings.
- They are watching adults' reactions to grief and will sometimes deny their own grief in order to protect an adults' feelings.
- They have a greater awareness of guilt and may feel they were responsible for the death by illogical reasoning (e.g., "Mommy died yesterday because I was naughty the night before").
- This is also the age of fear and fantasy and the child may personalize death as a monster, boogie man, etc.
- Children think more logically about death and begin to focus on rituals surrounding death and about the functions of dead bodies, such as do they need clothes and food.
- If the child is terminally ill, they often question "Why me?", they may feel they have done something wrong to deserve their illness and subsequent death, and frequently have a difficult time accepting that they are truly going to die.

9–12 years
- Child is aware of the finality of death and that death is common to all living things.
- Child may become fearful of his/her own death, which may cause psychosomatic symptoms to appear.
- The child is grieving more like an adult at this point and may try to deny feeling a sense of loss in order to just try to "get on with life."
- The terminally ill child is responsive to honest discussions (though it is still difficult to accept), to being included in decision making, and responds to open and honest discussions about what will be happening to their bodies.

Adolescence
- Adolescents are able to grieve more like adults do, with appropriate crying, sadness, confusion, somatic complaints, anger, denial of feelings and/or depression.

(cont.)

Table 38.1. (*cont.*)

- These powerful emotions may lead them to question their identity and the meaning of life.
- Interest in the occult, afterlife, and the rites of different cultures are not uncommon.
- They may feel social pressure to take on more responsibility and find themselves fulfilling the deceased parents' household duties.
- Members of the adolescent's peer group may not know how to handle the bereavement of one of their friends, leading to a sense of isolation for the bereaved adolescent.
- The terminally ill adolescent often has great difficulty with the physical assaults that the illness has on their body, and has a great need to feel in control of medical decisions. Tendencies to withdraw or reach out to others prior to death reflect how they responded to other stresses in their life prior to their illness.

What do bereaved children need?

- Adults who can respond to them with genuine caring, understanding, warmth, and empathy.
- Children should be told about death in a language appropriate for their age and development stage.
- Try to create opportunities for them to acquire knowledge and a vocabulary about death.
- Euphemisms and ambiguous answers are not helpful.
- Children need to be involved in the family's grieving process as much as possible and invited to express their feelings.
- Children need help understanding contradictions in the way people talk about death (e.g., Mommy is happier in Heaven; Your sister is asleep now and will be watching over you).
- Children need reassurance that their world has not disintegrated.
- Children need help to deal with anticipated additional losses (if other family members are also HIV-infected), secondary losses, such as new care providers, house moves, or a parent remarrying.
- It is important to keep the memory of the deceased person alive.
- One cannot replace the loss though it is important to also provide seeds of hope for a future with less emotional pain.

Grief in children who lose a parent

For children of any age, the loss of a parent is devastating and has long-lasting effects. When a youngster faces the loss of multiple family members, the impact extends for years into the future [5]. Parental loss creates uncertainty, instability, mistrust, isolation, feelings of abandonment, and fear of the future. For many, there has never been a stable family environment, so children may have serious concerns about who will care for them now.

In the USA, the majority of children infected with HIV are from communities of color [12], live in deteriorating urban centers, and as a result of poverty, and/or caretaker substance abuse, have limited access to medical resources, and few social supports. These risk factors create a compromised environment for children who are already vulnerable [5]. Many children who have lost a parent to AIDS have also lost other members of their families to drug addiction, violence, incarceration, and suicide. Helping restore a child's ability to invest in emotional relationships without excessive fear of future loss is the one of the greatest challenges to the professionals working with them [13].

Grief in children who lose a sibling

The childhood sibling bond has the potential to last longer than any other familial relationship [14], and when a sibling dies, a sense of abandonment is common. If the surviving child is also HIV-infected, the death of a sibling can be particularly frightening. For an uninfected child, losing a sibling may bring a complex mixture of feelings ranging from relief, to sorrow and guilt. A child can feel relieved that family circumstances may return to normal, followed by severe guilt for feeling this way or for escaping infection. Children who are not infected may have suffered from lack of parental attention. Professionals must be especially attentive to previous losses experienced and the sibling's, as well as the family's, reaction to the illness and death. It is necessary to know whether the sibling's HIV-infected mother has already died, or if the sibling anticipates this and/or other losses, and whether this child knows with whom he/she will live should the parent die. Age-appropriate information should be shared with the child, permanency plans made, and a support system identified swiftly and with compassion [15]. Support groups as well as individual counseling may also be of assistance in alleviating some of the fears and concerns that children experience. A list of national support groups available for affected children can be found in Table 38.2.

Recommendations for assisting grieving children

Clinicians need to explain death in simple, understandable and developmentally appropriate language. Ambiguity and euphemisms are not helpful. Children should be encouraged and given permission to take an active part in the grief process. Children must be reassured that their whole world has not been shattered, and they need help to deal with additional anticipated losses and secondary losses such as relocation of family due to moving, new care providers, new school or a parent remarrying. It is useful to learn the child's level of understanding and how that understanding evolves. Adults should be prepared to answer any questions openly and directly. Understanding and utilizing the strengths of each child's spiritual beliefs, rituals, and community is essential. For families whose first language is not English, communication with the child about any matter of importance should be done in the native language.

It is not uncommon for children to alternate between periods of mourning and periods of refusing to acknowledge the loss and pain [16]. It is natural for a child to

Table 38.2. Resources

National resources

Bereaved Children's Group
8119 Holland Road
Alexandria, VA 22306

Brothers and Sisters Together
Miami Children's Hospital
6125 SW 31st Street
Miami, FL 33155

The Camp Heartland Center
3326 East Layton Ave.
Cudahy, WI 53110

Centering Corporation
1531 N. Saddle Creek Rd
Omaha, NE 68104

Center for Grieving Children and Teenagers
819 Massachusetts Ave.
Arlington, Massachusetts 02476
http://www.childrensroom.org

Center for Sibling Loss
Southern Human Services
1700 West Irving Park Road
Chicago, IL 60613

Children's Hospice International
501 Slaters Lane, Suite 207
Alexandria, VA 22314

Compassionate Friends
P.O. Box 3693
Oakbrook, IL 60522-3696
http://www.compassionatefriends.org

Dougy Center
3909 SE 52nd
Portland, OR 97206

Fernside: A Center for Grieving Children
P.O. Box 8944
Cincinnati, OH 45208

Journey Program
c/o Children's Hospital
4800 Sand Point Way
Seattle, WA 98103

Kids Grieve Too
c/o Hospice of Red River
1316 South 23rd Street
Fargo, ND 58103

The Children's Legacy
P.O. Box 300305
Denver, CO 80203

National Childhood Grief Institute
3300 Edinborough Way, Suite 512
Minneapolis, MN 55435

National Pediatric and Family HIV
Resource Center
University of Medicine & Dentistry of NJ
15 South 9th Street
Newark, NJ 07107
email: NPHRC@daiid.umdnj.edu

SHARE – St. John's Hospital
800 E. Carpenter Street
Springfield, IL 62769

St. Francis Center
4880 A MacArthur Blvd.
Washington, DC 20007

Straight, Inc.
P.O. Box 21686
St. Petersburg, FL 33742

The Good Grief Program
Judge Baker Guidance Center
295 Longwood Avenue
Boston, MA 02115

Table 38.2. (*cont.*)

Resources

Camp Heartland
1845 N. Farwell, Suite 310
Milwaukee, WI 53202
www.campheartland.org
e-mail: helpkids@campheartland.org
ph: 800-724-HOPE

Center for Grieving Children and
Teenagers, Inc.
P. O. Box 306
Arlington, MA 02476
www.childrensroom.org
e-mail: info@childrensroom.org

Centering Corporation
7230 Maple Street
Omaha, NE 68134
www.centering.org
e-mail: centering@centering.org
ph: 402-553-1200

Children's Hospice International
901 North Pitt Street, Suite 230
Alexandria, V A 22314
www.chionline.org
e-mail: info@chionline.org
ph: 800-24-CHILD

The Children's Legacy
P. O. Box 300305
Denver, CO 80203

The Compassionate Friends, Inc.
P. O. Box 3696
Oakbrook, IL 60522-3696
www.compassionatefriends.org
ph: 877-969-0010

The Cove
Center for Grieving Children
134 State Street
Meriden, CT 06450
www.covect.org
ph: 800-750-COVE

The Dougy Center
P. O. Box 86852
Portland, OR 97268
www.dougy.org
e-mail: help@dougy.org
ph: 866-775-5683

Families Helping Families
The Jenna Druck Foundation
3636 Fifth Avenue, Suite 201
San Diego CA 92103
www.jennadruck.org

Fernside: A Center for Grieving Children
4380 Malsbary Road, Suite 300
Cincinnati, OH 45242
www.fernside.org
ph: 513-745-0111

St. Francis Center
4880 A MacArthur Blvd.
Washington, DC 20070

Journey Program
c/o Children's Hospital
4800 Sand Point Way
Seattle, W A 98103
ph: 206-987-2000

Judge Baker Guidance Center
295 Longwood Avenue
Boston, MA 02115

Kids and Teens Grieve, Too
c/o Hospice of Red River Valley
702 28th Avenue N
Fargo, ND 58102
ph: 701-237-4629

SuperSibs!
4300 Lincoln Ave, Suite I
Rolling Meadows, IL 60008
www.supersibs.org
ph: 866-444-SIBS

Table 38.2. (*cont.*)

Resources on the Internet
Growth House
http://www.growthhouse.org
Hospice Foundation of America
http://www.hospicefoundation.org
National Association for Home Care
http://www.nahc.org
Women, Children, and HIV
www.womenchildrenhiv.org
The Association for Death Education and Counseling
http://www.adec.org

avoid discussing a parent's death soon after the event, and denial or disinterest in the subject may be manifest in their behavior. When a child exhibits certain high risk signs or symptoms, referrals to a bereavement specialist may be warranted (see Table 38.3). Many behaviors may not appear for one to several years after the death.

The manner in which the surviving parent or relative responds to the child, the availability of social support, and subsequent life circumstances can influence whether a child develops bereavement-related problems [17]. Increased risk of developing behavioral problems is associated with a lack of continuity in the child's daily life after the death of a parent [18]. Numerous variables will influence this outcome, including how close a child is to either parent and the stability or instability of the child's home environment leading up to and surrounding the circumstances of the death. Maternal loss may have a more profound effect on a child than paternal loss [17]. For children as well as adults, death is not merely the loss of a person, but a dramatic change in a way of life [17].

Children try to maintain the relationship with the parent they have lost. Memorializing the person who died continues throughout an entire life [19]. Assisting the child to remember and maintain a connection to the deceased parent is important, and helps the child to express emotions that are difficult to voice. Memory books and videotapes are effective tools for bereaved individuals to use to remember their loved ones, validate their life together, and give personal meaning to past events.

Adult grief – grief in parents who lose a child to HIV/AIDS

Grief in adults usually consists of the passage through various stages identified by several theorists including Kubler-Ross [18] and Worden [19]. These stages can vary significantly but most grieving adults experience shock, denial, anger, bargaining, depression, and finally, acceptance.

Table 38.3. Indicators that the child may need to be referred for professional help

- Persistent anxiety about their own death
- Changes in appetite or sleep patterns
- Destructive outbursts, self-destructive behavior, acting-out (including attempts to become HIV-infected themself)
- Threats of hurting oneself or others
- Compulsive care giving
- Euphoria
- Unwillingness to speak about the deceased person (especially if a conflicted relationship existed)
- Expression of only positive or only negative feelings about the deceased person
- Inability or unwillingness to form new relationships
- Daydreaming – resulting in poor academic performance
- Stealing or hoarding household items
- Excessive separation anxiety and/or school phobia
- Withdrawal from peers or previously enjoyable activities
- Sudden unexplained change in behavior, attitude or mood

The period immediately prior to the death of a child is often confusing and overwhelming. One of the most important aspects of working with families at this stage is to allow them to enjoy the remaining time left with their child [22]. Healthcare providers should encourage families to decide where the child's final days will be spent and whether or not special measures to prolong life will be allowed. Help may be required to plan and pay for funeral arrangements.

The loss of a child is a devastating and life-altering experience. Parents often feel guilty about circumstances surrounding their infection and what they believe to be "failure" to save their child. Some HIV-infected parents describe a sense of relief that they lived long enough to care for, and comfort, their child. Others cannot tolerate or have the strength to cope with the loss of their child and do not pursue medical treatment for themselves.

Extensive literature on parental bereavement shows a high incidence of difficulty in parental emotional adjustment. Grieving parents may develop strained marital relationships, difficulties with parenting surviving siblings, and unresolved grief. Survivors often manifest serious medical problems, including hypertension, ulcers, somatic complaints, colitis, and obesity [23, 24]. In parents who are HIV-infected, it is important to differentiate these symptoms from manifestations of HIV disease. Many require psychiatric intervention following the death of a child [23, 25]. Factors associated with better adjustment include family participation in the care of a child, open discussion with the ill child about the illness and the dying process, a strong marital relationship and support system, and ongoing contact with the health care team [26]. Believing

Table 38.4. Interview questions of a school-age child or adolescent whose parent or sibling has died

Relationship with deceased

1. Can you tell me a little something about [cite person's name]?
2. What was your relationship like with [cite person's name]?
3. What kind of things did you do together?
4. Can you tell me a little something about [cite person's name} death?
5. Were you there? (If not) what had you heard?
6. Did you realize that [cite person's name] was sick enough to die?
7. Had you known that [cite person's name] had HIV/AIDS?
8. If yes, when had you learned this information?
9. Who told you?
10. What was your response when you first learned this?
11. Were you able to share this with anyone else?
12. Who knew the truth about [cite person's name] illness?
13. Does anyone else in your family have it?
14. (If the child is not also HIV-infected) Are you concerned that you might have it?
15. Before [cite person's name] died, were you able to tell him (her) the things you wanted to say?
16. (If no) What happened that you weren't able to say the things you wanted to say?
17. Is there anything that you wanted to do together that you didn't have a chance to do?
18. Do you have anything of [cite person's name] that you hold on to?
19. (If yes). Can you tell me about them?

Adjustment after death

20. I have talked to many other children who had a [cite relative's relationship to the child] die, and some of them are worried that they might have done something to cause the death. Does this worry you?
21. (If yes). Tell me about how this worries you.
22. Since [cite person's name] died, what has life been like for you?
23. What has life been like for your family (go through each significant person individually) since [cite person's name] died?
24. Other children have told me that sometimes when something bad like this happens, other things are also not going well for them either at school or at home. Has anything else not been going well for you?
25. (If yes) tell me about (each one).
26. Have you been through any other bad times like this before?
27. (If yes). Tell me about them – what helped you get through those times?
28. Tell me about your friends. (Trying to get a sense of quality of relationships and how these might have changed since the death.)
29. Now can you tell me about how you have been eating?
30. And sleeping? Has your sleeping changed? (If yes) Tell me about how it has changed. (Also get a sense of the kind of dreams he or she is having.)

(cont.)

Table 38.4. (*cont.*)

31. Tell me about your teacher(s). Do they know about [cite person's name] death? The nature of [cite person's name] illness?
32. How are you doing with your school work? Homework? Grades?
33. Have you been seeing a doctor for any health problems of your own?
34. (If yes) Tell me about that.
35. Do you think about dying too?
36. (If yes) What do you think about? (If they are suicidal, do an assessment for suicide risk.)
37. Is there something else that I haven't asked about?
38. Is there anything else you think I should know about how you are getting along?
39. (If yes). Tell me about that.
40. Do you have any questions that you would like to ask me?
41. (If yes) Go ahead.
42. Thank you for talking to me. If you have any questions or if you want to talk to me at any time, here is my card.

Source: Adapted from Sattler [14].

that one was able to care for, comfort, and communicate openly with the dying child positively affects the grief process.

Grief in parents who die before their child(ren)

One of the most difficult aspects of the illness for parents facing the possibility of dying before their children is the realization that they may not see their children grow to adulthood. Acknowledging that someone else will have to care for their children is often described as too painful to bear. Including children in future care planning and open discussions about their wishes may help the parent and the child. This is important for both practical and emotional reasons (see Chapter 39). Children want desperately to hold onto any part of their parent. Helping parents to create and leave concrete legacies for their children, in the form of letters or series of essays, life review books, drawings, audiotapes, portraits, or even videotapes or home movies is often therapeutic for the parent and especially helpful to the surviving child(ren) [27, 28].

Grandparents

Many grandparents have become the primary caretakers of two generations and they may witness the illness and eventual death of both their children and their grandchildren. A feeling of physical and emotional overload and overwhelming grief is common. Grandparents need a great deal of support, guidance, and education about HIV disease to deal with the losses they will be forced to encounter. Many express the sentiment that they have already raised their children, and resent that they are

Table 38.5. Books and reading materials for parents, children and professionals

Children's books

Agee, J. *A Death in the Family*. New York: Bantam, 1969.

Blackburn, L. B. *The Class in Room 44: When a Classmate Dies*. Omaha, NE: Centering Corporation, 1991.

Brack, P., Brack, B. *Moms Don't Get Sick*. Aberdeen: SD Melius Publishing, Inc., 1990.

Braithwaite, A. *When Uncle Bob Died*. London: Dinosaur Publications, 1982.

Bratman, F. *Everything You Need to Know When a Parent Dies*. New York: Rosen Group, 1992.

Brenna, B. *Year in the Life of Rosie Bernard*. New York: Harper & Row, 1971.

Buscaglia, L. *The Fall of Freddie the Leaf*. New Jersey: Charles B. Slack Inc., 1982.

De Paola, T. A. *Nana Upstairs and Nana Downstairs*. New York: Penguin, 1973.

Crawford, C. P. *Three-Legged Race*. New York: Harper & Row, 1974.

Draimin, B. H. *Coping When a Parent Has AIDS*. New York: Rosen Group, 1993.

Fitzgerald, H. *The Grieving Teen: A Guide for Teenagers and Their Friends*, 2000.

Girard, L. W. *Alex, the Kid with AIDS*. Morton Grove, Illinois: Albert Whitman and Co., 1991.

Gootman, M. E. *When a Friend Dies*. Minneapolis: Free Spirit Publishing, 1994.

Greene, C. C. *Beat the Turtle Drum*. New York: Viking, 1976.

Grollman, E. A. *Straight Talk About Death for Teenagers: How to Cope with Losing Someone You Love*, Boston, MA: Beacon Press, 1993.

Hichman, M. *Last Week My Brother Anthony Died*. Nashville, TN: Abingdon, 1983.

Holms, C. D. *Red Balloons, Fly High!* Warminster, PA: mar*co products, inc. 1997.

Johnson J., Johnson, M. *Where's Jess?* Omaha, NE: Centering Corporation, 1982.

Krementz, J. *How It Feels When A Parent Dies*. New York: Knopf, 1981.

Lee, V. *The Magic Moth*. New York: Seabury Press, 1972.

Linn, E. *Children Are Not Paper Dolls: A Visit with Bereaved Children*. Incline Village, NV: Publishers Mark, 1982.

McNamara, J. W. *My Mom is Dying: A Child's Diary*. Minneapolis: Augsburg Fortress, 1994.

Mellonie, B., Ingpen, R. *Lifetimes: The Beautiful Way to Explain Death to Children*. New York: Bantam, 1983.

Merrifield, M. *Come Sit by Me*. Toronto, Canada: Woman's Press, 1990.

Miles, M. *Annie and the Old One*. Boston: Little Brown, 1971.

Mills, J. C. *Gentle Willow A Story for Children about Dying*. New York: Magination Press, 1993.

Peterkin, A. *What About Me? When Brothers and Sisters Get Sick*. New York: Magination Press, 1992.

Powell, E. S. *Geranium Morning*. Minneapolis: Carolrhoda Books, 1990.

Richter, E. *Losing Someone You Love*. New York: Putnam, 1986.

Rofes, E. *The Kids' Book About Death and Dying*. Boston: Little, Brown, 1985.

Sanders, P. *Let's Talk About Death and Dying*. London: Aladdin Books, 1990.

Shriver, M. *What's Heaven?* Golden Books Publishing Co., 1999.

Sims, A. M. *Am I Still a Sister?* Slidell, Louisiana: Big A & Company / Starline Printing, Inc., 1986.

Starkman, N. *Z's Gift*. Seattle: Comprehensive Health Education Foundation, 1988.

Varley, S. *The Badger's Parting Gifts*. Mulberry Books, 1992.

Vigna, J. *Saying Goodbye to Daddy*. Morton Grove, Illinois: Albert Whitman and Co., 1991.

(cont.)

Table 38.5. (*cont.*)

Viorst, J. *The Tenth Good Thing About Barney.* New York: Atheneum, 1971.

White, E. B. *Charlotte's Web.* New York: Harper and Row, 1952.

Wiener, L., Best, A., Pizzo, P. *Be A Friend: Children Who Live With HIV Speak.* Morton Grove, Illinois: Albert Whitman and Co., 1994.

Williams, M. *The Velveteen Rabbit.* Garden City, NY: Doubleday, 1971.

Zim, H., Bleeker, S. *Life and Death.* New York: Morrow, 1970.

Books for parents

Fitzgerald H. *The Grieving Child*: A Parent's Guide. New York: Simon & Schuster, 1992.

Grollman, E. *Talking About Death.* Boston: Beacon Press, 1976.

Kander, J. *So Will I Comfort You.* Cape Town: Lux Verbi, 1990.

Kushner, H *When Bad Things Happen To Good People*, 1994

LeShan, E. *Learning to Say Goodbye.* New York: Macmillan, 1976.

Levang, E. *When Men Grieve: Why Men Grieve Differently, How You Can Help.* Minneapolis: Fairview Press, 1998.

Schaefer, D. Lyons, C. *How Do We Tell the Children? Helping Children Understand and Cope When Someone Dies* (revised edition). New York: Newmarket, 1988.

Schiff, H. *The Bereaved Parent.* UK:Souvenir Press, 1979.

Tasker, M. *How Can I Tell You? Secrecy and Disclosure with Children When a Family Member Has AIDS.* Bethesda, MD: Association for the Care of Children's Health, 1992.

Videotapes

A Child's View of Grief. Center for Loss and Life Transition. CO: Fort Collins, 1991.

A Family in Grief: The Ameche Story. Champagne, IL: Research Press, 1989.

How Children Grieve. Portland, OR: The Dougy Center.

Living with Loss: Children and HIV (Part 4 of the *Hugs Invited* series). Washington, DC: Child Welfare League of America, 1991

What do I Tell My Children? Wayland, MA: Aquarius Productions, 1990.

When Grief Comes to School. Bloomington, IN: Blooming Educational Enterprises, 1991.

With Loving Arms. Washington, DC: Child Welfare League of America, 1989.

Resources for healthcare providers

Baxter, G., Stuart, W. *Death And The Adolescent A Resource Handbook For Bereavement Support Groups In Schools.* Toronto: University of Toronto Press, 1999

Crowley, R., Mills, J. *Cartoon Magic: How to Help Children Dscover Their Rainbows Within.* New York: Magination Press, 1989.

Dougy Center Staff. *35 Ways to Help a Grieving Child.* Dougy Center, 1999.

Geballe, S., Gruendel, J., Andiman, W. *Forgotten Children of the AIDS Epidemic.* New Haven: Yale University Press, 1995.

Haasal, B., Marnocha, J. *Bereavement Support Group Program for Children: Leader's Manual.* Muncie, Indiana: Accelerated Development, Inc, 1990.

Lagorio, J. *Life Cycle Education Manual.* Solana Beach, CA: Empowerment in Action, 1991.

O'Toole, D. *Growing through Grief.* Burnsville, NC: Mt. Rainbow Publications, 1989.

Worden, J. W. *Grief Counseling and Grief Therapy: A Handbook for the Mental Health Practitioner.* Springer, 1982.

now forced to take on the responsibilities of raising another generation. Through an empathic response, and with help in obtaining individual, community, and group support, financial aid, and in-home support and respite care, these individuals can carry on their responsibilities while working through the painful consequences of AIDS and multiple deaths [29].

Conclusions

Even though access to and quality of therapy has improved greatly, the losses associated with AIDS will be with us for some time to come. Several psychotherapeutic interventions can assist families through the grief process. Healthcare providers must remember that bereavement is not a state that ends at a certain point in time, or from which one fully recovers [19]. Children need to appropriately express their emotions and develop a clear understanding of what has happened. Keepsakes, rituals, and other methods of preserving legacies are of utmost importance. Maintaining contact with the family after the death, especially on anniversaries, birthdays, and holidays is greatly appreciated. Positive, bereavement-related social support, and social interactions can help reduce depression in individuals who have suffered multiple losses. Lastly, helping the bereaved to continue with life and planning for the future is important for the healing process. Although the emotional losses are significant, the rewards of helping a child and/or family beyond their grief, are even greater.

REFERENCES

1. Osborn, J. Foreword. In Geballe, S., Gruendel, J., Andiman, W., eds. *Forgotten Children of the AIDS Epidemic*. New Haven: Yale University Press, 1995.
2. Goodkin, K., Blaney, N. T., Tuttle, R. S. *et al.*, Bereavement and HIV infection. *Int. Rev. Psychiatry* 1996;**8**:201–216.
3. Dane BO. Children, HIV infection, and AIDS. In Corr, C. A., Corr, D. M., eds. *Handbook of Childhood Death and Bereavement*. New York: Springer Publishing Company, 1996;51–70.
4. Elia, N. Grief and loss in AIDS work. In Winiarski, M. G., ed. *HIV Mental Health Care for the 21st Century*. New York: New York University Press, 1997;67–81.
5. O'Donnell, M. HIV/AIDS: *Loss, Grief, Challenge, and Hope*. Washington, DC: Taylor & Francis, 1996.
6. Scherr, L., Green, J. Dying, bereavement and loss. In Green, J., McCreaner, A., eds. *Counselling in HIV Infection and AIDS*, 2nd edn. Oxford: Blackwell Science, Ltd., 1996; 179–194.
7. The Working Committee on HIV, Children, and Families. *Families in Crisis*. New York: Federation of Protestant Welfare Agencies, 1997.
8. Fitzgerald, H. *The Grieving Child: A Parent's Guide*. New York: Simon & Schuster, 1992.
9. Pennells, S. M., Smith, S. C. *The Forgotten Mourners*. Bristol, PA: Jessica Kingsley Publishers, 1995.

10. Centers for Disease Control and Prevention (Feb. 22, 2001). *HIV/AIDS Surveillance Report*, **7**(1).

11. McKelvy, C. L. Counseling children who have a parent with AIDS or who have lost a parent to AIDS. In Odets, W., Shernoff, M., eds. *The Second Decade of AIDS: A Mental Health Practice Handbook*. New York: The Hatheleigh Company Limited, 1995;137–159.

12. Stahlman, S. D. Children and the death of a sibling. In Corr, C. A., Corr, D. M., eds. *Handbook of Childhood Death and Bereavement*. New York: Springer Publishing Company, 1996:149–164.

13. Fanos, J., Wiener, L. Tomorrow's survivors: siblings of HIV infected children. *J. Dev. Behav. Pediatr.*, 1994:**15**(3):S43–S48.

14. Siegel, K., Freund, B. Parental loss and latency age children. In Dane, B., Levine, C. eds. *AIDS and the New Orphans*. Westport, CT: Auburn House, 1994;43–58.

15. Silverman, P. R., Worden, J. W. Children's reactions in the early months after the death of a parent. *Am. J. Orthopsychiatry*, 1992;**62**(1):93–104.

16. Reese, M. F. Growing up: the impact of loss and change. In Belle, D., ed. *Lives in Stress: Women and Depression*. Beverly Hills, CA: Sage 1982; 65–88.

17. Silverman, P. R., Nickman, S., Worden, J. W. Detachment revisited: the child's reconstruction of a dead parent. In Doka, K. J., ed. *Children Mourning Children*. Washington, DC: Hospice Foundation of America, 1995; 131–148.

18. Kubler-Ross, E. *On Death and Dying*. New York: Macmillan Publishing Co, Inc., 1969.

19. Worden, J. W. *Grief Counseling and Grief Therapy: A Handbook for the Mental Health Practitioner*. New York: Springer, 1982.

20. Wiener, L., Fair, C., Pizzo, P. A. Care for the child with HIV infection and AIDS. In Armstrong, A., Goltzer, S. Z., eds. *Hospice Care For Children*. New York: Oxford University Press, 2001.

21. Kaplan, D. M., Grobstein, R., Smith, A. Predicting the impact of severe illness in families. *Health and Social Work*; 1976;**1**(3):71–82.

22. Tietz, W., McSherry, L., Britt, B. Family sequelae after a child's death due to cancer. *Am. J. Psychother.* 1977;**31**(3):417–425.

23. Binger, C. M., Ablin, A. R., Feuerstein, R. C., Kushner, J. H., Zoger, S., Mikkelsen, C. Childhood leukemia: emotional impact on patient and family. *N. Engl. J. Med.*, 1969;**280**(8): 414–418.

24. Wiener, L., Gibbons, M. Bereavement reactions in parents who have lost a child to HIV, unpublished manuscript.

25. Wiener, L. Helping a parent with HIV tell his or her children. In Aronstein, D., Thompson, B., eds. *HIV and Social Work: A Practitioner's Guide*. Binghamton, NY: Haworth Press, 1998: 327–338.

26. Taylor-Brown, S., Wiener, L. Making videotapes of HIV-infected women for their children. *Families in Society*, 1993;**74**(8):468–480.

27. Wiener, L., Septimus, A., Grady, C. Psychological support ethical issues for the child and family. In Pizzo, P. A., Wilfert, C. M., eds. Pediatric AIDS: *The Challenge of HIV Infection in Infants, Children, and Adolescents*, 3rd edn. Philadelphia: Lippincott Williams & Wilkins, 1998: 703–727.

28. Ingram, K. M., Jones, D. A., Smith, N. G. Adjustment among people who have experienced AIDS-related multiple loss: the role of unsupportive social interactions, social support, and coping. *Omega–J. Death Dying* 2001;**43**(4):287–309.

39 Legal issues for HIV-infected children

Carolyn McAllaster, J. D.

Duke University School of Law, Durham, NC

Introduction

HIV-infected children face a host of issues, many of which involve the legal system. These children often need to have future plans made for their care, or they may want to apply for government benefits or to participate in clinical trials. This chapter is designed to describe some common legal issues confronting the HIV-infected child in the USA. Each country will have different legal approaches to the subjects discussed in this chapter. The US legal response to the needs of HIV-infected children is illustrative of how one legal system has dealt with the issues discussed here.

Permanent custody planning for children

Introduction

Since the vast majority of HIV-infected children have a mother who is also infected, it is important that plans be made for a time when the mother either becomes unable to care for her child or dies. Permanency planning is the process by which plans are made for the long-term legal custody or adoption of children at risk of losing their custodial parent or guardian. Such plans are particularly important when the HIV-infected parent is a single parent.

The ideal custody plan includes the identification of a stable future guardian who: (a) already has a bond with the child; (b) has the physical, emotional, and financial ability to care for the child; (c) has a long-term commitment to the child; and (d) understands and is willing to meet the special needs of an HIV-infected child.

Obstacles to making permanent plans

HIV-infected parents face considerable obstacles to seeking the legal help necessary to make permanent plans for their children. Parents may deny the need for permanency

Handbook of Pediatric HIV Care, ed. Steven L. Zeichner and Jennifer S. Read.
Published by Cambridge University Press. © Cambridge University Press 2006.

planning, particularly during the asymptomatic phase of their illness. They may fear breaches of confidentiality relating to their HIV infection status. Clients may be intimidated at the prospect of dealing with an unknown lawyer or have trust issues surrounding the process. Many clients face transportation problems, financial constraints, or more immediate priorities that can interfere with their ability to make legally binding plans for their children. Healthcare professionals, case managers, and social workers can help by working collaboratively with attorneys to assist parents as they work through many of these issues.

Assessing the rights and responsibilities of non-custodial biological parents

When making long-term plans for an HIV-infected child, it is important to assess first the rights and responsibilities of the non-custodial parent. In some cases, the absent parent is a viable candidate for future custody of the child. If that is the case, plans should be made for a smooth transition of future custody to that parent should the custodial parent die or no longer be able to care for the child, by actively involving the non-custodial parent in the planning for a future change of custody. It may also be that the absent parent will consent to the custodial parent's plan to appoint a non-parent caregiver.

If it appears, however, that the absent parent is not an appropriate future caregiver for the child and might interfere with the implementation of an optimal plan, the custodial parent may want to consider terminating the absent parent's rights. The decision to terminate parental rights should not be made lightly. As a result of a court order terminating a parent's rights, the legal parent–child relationship is ended. Termination of parental rights involves not only a termination of the parent's right to seek custody or visitation, it also involves a termination of the parent's obligations, including child support, and terminates the child's right to collect benefits on his or her parent's record. For example, once a parent's rights are terminated, the child can no longer collect Social Security benefits to which he or she might be entitled as a result of an absent parent's death or disability. Before a decision to terminate is made, it is important to assess the effect on potential benefits for the child.

Assessing present and future benefits to which the child may be entitled

When developing a long-term custody plan for an HIV-infected child, it is important to evaluate the sources of financial support that may be available to the child both currently and once the plan is implemented. Depending on the family's financial situation and the child's health, the parent or HIV-infected child may be entitled to certain benefits, such as: temporary assistance for needy families (TANF), supplemental security income (SSI), social security disability income (SSDI), Medicaid, Food Stamps, Veteran's Administration Benefits, or state welfare benefits. When considering the permanent plan for the child, one must determine whether the benefits follow the child or are dependent on the status of the caretaker. For example, if the long-term plan involves the appointment of a non-relative as guardian for the child, that person would not be eligible for benefits which are limited to biological or adoptive parents or blood relatives of the child.

Powers of attorney for decisions relating to HIV-infected children

Many states allow custodial parents to sign a power of attorney authorizing another adult to make certain decisions regarding their minor child. For example, a typical power of attorney will authorize the adult to make healthcare decisions for the child. An HIV-infected parent who cannot be consistently available to make decisions for a child should consider signing such a power of attorney as a short-term measure. This may ensure that healthcare, schooling, and other decisions regarding the child are made in a timely manner. By signing a power of attorney, the parent is not relinquishing his/her rights to make decisions for the child. He/she is agreeing to share that power with another adult.

Guardianship arrangements

Guardianship laws vary from state to state. In many states, a guardian may be appointed while the parent is still alive. Although the procedures vary, they most certainly will require either consent or legal notification of any absent biological parent. Once appointed, the guardian can immediately make legal decisions on behalf of the child and the parent has the peace of mind of knowing that his/her choice of guardian is firmly established. Appointment of a guardian also has its disadvantages. The primary disadvantage is that the parent must relinquish custody and control over the child in order to have a guardian appointed. This is often a difficult and wrenching decision.

A parent may also opt to designate a guardian in his or her will. The designation takes effect only after the parent's death. If there is no surviving parent, the parent's nomination of a guardian in the will generally will be given deference. A guardianship designation in a will is not binding on the court, however, and only becomes effective if there is not a surviving parent. Furthermore, this method allows the parent to retain custody of the child, but does not effectively plan for the possibility that the parent, while still alive, will become unable to care for his or her child.

Several states [1] have now legislated solutions to the problem of requiring a parent to relinquish custody in order to make stable future plans for a child. These solutions allow HIV-infected parents to maintain custody of their children while at the same time solidifying a plan for the children's guardianship in the event the parent dies or becomes incapacitated. There are two types of alternative guardianships that have now been recognized in a minority of states – joint guardianships or standby guardianships. These laws allow a parent with a progressively chronic or terminal illness to have a guardian appointed while the parent is still alive and competent. Typically, the statutes do not require the parent to give up custody or legal decision-making authority, but allow the standby guardian to act legally for the child if the parent becomes mentally or physically incapacitated or dies. The statutes often also allow the parent to consent to sharing decision-making authority with the standby guardian. The standby or joint guardianship option gives the parent the flexibility of having someone who can step in to care for and make decisions for the child when the parent is unable to do so. During periods of good health, the parent can resume her parental role. The child may be able to stay with the parent throughout the parent's illness, while at the same time having the stability and security of knowing he or she will be cared for in the future.

None of the guardianship options discussed here results in a final termination of a biological or adoptive parent's rights. Rights to seek custody, visitation or child support remain, as does the child's right to inherit and collect benefits on the non-custodial parent's record.

Adoption

A parent may choose to relinquish her child for adoption. This difficult decision might be made because of the combined effect of a parent's declining health and the lack of an identifiable caretaker for the child. Once a child is adopted, the parental rights of the biological parents are terminated and the adoptive parent assumes all the rights and responsibilities of a biological parent. State adoption laws vary, but may or may not provide for contact between the child and the biological parent after the adoption is final. The child may also become ineligible for public assistance and/or Medicaid after being adopted. The Federal Adoption Assistance and Child Welfare Act of 1980 does make additional subsidies available to "special needs" children.

Foster care

Many HIV-infected children end up in the foster care system, either because their parent voluntarily places them in foster care or because of involuntary intervention by a child welfare agency based on a finding of abuse or neglect or in situations where a parent is unable to meet the needs of his or her child. In the case of a voluntary placement, the parent may be seeking a temporary respite from the child's care and may be able to regain custody after showing the ability to resume care of the child. In the case of an involuntary removal of the child from the home, the burden on the parent to regain custody will be higher and will be dictated in most situations by the terms of a court order.

Supplemental security income (SSI) for disabled children

Definition of disability

Low-income HIV-infected children may be eligible for SSI benefits. SSI is a federally financed and administered needs-based program that provides a monthly income benefit to disabled children, among others. Under welfare reform passed by Congress in August of 1996 [2] a child under age 18 would be considered disabled if he or she has a medically determinable mental or physical impairment that results in marked and severe functional limitations and that can be expected to result in death or which has lasted or can be expected to last for a continuous period of not less than 12 months.

The Social Security Administration publishes a list of HIV-related impairments, which include specific criteria about the level of severity that will be required for a child to be considered disabled [3]. An HIV-infected child applying for SSI benefits must either have one of the listed conditions or have a condition that is medically or functionally equivalent in severity to a listed condition.

Information needed to apply for SSI

Parents or guardians of disabled children can apply for SSI benefits by calling or visiting their local Social Security Office. In order to expedite the process, they should have the following information and documentation when they apply: the child's birth certificate and Social Security number, and records documenting the parent and child's income and assets. In order to document the severity of the child's disability, it also will be important to provide names, addresses, and phone numbers of the child's doctors and hospitals where s/he has received treatment, and the same information for teachers, childcare providers, counselors, social workers, and other professionals who have worked with the child. The parent also can expedite the process by providing copies of the child's medical records to Social Security. Parents who are considering filing an SSI claim on behalf of their child should keep a daily journal documenting specifically how the child's disability limits the child's day-to-day activities.

Presumptive disability

For children who are severely disabled, there are special provisions in the law which allow them to collect SSI benefits for up to 6 months while the formal disability decision is being made. If the child is later determined not to be disabled, the benefits do not have to be paid back.

Appeal process

If the initial SSI application is denied, the parent or guardian will receive a Notice of Denial of Benefits in the mail. The parent then has 60 days to appeal against the initial decision. The Notice will explain how to file an appeal. The appeal process has four steps: (a) reconsideration by a disability examiner; (b) a hearing before an administrative law judge; (c) social security appeals council review; and (d) appeal to federal court. A substantial number of initial social security determinations that are appealed are reversed at the hearing level, so for children with serious disabilities it is important to pursue the appeal process at least through the hearing level. If denied at the initial application step, it is generally advisable for the parents to seek legal representation from an attorney who specializes in handling SSI cases.

Consent to medical treatment for minor children

In general

It is generally required that a child's legal guardian consent to medical treatment for a child under age 18. There are exceptions to this general rule.

Emancipation

Many states recognize the emancipation of children under age 18 by statute or case law. Emancipation is typically recognized in situations where a minor has married, entered the armed services, or is living apart from parents and is financially independent [4]. Emancipation confers upon the child some or all of the rights and responsibilities of adulthood, depending on the state law where the minor child lives.

Laws allowing minors to consent to certain medical procedures

Many states also have laws which specifically allow minors to consent to their own medical treatment in certain enumerated situations, typically pregnancy, sexually transmitted diseases, birth control, and substance abuse [5].

Medical neglect: parental refusal to seek treatment

All states have a mechanism for overriding the requirement of parental consent for medical treatment where the child's life may be threatened or the parent's refusal to consent to medical treatment rises to the level of child abuse or neglect [6]. The child's parent or legal guardian ordinarily has the authority to make medical decisions on behalf of his or her child. In order to override that authority, the healthcare provider or social worker must seek a court order. In situations where the child's life may be threatened, the court can directly authorize the needed treatment. Where the refusal to seek medical treatment is not immediately life-threatening, but does constitute neglect, welfare agencies may seek legal custody from the court in order be able to give consent to the needed treatment.

Consent for participation in clinical trials

In order for an HIV-infected, non-foster child to participate in a clinical trial, it is necessary to obtain the consent of the custodial parent or legal guardian [7]. Clinical trials investigators must, in most circumstances, also obtain the assent of the children who enrol as subjects and who are capable of assenting [8]. In cases of children in foster care, the legal custodian is usually, but not always, the child welfare agency. Many states, however, do not allow children in the foster care system to participate as research subjects [9]. "Most child protection agencies . . . have only the authority to consent to 'standard' medical treatment for foster children" [10].

Conclusions

It is hoped that this chapter has provided a useful guide to those working with HIV-infected children regarding the basic US law that applies in the areas of custody planning, disability benefits, and consent to medical treatment for children. This chapter is designed to provide information illustrative of how one legal system has addressed the issues discussed here. The chapter should not be considered a substitute for legal advice from an attorney. For representation in individual cases or more detailed information, readers are urged to refer to the appendix in this book entitled "Selected legal resources for HIV-infected children." This Appendix lists on a state-by-state basis several organizations that provide direct legal services or referrals to HIV-infected individuals.

REFERENCES

1. Ark. Code Ann. § 28-65-221 (LexisNexis Supp. 2001); Cal. Prob. Code § 2105 (West Supp. 2002); Colo. Rev. Stat. Ann. § 15-14-202 (2) (Bradford Publishing 2001); Conn. Gen. Stat. §§ 45a-624 to 625 (West Supp. 2002); Fla. Stat. § 744.304 (West Supp. 2002); Ill. Comp. Stat. Ann ch. 755 § 5/11-5.3 (West Supp. 2002); Mass. Gen. Laws Ann. ch, 201 §§ 2A-2H (LexisNexis Supp. 2002); Md. Code Ann., Est. & Trusts §§ 13-901 to 908 (Lexis 2001); Minn. Stat. Ann. §§ 257B.01-257B.10 (West Supp. 2002); Neb. Rev. Stat. § 30-2608 (Lexis 2001); N. J. Rev. Stat. §§ 3B:12-67 to 78 (West Supp. 2001): N.Y. Surr. Ct. Proc. Act §§ 1726 (West 2001–2002); N.C. Gen. Stat. §§ 35A-1370 to 1382 (West 2000); Pa. Con. Stat. Ann. ch. 23 §§ 5601-5616 (West 2001); Va. Code Ann. §§ 16.1-349 to 355 (Michie 1999); W. Va. Code §§ 44A-5-1 (LexisNexis Supp. 2001); Wis. Stat. Ann. § 48.978 (West Supp. 2001).

2. Personal Responsibility and Work Opportunity Reconciliation Act of 1996, Pub.L.No. 104–193 (1996).

3. 20 C. F. R. pt. 404, subpt. P, App. 1, Part B, § 114.08 (2002).

4. See, for example, N. M. Stat. Ann. §§ 32A-21-1 to -21-7 (Michie 1999); Cal. Fam. Code § 7001 *et seq.* (West 1994).

5. See, for example, N.C.G.S. § 90-21.5 (West 2000).

6. Mookin R. H., Weisberg D. K. *Child, Family and State*, 3rd edn. Little, Brown and Company, 1995;558–561.

7. For research not involving greater than minimal risk, or for research involving greater than minimal risk but presenting the prospect of direct benefit to the individual subjects, the permission of only one parent is necessary. For research involving greater than minimal risk and no prospect of direct benefit to the subject, but likely to yield generalizable knowledge about the subject's disorder or condition, or for research not otherwise approvable which presents an opportunity to understand, prevent, or alleviate a serious problem affecting the health or welfare of children, the permission of both parents is required, "unless one parent is deceased, unknown, incompetent, or not reasonably available, or when only one parent has legal responsibility for the care and custody of the child." 45 C.F.R. § 46.408(b).

8. Assent is defined as "a child's affirmative agreement to participate in research. Mere failure to object should not, absent affirmative agreement, be construed as assent." 45 C.F.R. § 46.402(b). "In determining whether children are capable of assenting, the IRB shall take

into account the ages, maturity and psychological state of the children involved." 45 C.F.R. § 46.408(a).

9. *See* Martin & Sacks, Do HIV-Infected Children in Foster Care Have Access to Clinical Trials of New Treatments?, 5 AIDS *Pub Policy J.* 1990; **3**.

10. McNutt, The under-enrollment of HIV-infected foster children in clinical trials and protocols and the need for corrective state action. *Am. J. Law Med.* 1994; **231**.

Appendices

Appendix 1: I Formulary antiretroviral agents

Paul Jarosinski, Pharm.D.

Pharmacy Department
National Institutes of Health, Bethesda, MD

Formulary – Antiretroviral agents

Generic name (synonyms)/forms	FDA approved dose	Other doses	Comments
Nucleoside reverse transcriptase inhibitors			
Zidovudine (Retrovir®, AZT, ZDV)/100 and 300 mg tabs, 10 mg/ml oral solution, 10 mg/ml for iv infusion.	Neonates: 2 mg/kg po q6h or 1.5 mg/kg iv q6h 6 wk–12 years: 160 mg/m² (max 200 mg) po q8h >12 yo: 600 mg/day in two or three doses	Premature neonates: 2 mg/kg po or 1.5 mg/kg iv q12 h until 2 weeks of age then 2 mg/kg po q8h[a]	Can be taken without regard to food, only HIV antiretroviral available for iv infusion after dilution, not recommended for use with stavudine.
Zalcitabine (Hivid®, ddC)/ 0.375 and 0.750 mg tablets	No approved dose for < 13 yo Adult: 0.75 mg q8h	0.1 mg/kg q8h[a]	C_{max} decreased 40% and AUC 14% when given with food – significance unknown. Best given on an empty stomach. Not recommended for use with lamivudine and didanosine.

(cont.)

Formulary – Antiretroviral agents (*cont.*)

Generic name (synonyms)/forms	FDA approved dose	Other doses	Comments
Didanosine (Videx®, ddI)/ 25, 50,100, 150 mg chew tabs, 100/167/250 mg powder packets, 10 mg/ml oral solution, and 125/200/250/400 mg enteric coated tabs	Children ≥ 6 mo: 120 mg/m^2 bid Adult ≥ 60 kg: 200 mg (tablets)/250 mg (buffered powder) bid, 400 (EC) qd <60 kg: 125 mg (tablets)/167 mg (buffered powder) bid, 250 mg (EC) qd	Neonates < 90 days: 50 mg/m^2 q12h^a Ped dose: 90–150 mg/m^2 q12h^a	10 mg/ml buffered solution is stable for 30 days refrigerated, dose on empty stomach, two tablets required for sufficient antacid, children < 3 may require additional antacid with oral solution, EC daily tablet available for adults with compliance problems on bid (less optimal). Beware of interaction related to antacid content. Not recommended for use with zalcitabine.
Lamivudine (Epivir®, /Epivir-HBV, 3TC)/100, 150, and 300 mg tablet and 5 and 10 mg/ml solutions.	Children 3 mo–16 yo: 4 mg/kg bid–max 150 mg bid Adult: 150 mg bid or 300 mg qd	Neonate (<30 days): 2 mg/kg bid^a	Oral liquid is stable at room temperature, can be given without regard to food, not recommended for use with zalcitabine. 5 mg/ml solution and 100 mg tablet are marketed for HBV, but can be used for pediatric HIV treatment.

Drug	Dosing	Neonatal/Infant dose	Comments
Stavudine (Zerit®, Zerit XR, d4T)/15, 20, 30, 40 mg caps, 1 mg/ml solution, and 37.5, 50, 75, and 100 mg XR caps	Children < 30 kg: 1 mg/kg q12h; Adults 30 kg–<60 kg: 30 mg q12h, Adults ≥60 kg: 40 mg q12h; or 100 mg XR qd for ≥ 60 kg or 75 mg qd for < 60 kg (use of XR tablets has not be studied in children)	Neonatal dose under study in PACTG 332	Oral solution is stable for 30 days refrigerated, can be given without regard to food, XR (extended release) caps may be mixed with 2 tablespoons of yogurt or applesauce as long as beads are not chewed or crushed, not recommended for use with zidovudine.
Abacavir (Ziagen®, 1592U89)/ 300 mg tab and 20 mg/ml oral solution	Children 3 mo–16 yo: 8 mg/kg bid–max 300 mg bid; Adults: 300 mg bid	Infants (1–3 mo): 8 mg/kg bid is under study.	Oral solution is stable at room temperature, can be given without regard to food.
Emtricitabine (Emtriva®, FTC) 200 mg capsules	Adults 18 and over: 200 mg daily		Chemically related to lamivudine. May be taken with or without food.
Non-nucleoside reverse transcriptase inhibitors			
Nevirapine (Viramune®, NVP)/200 mg tablets and 10 mg/ml suspension	Children 2 mo or older: 4 mg/kg once daily × 14 days then 7 mg/kg bid (2 mo–<8 yo) or 4 mg/kg bid (>8 yo) – max 200 mg bid[b]; Adults: 200 qd × 14 days then bid	Neonatal dose (PACTG 356) under study[c] 120 mg/m² qd × 14d then 120–200 mg/m² bid, max 200 mg/dose[a]	Oral suspension is stable at room temperature, lead-in dose lessens occurrence of rash, new lead-in period required for any 7 day interruption in therapy, can be given without regard to food, induces 3A4 liver enzymes.
Delavirdine (Rescriptor®, DLV)/100 and 200 mg tablets	Not approved for children; Adults: 400 mg tid		100 mg tablet only can be dispersed in water, can be given without regard to food, separate from didanosine and any antacid by 1 hour, inhibits liver enzymes 3A4 and 2C9.

(cont.)

809

Formulary – Antiretroviral agents (*cont.*)

Generic name (synonyms)/forms	FDA approved dose	Other doses	Comments
Efavirenz (Sustiva®, Stocrin®, DMP266)/50, 100, and 200 mg capsules, 600 mg tablet, 30 mg/ml liquid in some countries	For children 3 yo and above 10–<15 kg 200 mg daily 15–<20 kg 250 mg daily 20–<25 kg 300 mg daily 25–<32.5 kg 350 mg daily 32.5 kg–<40 kg 400 mg daily ≥40 kg 600 mg	No information on dosing to younger children	Should be taken on an empty stomach preferably at bedtime to minimize side effects, induces liver enzymes 3A4, 2C9, and 2C19. For patients that cannot swallow the smallest capsule (50 mg), there are reports of opening the capsule for administration in food or liquids with grape jelly mentioned as effective in disguising the peppery taste.[a]
Nucleotide reverse transcriptase inhibitors			
Tenofovir (Viread®, PMPA prodrug)/ 300 mg tablets	Not approved for children Adult: 300 mg once daily	Children 4–18 yo: 175 mg/m² daily being studied at the NCI	No liquid formulation, tablets cannot be crushed or dissolved, should be taken with a meal.
Protease inhibitors			
Ritonavir (Norvir®, RTV)/100 mg caps and 80 mg/ml oral solution	For children 2 yo and above: 400 mg/m² bid starting at 250 mg/m² and increasing by 50 mg/m² q2–3d to full dose. Max dose = adult dose = 600 mg bid	Neonates: under study in PACTG 354	Oral solution (43% ethanol) is stable at room temperature, refrigerate capsules unless used w/in 30 days, take with food, unpleasant taste of solution may be minimized by chocolate, peanut butter, etc., potent inhibitor of 3A4 liver enzymes as well as 2D6 (check drug interactions).

Drug/formulation	Dose	Comments
200, 333, and 400 mg caps	Adults: 800 mg q8h	taken on an empty stomach not with an antacid or at the same time as didanosine, drink plenty of fluids – at least 1.5 liters per day for adult doses, inhibitor of 3A4 liver enzymes.
	hyperbilirubinemia. Older children: 350–450 mg/m^2 q8h+	
Nelfinavir (Viracept®, NFV)/250 and 625 mg tablets and oral powder	Children 2–13 yo: 20–30 mg/m^2 tid using the chart in the package insert. Children ≥ 23 kg get adult dose of 750 mg q12h. Alternate adult dose: 1250 mg bid	Oral powder may be mixed with water, milk, formula, and dietary supplements, administer with food, tablets may be dissolved in water or crushed, inhibitor of 3A4 liver enzymes.
Amprenavir (Agenerase®, AMP, VX-478, 141W94)/ 50 and 150 mg caps and 15 mg/ml solution	Neonates: 40 mg/kg q12h under study in PACTG 353 Children 4–12 yo or 13–16 yo and < 50 kg: 22.5 mg/kg bid or 17 mg/kg tid as solution, max 2800 mg/d or 20 mg/kg bid or 15 mg/kg tid as capsules, max 2400 mg/day. Children ≥ 50 kg and adults: 1400 mg bid as solution or 1200 mg bid as capsules	Oral solution is stable at room temperature, solution dose does not equal capsule dose, may be taken with or without food, avoid taking with high-fat meal, do not take vitamin E supplements, inhibitor of 3A4 liver enzymes.
Lopinavir/Ritonavir Kaletra®/ caps of 133/33 mg and 80/20 mg/ml oral solution.	Neonates: Not recommended in children ≤ 3 yo Children 6 mo–12 yo: 230/57.5 mg/m^2 bid (max 400/100 bid)^a Children 6 mo–12 yo (LPV/RTV)^d: 7–<15 kg: 12/3 mg/kg bid, 15–40 kg: 10/2.5 mg/kg bid, max 400/100 mg bid, >40 kg and adult: 400/100 mg bid	Oral solution contains 42% ethanol, capsules and solution should be refrigerated or used within two months if stored at room temperature, take with food, potent inhibitor of 3A4 liver enzymes as well as 2D6 (check drug interactions).

(cont.)

Formulary – Antiretroviral agents (*cont.*)

Generic name (synonyms)/forms	FDA approved dose	Other doses	Comments
Saquinavir (SQV, Invirase® 200 mg hard gel caps, Fortovase® 200 mg soft gel caps)	Not approved for children < 16 yo. Adult doses Invirase®: 600 mg tid Fortovase®: 1200 mg tid	Pediatric dose under study: 50 mg/kg q8h as single protease therapy or 33 mg/kg q8h with nelfinavir	Invirase® and Fortovase® may not be used interchangeably, Invirase® should be stored at room temperature and Fortovase® should be refrigerated or stored at room temperature and used within 3 months, should be taken with a meal, inhibitor of 3A4 enzymes.
Atazanavir (Reyataz®) 200 mg caps	Adult dose: 400 mg qd	There is insufficient data for a pediatric dosage recommendation	Take with food. Antacids (including didanosine tablets and powder) allowed ≥ 2 hours after atazanavir or ≥ 1 hour before. Notify doctor if white portion of eyes or skin yellows. Many drug interactions.
Fusion inhibitors			
Enfuvirtide (Fuzeon®, T-20)/ lyophilized powder reconstituted to 90 mg/ml	6–16 yo: 2 mg/kg sc bid (max dose 90 mg) Adults: 90 mg bid		Injections should be into upper arm, anterior thigh, or abdomen. 86% of patients have their first injection site reaction in first week of therapy. Injections should be not given in a site where there is a remaining reaction from a previous dose. Do not administer into moles, scars, navel, or bruises.

Dosing to prevent mother-to-child transmission of HIV is discussed earlier.

FDA = United States Food and Drug Administration.

PACTG = Pediatric AIDS Clinical Trial Group.

yo = years old.

N/V = nausea/vomiting.

C_{max} = Peak blood concentration.

AUC = Area under the curve (reflective of total absorption).

EC = Enteric coated tablet for once daily dosing.

Sc = subcutaneous.

[a] = Guidelines for the Use of Antiretroviral Agents in Pediatric HIV Infection, 12/14/01 edition.

[b] The FDA approved dose was based on pharmacokinetic modeling to achieve similar plasma concentrations as dosing of 150 mg/m². Nevirapine clearance is highest during the first two years of life and decreases gradually until reaching adult clearance around 12 years of age. The current FDA regimen results in an abrupt 43% decrease in dose on the eighth birthday that is not consistent with the gradual change in clearance. The majority of pediatric clinical studies were done with the 120 mg/m² dosing regimen.

[c] PACTG 356 dosing for neonates through 2 months of age: 5 mg/kg or120 mg/m² qd × 14 days then 120 mg/m² q12h for 14 days, then 200 mg/m² q12h.

[d] Two studies (NCI/PACTG) have now confirmed a significant incidence of renal toxicity at a 500 mg/m² pediatric dose. The optimal indinavir dose for children is somewhere between the 350 mg/m² dose in the NCI study and 450 mg/m² (10% below the 500 mg/m² dose).

[e] The FDA doses are extrapolated from the pediatric trials that were dosed on body surface area at LPV 230/ RTV 57.5 mg/m² bid.

II Formulary: Drugs for opportunistic infections associated with HIV

Paul Jarosinski, Pharm.D.

Pharmacy Department, National Institutes of Health, Bethesda, MD

Formulary: Drugs for opportunistic infections associated with HIV

Generic name (Synonyms)/dosage form	FDA approved dose	Other doses	Comments
Acyclovir (Zovirax®) 200 mg caps, 400 and 800 mg tabs, 40 mg/ml suspension	HSV 1, 2: 250 mg/m² iv q8h or (adults) 200 mg po q4h × 5 daily for 10 days. VZV: 500 mg/m² iv q8h or 20 mg/kg po qid (max is adult dose of 800 mg qid) × 5 days HZ: 500 mg/m² iv q8h and, in adults, 800 mg q4h × 5 daily for 7–10 days.	Oral HSV in children: 400 mg/m² po tid. Oral HZ in children: 20 mg/kg po qid (max dose 800 mg qid)	Crystallization of drug in renal tubules can lead to renal failure if hydration is not adequate especially with high iv doses for zoster.
Atovaquone (Mepron®) 250 mg tabs and 150 mg/ml suspension	PCP treatment: (13 yo–adult) 750 mg bid with meals for 21 days. PCP prophylaxis: (13–16 yo) 1500 mg qd with a meal.	PCP treatment and PCP/toxo prophylaxis: (3–24 months) 45 mg/kg per day and (1–3 mo or 2–12 yo) 30 mg/kg/d once daily	Must be taken with meals to maximize absorption, suspension must be shaken, drug interactions possible due to high protein binding (>99%) and metabolism. Effective for mild/moderate PCP in adults. May be taken by G6PD deficient patients.

Drug	Dosing	Comments
Azithromycin (Zithromax®) 250 mg cap, 600 mg tab, 20 mg and 40 mg/ml susp, 1 g single dose packet	MAC Prophylaxis (adults):1200 mg po q week MAC prophylaxis (children) 20 mg/kg (max 1200 mg) po q week or 5–10 mg/kg/dose (max 500 mg) qd (lower dose for prophylaxis/higher for treatment	Capsules should be taken on an empty stomach while the suspension and tablets can be taken without regard to food. Shake suspension before used. Can be refrigerated, but not required. Fewer drug interactions than clarithromycin.
Cidofovir (Vistide®) 75 mg/ml for iv infusion in 375 mg vials	CMV: 5 mg/kg iv q week × 2, then 5 mg/kg iv q2wk. Probenecid 2 gm po required 3 hour before each dose and 1 g 2 and 8 hours after each cidofovir dose.	Cidofovir should be given over 1 hour. Saline hydration required. Giving food before probenecid may reduce nausea.
Clarithromycin (Biaxin®) 250 and 500 mg tabs, 125 and 250 mg/ml susp, and 500 mg XL tabs	MAC prophylaxis (Children) 7.5 mg/kg (max 500 mg) bid, (adults) 500 mg bid MAC treatment (children) up to 12.5 mg/kg (max 500 mg) bid	May be given without regard to food. Shake suspension before use and do not refrigerate. Some drug interactions. XL (sustained release) form is not indicated for MAC therapy.
Clindamycin (Cleocin®) 75, 150, and 300 mg caps and 150 mg/ml inj in 2, 4, or 6 ml sizes	PCP treatment: 10 mg/kg iv (max 600 mg) q6h with primaquine 0.3 mg/kg (as base) po qd × 21 days	Effective to mild–moderate PCP in adults. Contraindicated in G6PD deficiency. Drug must be diluted and given iv over 30 minutes or more.

(cont.)

Formulary: Drugs for opportunistic infections associated with HIV (*cont.*)

Generic name (Synonyms)/dosage form	FDA approved dose	Other doses	Comments
Dapsone 25 and 100 mg tabs		PCP treatment: 2 mg/kg po daily (max 100 mg with 5 mg/kg trimethoprim po × 21d. PCP/toxo prophylaxis: (Children > 1 mo): 2 mg/kg qd (max 100 mg) or 4 mg/kg q week (max)	Effective to mild-moderate PCP in adults. Avoid in patients with G6PD deficiency. Do not give with antacids (e.g. didanosine) as this may significantly lower absorption. Toxo prophylaxis regimen must also include pyrimethamine 1 mg/kg qd plus leucovorin 5 mg po q3d.
Ethambutol (Myambutol®) 100 and 400 mg tablets	For TB with other agents: Children ≥ 13 yo: 15–20 mg/kg (1 g max) qd or 50 mg/kg (2.5 g max) 2 × per week. See CDC dosing chart for adults and children ≥ 15 yo or 40 kg.	For TB with other agents: Children 5–12 yo – 15–20 mg/kg (1 g max) qd or 50 mg/kg (2.5 g max) 2 × per week. May use in younger children if resistant to other agents,	Not recommended by manufacturer for children under 13 due to optic neuritis. Visual testing recommended before and monthly.
Famciclovir (Famvir®) 125, 250, and 500 mg tablets	HSV (adults): 125 mg bid × 5d Suppression of recurrent HSV (adults): 250 mg bid HZ (adults): 500 mg q8h × 7 d	Not tested in children	Start w/in 72 hours of rash onset. May be taken without regard to food.
Foscarnet (Foscavir®) 24 mg/ml inj in 250 ml or 500 ml bottles	CMV: 90 mg/kg q12h or 60 mg/kg q8h iv × 14–21 d induction, then 90–120 mg/kg iv qd. Acyclovir resistant HSV: 40 mg/kg iv over 1 hour q 8–12h × 2–3 weeks		IV solution must be diluted to 12 mg/ml or lower. 90 mg/kg dose given over 1.5–2 h and 60 mg/kg over 1 hr. Maintenance doses given over 2 hours. 90 mg/kg is preferred maintenance dose due to lower toxicity. Hydration is required.

Ganciclovir (Cytovene®, DHPG) 250 and 500 mg caps plus 500 mg vials for reconstitution	CMV: 5 mg/kg iv × 14–21 d induction, then 5 mg/kg iv qd or 6 mg/kg iv qd × 5 d per week or 1000 mg po tid or 500 mg 6x qd	Some clinicians use 5 mg/kg iv qd for 5 days/week for maintenance.	Infusion should be given over one hour with adequate hydration. Capsules should be taken with food, but absorption is still poor. Valganciclovir is preferred agent for oral dosing. Drug can cause birth defects in pregnant women. Causes elevation of didanosine levels and neutropenia with zidovudine.
Isoniazid (INH) 100, 300 mg tabs and 10 mg/ml solution and 100 mg/ml injection	Positive TB skin test or exposure: 10–15 mg/kg (max 300 mg) qd × 9 mo or 20–30 mg/kg (max 900 mg) twice weekly for 9 months, same dose for treatment in combination with other agents. Adult dose: 5 mg/kg per day (300 max) or 15 mg/kg (900 mg max) once, twice, or thrice weekly		Syrup should be shaken before use. Doses ideally given on an empty stomach.
Oseltamivir (Tamiflu®) 75 mg caps and 12 mg/ml suspension	13 yo and above: 75 mg bid × 5 d Children 1 yo and greater; ≤15 kg – 30 mg twice daily >15 to 23 kg – 45 mg twice daily >23 to 40 kg – 60 mg twice daily >40 kg – 75 mg twice daily		Inactivated influenza vaccine is the first choice for influenza prophylaxis. Treatment should begin within 2 days of onset of symptoms of influenza. The oral suspension should be shaken before use, stored in the refrigerator, and used within 10 days.

(cont.)

Formulary: Drugs for opportunistic infections associated with HIV (*cont.*)

Generic name (Synonyms)/dosage form	FDA approved dose	Other doses	Comments
Pentamidine Isothionate (Pentam®) 300 mg vial for reconstitution	PCP Treatment: 4 mg/kg iv/im qd × 21d, may switch to another agent po to complete 21d if clinically recovered. PCP prophylaxis (Children > 5 yo): 300 mg via Respirgard II nebulizer q month		Second choice drug for PCP treatment, iv route is preferred for treatment, administer iv over 60–90 minutes to avoid hypotension, use with caution with other nephrotoxic agents. Do not give with didanosine due to association with pancreatitis.
Primaquine 26.3 mg tablet		PCP treatment: 0.3 mg/kg (as base) po qd with clindamycin 10 mg/kg iv (max 600 mg) q6h × 21 days	Effective to mild–moderate PCP in adults. Contraindicated in G6PD deficiency. Each 26.3 mg tablet contains 15 mg primaquine base. Can be taken without regard to meals.
Pyrazinamide 500 mg scored tablet	For TB with other agents: 15–30 mg/kg (2 gm max) qd or 50 mg/kg (2 gm max) 2x/week. See CDC dosing chart for adults and children ≥ 15 yo or 40 kg.		
Rifabutin (Mycobutin®) 150 mg capsule	MAC prop (adults): 300 mg qd or 150 mg bid.	For TB with other agents: 5 mg/kg (300 mg max) qd or 2–3 × per week, children 5–6 mg/kg qd or 2 ×/wk	Patients with nausea may take 150 mg bid with food. May color body fluids brown–orange and permanently discolor soft contact lenses. Several drug interactions.

Drug	Dosing	Comments
Rifampin (Rifadin®) 150 and 300 mg caps, 600 mg powder for reconstitution.	Positive TB skin test or exposure: 10–20 mg/kg (max 600 mg) po/iv qd × 4–6 mo, same dose for treatment of TB in combination with other agents qd or 2 ×/week	For prevention in INH-resistant strains or intolerance. Given orally on an empty stomach. IV formulation available, but no liquid formulation available, but no liquid prep. Pharmacist can prepare 4-week suspension supply. May color body fluids brown–orange and permanently discolor soft contact lenses. Many drug interactions.
Streptomycin 1 g vials of 400 mg/ml	For TB with other agents: 20–40 mg/kg (max 1 g) qd or 20 mg/kg (max 1.5 g) 2 × per week, adults < 60 yo and children ≥ 15 yo or 40 kg: 15 mg/kg (1 g max) qd (5–7d per week) decreased to 2–3 × week after culture conversion.	Only available as im injection although there are reports of the IM injection being given intravenously, rotate injection sites, adults should not exceed total dose of 120 g.
Trimethoprim-Sulfamethoxazole (TMP/SMX, Bactrim®, co-trimoxazole, Septra®, and others)/as TMP 80 and 160 mg tab, 80 mg/ml inj, and 40 mg/ml suspension	PCP treatment: 15–20 mg/kg/day as TMP IV divided q6h × 21d, may complete treatment PO if clinically recovered. PCP prophylaxis: 75/375 mg/m² per day (TMP/SMZ) po bid three consecutive days/wk. Toxoplasma prophylaxis: same dose as PCP given qd. PCP prophylaxis: 75/375 mg/m²/d bid three times week on alternate days, bid every day, or double dose up to adult max (160/800) qd × 3 d per week.	TMP-SMX not used for PCP therapy in children less that 4–6 weeks due to displacement of bilirubin. Use with caution in those with renal or hepatic dysfunction, severe allergy or asthma, or G6PD deficiency when hemolysis could occur. Hydration is important especially with PCP doses to avoid crystalluria and stone formation.

(cont.)

Formulary: Drugs for opportunistic infections associated with HIV (*cont.*)

Generic name (Synonyms)/dosage form	FDA approved dose	Other doses	Comments
Trimetrexate (Neutrexin®, TMTX) 25 mg vial for reconstitution	PCP treatment (adults): 45 mg/m² iv qd × 21 d with leucovorin 20 mg/m² iv q6h × 21d (72 h after last TMTX)	Pediatric PCP treatment: 45 mg/m² iv qd × 21 d with leucovorin 20 mg/m² iv q6h × 21d (72 hr after last TMTX)	Salvage regimen for patients who fail or cannot tolerate TMP/SMX. Drug interactions exist related to 3A4 metabolism.
Valacyclovir (Valtrex®) 500 mg and 1 g tablets	HSV (adults): 1 gm bid × 10d Suppression of recurrent HSV (adults): 500–1000 mg qd HZ (adults): 1 gm tid × 7 d	Not tested in children	Start w/in 72 hours of rash onset.
Valganciclovir (Valcyte®) 450 mg tablets	CMV induction (adults): 900 mg bid × 21 day followed by 900 mg qd maintenance	No pediatric recommendations	A 900 mg dose of valganciclovir provides drug levels similar to a 5 mg/kg iv ganciclovir dose. Tablets should be taken with food. Drug can cause birth defects in pregnant women. Causes elevation of didanosine levels and neutropenia with zidovudine.

Appendix 2: National Institutes of Health sponsored clinical trials for pediatric HIV disease

J. G. McNamara, M.D.

NIAID Pediatric AIDS Clinical Trials Group Units – USA

ALABAMA
Children's Hospital of Alabama
University of Alabama at Birmingham
Department of Pediatrics, Infectious
  Diseases
1600 Seventh Avenue, CHB 309
Birmingham, AL 35233-0011
(205) 996-7790
Fax: (205) 996-2370

CALIFORNIA
University of California at Los Angeles
UCLA School of Medicine
Department of Pediatric Infectious
  Diseases, 22-442 MDCC
10833 Le Conte Avenue
Los Angeles, CA 90095-1752
(310) 825-5235
Fax: (310) 206-5529

University of California at San Diego
Department of Pediatrics, Division of
  Infectious Diseases
Clinical Sciences Bldg, Room 430
9500 Gilman Dr., Mail Code 0672
La Jolla, CA 92093-0672
(858) 534-7361
Fax: (858) 534-7411

University of California at San Francisco
UCSF, Moffitt Hospital, M-679
505 Parnassus Avenue, Box 0105

San Francisco, CA 94143-0105
(415) 476-2865
Fax: (415) 476-3466

FLORIDA
University of Miami School of Medicine
Division of Pediatric Infectious Diseases and
  Immunology
Batchelor Building, Room 296
1550 N.W. 10th Avenue
P. O. Box 016 960 D4-4
Miami, FL 33101
(305) 243-6676
Fax: (305) 243-5562

ILLINOIS
Chicago Children's Memorial Hospital
Division of Infectious Diseases
2300 Children's Plaza, Box 155
Chicago, IL 60614-3394
(773) 880-4757
Fax: (773) 880-3208

LOUISIANA
Charity Hospital of New Orleans
Tulane University School of Medicine
Pediatric Infectious Diseases
1430 Tulane Avenue
New Orleans, LA 70112-2699
(504) 988-5422
Fax: (504) 586-3805

MARYLAND

Johns Hopkins University Hospital
Department of International Health
615 North Wolfe Street, H Room W-5501
Baltimore, MD 21205-2103
(410) 955-1633
Fax: (410) 502-6733

MASSACHUSETTS

Children's Hospital of Boston
Infectious Diseases, Enders 6
300 Longwood Avenue
Boston, MA 02115-5724
(617) 355-6832
Fax: (617) 733-0911

University of Massachusetts Medical Center
Department of Pediatrics/ Molecular
   Medicine
Biotech II, Suite 318
373 Plantation Street
Worcester, MA 01605-2377
(508) 856-6282
Fax: (508) 856-5500

NEW JERSEY

New Jersey Children's Hospital
UMDNJ-New Jersey Medical School
Division of Pulmonary, Allergy,
   Immunology and Infectious Diseases
185 South Orange Ave., F570A
Newark, NJ 07103-2714
(973) 972-5066
Fax: (973) 972-6443

NEW YORK

Bronx-Lebanon Hospital Center
Pediatric ID Services
Department of Pediatrics, Milstein
   Bldg.-2C
1650 Selwyn Avenue
Bronx, NY 10457
(718) 960-1010
Fax: (718) 960-1011

Columbia Presbyterian Medical Center
Department of Pediatrics
630 West 168th Street
New York, NY 10032-3796

(212) 305-9445
Fax: (212) 342-5218

NORTH CAROLINA

Duke University Medical Center
Children's Health Center Erwin Road
DUMC PO Box 3461
Durham, NC 27710-T915
(919) 668-4857
Fax: (919) 416-9268

PENNSYLVANIA

Children's Hospital of Philadelphia
Division of Allergy, Immunity and Infectious
   Diseases
Abramson Research Bldg., Suite 1208
34th Street and Civic Ctr. Blvd.
Philadelphia, PA 19104-4318
(215) 590-3561
Fax: (215) 590-3044

PUERTO RICO

University of Puerto Rico
University Pediatric Hospital
4th Floor South
PO Box 365036
San Juan, PR 00936-5067
(787) 759-9595
Fax: (787) 767-4798

TENNESSEE

St. Jude Children's Research Hospital
Department of Infectious Diseases
332 North Lauderdale
Memphis, TN 38105-2794
(901) 495-2338
Fax: (901) 495-5068

TEXAS

Baylor College of Medicine
Texas Children's Hospital
Allergy/Immunology Service
Abercrombie Bldg., Room A380
6621 Fannin Street, MS 1-3291
Houston, TX 77030
(832) 824-1319
Fax: (832) 825-7131

NIAID Pediatric AIDS Clinical Trials Group Units – International

SOUTH AFRICA

Red Cross Children's Hospital
University of Cape Town
Department of Pediatrics and Child Health
46 Sawkins Road
Rondebosch
Cape Town, South Africa, 7700
+27 21 685 4103
Fax: +27 21 689 5403

Chris Hani Baragwanath Hospital
Pediatrics Department
Harriet Shezi Clinic
P.O. Bertsham, 2013
Soweto, Johannesburg, South Africa
+27 82, 330 0882
Fax: +27 11 7938 7785

Chris Hani Baragwanath Hospital
Perinatal HIV Research Unit
Old Nurses Home, West Wing 12th Fl.
Old Potch Road
P.O. Bertsham 2013
Soweto, Johannesburg, South Africa
+27 11 989 9707
Fax: +27 11 989 9762

Tygerberg Children's Hospital
KID-CRU, J8
Stellenbosch University
Fancie vanZyl Ave.
Tygerberg 7505
South Africa
+27 21 938 4219
Fax: +27 21 938 4153

THAILAND

Siriraj Hospital
Mahidol University
Pediatric Infectious Diseases
Department of Pediatrics, Faculty of
  Medicine
2 Prannok Rd, Bangkoknoi
Bangkok 10700, Thailand
+66 2 418 0545
Fax: 66 2 418 0544

Institute for Research Development
Perinatal HIV Prevention Trials
57/2 Faham Road
Chiang Mai, Thailand
+66 (0) 538 4270
Fax: +66 (0) 538 4269

NICHD Clinical Trials Network Sites

CALIFORNIA

Los Angeles County/USC Medical Center
Maternal Child Program
Health Science Campus (CHB-HSC)
1640 Marengo Street
Los Angeles, CA 90033
(323) 226-6447 and 226-5068
(323) 226-8362 and 226-5960 Fax

COLORADO

University of Colorado Health Science
  Center
Department of Pediatrics

Infectious Disease Section
4200 East Ninth Avenue
Campus Box C227
Denver, CO 80262
(303) 315-4620
Fax: (303) 315-7909

CONNECTICUT

Yale University School of
  Medicine
Department of Pediatrics
Division of Infectious
  Diseases

420 LSOG, PO Box 3333
333 Cedar Street
New Haven, CT 06510-8064
(203) 785-4730
Fax: (203) 785-6961

DISTRICT OF COLUMBIA
Howard University Hospital
Department of Pediatrics
2041 Georgia Avenue, NW
Corridor 6N, Room 6E15
Washington, DC 20060
(202) 865-4583
Fax: (202) 865-7335

Children's National Medical Center
Special Immunology Service
111 Michigan Avenue, NW (WW 3.5-105)
Washington, DC 20010-2970
(202) 884-2980 and (202) 884-2837
Fax: (202) 884-3051

FLORIDA
South Florida Children's Diagnostic &
    Treatment Center
1401 South Federal Highway
Ft. Lauderdale, FL 33316
(954) 728-1017
Fax: (954) 712 5072

University of Florida Health Science Center
Pediatric Infectious Diseases/Immunology
653-1 West 8th Street
Jacksonville, FL 32209
(904) 244-3051
Fax: (904) 244-5341

University of Florida College of Medicine
Department of Pediatrics
1600 S.W. Archer Road
PO Box 100296
Gainesville, FL 32610-0296
(352) 392-2691
Fax: (352) 846-1810

University of South Florida Physicians
    Group
College of Medicine
Department of Pediatrics

17 Davis Boulevard, Suite 313
Tampa, FL 33606-3475
(813) 259-8800
Fax: (813) 259-8805

ILLINOIS
University of Illinois College of Medicine
Department of Pediatrics, M/C 856
840 S. Wood Street
Chicago, IL 60612
(312) 996-6711
Fax: (312) 413-1526

MICHIGAN
The Childrens Hospital of Michigan
Division of Clinical Immunology and
    Rheumatology
3901 Beaubien Boulevard
Detroit, MI 48201
(313) 993-8794 and (313) 745-4450
Fax: (313) 993-3873

NEW YORK
Harlem Hospital Center
Department of Pediatrics
506 Lenox Avenue, Room 16-119
New York, NY 10037
(212) 939-4040
Fax: (212) 939-4048

Children's Hospital at Suny Downstate
Department of Pediatrics
450 Clarkson Avenue, Box 49
Brooklyn, NY 11203
(718) 270-3185
Fax: (718) 270-1354

Jacobi Medical Center
Family Based HIV Services
JACP-5C-15
1400 Pelham Parkway South
Bronx, NY 10461
(718) 918-4903
Fax: (718) 918-4699

New York University of Medicine
Department of Pediatrics
550 First Avenue, Room 8W51
New York, NY 10016

(212) 263-6426
Fax: (212) 263-7806

SUNY Health Science Center at
  Stony Brook
Department of Pediatric Infectious Disease
HSC – T09-030
Stony Brook, NY 11794-811
(631) 444-7692
Fax: (631) 444-7248

SUNY Upstate Medical University
Division of Infectious Diseases
750 East Adams Street
Syracuse, NY 13210
(315) 464-6331
(315) 464-7564

University of Rochester
Strong Memorial Hospital
Department of Pediatrics
601 Elmwood Avenue, Box 690
Rochester, NY 14642
(585) 275-0588 and (585) 275-8760
Fax: (585) 273-1104

PUERTO RICO
Centro Medico
San Juan City Hospital
Padiatrics Department
PMB # 128 G.P.O., Box 70344
San Juan, PR 00936
Puerto Rico
(787) 764-3083 and (787) 274-0904
Fax: (787) 751-5143

WASHINGTON
University of Washington
Children's Hospital and Regional
Medical Center
Department of Pediatrics
4800 Sand Point Way, NE, 8G-1
Seattle, WA 98105
(206) 528-5140
Fax: (206) 527-3890

BAHAMAS
Princess Margaret Hospital
Shirley Street, PO Box 3730/N17 84

Nassau, Bahamas
Bahamas
(242) 322-2839
Fax: (242) 356-2893

BRAZIL
Servico de Doencas Infecciosas – HUFF
Av. Brigadeiro Trompowski
S/N Ilha do Fundao
Rio de Janeiro, CEP 21941-590
Brazil
55-21-562-61-48/49
Fax: 55-21-2562-6191

Hospital dos Servidores do Estado – RJ
Servico de Doencas Infecciosas e
  Parasitarias
Rua Sacadura Cabral
178 Anexo IV 5° Andar
Saude, Rio de Janeiro, CEP 20221-161
Brazil
55-21-535-0493
Fax: 55-21-535-0493

Universidade Federal de Minas Gerais
Escola de Medicina
Av. Alfredo Balena 90-4 Andar
Belo Horizonte, Minas Gerais,
  CEP 30130-100
Brazil
55-31-3248-9822
Fax: 55-31-3273-0422

Universidade de Sao Paulo
Hospital das Clinicas da Faculdade de
  Medicina de Ribe
Av. Bandeirantes 3900
Ribeirao Preto, Sao Paulo, CEP 14049-900
Brazil
55-16-6330-136
Fax: 55-16-6022-700
Instituto de Infectologia Emilio Ribas
Av. Dr. Arnaldo 165-2 Andar-Sala 218
Sao Paulo, Sao Paulo, CEP 01246-900
Brazil
55-11-3085-0295
Fax: 55-11-3061-2521

Appendix 3: Selected HIV-related internet resources

Leslie K. Serchuck, M.D.

Pediatric, Adolescent & Maternal AIDS Branch, NICHD/NIH, Rockville, MD

General AIDS information

AIDS info

http://www.aidsinfo.nih.gov

US Government sponsored portal with links to treatment guidelines and clinical trials (see below).

HIV InSite

http://hivinsite.ucsf.edu

A project of the University of California, San Francisco AIDS Program at San Francisco General Hospital and the UCSF Center for AIDS Prevention Studies. This is a comprehensive website for HIV and AIDS. This site also contains the AIDS Knowledge Base: an electronic textbook on AIDS and HIV that is frequently updated, with summaries of recent research on HIV and AIDS.

Johns Hopkins University AIDS Service

http://www.hopkins-aids.edu/

A wide-ranging collection of resources from Johns Hopkins University. Includes treatment updates, guidelines, plus full text of the AIDS handbook, *Medical Management of HIV Infection*, as well as a bimonthly newsletter, *The Hopkins HIV Report*.

Division of AIDS, National Institute of Allergy and Infectious Diseases, National Institutes of Health

http://www.niaid.nih.gov/daids/

Links to treatment and prevention information, publications and meetings; vaccine, prevention, and treatment networks, and the Comprehensive International Program of Research on AIDS (CIPRA). Funding opportunities for both United States and international investigators, including those in poor countries with large HIV burdens.

United States Centers for Disease Control and Prevention

http://www.cdc.gov/

The CDCs website and its HIV homepage http://www.cdc.gov/hiv/dhap.htm, the definitive US source for epidemiologic information, downloadable publications and slide sets.

(*Note*: The manufacturers of antiretrovirals, HIV diagnostics, and agents for AIDS-related opportunistic infections maintain websites with information pertaining to their products. These are often country specific, but can generally be easily found using the popular search engines.)

United States Food and Drug Administration

http://www.fda.gov/

Information about drug regulation and development.

AEGIS: AIDS Education and Global Information System

http://www.aegis.com/

This website features newsletters, HIV news from newspapers and wire services, and search capability for all documents. Contains an extensive publication library and many links.

AIDS Clinical Research Information Center

http://www.critpath.org/aric/

Contains an AIDS basic science information library and information and resources for People with AIDS (PWAs).

HIV Medicine Association

http://hivma.org

An organization of medical professionals caring for HIV-infected patients and a part of the Infectious Diseases Society of America. Site has links to IDSA practice guidelines and other resources.

International Association of Physicians in AIDS Care

http://www.iapac.org

This site is devoted to education of physicians and other healthcare providers. It advocates for the faster development and approval of treatments, vaccines and technologies for the prevention and treatment of HIV/AIDS and provides good clinical information.

Project inform

http://www.projinf.org/

A national, non-profit, community-based organization which provides information on diagnosis and treatment of HIV disease to HIV-infected individuals, their caregivers, and their healthcare and service providers. Project Inform provides excellent Fact Sheets and a frequently published journal *PI Perspective* which provides information from the most recent clinical trials and discussion regarding state of the art treatment and research issues. The site is in Spanish and English.

Medscape

http://www.medscape.com/hiv-aidshome

A commercial website with up-to-date information on HIV/AIDS as well as numerous other specialties. Contains international homepages as well.

Gay men's health crisis

http://gmhc.org

Focus mainly on gay men, which may be helpful for gay adolescents, but also includes useful information on a variety of treatment-related topics, and educational information on HIV infection and AIDS pathogenesis for non-medical personnel.

All the virology on the WWW

http://www.virology.net

Site for virology resources on the web, with links to virology and microbiology courses, dictionaries, and specific virus sites (including emerging viruses and HIV/AIDS among numerous others).

Treatment centered sites

AIDS info

http://www.aidsinfo.nih.gov

Provides Guidelines federally approved including *Guidelines for Use of Antiretroviral Agents in Adults and Adolescents* and *Guidelines for Use of Antiretroviral Agents in Pediatric Infection*. ATIS is staffed by bilingual (English and Spanish) health information specialists who answer questions on HIV treatment options.

AIDS treatment data network

http://www.atdn.org/

National, not-for-profit, community-based organization. Extensive, comprehensive and up-to-date informational databases about AIDS treatments, research studies, services, and accessing care. Available in English and Spanish.

HIV-druginteractions.org

http://www.HIV-druginteractions.org

A service of the University of Liverpool, Department of Pharmacology and Therapeutics features interactive drug interaction queries for antiretrovirals

The Body

http://www.thebody.com/

A multimedia AIDS and HIV information resource. Its focus is on providing information for prevention and treatment of HIV infection but it includes some information on biology and immunology of HIV. The site features answers by experts to questions about AIDS and HIV.

Critical path AIDS project

http://www.critpath.org/

Critical path AIDS project was founded by persons with AIDS (PWAs) to provide treatment, resource, and prevention information in wide-ranging levels of detail – for researchers, service providers, treatment activists, and other PWAs. AIDS prevention, treatment, and referral information is available. Important site for patients and activists. Many links.

Clinical trials

AIDS info

http://www.aidsinfo.nih.gov/

US Government-sponsored site containing current information on federally and privately sponsored clinical Pediatric and Adult clinical trials open to accrual. Includes both treatment and prevention trials. Also contains links to treatment guidelines. Available in Spanish.

ClinicalTrials.gov

http://www.clinicaltrials.gov/

The US National Institutes of Health, through its National Library of Medicine, has developed ClinicalTrials.gov to provide patients, family members and members of the public current information about clinical research studies for many diseases. The site currently contains thousands of clinical studies sponsored by the National Institutes of Health, other Federal agencies, and the pharmaceutical industry worldwide. Studies listed in the database are conducted primarily in the United States and Canada, but include locations in about 70 countries.

AIDS/HIV Treatment Directory (AMFAR)

http://www.amfar.org

The American Foundation for AIDS research. Contains information about conferences, grants, and a link to the AmFAR treatment directory, including information about treatment strategies and clinical trials.

The National Cancer Institute HIV and AIDS Malignancy Branch

http://www.aidstrials.nci.nih.gov

Links to the clinical trials in the HIV and AIDS Malignancy Branch, for both adults and children.

National Institutes of Health Vaccine Research Center

http://www.niaid.nih.gov/vrc/

Basic and clinical research toward the development of vaccine for AIDS and other diseases. Enrolling patients in prophylactic and therapeutic vaccine clinical trials.

CENTER WATCH- Clinical Trials Listing Service

http://www.centerwatch.com/

A commercial web site offering a variety of information related to clinical trials in many disease areas. The site is designed to be a resource both for patients interested in participating in clinical trials and for research professionals.

International AIDS resources

UNAIDS- The Joint United Nations Programme on HIV/AIDS

http://www.unaids.org

Links to publications, surveillance and response, WHO Initiative on HIV/AIDS and Sexually Transmitted Infections (HSI). Also contains news, upcoming events and publications for the international community. Includes up-to-date country-specific HIV/AIDS statistics. Information is provided in English, Spanish and French.

International AIDS Society

http://www.ias.se/

The International AIDS Society, a leading international professional society devoted to HIV/AIDS.

Global Fund to Fight AIDS, Tuberculosis and Malaria

http://www.theglobalfund.org/

International organization that collects and disburses funds to fight these serious infectious diseases in poor countries.

Pan American Health Organization (PAHO)

http://www.paho.org

PAHO is a UN agency. This site provides AIDS information by region from throughout Latin America and the Caribbean.

International AIDS Vaccine Initiative

http://www.iavi.org

Provides funding globally directed toward the development of an AIDS vaccine.

Gates Foundation

http://gatesfoundation.org

An important source of funding for HIV-related research globally.

Canadian HIV Trials Network

http://www.hivnet.ubc.ca/e/home

Links to Canadian clinical trials.

Conasida

http://www.ssa.gob.mx/conasida

This is the Mexican government health ministry HIV/AIDS server. This site is in Spanish.

The Body-International HIV/AIDS Service Organizations and Resources

http://www.thebody.com/hotlines/internat.html

Includes international health organizations and resources and sites by region. Includes sites from Africa, Latin America, Asia, Russia, Europe and Canada.

International Council of AIDS Services Organizations (ICASO)

http://www.icaso.org/

ICASO is a global network of non-governmental and community-based organizations. It has Regional Secretariats in Africa, Asia/Pacific, Europe, Latin America and the Caribbean, and North America.

Asian AIDS resources

http://www.utopia-asia.com/aids.htm

HIV/AIDS in the Asia/Pacific Region. Includes China, Thailand, Vietnam and many others.

AIDS map

http://www.aidsmap.com/

British HIV site, also with information on AIDS topics for continental Europe, Africa, and Asia.

Avert

http://www.avert.org/

A UK AIDS charity.

Pediatric AIDS resources

AIDS Alliance for Children, Youth & Families

http://www.aidspolicycenter.org/

The Alliance is a leading advocate for children, youth, and families affected by HIV/AIDS. Its' mission includes policy analysis, advocacy, education, and training.

The Elisabeth Glaser Pediatric AIDS Foundation

http://www.pedaids.org/

This foundation is a non-profit organization that is an important funding source for pediatric AIDS research globally.

National Pediatric and Family HIV Resource Center

http://www.pedhivaids.org/

Non-profit organization serving professionals. Offers consultation, training, teaching.

Research-oriented sites

Guide to NIH HIV/AIDS Information Services

http://www.sis.nlm.nih.gov/aids/hiv.html

The National Library of Medicine and Office of AIDS Research on-line guide containing data about HIV/AIDS information-related activities at the National Institutes of Health, along with selected Public Health Service offerings. Links to all institutes at the NIH are provided.

National Library of Medicine- PUBMED

http://gateway.nlm.nih.gov/

The National Library of Medicine Gateway to bibliographic and consumer health resources. Provides free access to the MEDLINE medical literature database through PubMed, and access to online versions of selected biomedical texts, online nucleic acid and protein sequence analysis tools, and online compilations of genetic information. Extensive links to voluminous collections of biomedical data. Links available to MedlinePlus, health information for consumers.

HIV Nucleic Acid Sequence and Immunological Databases
http://www.hiv-web.lanl.gov/
The HIV databases contain data on HIV genetic sequences, immunological epitopes, drug resistance-associated mutations.

NCI Drug Resistance Program
http://www.home.ncifcrf.gov/hivdrp/
The National Cancer Institute Drug Resistance Program, researching the mechanisms and implications of HIV drug resistance.

Harvard AIDS Institute
http://www.hsph.harvard.edu/hai/
The Institute has targeted four primary research areas related to HIV/AIDS: Basic Science (including molecular biology, virology and vaccines); Clinical Science (including pathogenesis and treatments); Epidemiology/Public Health and Prevention; Social Science and Policy.

Death and bereavement

Association for Death Education and Counseling
http://www.adec.org/
ADEC is an international, multidisciplinary organization dedicated to improving the quality of education, counseling, and care-giving pertaining to dying, death, grief, and loss.

Growth House
http://www.growthhouse.org
This site provides public education and resources about hospice and home care, palliative care, pain management, death with dignity, bereavement, and related end of life topics. Includes international resources. Grief sites are devoted to grief and bereavement, and include special pages for bereaved families, natal and infant loss, and helping children with grief and serious illness.

Hospice Foundation of America
http://www.hospicefoundation.org
HFA promotes hospice care and works to educate professionals and the families they serve in issues relating to caregiving, terminal illness, loss, and bereavement.

National Association for Home Care

http://www.nahc.org

This is the virtual headquarters of the National Association for Home Care (NAHC). Since its inception in 1982, NAHC has remained committed to serving the home care and hospice industry, which provides services to the sick, the disabled, and the terminally ill in the comfort of their homes.

Appendix 4: Selected legal resources for HIV-infected children[1]

Carolyn McAllaster, J. D.

ALABAMA
AIDS Task Force of Alabama, Inc.
Post Office Box 55703
Birmingham, AL 35255
(205) 324-9822
Legal referrals provided

ALASKA
Alaskan AIDS Assistance Association
1057 West Fireweed Lane, #102
Anchorage, AK 99503
(907) 263-2050
Legal referrals provided
Bform documents with notary on site.

ARIZONA
AIDS Project Arizona
1427 N. 3rd Street, Suite 125
Phoenix, AZ 85004
(602) 253-2437
Legal referrals provided; estate planning & documents with notice

HIV/AIDS Law Project (HALP)
Maricopa County Bar Association
Volunteer Lawyers Program
305 S. 2nd Avenue
Phoenix, AZ 85003
(602) 258-3434, ext. 282;
    1-800-852-9075, ext 282

Direct legal services provided; legal referrals provided

ARKANSAS
Arkansas AIDS Foundation
518 East 9th Street
Little Rock, AR 72202
(501) 376-6299
Legal referrals provided

CALIFORNIA
North Coast AIDS Project 529 I Street
Eureka, CA 95501
(707) 268-2132
Legal referrals provided

Central Valley AIDS Team
416 West McKinley
Fresno, CA 93728
(559) 264-2437
Legal referrals provided

The Barristers AIDS Legal Services
1313 North Vine
Los Angeles, CA 90028
(323) 993-1640
Legal referrals provided

HIV/AIDS Legal Services Alliance Inc. (HALSA)

---

[1] A primary resource for this compilation was the Directory of Legal *Resources for People with AIDS and HIV*, 2nd edn. ABA, AIDS Coordination Project, 1997.

3550 Wilshire Blvd., Suite 750
Los Angeles, CA 90010
(213) 201-1640
Legal referrals provided
Direct legal services provided

The Los Angeles Free Clinic Legal
Dept.
8405 Beverly Boulevard
Los Angeles, CA 90048
(323) 655-2697
Direct legal services provided

Los Angeles Gay and Lesbian Center
Legal Services Department
1625 North Schrader Boulevard
Los Angeles, CA 90028
(323) 993-7670
Direct legal services provided

Desert AIDS Project Legal Services
1695 N. Sunrise Way, Bldg. 1
Palm Springs, CA 92262
(760) 323-2118
Legal referrals provided
Direct legal services provided

AIDS Service Center
1030 South Arroyo Parkway
Pasadena, CA 91105
(818) 441-8495; (626) 441-8495
Legal referrals provided

AIDS Legal Referral Panel of the
San Francisco Bay Area
205 13th St.
San Francisco, CA 94104
(415) 291-5454
Legal referrals provided
Direct legal services provided

Legal Services for Prisoners with
Children
Women Prisoners with
HIV/AIDS Project
100 McAllister Street
San Francisco, CA 94102
(415) 255-7036

San Francisco AIDS Foundation
Financial Benefits Advocacy
Program
1 Sixth St.
San Francisco, CA 94103
(415) 487-8000
Legal referrals provided
Direct legal services provided
Require clients to be 18 years old

AIDS Legal Services
111 West St. John Street, Suite 315
San Jose, CA 95113
(408) 293-3135
Direct legal services provided
Legal referrals provided

Community Services AIDS Program
1601 East Hazelton Avenue
Stockton, CA 95201-2009
(209) 468-2235
Case management services

Valley HIV/AIDS Center
6850 Van Nuys Boulevard, 110
Van Nuys, CA 91405
(818) 908-3840
Legal referrals provided

AIDS Care Legal Clinic
73 North Palm Street
Ventura, CA 93001
(805) 643-0446
Legal referrals provided

COLORADO
Boulder County AIDS Project Pro Bono
Attorney Team
2118 14th Street
Boulder, CO 80302
(303) 444-6121
Direct legal services provided

Southern Colorado AIDS Project
1301 S. 8th Street, Suite 200
Colorado Springs, CO 80906
(719) 578-9092
Legal referrals provided

Southern Colorado AIDS Project
1301 South 8th Street, Suite 200
Colorado Springs, CO 80906
(719) 578-9092
Legal referrals provided

Colorado AIDS Project Legal Program
701 East Colfax Avenue, Suite 212
Denver, CO 80203
(303) 837-1501
Legal referrals provided

The Legal Center for People with
    Disabilities and Older People
HIV/AIDS Legal Program
455 Sherman Street, Suite 130
Denver, CO 80203
(303) 722-0300
Direct legal services provided
Legal referrals provided

CONNECTICUT
AIDS Legal Network for
    Connecticut
80 Jefferson St.
Hartford, CT 06106
(860) 541-5000
Legal referrals provided
Direct legal services provided

DISTRICT OF COLUMBIA
District of Columbia School of
    Law
HIV/AIDS Legal Clinic
4200 Connecticut Avenue, NW
Washington, DC 20008
(202) 274-7330
Direct legal services provided

Whitman-Walker Clinic
Legal Services Department
1701 14th Street
Washington, DC 20009
(202) 939-7627
Direct legal services provided

FLORIDA
Comprehensive AIDS Project
2222 West Atlantic Avenue

Delray Beach, FL 33445
(561) 274-6400
Legal referrals provided
Direct legal services provided

Jacksonville Area Legal Aid, Inc.
Ryan White Legal Project
126 W. Adams Street
Jacksonville, FL 32202
(904) 356-8371
Direct legal services provided

AIDS Help, Inc.
Post Office Box 4374
Key West, FL 33041
(305) 296-6196
Legal referrals provided

Legal Services of Greater Miami, Inc.
AIDS Legal Advocacy Project
3000 Biscayne Boulevard, Suite 500
Miami, FL 33137
(305) 576-0080
Direct legal services provided

Big Bend Comprehensive AIDS Resources,
Education & Support, Inc.
Post Office Box 14365
Tallahassee, FL 32317
(904) 656-AIDS
Legal referrals provided

Legal Aid Society of Palm Beach County
HIV/AIDS Legal Project
423 Fern Street, Suite 200
West Palm Beach, FL 33401
(561) 655-8944, Ext. 286
Direct legal services provided

GEORGIA
Atlanta Legal Aid Society
AIDS Legal Project
151 Springs Street, NW
Atlanta, GA 30303
(404) 614-3969
Legal referrals provided
Direct legal services
    provided

AIDS Law Project of Middle
 Georgia
111 Third Street, Suite 230
Macon, GA 31202
(912) 751-6261
Legal referrals provided
Direct legal services provided

HAWAII
Hawaii State Bar Association
Lawyer Referral & Information
 Service
1132 Bishop St., Suite 906
Honolulu, HI 96813
(808) 537-1868
Legal referrals provided

ILLINOIS
AIDS Legal Council of Chicago
188 W. Randolph St., Suite 2400
Chicago, IL 60601
(312) 427-8990
Direct legal services provided; legal
 referrals provided

Lambda Legal Defense & Education
 Fund, Inc.
Midwest Regional Office
11 East Adams, Suite 1008
Chicago, IL 60603
(312) 663-4413
Legal contacts provided
Direct legal services provided for
 precedent setting cases, often appellate
 level cases
Legal Assistance Foundation, Inc. of
 Metropolitan Chicago
HIV/AIDS Project
111 W. Jackson. Suite 300
Chicago, IL 60604
(312) 347-8309
Legal referrals provided
Direct legal services
 provided

Cook County Legal Assistance Foundation,
 Inc.
AIDS Advocacy Project
828 Davis Street, Suite 201
Evanston, IL 60201-4489
(847) 475-3703
Legal referrals provided
Direct legal services provided

Springfield AIDS Resource Association
1315 North Fifth
Springfield, IL 62702
(217) 523-2191
Legal referrals provided

INDIANA
AIDS Task Force, Inc.
2124 Fairfield Avenue
Fort Wayne, IN 46802
(219) 744-1144
Legal referrals provided

Indiana HIV Advocacy Program
3951 North Meridian Street, Suite 200
Indianapolis, IN 46208
(317) 920-3190
Legal referrals provided
Direct legal services provided

Legal Services Organization of Indiana, Inc.
HIV/AIDS Legal Project
151 North Delaware, 18th Floor
Indianapolis, IN 46204
(317) 631-9410
Direct legal services provided

AIDS Ministries/AIDS Assist
Post Office Box 11582
South Bend, IN 46634
(219) 234-2780
Legal referrals provided
Direct legal services provided

IOWA
University of Iowa College of Law
AIDS Representation Project

Iowa City, IA 52242-1113
(319) 335-9023
Legal referrals provided
Direct legal services provided

KENTUCKY
AIDS Volunteers, Inc.
AIDS/HIV Legal Project
Post Office Box 431
Lexington, KY 40588
(859) 225-3000
Legal referrals provided

Legal Aid Society
HIV/AIDS Legal Project
810 Barret Avenue, Room 301
Louisville, KY 40204
(502) 574-8199
Direct legal services provided
Legal referrals provided

LOUISIANA
AIDS Law of Louisiana, Inc.
mailing address:
Post Office Box 30203
New Orleans, LA 70190

physical address:
144 Elk Place, Suite 1530
New Orleans, LA 70112
(504) 568-1631; 1-800-375-5035
Legal referrals provided
Direct legal services provided

MAINE
The AIDS Project, Inc.
615 Congress Street
Post Office Box 5305
Portland, ME 04101
(207) 774-6877
Legal referrals provided

MARYLAND
Health Education Resource Organization
   (HERO)
1734 Maryland Avenue
Baltimore, MD 21201

(410) 685-1180
Direct legal services provided

University of Maryland Law School
AIDS Legal Clinic
500 West Baltimore Street
Baltimore, MD 21201-1786
(410) 706-8316
Legal referrals provided
Direct legal services provided

MASSACHUSETTS
AIDS Action Committee
131 Clarendon Street
Boston, MA 02116
(617) 450-1250
Legal referrals provided

Gay & Lesbian Advocates & Defenders
AIDS Law Project
294 Washington Street, Suite 740
Boston, MA 02108
(617) 426-1350
Legal referrals provided
Direct legal services provided

North Shore AIDS Project
67 Middle Street
Gloucester, MA 01930
(978) 283-0101
Legal referrals provided

AIDS Law Clinic
122 Boylston Street
Jamaica Plain, MA 02130
(617) 522-3003
Legal referrals provided
Direct legal services provided

MICHIGAN
Wayne County Neighborhood
   Legal Services
AIDS Law Center
51 W. Hancock St., Suite 345
Detroit, MI 48201
(313) 832-8730
Direct legal services provided

Michigan Protection and Advocacy
Service, Inc.
HIV/AIDS Advocacy Program (HAAP)
106 West Allegan, Suite 300
Lansing, MI 48933
(517) 487-1755
Legal referrals provided
Direct legal services provided

MINNESOTA
Minnesota AIDS Project Legal
Program
1400 Park Avenue South
Minneapolis, MN 55404
(612) 341-2060
Legal referrals provided
Direct legal services provided

MISSOURI
Legal Aid of Western Missouri
AIDS Legal Assistance
1005 Grand, Suite 600
Kansas City, MO 64106
(816) 474-6750
Direct legal services provided

Legal Services of Eastern Missouri,
Inc.
AIDS Project
4232 Forest Park Avenue
St. Louis, MO 63108
(314) 534-4200, ext. 1224
Direct legal services provided
Legal referrals provided

St. Louis University School of Law
Health Law Clinic
3700 Lindell Boulevard
St. Louis, MO 63108
(314) 977-2778
Direct legal services provided

MONTANA
Butte AIDS Support Services
25 West Front Street
Butte, MT 59701
(406) 723-6507

NEVADA
Aid for AIDS Nevada
2300 South Rancho, Suite 211
Las Vegas, NV 89102
(702) 382-2326
Legal referrals provided

Nevada AIDS Foundation
P. O. Box 478
Reno, NV 89504
(702) 329-2437
Legal referrals provided

NEW HAMPSHIRE
Merrimack Valley AIDS Project, Inc.
Post Office Box 882
Concord, NH 03302
(603) 226-0607

Greater Manchester AIDS Project
Post Office Box 59
Manchester, NH 03105
(603) 623-0710
Legal referrals provided

NEW JERSEY
Hyacinth AIDS Foundation
78 New Street, 2nd Floor
New Brunswick, NJ 08901
(732) 246-0204
Legal referrals provided
Direct legal services provided

NEW MEXICO
AIDS Law Panel
Post Office Box 22251
Santa Fe, NM 84502
(505) 982-2021
Legal referrals provided
Direct legal services provided

NEW YORK
Bronx AIDS Services
Legal Advocacy Program
2633 Webster Ave
Bronx, NY 10458
(718) 295-5690
Legal referrals provided
Direct legal services provided

Brooklyn Legal Services Corp. B HIV Project
105 Court Street
Brooklyn, NY 11201
(718) 237-5546
Direct legal services provided

Nassau/Suffolk Law Services
    Committee, Inc.
David Project
1757 Veteran=s Highway, Suite 50
Islandia, NY 11722
(516) 232-2400
Direct legal services provided
Legal referrals provided

Queens Legal Services Corporation
HIV Advocacy Project
89-00 Sutphin Boulevard
Jamaica, NY 11435
(718) 657-8611
Legal referrals provided
Direct legal services provided

AIDS Service Center of Lower
    Manhattan
80 Fifth Avenue, 3rd Floor
New York, NY 10011
(212) 645-0875
Legal referrals provided
Direct legal services provided

The Family Center
66 Reade Street
New York, NY 10007
(212) 766-4522
Direct legal services provided
Legal referrals provided

Gay Men's Health Crisis
Legal Services Department
119 West 24th Street
New York, NY 10011
(212) 367-1040
Legal referrals provided
Direct legal services provided

HIV Law Project
161 William Street, 17th Floor

New York, NY 10038
(212) 674-7590
Direct legal services provided

Lambda Legal Defense & Education
    Fund, Inc.
120 Wall Street, Suite 1500
New York, NY 10005
(212) 809-8585
Legal referrals provided
Impact litigation

Public Interest Law Office of
    Rochester
80 St. Paul Street, Suite 701
Rochester, NY 14604
(716) 454-4060
Direct legal services provided
Legal referrals provided

Volunteer Legal Services Project of
    Monroe County
80 St. Paul Street, Suite 640
Rochester, NY 14604
(716) 232-3051
Legal referrals provided
Direct legal services provided

Project Hospitality
Legal Advocacy Program
100 Park Avenue
Staten Island, NY 10302
(718) 448-1544, ext. 118
Direct legal services provided
Legal referrals provided

AIDS Law Project
472 South Salina Street, Suite 300
Syracuse, NY 13202
(315) 475-3127
Direct legal services provided
Legal referrals provided

Westchester/Putnam Legal
    Services
4 Cromwell Place

White Plains, NY 10601
(914) 949-1305
Direct legal services provided

NORTH CAROLINA
AIDS Legal Assistance Project
Duke School of Law
Box 90360
Durham, NC 27708
(919) 613-7169
Direct legal services provided

OHIO
Columbus AIDS Task Force
751 Northwest Blvd.
Columbus, OH 43212
(614) 299-2437
Legal referrals provided

Toledo Bar Association
AIDS Assistance Committee
311 North Superior
Toledo, OH 43604
(419) 693-4433
Legal referrals provided
Direct legal service provided

OKLAHOMA
Legal Services of Oklahoma, Inc.
HIV/AIDS Legal Resources
    Project
2901 N. Classen Boulevard,
    Suite 110
Oklahoma City, OK 73106
(405) 524-4611
Direct legal services provided
Legal referrals provided

OREGON
Multnomah County Legal Aid
    Service
700 SW Taylor Street, Suite 300
Portland, OR 97205
(503) 224-4086
Direct legal services provided

PENNSYLVANIA
AIDS Law Project of Pennsylvania
1211 Chestnut Street, Suite 600
Philadelphia, PA 19107
(215) 587-9377
Direct legal services provided
Pittsburgh AIDS Taskforce
905 West Street, 4th Floor
Pittsburgh, PA 15221
Columbus, OH 43212-3856
(412) 242-2500
Legal referrals provided
Direct legal services provided

RHODE ISLAND
AIDS Project of Rhode Island
232 West Exchange Street
Providence, RI 02903
(401) 831-5522
Legal referrals provided

SOUTH CAROLINA
Lowcountry AIDS Services
Legal Clinic
501 Manley Avenue
Charleston, SC 29405
(843) 747-2273
Direct legal services provided

TEXAS
AIDS Services of Austin
Post Office Box 4874
Austin, TX 78765
(512) 458-2437
Legal referrals provided
Direct legal services provided

Dallas Legal Hospice
390 West Seventh St.
Dallas, TX 75208
(214) 941-2600
Direct legal service provided

La Fe CARE Center
1505 Mescalero
El Paso, TX 79925
(915) 772-3366
Direct legal service provided

AIDS Outreach Center Legal Network
801 West Cannon
Fort Worth, TX 76104
(817) 355-1994
Direct legal services provided

Houston Volunteer Lawyers Program, Inc.
AIDS Project
806 Main St., 16th Floor
Houston, TX 77002
(713) 228-0735
Legal referrals provided
Direct legal services provided

UTAH

Utah AIDS Foundation
1408 South 1100 East
Salt Lake City, UT 84105
(801) 497-2323
Legal referrals provided

VERMONT

AIDS Project of Southern Vermont
Post Office Box 1486
Brattleboro, VT 05302
(802) 254-8263
Legal referrals provided

VIRGINIA

Whitman-Walker Clinic
Legal Services Department
5232 Lee Highway
Arlington, VA 22207
(703) 237-4900
Legal referrals provided
Direct legal services provided

AIDS/HIV Services Group
Post Office Box 2322
Charlottesville, VA 22902
(804) 979-7714
Legal referrals provided

WASHINGTON

Volunteer Attorneys for Persons with AIDS

(VAPWA)
AIDS Legal Access
900 Fourth Avenue, Suite 600
Seattle, WA 98164
(206) 340-2584
Legal referrals provided
Direct legal services on an emergency basis.

WEST VIRGINIA

Charleston AIDS Network
Post Office Box 1024
Charleston, WV 25324
(304) 345-4673; 1-888-455-4673
Legal referrals provided

WISCONSIN

AIDS Resource Center of Wisconsin
1212 57th Street
Kenosha, WI 53141
(262) 657-6644
Legal referrals provided
Direct legal services provided

Madison AIDS Support Network
Legal Services Program
600 Williamson Street
Madison, WI 53703
(608) 252-6540
Legal referrals provided
Direct legal services provided

AIDS Resource Center of Wisconsin
Legal Services Program
820 N. Plankinton Avenue
Milwaukee, WI 53203
(414) 225-1578; 1-800-878-6267
Direct legal services provided

AIDS Law, Education, Research and Training
("ALERT")
Legal Aid Society of Milwaukee, Inc.
229 E. Wisconsin Ave., Suite 200
Milwaukee, WI 53202
(414) 765-0600
Direct legal services provided

Index

Note: page numbers in *italics* refer to figures and tables.